NURSING
ETHICS

FIFTH EDITION

Ian E. Thompson BA(Hons) PhD

Former Professor of Ethics and Philosophy,
University of Notre Dame Australia, Fremantle, Western Australia,
Honorary Research Fellow, School of Social and Political Studies,
University of Edinburgh, Edinburgh, UK

Kath M. Melia BNurs(Manc) PhD

Head of School of Health in Social Science, College of Humanities and Social Science,
University of Edinburgh, Edinburgh, UK

Kenneth M. Boyd MA BD PhD FRCPEd

Professor of Medical Ethics, Medical School, University of Edinburgh, and General Secretary,
Institute of Medical Ethics, Edinburgh, UK

Dorothy Horsburgh RGN RNT RCNT BA (Hons) MEd PhD

Lecturer, School of Acute and Continuing Care Nursing, Napier University, Edinburgh, UK

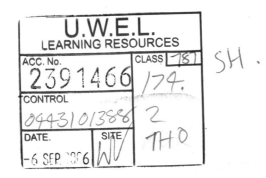

CHURCHILL
LIVINGSTONE

ELSEVIER

EDINBURGH LONDON NEW YORK OXFORD PHILADELPHIA ST LOUIS SYDNEY TORONTO 2006

CHURCHILL
LIVINGSTONE
ELSEVIER

© Longman Group Limited 1983
© Longman Group Limited 1988
© 1994 Pearson Professionals Ltd
© 2000 Harcourt Publishers Ltd
© 2006, Elsevier Limited. All rights reserved.

The rights of Ian E. Thompson, Kath M. Melia, Kenneth M. Boyd, and Dorothy Horsburgh, to be identified as authors of this work have been asserted by them in accordance with the Copyright, Designs and Patents Act 1988

First edition 1983
Second edition 1988
Third edition 1994
Fourth edition 2000
Fifth edition 2006

ISBN-10; 0 443 10138 8
ISBN-13; 978 0 443 10138 0

British Library Cataloguing in Publication Data
A catalogue record for this book is available from the British Library

Library of Congress Cataloging in Publication Data
A catalog record for this book is available from the Library of Congress

Notice
Medical knowledge is constantly changing. Standard safety precautions must be followed, but as new research and clinical experience broaden our knowledge, changes in treatment and drug therapy may become necessary or appropriate. Readers are advised to check the most current product information provided by the manufacturer of each drug to be administered to verify the recommended dose, the method and duration of administration, and contraindications. It is the responsibility of the practitioner, relying on experience and knowledge of the patient, to determine dosages and the best treatment for each individual patient. Neither the Publisher nor the editors or contributors assume any liability for any injury and/or damage to persons or property arising from this publication.

The Publisher

ELSEVIER your source for books, journals and multimedia in the health sciences
www.elsevierhealth.com

Working together to grow libraries in developing countries
www.elsevier.com | www.bookaid.org | www.sabre.org

ELSEVIER   BOOK AID International   Sabre Foundation

The Publisher's policy is to use paper manufactured from sustainable forests

Printed in the UK

NURSING
ETHICS

For Churchill Livingstone:

Senior Commissioning Editor: Ninette Premdas
Development Editor: Mairi McCubbin
Project Manager: Morven Dean
Design Direction: Sarah Russell
Illustrations Manager: Bruce Hogarth

Contents

Preface and acknowledgements

We were pleased, though challenged, when the publishers, Elsevier Limited, decided that a fifth edition of *Nursing Ethics* was called for, to meet rising demand and to meet the challenges of changing conditions in healthcare in the 21st century. The continued interest in and positive feedback on the book has given us satisfaction as authors, and made us feel part of a growing community of interest in the ethics of healthcare and in nursing ethics around the world. We begin, therefore, by acknowledging our readers, those who have purchased and read the book, and have given positive feedback to the publishers and to us individually. Their criticisms have been most helpful, especially their constructive suggestions about ways to improve the book. We only hope we have gone some way towards meeting their expectations.

It is hard to believe that a full quarter of a century has passed since the publication of the first edition of *Nursing Ethics*. Our brief for that first edition was to write a 'short, popular, readable introduction to ethics for nurses'. The fact that the fourth and fifth editions have grown in size and scope partly reflects the growth of interest in nursing and healthcare ethics over the past 25 years, but it has also been demanded by the widening of the scope of debate about ethics in healthcare, and the book's recommendation by WHO for use in Project 2000. However, it is the quality of the feedback we have received from teachers and students of nursing and allied health professions, in particular, that has challenged and motivated us to undertake the arduous and time-consuming task of revising and updating *Nursing Ethics* for the fourth time. It is the faith that they have placed in us that has driven us to undertake a more comprehensive revision, and a complete rewrite, in some cases, of material in the fourth edition. This has been rewarding too, as it has forced us to re-engage with the task of evaluating our own work, and to research how it needed to be updated. We clearly have an obligation, as authors, to practise what we preach, by evidencing our commitment to continuous quality improvement by the way we address our task as author/editors.

In particular we wish to acknowledge with thanks the contribution of the team of academic teachers who reviewed and commented in detail on the strengths and weaknesses of the fourth edition, at the invitation of Elsevier. These reviewers were:

Nina Hallowell, Lecturer in Social Sciences and Public Health, University of Edinburgh
Jean Harbison, Lecturer, Health and Nursing, Queen Margaret University College, Edinburgh
Alice Kiger, Director, Centre for Advanced Studies in Nursing, Aberdeen University
Cheryl Tringham, Teaching Fellow, Department of Nursing & Midwifery, University of Stirling.

Dorothy Horsburgh's agreement to assist us with the revision and updating of the text as an author has reinvigorated the editorial team, and has brought a new sense of vision and energy to our task. The result is a book that has been more extensively revised and rewritten than we intended when we set out. We trust that this will make the fifth edition of *Nursing Ethics* more relevant to the changing world of contemporary healthcare. We hope it will help broaden and deepen the debate about ethics in healthcare by making it more directly applicable to the practical concerns of nurses and front-line practitioners. If we have achieved this aim, then the book should also be more useful as a teaching text, and as a reference book for nurses and other health practitioners involved in management, research and policy development.

Our special thanks to Rowan Thompson, for the contribution of his artwork to illustrate the different models of carer/client relationships, and different models of management, and so enliven the text.

We appreciate the confidence shown in us by the publishers, Elsevier, and in particular wish to thank Mairi McCubbin and Ninette Premdas for the patience and understanding, professional support and encouragement they have shown in the long process of appraising and refining, editing and preparing this fifth edition for publication.

Once again, we dedicate this edition to our nearest and dearest, without whose support we could not have begun, continued and finished the arduous task of preparing this fifth edition of *Nursing Ethics*. We commend it to you, acknowledging that its limitations are ours, and that its strengths lie in the ongoing dialogue we have had with our own students, and with others we have been invited to teach, and most especially with our academic colleagues and fellow teachers, who are also concerned with ethics and striving for excellence in healthcare.

Ian E. Thompson
Kath M. Melia
Kenneth M. Boyd
Dorothy Horsburgh
Edinburgh, 2005

Introduction – ethics in nursing, continuity and change

AIMS

To provide an overview of the rationale for the book, its content and format.

ETHICS IN NURSING TODAY

Our purpose in writing a fifth edition of this book is to respond to some of the changes that have occurred both locally and globally during the past decade. Whilst we will address recent issues that have impacted on ethical issues in nursing practice, we will also focus on areas of perennial relevance. The remit of the book is therefore to address both change and continuity.

The intention is that this new edition will have a fairly broad readership within nursing and be of relevance to practitioners throughout their career, rather than at one specific point within it. The content is therefore aimed at nurses from senior under-graduate level through to registered practitioners, postgraduate students and those who teach nursing ethics. As nursing is a practice-based occupation we have tried to ensure that our discussion focuses on examples that practitioners will recognise as relevant to their everyday ethical decision-making. We therefore take nursing *practice* as our starting point and subsequently use *theory* to inform and develop the discussion. Our intention in this introductory chapter is to 'set the scene' for the reader and to provide our rationale for the book's content and format.

Issues of health and disease and what is good and bad for us are closely linked, so the discussion of healthcare and discussion of ethics cannot really be separated from each other. Before we come to the discussion of ethical rules, rights and duties, ethics is most fundamentally concerned with the conditions for human flourishing and what factors and forces militate against our well-being. Not surprisingly, the World Health Organization (1947) defines health as 'complete mental, physical and social well-being, and not just the absence of disease or infirmity'. This makes the issue of health a matter that links closely with our most fundamental life values and life choices.

To a greater or lesser degree we are all concerned about our own health. Of course, the extent to which it is the primary focus of our attention will depend on our circumstances, and whether we are well, injured or sick at the time. However, our health will always be of vital importance to us, as health of body and mind are important in enabling us to work, to support ourselves and to achieve our life goals. We are also bound to be concerned about health services, on our own behalf or that of others, because we will all require healthcare at some point in our lives – whether at birth, during the course of our development, or when we face crises in adult life, problems with reproduction, mental health, old age and physical frailty, or when we are dying. Again, not surprisingly, the United Nations, in formulating its *Universal Declaration of Human Rights* (1948), recognised access to adequate healthcare as a fundamental human right, and imposed on all member states a moral obligation to attempt to provide healthcare for all their citizens, without discrimination or regard to wealth or status.

Given our personal desire for good health, and our need for reliable and accessible healthcare provision when our circumstances demand it, we cannot really avoid making personal value choices relating to our health – ethical choices related to our choice of lifestyles, to our own health promotion and health protection. As consumers of health services, citizens and taxpayers, we are likely to, and perhaps ought to, take part in the public debate about the just and equitable allocation of healthcare resources. These economic and political choices are fundamentally ethical choices about the kind of society in which we want to live and the quality of life of all its citizens. The demand that health professionals and all employed in health services should be publicly accountable for the decisions they make, for their use of scarce healthcare resources and for the quality of their professional and clinical services, arises out of public recognition that health and the quality of healthcare is a legitimate concern of everybody.

While ethics has always played a part in professional and political debate about healthcare, during the past century ethics has achieved a new prominence in the public media worldwide – in state-sponsored health education, through the treatment of health issues in magazines, in radio and television documentaries, and in soap operas. Programme producers have discovered that coverage of health issues, and problems related to healthcare provision, attracts big audiences. While popular television tends to focus on dramatic situations demanding life and death decisions, there is increasing coverage of more general ethical and political issues related to healthcare delivery: e.g. the length of waiting lists and professional malpractice, dilemmas of resource allocation, quality of life issues for people who have high dependency, the need for rigorous evaluation of the effectiveness of treatments, and credible performance indicators on the quality of services.

These developments have meant that nurses and other health professionals have had to be better informed about ethics and ethical issues in their work so as to be able to deal with the questions of an increasingly informed and critical public – especially the worries of their 'patients', 'clients' or 'customers'. In addition, the more critical breed of healthcare 'consumers' (including politicians and taxpayers) increasingly demand that health professionals are more accountable – that they can justify their decisions and actions on both clinical and ethical grounds. To meet this demand for a professionally and ethically accountable workforce, nurses, like other health professionals, have had to become better informed about ethics in healthcare generally and in their own areas of responsibility in particular. They have also had to become more skilled in applied ethics. Having ethical convictions or being knowledgeable about ethics is no longer sufficient. To be adequately accountable, nurses have to be not only clinically competent, but also able to demonstrate competence in:

- clarifying values and goals for sound evaluation of their work against clear objectives
- ethical decision-making and the ability to give a sound rational justification for decisions
- developing ethical policy and standards for the strategic management of resources.

The nature of healthcare provision is such that decisions made and the treatment and care provided (or withheld) may alter the duration and quality of the lives of the individuals who experience it. In this book, we argue that the relationship of nursing to the health and well-being of recipients renders nursing itself a moral enterprise. We cannot separate off some elements of nursing practice as morally significant and others as morally neutral. *All* decisions in healthcare, and actions taken or omitted, inevitably raise questions about the beneficial or harmful effects they have upon recipients, and questions about individual rights and justice and equity for all. Moral choice is an integral, and inescapable, part of *everyday* life. For nursing ethics to simply focus on life and death dilemmas clouds the fact that the majority of moral issues faced by nurses are encountered by them in their routine practice and treatment of patients. Important value judgements and moral decisions also have to be made by nurses in their management of resources in healthcare settings, on behalf of the community.

CHANGES WITH A BEARING ON NURSING ETHICS

In discussing the scope of ethics as it relates to nursing and healthcare there are several other factors that should be taken into consideration, namely:

- *Changes in demography both worldwide and locally, including the dislocation of people and changes in population distribution.* When these changes result from violent conflict, nurses will be involved in the care of individuals who have been physically and mentally traumatised. Caring for diverse client groups requires nurses to demonstrate enhanced awareness of cultural differences in order to optimise healthcare delivery.
- *Changes in epidemiology – in the pattern and distribution of diseases both 'old' and 'new', like tuberculosis, malaria, or HIV/AIDS and new drug-resistant hospital-acquired infections.* These changes raise important issues of prevention as well as care and cure. Conditions, such as obesity, may predispose people to developing other diseases such as hypertension and type 2 diabetes mellitus. Epidemiological evidence about risk factors raises questions as to whether it is ethically justifiable to intervene in people's lives in order to reduce morbidity and increase longevity. At what point then should nurses intervene with people who put themselves at risk because of their lifestyles? Other questions that arise relate to whether healthcare resources should be aimed at achieving the greatest benefit for the majority of people or whether the specific health needs of individuals should be met first.
- *Changes in the focus of healthcare delivery from hospital to community settings, encouraged by the World Health Organization (WHO) and made possible by new technology.* These changes provide opportunities for nurses to work outside hospital settings, but may increase their individual responsibility and accountability for care provision. Closure of institutions caring for people who have mental health problems and learning disabilities, for example, has raised new ethical issues around the responsibility of nurses for ensuring the safety and well-being of these people (and others connected with them) in community settings.
- *The impact of globalisation of trade and communications, and the emergence of multinational pharmaceutical companies and healthcare providers.* Globalisation has opened up new possibilities for nurses, including new opportunities for training, working for international agencies and scope to sell their labour and expertise to multinational companies and healthcare providers. Nurses need to ensure that their professional standards and practice are not compromised by commercial interests; but they should also reflect on whether by seeking better paid employment in the more industrialised societies, they are not contributing to the 'brain-drain' and impoverishment of their own countries.
- *The impact of the new technologies and developments (e.g. in genetic engineering and nanotechnology) which*

are likely to change the way healthcare is delivered. In their own interests and that of their patients, nurses have a moral responsibility to be well informed about these developments and their implications for nursing care. On the one hand, they may need to adapt their working practices and be willing to be more flexible in the way they deliver care to people. On the other hand, nurses need to respond to these in a way that will ensure decision-making is both clinically sound and ethical, being concerned always for the well-being and protection of patients.

- *The impact of new national and international contracts and agreements – e.g. WHO policy, the European Union Working Time Directive, or the NHS Direct/NHS24 nurse-led patient services within the UK.* These, and other changes may lead to an 'expansion' of nurses' roles, and better working conditions, but nurses have a responsibility to ensure that these developments do not harm patients but rather serve for their benefit.

Such demographic changes, and the implications of these for providers and recipients of nursing care, have received increasing attention in the nursing press in recent years, as has the relocation of care from institutional to community settings. However, discussion of the latter by the general media has frequently focused upon a perceived threat to public safety, rather than encouraging public debate about what forms of care are most beneficial to patients. Here nurses, as responsible professionals with particular knowledge and expertise, cannot abrogate their responsibility to contribute constructively to debate about the various possible forms of healthcare provision and their impact on patients.

In an era of increasing globalisation, in terms of international trade, cooperation and conflict, nursing itself has become part of a global healthcare workforce. As teachers and practitioners there is a need to 'think globally' as well as 'act locally'. There is, however, uncertainty about future trends and the unpredictability of world health needs has been reinforced by the global HIV/AIDS pandemic, the re-emergence of malaria and tuberculosis in drug-resistant forms, affecting both developed and developing countries, and the recent outbreak of severe acute respiratory syndrome (SARS). The sanguine expectation that diseases such as polio or smallpox might be completely eradicated appears premature. Healthcare provision is also complicated by the fact that drug companies, by the (legal) use of patents, wield the ability to influence decisions as to which countries, and individuals, receive treatments. However, recent developments, due to public pressure, suggest that commercial interests may be overridden by a new political will in G8 countries, to ensure greater equity in access to therapeutic drugs, in a concerted attempt to address world poverty.

PREPARATION FOR PRACTICE

The student nurse experience has changed in many respects over the past 15 years. The demographic profile of entrants to nursing in the UK has altered considerably over this period. Women continue to outnumber men (although within higher grade posts men continue to outnumber women), but the average age and socio-economic profile of entrants has changed. The average age on entry to an undergraduate nursing programme within the UK is now mid to late twenties. This means that many entrants have a wider range of life experience than was previously the case and students frequently have domestic and financial commitments that require them to undertake paid employment while undergoing their education and training.

The environment in which programmes of preparation for practice are undertaken has changed. In 1992 many polytechnics in the UK acquired university status and these are the establishments within which the majority of nursing students now undertake their education programmes, and now at diploma or degree, rather than certificate, level. This has impacted on the ratio of theory to practice in nurse training. Students previously spent approximately 20% of their time on theory and 80% in practice placements. This figure now approximates to a ratio of 50:50 theory/practice. Locations for health and social care, previously focused upon institutions, have now changed considerably. Hospital admissions generally are of shorter duration than they were previously, with patients being rapidly discharged home, or to other community-based settings. Hospitals are now consequently the reserve of larger numbers of acutely ill patients who require considerable assistance with the basic activities of living as well as technical support. Care of patients by primary care teams, within community settings, is more widespread and intensive than 20 years ago, and nurses experience practice placements in areas that differ in many significant respects from those previously used.

Many developments over the past three decades have affected healthcare provision and raised new questions for nursing ethics such as demographic trends referred to earlier, e.g. an ageing population with proportionately fewer younger people available to support the elderly and sick. Technological advances which have significant social and ethical implications have taken place in many fields, for example new reproductive technologies, the mapping of the human genome, genetic screening and the developments in the field of immunology and organ transplants. Challenges have also emerged for practitioners in relation to hospital-acquired infections (HAIs) that prove resistant to most antibiotic therapy and whose cause is directly linked to inadequate standards of hospital hygiene – which are not merely the responsibility of healthcare staff but the result of policies of privatisation of cleaning services and changing political priorities within the UK.

Porter (1997, p. 595) summed up the state of healthcare at the end of the 20th century:

> Basic research, clinical science and technology working with one another have characterised the cutting edge of modern medicine. Progress has been made. For almost all diseases something can be done; some can be prevented or fully cured. Nevertheless, a century which has brought the most intense concentration of attention and resources on medical research ends with many of the major killers of western society – particularly heart and vascular disease, cancer, and chronic degenerative illnesses – largely incurable and in many cases increasing in incidence.

Additional to the major health problems cited by Porter, we have pointed out that there is an ever-increasing number of people in westernised societies who are obese, with the attendant risk of developing disorders such as: type 2 diabetes mellitus, osteo-arthritis and some forms of cancer. Political, economic and societal changes all impact on healthcare and provide us with some indication of future require-ments for health service provision and the place that nursing will occupy within it.

PROFESSIONAL ACCOUNTABILITY AND THE LAY PERSPECTIVE

As the demands on the healthcare system have continued to grow, and show no signs of abating, so has the importance of cost-effectiveness and efficiency. Accountability for clinical practice is partly driven by public demand for professional openness and an increasing appetite for litigation. A more educated public and a society in which watchdog organisations, lobbying and whistle-blowing are commonplace mean that healthcare is delivered under much greater public and media scrutiny than was once the case. For healthcare professionals there is increased emphasis on evidence-based practice. This is partly to be able to demonstrate to a critical public and politicians that

their work brings beneficial outcomes for patients, but this drive for evidence is also a demand of any soundly based scientific practice.

Public attitudes to the occupations classed as professions have been less supportive and more critical of them, at least in some respects, than was previously the case. Gradual societal changes, in conjunction with specific events such as those that led to the Royal Liverpool Children's Inquiry (HM Government 2001a), the inquiry into the management of care of children receiving complex heart surgery at the Bristol Royal Infirmary (HM Government 2001b), the case of Harold Shipman GP (Shipman Inquiry: HM Government 2005a), and a series of highly publicised professional misconduct cases, have resulted in greater awareness by the public that their trust in, and reliance on, professional opinion cannot be unquestioning. While trust in professional integrity and advice has been a strength of the system in the past, it is a weakness when it allows professionals to take advantage of that trust and dependence on their authority.

In the past 35 years, particularly since the World Health Assembly at Alma Ata in Russia in 1978, discussion about healthcare has moved from being a disease and medically dominated debate to one which takes more account of behavioural and social dimen-sions of health, and the lay view of health and illness in particular. The World Health Assembly's Alma Ata Declaration reaffirmed the wider definition of health included in the original 1947 WHO definition, recognising the need to shift priorities from a 'medical model' to a 'community health model', and from an emphasis on hospital medicine to primary care health and nursing services (WHO 1978).

The emergence of a plethora of self-help groups, and growth in popular interest in 'alternative medicine', presents a challenge to nurses and nursing as a profession. WHO, in noting these trends, has emphasised the key role that nurses can play here in the provision of sound health education and in teaching; and in transferring skills to lay people to enable them to do more at home and in the community to help themselves. Nurses too can help address the problems of delivering health services to the growing world population, especially where resources are constrained and limited, as in developing countries.

Developments within the field of medical sociology and sociological research demonstrate this shift away from naive dependence on medical science (e.g. Mackay et al 1998). Highly influential in this process was Stacey's call for a move from medical sociology to the sociology of health and illness (Stacey & Homans 1978). This was motivated by the belief that an understanding of health and illness would be better served by a move away from a medically oriented study of disease and illness behaviour, to one where more attention is given to the social factors that influence health and illness.

The Nursing and Midwifery Council (NMC) and General Medical Council have responded to pressure by increasing the lay membership of their councils. This has been beneficial and educative for both nurses and the lay people involved, but the extent to which lay members are truly 'representative' of the general population is debatable. Research by Davies (2001), for example, found that lay members within the UK are drawn from a narrow band of the population, the majority being white, middle-aged males with high socio-economic status.

'NURSING' ETHICS OR 'HEALTHCARE' ETHICS?

It has been argued that the divisions between medical ethics, nursing ethics and the ethics of the various paramedical professions are unhelpful in promoting collaborative activity in healthcare delivery, and that we should move towards an inclusive and generic ethics of healthcare. It is possible to maintain that a wider concept of healthcare ethics would help to ensure that the central emphasis is on the patient or client, rather than the doctor or nurse. Indeed, we suggested in the 4th edition of this book that the debates about ethics would benefit from a similar shift of emphasis – in this case away from a focus on medical and nursing ethics towards a more patient-centred healthcare ethics.

In this edition, however, we maintain the position that there is a place for the specific study of nursing ethics, because nurses occupy a specific place in the division of labour within healthcare. As long as this remains the case, adoption of a kind of ecumenical approach to 'healthcare ethics' does not do justice to the specific responsibilities of nurses. Whilst some issues that we discuss are pertinent to other health practitioners, there are specific issues that impact upon nurses and their practice. Clearly, each group of healthcare professionals contributes its own particular insights, values and ethical stances to healthcare. Consequently, the codes of conduct for each profession are slightly different. While these must embody the same general ethical principles that are applicable to all the caring professions, they must also relate to the specific responsibilities of each occupational group. If ethical debate is too global and aspirational, it may be of limited practical benefit to individual professionals in their own work. Ethics is essentially a practical discipline or 'practical science' – as Aristotle

maintained. If ethics does not relate meaningfully to the occupationally specific tasks and responsibilities of each group then it will be of little practical value – regardless of whether they have a 'customer focus' or are directed more at the needs of the recipient of healthcare than its providers. Whilst the boundaries of professional responsibility and roles in the division of labour may change, and the Health Professions' Council in the UK may assume an increasing and overarching influence in forthcoming years, the risk is that a too broad-based 'healthcare ethics' will not make allowances for the differences, as well as similarities, in the healthcare professions' relationships with their clients. There is a risk that ethics becomes applicable to everything in general and nothing in particular.

During the past 30 years nursing has made a determined effort to identify and produce a body of knowledge that it can call its own. Developments in the sociology of health and illness have been significant for the development of nursing as an academic discipline. In this, the focus upon the individual patient has become paramount. These developments fit well with the growing interest in, and educational emphasis upon, nursing ethics.

For this reason, among others discussed below, the title of this book remains unchanged. This does not imply that its content is irrelevant to those in other healthcare professions. On the contrary, we believe not only that the analysis and discussion of general issues in healthcare in this book will be of interest to all other health professions, but also that by clarifying the particular dimensions of nursing responsibility and examining the ethical aspects of nursing practice this will throw into relief the different aspects of practice that are of concern to other professions as well. While the primary focus of the book will be upon ethical issues raised by the specific nature of nursing work, as we move towards greater interprofessional collaboration and teamwork our hope is that this book may contribute to better understanding of the core values that define the ethos and practice of nursing.

CHANGE AND CONTINUITY

As authors we have attempted to ensure the book is relevant to the contemporary scene and while we look to the future, we must also seek to preserve what has served us well in the past. Tradition and innovation always remain in tension with one another in any living, developing moral community. This is reflected in the changing ways in which we view individuals and their rights and responsibilities relative to other people and the community at large in different cultures at different times. The processes by which a community maintains its common values and goals are as important to its continuation as a moral community as is the need for innovation and adaptation to change. This applies as much to nursing as to any other community. Kant pointed out, in his great 18th century work on the foundations of ethics (Paton 1969), that the *concept of a person* (or responsible moral agent) and the *concept of a moral community* (a body of people who share common principles) are logically connected, and both concepts are necessary for, and presupposed in, any discussion of ethics.

Developments and changes in nursing, and in society, involve challenges to the existing definition of nursing and may result in its redefinition, and this has an impact on the scope and nature of 'nursing ethics'. It is a sign of vitality in nursing that it is not stuck in a particular image of the nurse, despite the stereotypical caricatures sometimes depicted in the media. Nurses continue to debate the nature and role of nursing, both within the profession and also in dialogue or competition with medicine and other health professions. Nurses additionally engage with society as a whole, as they strive to change public expectations and break out of the confines of an oppressively patriarchal past. Nursing ethics, now and in the future, will have to grapple with gender-related politics in a profession where women continue to predominate numerically, but where, in proportion to their numbers, men continue to enjoy disproportionate power and influence.

This reflection on past experience and attempt to discern the most appropriate way to move forward into the future is in some ways a model of ethical decision-making itself, for we make decisions based on *evaluative* judgements – we evaluate the past, assess the needs of the present and project ourselves forward into the uncertainty of the future. We apply our own values as we examine how the current context is shaped by the past, confront challenges in the present and develop strategies to deal effectively with these in the future. We must identify, and strive to achieve, the specific goals that are implied in our choice of *values* in the first place. Sound ethics must involve giving a proper weight to tradition and past experience in making judgements, but ethical decision-making is not retrospective, it must be prospective. It requires the courage to move forward into the future, to engage with uncertainty and unpredictability. Ethics cannot be solely reactive to the demands of the past, to established conventions, rules and practice. Ethical competence requires the knowledge, skills and confidence to be proactive, to take risks and accept responsibility for difficult decisions.

Although nursing, as the activity of caring for those who are sick, injured, weak and vulnerable, is as old as human society itself, as a formally recognised profession it has a short history. If the pace of change in the past century is anything to go by, it is likely that the rate of change in the future is likely to continue, or to accelerate. Nursing, throughout its history, has had to adapt to changing social conditions, changes in patterns of morbidity and mortality, advances in medicine and applied medical technology, changes in the modes of healthcare delivery, and associated changes in the roles and responsibilities of nurses in healthcare policy and administration. As an occupational group, nurses have proved remarkably resilient in their ability to adapt to change. This has perhaps been a distinctive mark of their professionalism and commitment to vocational ideals.

Social, demographic, economic and epidemiological changes have brought challenges to nurses, to improve, and expand upon, their knowledge and repertoire of skills; but they have also brought additional challenges of an ethical nature – both in terms of new problems to be addressed and in terms of increased personal and professional moral responsibility. Nursing ethics itself has undergone a revolution from a focus on nursing etiquette in the early 1900s to a serious exploration of the knowledge and skills required by nurses to enable them to bring the same professionalism to their ethical decision-making that they seek to apply to their clinical, educational and managerial roles. Partly as a result of the move of nursing into the higher education sector, nursing ethics has been a rapidly developing area of professional study, and nurses in their own right are increasingly making a significant contribution to academic debate, research and teaching in the subject area.

THE PERENNIAL AND CURRENT ISSUES IN NURSING

In the attempt to be contemporary and relevant, to address the extraordinary challenges presented by new developments (e.g. in genetic engineering), there is a risk that we will fail to address the ordinary routine issues and ethical problems that all nurses must face. Some issues lose their topicality over time, due to attention shift, to media manipulation of public interest or to 'resolution' of the issue. We attempt in this book to identify and discuss some of the new problems confronting nurses at the frontiers of medical advance and research, but are convinced that we must not neglect the everyday moral problems which are perennially part of the care and treatment of people made vulnerable by mental or physical health problems. Whilst the moral problems encountered on a daily basis for the majority of practitioners are not 'life and death' issues, decisions made may impact significantly upon patients' quality of life.

Life is characterised by both continuity and change and, while we must address the challenges of the present and future, there are certain features of human life and the human condition that are perennial. For example, the processes and problems, pleasure and suffering related to birth, maturation, adulthood, reproduction, parenting, maintenance of physical and mental health, ageing and death apply to all human beings. While individuals may change, for good or ill, it is questionable whether human nature changes. The problems inherent in making sense of life, of pain and suffering, of facing death and bereavement, and the quest for happiness remain, despite scientific and social advancements. With the publication of *Health for All in the 21st Century* (WHO 1999b) we were faced with the challenge of where nursing should be going. The role of nursing in the healthcare systems of the 21st century is likely to preserve many features of its past – insofar as supporting patients through experiences of altered health state to achieve some resolution of their health problems, or accommodation to them, will remain a major feature of nursing work.

Within the UK, expansion of health services in the form of NHS Direct and NHS24 (Scotland) means that nurses and paramedical staff play an increasing role as the first point of contact for those seeking healthcare advice and will provide a gateway to appropriate services. The General Medical Services contracts mean that 'out of hours' services may be delivered in ways that are different from the past, as the pattern of work by health professionals changes in accordance with the European Union Working Time Directive, which stipulates a maximum number of working hours per week. As junior medical staff commonly exceed this number of hours, compliance with the EU legislation necessitates employment of larger numbers of staff at this grade than currently exist, to meet society's needs. Recruitment drives are unlikely, at least in the short term, to cover this labour shortfall, thus necessitating delegation of some of the workload at present dealt with by junior medical staff to others, e.g. to nurses. This 'solution' has already been implemented in some areas. Nursing has a history of role expansion in relation to tasks previously deemed to be 'medical work' and this has the potential to develop further. It would be over-sanguine to regard these alterations in working practice as providing unqualified benefits either to health professionals or to society. There

are questions of an ethical nature to be addressed concerning the overall benefit or detriment to healthcare resulting from current trends in health policy and the 'Agenda for Change', including the role expansion and extension of responsibility for nurses and others. Nurses should be wary of enthusiastic 'colonisation of territory' that medicine is willing to relinquish, as this may not invariably be in the short-, or long-term interests of either care recipients or practitioners.

THE RELEVANCE OF RESEARCH IN NURSING AND APPLIED ETHICS

Research is never value-neutral. We may begin with the apparently neutral question: 'Can this project be undertaken?' (i.e. methodologically and logistically). However, we soon have to proceed to the question 'Should or ought this research be undertaken?' (i.e. ethically). Once research is commenced, we are confronted by a whole series of further ethical questions related to obtaining informed consent from research subjects, confidentiality of records, risks and benefits and the value of the research to society as a whole – matters in relation to which nurse researchers would have to satisfy their Research Ethics Committees that they have provided adequate safeguards. Epistemological questions about the scientific quality of the research and the methods used are also implicitly ethical, in that they affect the legitimacy of the research, with reference to the propriety of the means used and the costs and benefits of its practical outcomes.

Research is an area in which issues have sometimes been unhelpfully dichotomised. A quantitative paradigm, in which hypotheses are tested and an attempt made to establish cause-and-effect relationships statistically, is associated with a scientific medical model that purports to be value-free. Randomised controlled trials (RCTs) have been referred to as constituting a 'gold standard', against which all other research approaches in healthcare are to be evaluated. A quantitative approach aims to use sufficiently large numbers to enable generalisation of findings from the study group to be applied to the population at large. Qualitative research methods are characterised by in-depth, non-numerical, exploration of the area under study (frequently by observation, interview or a combination of these) and the art of qualitative research lies in the interpretation of the evidence. The purpose of qualitative work is to elicit meaning, and possibly generate theory, from rigorous analysis of the data. Quantitative research has frequently been justify our ethical decisions. The authors set out to avoid the problems of either a simple *deductivist* approach based on ethical theory, or an *inductive* approach based on individual case studies or casuistry, by advocating a *coherence theory of justification*. However, the way in which they categorise different approaches to justification, and the heavy emphasis given to moral theory in the succeeding chapters reinforce an overly theoretical approach to justification of ethical beliefs and policies, rather than addressing the practical task of making sound ethical decisions and being able to give a reasonable account of how we reached our conclusions in a particular case. We argue that two different levels or types of 'justification' are being confused and conflated here, namely the first-order level of moral judgement at which we may have to *justify specific decisions or actions* to someone else (e.g. the decision to sedate a *specific* patient who is disturbed); and the second-order level of 'moral judgement' where we are concerned to *justify our general approach* to *types* of situations of this kind (i.e. in defining our general policy on sedating patients).

Debate about theories of moral development and methods of developing skills in moral reasoning have been given greater emphasis in nursing curricula due to the requirement of the UK NMC, for example, that ethics should permeate all undergraduate programmes. Kohlberg (1973, 1976, 1984) put forward a theory of moral development and claimed there are gender differences in the way individuals progress through his various stages. Gilligan's critical response to Kohlberg (Gilligan 1982, 1993), and the controversy which developed, stimulated much research on whether there are significant gender differences in the pattern of moral development and moral reasoning between the sexes.

This work has been considered by some authorities to be of particular relevance to nursing, in its role as a caring profession and in relation to gender issues and medical dominance in healthcare. Writers have tended to set up the *caring* role of nursing and the *curing* activity of medicine in opposition to one another, whereas in reality care and cure are not polar opposites, and medicine and nursing have to combine elements of both. Some writers have also attempted to demonstrate a link between the alleged care/cure dichotomy and the gendered stereotyping of the two occupational groups. Controversies about the ethics of care and the philosophical exploration of the nature of caring, as distinct from a more rational justice ethic, are not new. They have their parallels in the biblical Old Testament controversies about the respective demands of justice and mercy, and the New Testament ones concerning the respective demands of law on the

one hand, and love on the other. Nor is the debate entirely new to healthcare, where issues such as the relation of care and cure, and of medicine as an art to medicine as a science, and the contribution of caring to therapy and the healing process, are almost as old as medicine itself. This kind of controversy has been part of an ongoing debate in nursing too, about the role of knowledge and technical skills, and their relation to the delivery of effective nursing care.

There are several ways in which the focus on 'caring ethics' has influenced ethical debate in nursing. *First*, the cure/care dichotomy has been used here, as in the past, to distinguish the 'objective and scientific medical model' of health from 'a more personal nursing perspective'. In this way, it has often become the focus, or a central theme, in claims made for a specialised body of nursing knowledge, or arguments for the application of distinctive methods of research to nursing. *Second*, it has generated a whole body of literature by feminist writers, analysing the pattern of ethics and relationships in hospitals and other healthcare institutions, as constructed on a pattern of a type of 'master discourse' that is patriarchal, impersonal and determined by a 'justice perspective', to which another type of discourse, the 'caring perspective' of the nurse, must be opposed. *Third*, it has raised some interesting questions about the nature of ethics itself and whether the pursuit of a universal framework of principles, rights and duties is to be preferred to a more phenomenological and existentially grounded approach which attends to the specific situation, particular relationships and the demands inherent in the exercise of personal moral responsibility.

A 'postmodernist' feminist approach to ethics identifies traditional philosophical ethics as 'patriarchal' and, with its emphasis on universal principles and rational justice, as driven by a 'will to control' the world and other people (particularly women). In opposition to this, the 'caring perspective' of feminist ethics is recommended, because it avoids the 'totalising' and 'dominative critical' approach of a 'masculinist' ethic (Gilligan 1982, 1993). In place of an attempt to base ethical decision-making on universal rational principles and logical methods of problem-solving (allegedly the natural tendencies of the 'master discourses' of men), we are urged to listen to the 'different voice' of feminine sensibility, with its emphasis on 'narrative and contextual accounts, that encourage respect for the differences between persons and sensitivity to the complexity of our interconnections' (Bowden 1997, p. 10).

At best, the plethora of research generated by the work of Kohlberg and Gilligan has reinforced the fact

contrasted with qualitative approaches, with the former being seen as 'objective' and the latter as involving value judgements and being more 'subjective'. Rather than making inappropriate comparisons between quantitative and qualitative approaches, a more constructive approach might be to stipulate that the research method selected in conducting a piece of research should be driven by the research question, rather than by an ideological commitment to one research paradigm over another.

'Evidence-based practice' is an essential prerequisite for ensuring medically and scientifically sound practice and good quality patient care. Unlike purely academic research, evidence-based practice is essentially a form of operational research and should be an integral part of everyday professional work. It involves building in evaluation to all aspects of routine nursing care and the systems that support it. Here, tension may arise in trying to achieve a balance between the demands of 'effectiveness', particularly in economic terms, and maintenance of quality standards in meeting patient needs. Nursing, like other professions in healthcare, must be concerned with the quality of care but is also under pressure to produce value for money. The nursing profession exists in order to provide a public service and so there is a need to balance the costs and benefits of various forms of service provision with the demands for effectiveness and efficiency. Nurses often find themselves caught in the middle, having to advocate for and defend the rights of individual patients in the face of arguments that are directed to achieving the best overall outcomes. The same tensions also exist within the private healthcare sector, in which profit margins require to be optimised, and may even take more acute forms where people cannot afford the treatment options offered to them. As a policy, 'customer choice' may become a 'Hobson's choice' for both consumers and practitioners!

The rapid changes in nursing practice over the past half century, with the development of tertiary level education and training for nurses, and the establishment of nursing as a recognised subject of academic study and research, necessitates that discussion of ethics in nursing takes proper account of the advances in nursing research. Nursing now has a body of applied research in its own right. The application of the behavioural and social sciences, as well as the clinical sciences, to the study of the theory and practice of nursing has changed the profession's perception and understanding of itself and the image of nurses in society. Nursing research has become multidimensional, ranging from research into the efficacy of nursing procedures routinely used in patient care,

through studies of nurse–patient communication, the social dynamics of hospitals and life on a hospital ward, to research undertaken in order to establish appropriate indicators for appraisal of nursing performance, quality assurance and the economics of nursing within the context of hospital and community-based healthcare. As in any other research involving human subjects, directly or indirectly, nursing research must be subject to objective monitoring in order to maintain rigorous scientific and ethical standards. In this connection, the experience of nurses is increasingly sought on ethics of research committees dealing with both clinical and administrative practice in healthcare. The role of ethics committees with their attendant bureaucracy is, however, currently under scrutiny, as their remit is deemed by some researchers to overstep the level of scrutiny required to ensure protection of potential participants and instead may impede commencement and the conduct of valuable research. If it is the case that overzealous bureaucracy is hampering ethically justifiable healthcare research that may benefit patients then this, in itself, does require critical review and the development of more appropriate ethical policy and procedures. It does not mean allowing researchers, or their funding bodies, to dictate how ethical and scientific review of research proposals is to take place.

The relationship of ethics to research does not, of course, relate solely to the conduct of formal research studies, but extends to the fundamental requirement that nursing practice be based, wherever possible, upon sound evaluation of practice and credible evidence, rather than on anecdotal evidence, and customary practice.

TEACHING ETHICS IN NURSING

Since the emergence of nursing as a recognised occupation within the past 160 years, nursing ethics has undergone a revolution, both in the perception of its form and scope, and in the sophistication of the debate among nurses themselves. Nursing ethics has left behind the view that ethics is simply a matter of observing the right social etiquette, or the view that ethics is simply a matter of adherence to a disciplinary code, or that nursing ethics is just an echo of biomedical ethics. We believe that nurses have come to recognise that ethics is central to their profession as a caring profession; that the moral 'virtues' are fundamental theoretical and practical competencies required by nurses to perform effectively and well in their occupation. Furthermore, that ethics encompasses all levels of nursing services and their delivery – the values and standards of nursing practice, nursing management, and the collaboration of nurses with other professions in the organisation and delivery of healthcare services generally. Acknowledgement of the importance of nursing ethics is reflected in, and is in turn promoted by, official policy recognition. In the UK, the NMC (2005a) stipulates that teaching of ethics must be integrated into all undergraduate nursing programmes. In postgraduate nursing programmes, there has been increased time and attention given to ethics. Specialised units dealing with various aspects of ethics have been developed, and many nurses have now acquired formal training and qualifications in ethics. Associated with these developments, there is a growing body of academic and practical research literature on nursing and healthcare ethics, contributed to by a variety of experts in law, ethics, behavioural and social sciences and nursing (for website links related to this topic, please see http://evolve.elsevier.com/Thompson/ nursing ethics).

There has been a shift in both the form and content of the debate about ethics in nursing. This has been driven not only by research and the changes in healthcare mentioned earlier, but also by the needs of nurses themselves. As they have taken on greater responsibility in decision-making and new clinical roles they have demanded assistance to meet the challenges with which they find themselves confronted. This book was written originally in response to such demands, and in its various editions we have attempted to keep pace with changes in nursing and healthcare. In this edition we seek to highlight how these changes have exerted a direct influence on the nature of ethical debates within nursing. It is important for the profession to have an understanding of where nursing has come from and some view of the direction in which it is moving, if nurses are to be equipped to take an informed and responsible part in contemporary ethical debate. Nurses require up-to-date knowledge and understanding of the implications for nursing practice of biomedical, technical and scientific innovations, but also, more fundamentally, relevant skills in applied ethics. These include: skills in clarifying and differentiating personal, professional and organisational values; skills in systematic methods of ethical decision-making; and skills in setting practical ethical standards and policy within their own teams and institutions. As we progress into the 21st century, study of the ethical issues of particular importance in nursing cannot be divorced from the wider debate about the ethics of healthcare generally. In fact the better nurses understand ethics from the point of view of their own

profession and practice, the better they will be able to contribute to this debate.

Research on ethics in nursing and the effectiveness and/or ineffectiveness of various approaches to teaching ethics in nursing is still relatively new, but recent work in this area is taking the discussion beyond the anecdotal, or the opinionated grandstanding of untried theories, into an era of more systematic application of tried and tested methods of appraisal adapted from other human sciences. From educational research, and health education research in particular, nurses and others have begun to apply objective measures to appraise education and skills training in ethics, in both formative and summative evaluation. This book attempts to apply what has been learned from these sources to the way our material is presented and teachers are offered some practical guidance on appropriate methods.

Since 1980 when the first edition of this book was published, the previously exclusive focus on 'medical ethics' has given way to a recognition that nursing ethics represents a proper domain of study in its own right. There have been changes in the range of 'fashionable' issues which have been the centre of ethical debate in nursing, and a related shift from a narrow focus on clinical nursing ethics to study of the many levels at which nurses exercise moral responsibility – including critical study of the whole culture and organisation of nursing management and service delivery. Our own attempts to apply adult education and group learning methods to ethics teaching in healthcare have been part of ongoing research on educational methodology as applied to nursing, and this has led to some revolutionary new approaches to teaching and learning. We have progressed from segregated and didactic courses to multidisciplinary, interactive and participative learning; and from an overly theoretical approach to ethics to a focus on case-based, self-directed and experiential learning in appropriate learning environments. Further, as nurses have increasingly acquired familiarity with literature in ethics, nursing and healthcare, so there has been more emphasis on wider familiarity with logic, epistemology (or theory of knowledge) and philosophy of science as well as philosophical ethics.

The challenge in teaching ethics is not to teach a body of rules that may change, or doctrines that will inevitably go out of fashion, and be superseded by new rules and new teaching. The pedagogical challenge is to find ways to help people develop practical understanding of the ideals and standards of the profession. and to equip them with the necessary tools or decision-making skills for responsible practice. These skills should enable them to apply

general principles intelligently in a context-sensitive way, to ensure competent and confident selection of the right means to achieve good outcomes, and accept public accountability for their actions. By doing this we are essentially concerned with teaching what Aristotle called prudence or practical wisdom as the foundation for responsible moral living and sound ethical decision-making, namely, the informed and skilful ability to apply general principles to the demands of particular situations, so that we choose the most effective means to achieve the best possible outcome.

The task of teaching practical ethics cannot be achieved by a textbook, however good. It requires the maieutic skills of the intellectual midwife (Plato 1984), the educator's skill to nurture and draw out the potential of the trainee; the counsellor's skill to assist students to develop their capacity for reflection on practice; the ability to identify good practice and to imitate positive role models – in the interests of improving their performance as nurses. These pedagogical skills are all necessary to provide relevant support and a practical context in which learners can practise and master the skills they require to be competent moral agents. In particular, we argue that nurses need to develop the core skills mentioned above, namely:

- skills in clarifying values applicable to the different levels of nursing operations
- skills in systematic and problem-solving approaches to ethical decision-making
- skills in collaborating with others to determine sound ethical standards or policy.

This book is not intended as a training manual for those responsible for the education and training of nurses. That is a task for a different kind of publication. However, we have stated learning outcomes for each chapter and, based on our experience of teaching ethics, we have provided suggestions for methods that may be of assistance to teachers (suggestions for teaching strategies may be found at the website that accompanies this book: http://evolve.elsevier.com/ Thompson/nursing ethics).

THE PLACE OF MORAL THEORY IN PRACTICAL NURSING ETHICS

Ethics, as Aristotle observed over 2000 years ago, is a *practical science*. It is practical in two senses: first, it must be rooted in actual practice, and second, it must help us to make more soundly based decisions so as to deal effectively with real problems in life. If a book on

nursing ethics is to be practical in the first sense, then it must address the specific context of nursing practice and deal with the specific problems faced by nurses. For this reason we have not attempted to write a book for nurses on general moral philosophy, but we have sought deliberately to address the specific contexts of nursing practice and nursing experience directly. If ethics is to be practical in the second sense, then it must help nurses develop the practical wisdom and skills that will enable them not only to become more competent in decision-making, but also to develop as responsible moral agents. For this reason, general discussion of moral theory is kept to a minimum, and emphasis is placed on dealing with cases and the management of problems taken from the realities of nursing practice.

Given queries from a number of reviewers as to why ethical theory is not dealt with at the beginning and is left to the final chapters of the book, it may be helpful to provide the rationale for our approach. Moral philosophy is preoccupied with moral theory, rather than practical decision-making. It seeks to explain concrete moral experience, not in its everyday occurrence, but in terms that are generalisable. If we start off from a moral theory perspective, then we tend to see the justification for specific ethical decisions as requiring to be based on one or another of the classical moral theories. This seems to us to be misguided – partly for practical pedagogical reasons and partly for philosophical reasons. From the pedagogical perspective, our experience is that attempting to teach moral theory to medical and nursing students in a vacuum is not of interest to the majority, whose need and desire is for practical assistance in their day-to-day decision-making. The philosophical objections are similar to Aristotle's insofar as he maintains that ethics is a practical discipline requiring the development of practical skills. Alternatively, we might apply to ethics Marx's general claim that 'praxis drives theoria' and argue that moral theory arises out of reflection on everyday experience of action and decision-making, rather than the other way around, and that justifying general ethical policy and justifying specific moral judgements or actions are different kinds of activity.

A number of influential textbooks on nursing ethics have adopted the approach that in order to justify moral judgements we need prior knowledge of ethical theory (e.g. Davis & Aroskar 1983, Tschudin 1986, Kerridge et al 1998). This seems contrary to both common sense and the traditions of ethical realism. Even Beauchamp & Childress (2004), in their widely used textbook on biomedical ethics, seem to presuppose that we need understanding of philosophical categories and moral theory in order to be able to

contrasted with qualitative approaches, with the former being seen as 'objective' and the latter as involving value judgements and being more 'subjective'. Rather than making inappropriate comparisons between quantitative and qualitative approaches, a more constructive approach might be to stipulate that the research method selected in conducting a piece of research should be driven by the research question, rather than by an ideological commitment to one research paradigm over another.

'Evidence-based practice' is an essential prerequisite for ensuring medically and scientifically sound practice and good quality patient care. Unlike purely academic research, evidence-based practice is essentially a form of operational research and should be an integral part of everyday professional work. It involves building in evaluation to all aspects of routine nursing care and the systems that support it. Here, tension may arise in trying to achieve a balance between the demands of 'effectiveness', particularly in economic terms, and maintenance of quality standards in meeting patient needs. Nursing, like other professions in healthcare, must be concerned with the quality of care but is also under pressure to produce value for money. The nursing profession exists in order to provide a public service and so there is a need to balance the costs and benefits of various forms of service provision with the demands for effectiveness and efficiency. Nurses often find themselves caught in the middle, having to advocate for and defend the rights of individual patients in the face of arguments that are directed to achieving the best overall outcomes. The same tensions also exist within the private healthcare sector, in which profit margins require to be optimised, and may even take more acute forms where people cannot afford the treatment options offered to them. As a policy, 'customer choice' may become a 'Hobson's choice' for both consumers and practitioners!

The rapid changes in nursing practice over the past half century, with the development of tertiary level education and training for nurses, and the establishment of nursing as a recognised subject of academic study and research, necessitates that discussion of ethics in nursing takes proper account of the advances in nursing research. Nursing now has a body of applied research in its own right. The application of the behavioural and social sciences, as well as the clinical sciences, to the study of the theory and practice of nursing has changed the profession's perception and understanding of itself and the image of nurses in society. Nursing research has become multidimensional, ranging from research into the efficacy of nursing procedures routinely used in patient care, through studies of nurse–patient communication, the social dynamics of hospitals and life on a hospital ward, to research undertaken in order to establish appropriate indicators for appraisal of nursing performance, quality assurance and the economics of nursing within the context of hospital and community-based healthcare. As in any other research involving human subjects, directly or indirectly, nursing research must be subject to objective monitoring in order to maintain rigorous scientific and ethical standards. In this connection, the experience of nurses is increasingly sought on ethics of research committees dealing with both clinical and administrative practice in healthcare. The role of ethics committees with their attendant bureaucracy is, however, currently under scrutiny, as their remit is deemed by some researchers to overstep the level of scrutiny required to ensure protection of potential participants and instead may impede commencement and the conduct of valuable research. If it is the case that overzealous bureaucracy is hampering ethically justifiable healthcare research that may benefit patients then this, in itself, does require critical review and the development of more appropriate ethical policy and procedures. It does not mean allowing researchers, or their funding bodies, to dictate how ethical and scientific review of research proposals is to take place.

The relationship of ethics to research does not, of course, relate solely to the conduct of formal research studies, but extends to the fundamental requirement that nursing practice be based, wherever possible, upon sound evaluation of practice and credible evidence, rather than on anecdotal evidence, and customary practice.

TEACHING ETHICS IN NURSING

Since the emergence of nursing as a recognised occupation within the past 160 years, nursing ethics has undergone a revolution, both in the perception of its form and scope, and in the sophistication of the debate among nurses themselves. Nursing ethics has left behind the view that ethics is simply a matter of observing the right social etiquette, or the view that ethics is simply a matter of adherence to a disciplinary code, or that nursing ethics is just an echo of biomedical ethics. We believe that nurses have come to recognise that ethics is central to their profession as a caring profession; that the moral 'virtues' are fundamental theoretical and practical competencies required by nurses to perform effectively and well in their occupation. Furthermore, that ethics encompasses all levels of nursing services and their delivery – the values and standards of nursing practice, nursing management, and the collaboration of nurses with other professions in the organisation and delivery of healthcare services generally. Acknowledgement of the importance of nursing ethics is reflected in, and is in turn promoted by, official policy recognition. In the UK, the NMC (2005a) stipulates that teaching of ethics must be integrated into all undergraduate nursing programmes. In postgraduate nursing programmes, there has been increased time and attention given to ethics. Specialised units dealing with various aspects of ethics have been developed, and many nurses have now acquired formal training and qualifications in ethics. Associated with these developments, there is a growing body of academic and practical research literature on nursing and healthcare ethics, contributed to by a variety of experts in law, ethics, behavioural and social sciences and nursing (for website links related to this topic, please see http://evolve.elsevier.com/Thompson/ nursing ethics).

There has been a shift in both the form and content of the debate about ethics in nursing. This has been driven not only by research and the changes in healthcare mentioned earlier, but also by the needs of nurses themselves. As they have taken on greater responsibility in decision-making and new clinical roles they have demanded assistance to meet the challenges with which they find themselves confronted. This book was written originally in response to such demands, and in its various editions we have attempted to keep pace with changes in nursing and healthcare. In this edition we seek to highlight how these changes have exerted a direct influence on the nature of ethical debates within nursing. It is important for the profession to have an understanding of where nursing has come from and some view of the direction in which it is moving, if nurses are to be equipped to take an informed and responsible part in contemporary ethical debate. Nurses require up-to-date knowledge and understanding of the implications for nursing practice of biomedical, technical and scientific innovations, but also, more fundamentally, relevant skills in applied ethics. These include: skills in clarifying and differentiating personal, professional and organisational values; skills in systematic methods of ethical decision-making; and skills in setting practical ethical standards and policy within their own teams and institutions. As we progress into the 21st century, study of the ethical issues of particular importance in nursing cannot be divorced from the wider debate about the ethics of healthcare generally. In fact the better nurses understand ethics from the point of view of their own profession and practice, the better they will be able to contribute to this debate.

Research on ethics in nursing and the effectiveness and/or ineffectiveness of various approaches to teaching ethics in nursing is still relatively new, but recent work in this area is taking the discussion beyond the anecdotal, or the opinionated grandstanding of untried theories, into an era of more systematic application of tried and tested methods of appraisal adapted from other human sciences. From educational research, and health education research in particular, nurses and others have begun to apply objective measures to appraise education and skills training in ethics, in both formative and summative evaluation. This book attempts to apply what has been learned from these sources to the way our material is presented and teachers are offered some practical guidance on appropriate methods.

Since 1980 when the first edition of this book was published, the previously exclusive focus on 'medical ethics' has given way to a recognition that nursing ethics represents a proper domain of study in its own right. There have been changes in the range of 'fashionable' issues which have been the centre of ethical debate in nursing, and a related shift from a narrow focus on clinical nursing ethics to study of the many levels at which nurses exercise moral responsibility – including critical study of the whole culture and organisation of nursing management and service delivery. Our own attempts to apply adult education and group learning methods to ethics teaching in healthcare have been part of ongoing research on educational methodology as applied to nursing, and this has led to some revolutionary new approaches to teaching and learning. We have progressed from segregated and didactic courses to multidisciplinary, interactive and participative learning; and from an overly theoretical approach to ethics to a focus on case-based, self-directed and experiential learning in appropriate learning environments. Further, as nurses have increasingly acquired familiarity with literature in ethics, nursing and healthcare, so there has been more emphasis on wider familiarity with logic, epistemology (or theory of knowledge) and philosophy of science as well as philosophical ethics.

The challenge in teaching ethics is not to teach a body of rules that may change, or doctrines that will inevitably go out of fashion, and be superseded by new rules and new teaching. The pedagogical challenge is to find ways to help people develop practical understanding of the ideals and standards of the profession. and to equip them with the necessary tools or decision-making skills for responsible practice. These skills should enable them to apply general principles intelligently in a context-sensitive way, to ensure competent and confident selection of the right means to achieve good outcomes, and accept public accountability for their actions. By doing this we are essentially concerned with teaching what Aristotle called prudence or practical wisdom as the foundation for responsible moral living and sound ethical decision-making, namely, the informed and skilful ability to apply general principles to the demands of particular situations, so that we choose the most effective means to achieve the best possible outcome.

The task of teaching practical ethics cannot be achieved by a textbook, however good. It requires the maieutic skills of the intellectual midwife (Plato 1984), the educator's skill to nurture and draw out the potential of the trainee; the counsellor's skill to assist students to develop their capacity for reflection on practice; the ability to identify good practice and to imitate positive role models – in the interests of improving their performance as nurses. These pedagogical skills are all necessary to provide relevant support and a practical context in which learners can practise and master the skills they require to be competent moral agents. In particular, we argue that nurses need to develop the core skills mentioned above, namely:

- skills in clarifying values applicable to the different levels of nursing operations
- skills in systematic and problem-solving approaches to ethical decision-making
- skills in collaborating with others to determine sound ethical standards or policy.

This book is not intended as a training manual for those responsible for the education and training of nurses. That is a task for a different kind of publication. However, we have stated learning outcomes for each chapter and, based on our experience of teaching ethics, we have provided suggestions for methods that may be of assistance to teachers (suggestions for teaching strategies may be found at the website that accompanies this book: http://evolve.elsevier.com/Thompson/nursing ethics).

THE PLACE OF MORAL THEORY IN PRACTICAL NURSING ETHICS

Ethics, as Aristotle observed over 2000 years ago, is a *practical science*. It is practical in two senses: first, it must be rooted in actual practice, and second, it must help us to make more soundly based decisions so as to deal effectively with real problems in life. If a book on nursing ethics is to be practical in the first sense, then it must address the specific context of nursing practice and deal with the specific problems faced by nurses. For this reason we have not attempted to write a book for nurses on general moral philosophy, but we have sought deliberately to address the specific contexts of nursing practice and nursing experience directly. If ethics is to be practical in the second sense, then it must help nurses develop the practical wisdom and skills that will enable them not only to become more competent in decision-making, but also to develop as responsible moral agents. For this reason, general discussion of moral theory is kept to a minimum, and emphasis is placed on dealing with cases and the management of problems taken from the realities of nursing practice.

Given queries from a number of reviewers as to why ethical theory is not dealt with at the beginning and is left to the final chapters of the book, it may be helpful to provide the rationale for our approach. Moral philosophy is preoccupied with moral theory, rather than practical decision-making. It seeks to explain concrete moral experience, not in its everyday occurrence, but in terms that are generalisable. If we start off from a moral theory perspective, then we tend to see the justification for specific ethical decisions as requiring to be based on one or another of the classical moral theories. This seems to us to be misguided – partly for practical pedagogical reasons and partly for philosophical reasons. From the pedagogical perspective, our experience is that attempting to teach moral theory to medical and nursing students in a vacuum is not of interest to the majority, whose need and desire is for practical assistance in their day-to-day decision-making. The philosophical objections are similar to Aristotle's insofar as he maintains that ethics is a practical discipline requiring the development of practical skills. Alternatively, we might apply to ethics Marx's general claim that 'praxis drives theoria' and argue that moral theory arises out of reflection on everyday experience of action and decision-making, rather than the other way around, and that justifying general ethical policy and justifying specific moral judgements or actions are different kinds of activity.

A number of influential textbooks on nursing ethics have adopted the approach that in order to justify moral judgements we need prior knowledge of ethical theory (e.g. Davis & Aroskar 1983, Tschudin 1986, Kerridge et al 1998). This seems contrary to both common sense and the traditions of ethical realism. Even Beauchamp & Childress (2004), in their widely used textbook on biomedical ethics, seem to presuppose that we need understanding of philosophical categories and moral theory in order to be able to justify our ethical decisions. The authors set out to avoid the problems of either a simple *deductivist* approach based on ethical theory, or an *inductive* approach based on individual case studies or casuistry, by advocating a *coherence theory of justification*. However, the way in which they categorise different approaches to justification, and the heavy emphasis given to moral theory in the succeeding chapters reinforce an overly theoretical approach to justification of ethical beliefs and policies, rather than addressing the practical task of making sound ethical decisions and being able to give a reasonable account of how we reached our conclusions in a particular case. We argue that two different levels or types of 'justification' are being confused and conflated here, namely the first-order level of moral judgement at which we may have to *justify specific decisions or actions* to someone else (e.g. the decision to sedate a *specific* patient who is disturbed); and the second-order level of 'moral judgement' where we are concerned to *justify our general approach* to *types* of situations of this kind (i.e. in defining our general policy on sedating patients).

Debate about theories of moral development and methods of developing skills in moral reasoning have been given greater emphasis in nursing curricula due to the requirement of the UK NMC, for example, that ethics should permeate all undergraduate programmes. Kohlberg (1973, 1976, 1984) put forward a theory of moral development and claimed there are gender differences in the way individuals progress through his various stages. Gilligan's critical response to Kohlberg (Gilligan 1982, 1993), and the controversy which developed, stimulated much research on whether there are significant gender differences in the pattern of moral development and moral reasoning between the sexes.

This work has been considered by some authorities to be of particular relevance to nursing, in its role as a caring profession and in relation to gender issues and medical dominance in healthcare. Writers have tended to set up the *caring* role of nursing and the *curing* activity of medicine in opposition to one another, whereas in reality care and cure are not polar opposites, and medicine and nursing have to combine elements of both. Some writers have also attempted to demonstrate a link between the alleged care/cure dichotomy and the gendered stereotyping of the two occupational groups. Controversies about the ethics of care and the philosophical exploration of the nature of caring, as distinct from a more rational justice ethic, are not new. They have their parallels in the biblical Old Testament controversies about the respective demands of justice and mercy, and the New Testament ones concerning the respective demands of law on the one hand, and love on the other. Nor is the debate entirely new to healthcare, where issues such as the relation of care and cure, and of medicine as an art to medicine as a science, and the contribution of caring to therapy and the healing process, are almost as old as medicine itself. This kind of controversy has been part of an ongoing debate in nursing too, about the role of knowledge and technical skills, and their relation to the delivery of effective nursing care.

There are several ways in which the focus on 'caring ethics' has influenced ethical debate in nursing. *First*, the cure/care dichotomy has been used here, as in the past, to distinguish the 'objective and scientific medical model' of health from 'a more personal nursing perspective'. In this way, it has often become the focus, or a central theme, in claims made for a specialised body of nursing knowledge, or arguments for the application of distinctive methods of research to nursing. *Second*, it has generated a whole body of literature by feminist writers, analysing the pattern of ethics and relationships in hospitals and other healthcare institutions, as constructed on a pattern of a type of 'master discourse' that is patriarchal, impersonal and determined by a 'justice perspective', to which another type of discourse, the 'caring perspective' of the nurse, must be opposed. *Third*, it has raised some interesting questions about the nature of ethics itself and whether the pursuit of a universal framework of principles, rights and duties is to be preferred to a more phenomenological and existentially grounded approach which attends to the specific situation, particular relationships and the demands inherent in the exercise of personal moral responsibility.

A 'postmodernist' feminist approach to ethics identifies traditional philosophical ethics as 'patriarchal' and, with its emphasis on universal principles and rational justice, as driven by a 'will to control' the world and other people (particularly women). In opposition to this, the 'caring perspective' of feminist ethics is recommended, because it avoids the 'totalising' and 'dominative critical' approach of a 'masculinist' ethic (Gilligan 1982, 1993). In place of an attempt to base ethical decision-making on universal rational principles and logical methods of problem-solving (allegedly the natural tendencies of the 'master discourses' of men), we are urged to listen to the 'different voice' of feminine sensibility, with its emphasis on 'narrative and contextual accounts, that encourage respect for the differences between persons and sensitivity to the complexity of our interconnections' (Bowden 1997, p. 10).

At best, the plethora of research generated by the work of Kohlberg and Gilligan has reinforced the fact that, as with all human learning, the processes of moral reasoning are complex and multifactorial. While the empty formalism and impersonal nature of rationalist ethics invite criticism, and an emphasis on the concrete and particular needs of any given situation is important, it must also be argued that the great moral philosophers have all sought to give due weight to the emotions and to people's desires and loves. To suggest otherwise is a caricature rather than an accurate representation of traditional moral theory, and lacks historical veracity. Different approaches to ethics will be discussed and a variety of models for practical decision-making examined in the final two chapters of this book, to avoid 'putting the cart before the horse'.

Because we believe that ethics is essentially a practical discipline, we have deliberately proceeded *a posteriori* rather than *a priori*; that is, we have started with nurses' ordinary moral experience rather than with theory, in order to show how moral theories seek to explain, after the event, why difficulties arise in moral practice. The traditional approach has been to set out various moral theories, with generalised and 'typical' examples to illustrate how they might apply to these, and the implication of this approach is that practical decision-making should 'fit' with one, or more, of these theories. We believe, however, that this approach assumes that theory precedes action, rather than that theory arises out of our experience of life, of trial and error, that we arrive at general theories, on the basis of particular experience/s. In putting theoretical considerations first we are then faced with the twin difficulties of how to justify our choice of moral theory and how to relate the theory or theories back to actual practice. This is contrary to common sense experience, whereby the majority of people manage to make reasonably competent moral decisions in blissful ignorance of moral philosophy, unaware of the content of classical moral theories, or even their names! Our experience is that students have no difficulty recognising ethical problems or dilemmas, but have considerable difficulty getting their heads around the various ethical theories. We believe with Aristotle that we should start with people's ordinary experience and work towards clarification of decision procedures and ethical policy, rules or theory. This demands critical reflection on actual practice, on the contextual issues, instrumental means and desired outcomes of actions.

If we begin the teaching of ethics with instruction in moral philosophy and critical study of the various ethical theories debated by philosophers through the ages, the illusion is created that moral theory is directly applicable to or relevant to ethical decision-making. Moral theory only becomes relevant when we are faced with disputes about the general rationale for our moral rules, or conflicts of ethical policy, or ideological differences between people. When we are involved in dispute about ethical policy, we may appeal to higher-level moral theories in order to justify our overall moral position. It would not be considered necessary, or appropriate, in justifying a specific action or decision to a court or enquiry, to say, for example: 'I gave the dying patient an overdose of diamorphine because I am a utilitarian, and one must minimise pain and maximise happiness!' or 'I told the patient that he was dying because I am a deontologist, and one has a duty to tell the truth, regardless of consequences!'

In theoretical debate, far removed from situations in which we have to make real decisions, we may engage in discussion of the relative merits of these different ethical theories as a means of justifying or explaining why we opt for certain general policies or rules of action, but this type of theoretical exercise has seldom, in our experience, been perceived as relevant by students of practice-based professions. Indeed, when challenged to explain or justify a specific moral decision to a friend, to a manager, or before a formal enquiry, then the normal expectation would comprise an outline of:

- *what* the main facts of the case were
- *which* principles or rules we applied to the problem
- *why* we acted as we did, i.e. what goal or purpose we set out to achieve
- *how* we chose the means or methods used to achieve the goal
- *what consequences* we anticipated on the basis of past experience
- *whether or not* our action was successful in reaching its intended goal.

Such an explanation or justification for an action would normally suffice to satisfy a court and our standard tests of a responsible person's ability to give a coherent account of what they have done, why they acted as they did, and whether or not their desired outcome was achieved.

We believe then that the proper place for ethical theory, and debate about the strengths and weaknesses of different ethical theories, is not in determining or justifying specific decisions or actions, but rather that moral theory becomes relevant when we come to justify rules or policies. The relevance of ethical theory to practical action is limited, as most students find when they emerge from the lecture theatre into the realities of practice. However, when the basis for our assent to rules, trust in authority, or our general ethical approach to problems is challenged, then the relevance of ethical theory becomes apparent. Another way of expressing this is to say that debate about ethical theory belongs to the *second-order* level of debate about ethics in general, rather than to debate about the rights and wrongs of a particular action, or even whether a specific action is good or bad.

The consequence of placing the primary emphasis in teaching on ethical theory is that it creates, or reinforces, the belief that everything in ethics is contestable, and simply a matter of opinion (or rhetorical debate about our opinions). To the degree that this happens, it encourages the view that ethical decision-making is either so difficult that it must be left to experts, or an area where 'anything goes' (and where one person's opinion is just as good as another's). The object of teaching ethics, as distinct from moral theory or moral philosophy, is to help people reach ethically sound and justifiable decisions and to develop relevant life skills to operate with confidence as responsible moral agents. Instead of 'putting the cart before the horse', we advocate working up to and ending with moral theory, rather than beginning with it, for we start where Aristotle suggests we should, with everyday practice, rather than in the speculative world of theory.

COMPETENCY-BASED TRAINING AND VIRTUE ETHICS

One crucial lesson we have learned from the debate about the nature of nursing ethics, and from personal experience in teaching ethics, is that the question of *how* ethics is taught may be of greater importance than *what* is taught. In line with concern in other areas with defining competence and the competencies required of nurses to practise, more attention needs to be given not only to how we create the sort of learning opportunities and environments where nurses can acquire the knowledge and skills in ethics to make competent decisions, but also to how we can ensure that student nurses develop the personal attributes or competencies that will make them confident and responsible moral agents. Here the revival of interest in, and increasing influence of, virtue ethics in academic circles, and even in the business world, reflects a growing awareness that in appraising our own or other people's performance, it is not enough to assess people's theoretical knowledge of ethics. The extent to which individuals acquire and internalise the core skills in applied ethics, and the ease with which they use them in practice, is of equal, or greater, importance.

The acquisition of both scientific knowledge and practical expertise is not sufficient to ensure that we can act responsibly as moral agents. Neither is it sufficient that we are good decent people with a capacity for self-insight and self-mastery, courage and integrity, or that we show respect and deal fairly with others, for if we do not have the necessary professional competence, we can be of little help to people in need. Professional integrity or competence requires a balance between the former, which Aristotle called the *intellectual virtues*, and the latter, which he called the *moral virtues*. What he believed holds them together is *prudence* or *practical wisdom* which not only enables us to integrate theory and practice and to apply our expertise in a responsible ethical way for the benefit of ourselves and others, but also represents the only way in which we can achieve the kind of consistent and coherent moral character that we refer to when we speak of the virtuous, integrated person (Thomson 1976).

Throughout this book we take an approach that draws upon the arguments of ethics and philosophy, on the one hand, and evidence taken from nursing research and experience, on the other. We base our arguments on real cases and situations drawn from the everyday practice of nursing, but we have also sought to interpret these in the light of normative theories. This is not surprising, for there is no human science that is value-free. The normative questions asked by the philosophy of nursing, concern both what nursing is and what it ought to be. In a sense, every answer we give to the question 'What is nursing?' is implicitly normative. Here the task of philosophy is, as has often been said, to make the implicit explicit; that is, its task is to make the values presupposed in a particular operational definition of nursing clear, to examine these critically and to determine their adequacy. Conversely the question 'What is nursing?' cannot be asked without regard to the facts, without taking account of the history of nursing, and the evidence of where it stands today, and the future directions that it may take. Thus, our focus within the book is practical, and we seek to 'walk the talk' with our readers through consideration with them of some of the options it is necessary to consider in real life. We have aimed to emphasise the relevance of ethics to those whose daily work experience requires them to make decisions that impact upon the quality, as well as duration, of people's lives.

STRUCTURE OF THE BOOK

Besides this introduction, the book has been divided into five parts:

Part 1: Cultural issues, methods and approaches to nursing ethics

We start by attempting to place the study of ethics in nursing in its historical context in relation to the development of professions generally and of nursing in particular. We also emphasise the changing nature of cultural values and priorities. This leads on to a chapter in which we examine what is involved in defining nursing ethics, first, in terms of the various relationships of power and responsibility between nurses and patients and between nurses and other professions, including the public; and secondly by seeking to clarify some fundamental distinctions and conceptual issues involved in the definition of ethics, both in theoretical and practical terms.

Part 2: Socialisation, professionalisation and nursing values

A fundamental presupposition of the approach adopted in this book is that ethics cannot be studied in isolation or abstraction from the behavioural and social sciences (in fact ethics used to be the umbrella term used to cover these sciences, including economics!). Hence, Part 2 is concerned to explore a number of issues from a sociological perspective that have a crucial bearing on nursing ethics. These are respectively: what is entailed in becoming a nurse and being a member of the profession of nursing; the division of labour in healthcare and how the scope of power, responsibility and accountability are defined in practice; and finally, what is meant by professional responsibility and accountability in nursing.

Part 3: Nursing ethics – issues in clinical practice

In this section we start with an examination of the issues that are most commonly cited in the popular media and nursing press as typical moral dilemmas, and consider whether or not these should be the main focus for nursing ethics. While these issues – abortion, euthanasia, truth telling, compulsory psychiatric treatment – are all important and of perennial relevance to general discussion of ethics in healthcare, we have

argued that there are a number of other issues to which nurses should direct their attention. In Chapters 7 and 8, and Chapters 9 and 10 in Part 4, we have taken a number of cases from everyday practice to illustrate the different kinds of ethical responsibility that nurses have to exercise. These relate to: dealing directly with patients, ward management, working in multi-disciplinary teams, the different roles of nurses in prevention and providing nursing care, the responsibilities of nurses in management and in policy-making and public accountability for healthcare resources.

Part 4: Ethics in nursing management, research and teaching

As indicated above, this section continues the discussion of issues raised for nurses in everyday practice at a variety of levels, but the focus is different. Whereas the typical dilemmas in Part 3 arise because of perceived conflicts between the demands of the nurse's duty of care for patients and respect for patients' rights, the typical dilemmas in Part 4 relate to concern for the common good and public account-ability, in which the conflicts that arise relate to the tensions between the demands for justice and equity in access to healthcare on the one hand and either practitioners' duty of care for their patient/s or the rights of patients themselves. The issues covered relate to nurses' responsibilities for resource allocation, competent and fair management, for sound basic and operational research to underpin sound nursing practice and patient care, and to ensure that there is a reliable evidence base for performance appraisal.

Part 5: Ethical decision-making and moral theory

In this final section we return to the issues discussed in this Introduction, namely how we justify ethical decisions, as distinct from ethical policy or rules, and examine the usual range of classical moral theories, namely, deontology, axiology and teleology and a number of variants of these classical theories, e.g. utilitarianism and virtue ethics.

Website

Useful web links and Chapter teaching notes can be found on this site:
http://evolve.elsevier.com/Thompson/nursingethics/

further reading

Baggott R 2004 Health and healthcare in Britain, 3rd edn. Palgrave Macmillan, Basingstoke

Beauchamp T, Childress J 2004 Principles of biomedical ethics, 5th rev edn. Oxford University Press, Oxford

Bowden P 1997 Caring: gender-sensitive ethics. Routledge, London

Harrison M I 2004 Implementing change in health systems: market reforms in the United Kingdom, Sweden, and the Netherlands. Sage Publications, London

Kerridge I, Lowe M, McPhee J 1998 Ethics and law for the health professions. Social Science Press, Katoomba, NSW, Australia

Melia K M 1994 The task of nursing ethics. Journal of Medical Ethics 20(4):7–11

PART 1

Cultural issues, methods and approaches to nursing ethics

Nursing ethics: historical, cultural and professional perspectives

1

AIMS

This chapter has the following aims:

1. To help situate current debate about nursing and nursing ethics in the wider context of the development of healthcare and the professions in the modern period, since the Enlightenment and in the 20th century

2. To clarify some of the preconceptions we have about the nature of a profession and to examine changing popular attitudes towards the traditional professions, including nursing

3. To explore the basis for the alleged loss of public trust in the professions, particularly of medicine and indirectly in other healthcare professions

4. To clarify and examine the factors contributing to the evolution of ethics and the foundations of ethics as a separate philosophical discipline

5. To consider the perennial concerns of ethics in the light of cultural diversity and changing personal and social values, and the related question of relativism in ethics

6. To begin to explore the constitutive and regulative principles of ethics as providing us with a basis for the evaluation and appraisal of human action and social conduct.

LEARNING OUTCOMES

When you have read and worked through this chapter, you should be able to:

- Give a reflective account of the place of the professions in the wider context of modern culture and be able to discuss the relevance of these considerations to healthcare practice
- Demonstrate an understanding of the ambivalent attitudes of the public to the professions generally, and to the healthcare professions in particular
- Articulate some of the things that the professions can do to change public attitudes to nursing and the health professions and to improve the public's confidence in them
- Discuss the wider connections of ethics with religion, philosophy and social customs, and how it differs from these as a legitimate area of study in its own right
- Demonstrate understanding of the significance of diversity in cultural and ethical values, and how ethics might be defended against ethical relativism.

Part A Nursing, professions and history

INTRODUCTION

Nursing ethics does not exist in a social or historical vacuum. The formal and public aspects of nursing ethics – a code of conduct, educational requirements and a regulatory body, for example – are characteristic features of many professions. Like nursing, these professions also have been shaped by historical developments in both the recent and the more remote past.

Human history is never-ending and ever-changing. From the perspective of the present, the past is often thought of as what we, or our society, or our profession, have 'got past' – ways of living that have been left behind in the march of economic, or scientific, or educational progress. Each new generation usually finds some aspects of the previous generation's way of living unsatisfactory, and seeks to change, improve or modernise society. Through revolution, reforms, or slow incremental change in people's daily habits, earlier ways of living are left behind. Thus the past, especially as it becomes more remote, comes to seem like 'a foreign country', whose inhabitants and their curious ways we view from the present, rather as tourists do when abroad.

To see the past of our own society or profession in this way, however, can be to misunderstand both the past and ourselves. There is continuity as well as change in history; and just as events which happened in our individual infancy can colour our emotions and attitudes in adult life, so developments in a profession's past can colour how it is regarded by its members and by others outside the profession. If we do not understand how events in our own early life still influence us, then we may act in ways that seem inexplicable to us. Something similar may be true of professions.

The word 'nurse', for example, had a long history before it eventually came to mean a member of the modern nursing profession. It derives from the Latin verb *nutrio*, 'to nourish', and in that language was used to refer both to animals suckling their young and to humans tending plants or a fire. At some point the Latin noun *nutrix*, 'a nurse' or 'foster-mother', was formed from *nutrio*. A similar development is first recorded in the English language around a thousand years ago, when the noun 'nurse' appears as a shortened version of the verb 'to nourish'. In English, as in Latin earlier, the new noun was originally used to refer to a woman who breastfed a baby.

(This derivation from an existing word of a new term with a more precise reference is characteristic of the way language grows, using similes and metaphors to develop and differentiate new and more precise meanings from older and more general ones. Most scientific terms, for example, are 'dead metaphors': they have been adapted, that is, from one or more existing words which came closest to capturing, but themselves never quite captured, what the new term more precisely refers to.)

Looking back from the present, the association of nursing with breastfeeding sounds like one of those aspects of a past way of living that is no longer relevant to modern life. More relevant to the modern nursing profession, perhaps, are its historical associations with 'professed' religious communities who cared for the dying and the sick poor in the Middle Ages, or the creation of a reformed and regimented workforce to meet the needs of military medicine and modern hospitals in the 19th century, or again the emergence of increasingly specialised and technical roles for nurses, male as well as female, in the 20th century hospital and community. Yet while the original association of 'nurse' with 'nourishing' in its literal breastfeeding sense is no longer relevant to the modern nursing profession, 'nourishing' remains a powerful and perhaps irreplaceable metaphor for much of what the public expects, and many patients receive, from skilled and caring nurses. To nourish vulnerable persons, just as to nourish tender plants, requires both skill, and 'care' in all its senses.

Like persons, professions do not spring from nowhere, fully and finally formed. They become what they are in their relationships with one another, their patients or clients, and the wider society, and they continue to develop and change in the context of these relationships. Other social, cultural or economic developments moreover, set in train centuries ago, and at that time with no obvious relevance to the professions, may eventually have significant consequences for them, consequences that often are unknown until they actually arrive.

Among such developments in the present and recent centuries are scientific and technological advances, industrialisation, urbanisation and globalisation. They also include changing popular expectations which support or challenge the place of professions in society, and can have important implications for their future.

This section discusses some of these developments, particularly those related to:

- the history and logic of professionalism
- the growth of modern professions
- popular expectations of professions
- an alleged public loss of trust in professionals in the context of modernity, and
- how professionals might respond to current challenges.

THE HISTORY AND LOGIC OF PROFESSIONALISM

The need for a division of labour between different occupations has been recognised from the earliest historical times. The emergence of professions in the modern sense is more recent, however. By the end of the Middle Ages, not long after the word 'nurse' had entered the English language, the word 'profession' was used to refer to secular occupations (such as the military and the theatrical) as well as religious vocations or 'callings'. But it was not until around the 17th century that barristers, physicians and clergy began to be distinguished from other occupations and accorded a special status as the 'ancient' or 'learned' professions of law, medicine and the Church. Even then, this status was not accorded to all lawyers, doctors or ministers of religion, and it was not until the 19th and 20th centuries that professions in the modern sense emerged. When they did so, they included many more than the three ancient ones.

What distinguishes modern professions from other occupations? According to the sociologist Eliot Freidson, a profession is 'an organized occupation [which] gains the power to determine who is qualified to perform a defined set of tasks, to prevent all others from performing that work, and to control the criteria by which to evaluate performance' (Freidson 2001, p. 12). Freidson argues that there are three distinct 'logics' by which occupations today are organised and controlled. These are the *logic of the market*, of *managerialism*, and of *professionalism*.

The *logic of the market* is that the wishes of consumers determine the work people do: workers in the market are there primarily to earn a living, and the particular work they do is secondary.

The *logic of managerialism* is similar, except that here it is not the wishes of consumers but the production plans of managers that control the work people do. 'Since tasks and positions in firms are subject to change as productive means and ends change, commitment by workers to any particular job and body of knowledge is obstructive and therefore undesirable' (Freidson 2001, p. 109).

In *professionalism*, by contrast, the work people

do and the criteria for evaluating performance are determined by the profession itself. The 'logic' of this is that complex professional work requires the exercise of knowledge, skills and discretionary judgement, the development of which in turn requires the long-term commitment of professionals and their professional bodies to their particular sphere of work and to the advancement of their particular body of knowledge. Professional organisation provides a 'shelter' from those demands of market or managerial logic which would hinder that development by subordinating that commitment to the vagaries of consumer demand or managerial targets. Contrary to the claim (made for example by Adam Smith in the 18th century and George Bernard Shaw in the 20th) that professions are conspiracies against the public, professions provide a 'shelter' for the growth and development of knowledge and skills which benefit the public.

The respective 'logics' of professionalism, managerialism and the market, Freidson emphasises, are 'ideal-types': in real life each has some admixture of the others. Markets are managed, managers must heed the market, and professions cannot be entirely sheltered from market or managerial logic. In practice, moreover, any profession's claim to a monopoly in its own occupational sphere requires recognition by its clients and the public that this is the most effective way of meeting the needs that the profession claims to serve.

Agreeing to these professional claims, Freidson argues, may make good sense. 'In light of the large gap between specialized knowledge and the capacity of non-specialists to deal with it intelligently, let alone the massive and sophisticated commercial efforts to manipulate choice, it is sometimes reasonable to restrict consumer choice to credentialed workers.' As other sociologists have observed, he notes, 'professional licensure is a theoretical solution to certain organizational problems which are intrinsic to any complex society' (Freidson 2001, p. 206).

THE GROWTH OF MODERN PROFESSIONS

On Freidson's interpretation then, professionalism is an organisational logic, alongside those of the market and managerialism, which complex modern societies require to meet many of their vital needs.

Historically, society's recognition of this can be illustrated by the proliferation of professional, or 'qualifying', associations in 19th century Britain. According the historian Harold Perkin, their growth,

> was led by the Institution of Civil Engineers in 1818, the Law Society in 1825, the Institute of British Architects in

1834, the Institute of Actuaries in 1848, and the General Medical Council in 1858. By 1880 there were 27 qualifying associations, by 1900 48, by 1918 75, by 1939 121, and by 1970 167. (Perkin 2004)

During this period, Perkin argues, England was transformed from a society dominated by class-based interests to one increasingly dominated by professionals. These included not only professionals who provided specialised services to individuals or corporations, but also professional managers in the private as well as public sectors, and a growing proportion of professional politicians, increasingly drawn from other professions rather than from landed, business or working-class interests. During the 20th century, and especially during its two world wars, politics, the economy, the welfare state and the health service in Britain were largely managed by professional elites of specialised experts.

In the late 20th century, however, there was a 'backlash' against this 'professional society' (Perkin 1990, pp. 472ff.). The notion of professions as conspiracies against the public was revived by figures as different as the radical thinker Ivan Illich and the conservative politician Margaret Thatcher. The privileges of professionalism were attacked in the name both of the public interest and of the free market. However, much of this, Perkin argues, in fact was an attack on the public sector professions by private sector professionals and their professional allies in politics and the media. The attack was fuelled by media revelations of 'scandals' involving individual members of the traditional and public sector professions, not least medicine and the Church. But the private sector professionals themselves also came under attack as various corporate malpractices were revealed. By the beginning of the 21st century, it was evident that if, as politicians and the media often proclaimed, there was now a lack of public trust in professionals, there was an even greater lack of public trust in politicians and the media.

Loss of trust

What were the reasons for the late 20th century loss of public trust in professionals? According to Perkin, one reason was 'the condescension of professionalism'. The 'Achilles' heel of professionalism' in the 19th and 20th centuries, he suggests, was

> individual arrogance, collective condescension to the laity and mutual disdain between the different professions. On all three levels professionalism was weakened by its own vanity and elitism, which often infuriated other individuals, classes and rival professions. (Perkin 1990, p. 390)

This is a large generalisation, but there is some truth to it. Members of the nursing profession may recognise this in their relations with the medical profession, and members of both in their relations with professional managers or professional politicians.

On the other hand, the alleged loss of trust is not necessarily all that critics of the professions represent it to be. The nursing profession, for example, has not been subject to nearly as much public criticism in this respect as the medical profession has been. Or again, 'public opinion' on loss of trust in the professions is not reflected in the highly favourable opinions expressed by many individual members of the public about the professionals, especially doctors and nurses, with whom they actually come into contact. As the philosopher Onora O'Neill has pointed out:

> Loss of trust, it seems, is often reported by people who continue to place their trust in others; reported perceptions about trust are not mirrored in the ways in which people actually place their trust. (O'Neill 2002, p. 9)

Even the media, apparently, are ambivalent on this issue. As Freidson observes:

> It is no accident that for well over a century in the iconography of popular media it is professionals who are the 'crusaders' seeking Justice, Health, Truth, and Salvation. While it is common to see physicians and lawyers, scientists and professors, and sometimes journalists and politicians in that principled role one does not see bankers, stockbrokers, or business executives. (Freidson 2001, pp. 221ff.)

To try to understand this conflicting evidence about loss of trust a little better, it may be helpful to enlarge the focus, and consider, beyond the rise of professional society in the 19th and 20th centuries, the larger context of what is now often described as 'modernity' – the modern world as many people, including many nurses and many patients, now think of and experience it.

MODERNITY

'Modernity' can be described as the amalgam of ideas and practices largely taken for granted as the background to everyday life today in developed countries, not by everyone all of the time, but by most people most of the time. These ideas and practices are not necessarily shared by the majority of people worldwide today. For example, many people in Asian and African societies are culturally unsympathetic to or positively reject what they perceive to be the values of European or North American modernity. Paradoxically the cultural values they seek to defend may be closer to the communitarian values of Europe in the past, than to the more individualistic ones of today. Even those who regard the idea of modernity favourably may interpret what it means for their own society in a variety of different ways, for example accepting the advantages of modern science, technology and healthcare, while rejecting the values of cultural and religious pluralism or liberal democracy.

In the 21st century world, then, there are many different ways of being modern. Nor is it any longer as obvious as it seemed in 19th century Europe (whose intellectual elites often contrasted their own 'superior' ideas and practices with those of more 'primitive' societies), that a 'modern' view of the world is necessarily closer to the truth than a 'traditional' view. In terms of scientific knowledge and technological mastery, the 21st century is superior to the 12th. But many of the prevailing assumptions and expectations, about individuals, society and life generally, which are taken for granted by many people in liberal democracies are no less selective and socially constructed than those of earlier or other societies.

Central to the modernity of liberal democracies is a rejection of the hierarchical and deferential societies of their past. In this idea of modernity, the philosopher Charles Taylor suggests, everyone is expected to have (i) an equal claim on a political economy whose aim is mutual benefit and (ii) an equal say in a public sphere where the people are sovereign (Taylor 2004). A major difficulty with this view of modernity, however, is that it embodies significant internal tensions, notably between the desires of individuals and the common good, and between the views of minorities and the general will. This means that no political economy can satisfy all the claims of all individuals, and if every individual is given an equal say in the public sphere, it may be impossible to discern what the sovereign people want.

The difficulties caused by these tensions have been partially resolved, of course, by the creation of representative institutions of government. Where these are responsive to the needs and wishes of a sufficient proportion of individuals and interest groups they can make the status quo seem preferable to a revolutionary crisis – in which the internal tensions of modernity could explode in socially destructive ways. But this degree of social stability is generally achieved at the cost of leaving other individuals and interest groups (including many in developing countries) believing that their claims have not been met, and that their voices have not been heard as they ought to have been. It is also often achieved at the cost of a lack of transparency in political decision-making which leaves the decision-makers open to the charge by their critics that they are untrustworthy.

Problems of this kind are particularly difficult for large modern representative democracies. In families or small communities, skilled mediation may sometimes enable individuals, having made their claims and had their say, to moderate their respective claims and achieve what all regard as a just compromise. Where whole populations are involved, however, the number and variety of possibly conflicting claims and voices to be heard often make the ideals embodied in Western modernity impossible to achieve.

Matters may be especially difficult when the scientific, social or economic aspects of the choices under discussion are complex or uncertain, as they often are, for example, in current debates about future directions in healthcare. In order fully to appreciate what is at stake for present and future generations, may require either a lengthy education in the subject, or a scientific willingness to tolerate uncertainty until further evidence emerges. Such an education, however, may well not be a practical possibility for many individuals who believe they should have a say in the matter, and those who believe that their vital interests are at stake in the choices to be made may well find such uncertainty difficult to accept.

Informed public debate about the issues involved in health choices, for example, often is highly dependent on what individuals can glean from the media, or the internet. While reliable information can be extracted from such sources, most individuals, including the most highly educated, may well have difficulty in distinguishing between what is and is not reliable information on subjects of which they have no first-hand knowledge or experience. When that is the case, the media cannot necessarily be relied on as a guide to what is reliable.

Part of the reason for the unreliability of the media, as Onora O'Neill has pointed out (O'Neill 2002, pp. 165ff.), is that unlike other professions whose conduct is regulated, and unlike politicians who can be voted out of office, the media (with the exception of some public broadcasting bodies) are largely unregulated and unlikely (outside the law of libel) to suffer any penalties for circulating misleading information. While much that contributes valuably to public debate can be found in the writing of conscientious reporters, the media's freedom to select, neglect, spin and in some cases even invent news is all-too-often abused, as anyone will know who works in a hospital where a real or imagined 'scandal' has been 'exposed'. When the media claim to be speaking in the name of 'the people', moreover, this all-too-often obscures or misrepresents what the people actually might have concluded, had they been more accurately and impartially advised.

SCAPEGOATING

In this interpretation of modernity, then, everyone is expected to have an equal claim on a political economy whose aim is mutual benefit, and an equal say in a public sphere where the people are sovereign. But on many occasions it may simply not be possible for all of these often conflicting expectations to be satisfied. Yet the general expectation is that they ought to be satisfied, and that because they ought to be, they can be.

The question then is, by whom ought they to be satisfied? One answer to this is that no individual or institution on its own has the power to satisfy all of these expectations, and indeed that failure to satisfy all of them cannot be attributed to any human agency, but is simply an aspect of the human condition. If that is correct, the best chance of satisfying as many of these expectations as possible is to seek an agreed compromise between moderated claims on the model of mediation mentioned above. For the reasons stated there, however – the sheer number and variety of possibly conflicting claims and voices to be heard – such compromise can be very difficult to achieve. Moreover, because power is perceived to be distributed unevenly between different individuals and institutions, those who believe themselves to have less power than others may be reluctant to agree to any compromise, lest it leave them even more disadvantaged.

When, as is normally the case, power is perceived to be distributed unevenly, there is frequently a tendency for what Charles Taylor calls 'one of the more disquieting features of modernity' to surface (Taylor 2004, p. 138). This is the phenomenon of scapegoating, or seeking someone on whom to pin the blame for failure to satisfy what may be unrealistic expectations.

Scapegoating in fact is a very ancient response to the tensions of existence, apparently with deep roots in the human psyche (Girard 1986). But its prevalence in contemporary society is particularly challenging to the professions, which have often claimed the competence and expertise necessary to manage the needs of society successfully. One way of trying to defend this claim, commonly resorted to when management fails and expectations are unsatisfied, is for a particular individual or institution to be identified as being to blame and requiring to be punished by being removed from power. For example, media coverage of the spread of MRSA, or other hospital-acquired infections,

has led to nurses or nurse management being scapegoated – leading to calls for the reinstatement of old-fashioned 'Matrons' or blaming its spread on academically trained nurses! This is often done with the explicit or implicit promise that those who replace the discredited individual or institution will 'ensure that this never happens again'; and in many instances the promise is buttressed by new and more detailed legislation, guidelines, and procedures for micro-management. On a broader political level, press reports of threatened pandemics caused by the SARS virus, or avian influenza ('bird flu') can create public panic and lead to the scapegoating of governments and the WHO, as well as health professionals in particular countries.

RESPONDING TO CURRENT CHALLENGES TO PROFESSIONALISM

Contemporary claims about 'loss of trust' in professionals appear to belong to the same set of expectations as does scapegoating. In a culture in which, when things go wrong, people are unsatisfied until blame can be pinned on some individual or institution, professionals are especially vulnerable. By the very nature of their work, professionals can never guarantee success in their management of the needs of individuals and society. This is because the exercise of discretionary judgement is essential to professional work, and because judgement is inherently fallible. Professionals thus will never be able to satisfy all people all of the time, and when cases of real or alleged professional inefficiency, negligence or misconduct are uncovered, especially with extensive media publicity, the logic and values of professionalism are likely to face renewed challenges.

When such challenges arise, there is a risk that professionals may be tempted to doubt whether it is worth the effort of standing by the logic and values of professionalism and instead may take refuge in the logic and values of consumerism or managerialism, in particular the 'individual pursuit of material self-interest and the standardization of professional work'. To avoid further public criticism, surgeons may begin to practise defensively, avoiding high-risk operations, for example, or nurses may decide to work to rule. For professionals to adopt such practices however, as Freidson observes, is precisely what most effectively undermines public trust in them (Freidson 2001, p. 181).

A significant challenge to professionalism today therefore is how to resist inappropriate incursions of consumerism and managerialism into the professional sphere. But it is also how do to this in ways that gain public understanding of the need for professional judgement, fallible though it may be, and of the benefits and inevitable risks involved. It is doubtful whether this can be achieved by reiteration of mission statements, or by public protestations of professional virtue. Their effect, like that of over-regulation and ever-increasing micromanagement, may well be counterproductive, leading those who are already sceptical about the professions to become even more so.

On the other hand, as has already been suggested, there is often a considerable mismatch between 'public opinion' about 'loss of trust' in professionals, and the highly favourable opinions expressed by many individual members of the public about the professionals with whom they actually come into contact. This suggests that the most effective way to maintain trust in fallible professionals, is for professionals, individually and collaboratively, to continue doing what most already do – acting in their patients' best interests, being honest about their limitations, trying wherever possible to improve their practice, and thereby giving their patients even better reasons to think well of them. The fact that public opinion surveys consistently rate nurses highly in terms of public trust and esteem may give nurses cause for satisfaction. This may partly be due to the fact that nurses are nearer to patients (and their families) and in a better position to understand them and their needs. This also may be explained by the fact that nurses are currently seen to be in a subordinate position to doctors and health service managers and that the latter should be blamed when things go wrong. However, as nurse practitioners take on more responsibility and autonomy as professionals in their own right, they will be exposed to more direct criticism by patients and the public.

According to the medical historian Laurence McCullough, the main components of professionalism are competence, commitment to the client's interests over the professional's own, and an understanding that being a professional is a public trust. In a culture 'that celebrates the pursuit of self-interest', he argues, professionals remain 'accountable to the worthwhile and therefore durable ideas of the past' – embodied in these aspects of professionalism (McCullough 2004). In the 21st century era of interprofessional and professional–patient/client partnership, the challenge is to turn that rhetoric into reality, not by a pendulum swing from condescending paternalism to uncaring

consumerism or managerial standardisation, but by finding the means that in practice best meet the expectations of all parties to the partnerships involved.

In this social and historical context, a significant question for the nursing profession may be to determine what, among its own 'durable ideas of the past', best corresponds to 'Justice, Health, Truth and Salvation', which Freidson has identified as the 'transcendent values' of the legal, medical, academic and religious professions. It was suggested above that 'nourishing' and 'nurturing', from which the English word 'nursing' comes, remain as powerful and perhaps irreplaceable metaphors for much of what the public expect, and many patients receive, from skilled and caring nurses. To nourish is not simply to provide someone with food but, with knowledge, skill and tenderness, to do whatever is needed to build up their strength, encourage their growth, and restore their health and independence. To nourish, in other words, is to do precisely what Henderson's classic definition of nursing's function prescribes.

> To help people, sick or well, in the performance of those activities contributing to health or its recovery (or a peaceful death) that they would perform unaided if they had the necessary strength, will or knowledge. It is likewise the function of nursing to help people gain independence as rapidly as possible. (Henderson 1996, p. 4)

As a 'transcendent value' of nursing, on which the profession, patients and the public might agree, 'nourishing' therefore has a strong claim to be regarded as at the historical heart of nursing ethics.

In 2005, the following statement appeared in an advertisement on the Singapore National Healthcare Group Health Professionals' website.

> You know you're meant to be a nurse when you feel in the very depths of your being that nursing is the balm that will nourish your restless spirit. It is what you have to do in order to feel complete. (Anon 2005)

The language of this advertisement may not be that which all nurses would wish to use, and its sentiment may need to be complemented by the astringent comment of another healthcare professional that 'the kindest form of care is competence'. But when reflecting on nursing in modernity, where many social and economic exchanges are regarded as zero-sum games in which one person's gain is another's loss, it may not be inappropriate to be reminded that to be nourishing can also be nourishing.

Part B Foundations of ethics — religious, cultural and philosophical

SOURCES OF INSPIRATION FOR ETHICS

In almost every human culture, the connection between religion and ethics has been very close, and many people still assume that the roots of ethics are in religion. Some people would go so far as to claim that there is a necessary connection between them – that there must be a divine source and guarantee for the authority of the moral law, and that without religion there can be no ethics. Alternatively, some anti-religious thinkers have maintained that if God is dead, or there is no God, then there is no pre-established moral law or ethical principles, and we have to make up our own morality. For example, in the 19th century Dostoevsky has Ivan Karamazov say: 'If God does not exist, then everything is licit' (Dostoevsky 1957, Pt 1 Bk 1, Ch. 6) and Nietzsche asserts in his work *The Gay Science* that 'God is dead' (Nietzsche 1954); and Sartre in the 20th century makes a similar point in his *Existentialism and Humanism* (Sartre 1948).

Now while there is plenty of historical evidence for the association between religion and ethics in most known cultures, the emergence of independent ethical thought from within religious traditions and culture can also be shown in the tension between philosophers or prophets on the one hand and the guardians of the religious traditions of the people, on the other. We see this in the case of Socrates' critique of traditional Greek polytheistic religion, of Confucius in relation to Chinese Taoism, of Buddha in relation to Indian Hinduism, and the critical stance of the Old Testament prophets and Jesus in relation to the religious law and practices of the Jews (see Hick 1990, Chs 1–4, Davies 2000, Pt VI).

Because ethics springs out of the social customs and religious traditions of a country, this does not imply that ethics is confined to the boundaries of that culture. On the contrary, because ethics is a reflective discipline (as the rational science of morals), it involves critical exploration of the fundamental questions of human life – the questions of the meaning of being and what values should ultimately determine our individual lives and social goals. As a philosophical discipline, ethics involves both a quest and a continual questioning. It is a spiritual quest, in the sense that it is a quest for the ultimate meaning and purpose of human life. It also necessarily involves questioning the traditions imposed on us by family, religion and society. For, as we have seen, we cannot develop as mature human beings or independent moral agents unless we make a personal commitment to a set of values and a corresponding way of life. This may involve a personal re-appropriation of the religious vision and values of our upbringing, or it may involve rejection or adaptation of our inherited cultural traditions to our own needs and times. Either way this requires critical questioning and serious commitment to the quest for truth. As Heidegger said: 'Questioning is the piety of philosophy!'

Many ethical traditions around the world appeal to 'the gods', 'God' or 'the ancestors' as the source and inspirational foundation of morality. These 'divine command theories', as they are called, either appeal directly to divine revelation to justify ethical rules or commandments, or claim that the earthly representative/s of the Deity have the ability to communicate moral truth to us. Alternatively, within the traditions of religious ethics, it is argued that the order we perceive in the world and try to imitate in human society is a divinely created moral order, and that this order is discernible by human reason. By applying our reason to understand the basis of the given order in the world, we are led to understand how we can be happy or lead fulfilled lives, namely, if we live in accordance with the built-in moral imperatives of this created order and our own given nature (Frankena 1973).

We will have more to say about the issues raised by such ethical theories in the final chapter, but it is important to note in this chapter that ethics is not simply concerned with the regulation of conduct. It is also concerned with the deepest human longings and our quest for physical, mental and spiritual fulfilment as human beings. For nurses, as for other human beings, concern with ethics is part of a larger quest for spiritual and moral truth. The importance of the study of ethics for nurses is not merely for the knowledge it gives of moral rules and codes of conduct, or the skills we learn in clarifying our values, in ethical decision-making and setting standards. To study ethics is to engage with some of the most profound questions asked by human beings.

Nurses often ask for training in how to give 'spiritual support' to patients faced with various kinds of personal distress, unrelieved pain or terminal illness. Here training in listening skills may be more important that attempting to tell people what they should think or believe. Counselling patients in these contexts is less about giving answers, than learning how to listen attentively to people's questions, needs and personal stories, and helping them to discover their own solutions to their problems. If 'answers' are demanded, this requires more than anything else that we are honest with ourselves and our patients — honest about the difficult and painful nature of the quest for meaning and purpose in human life, or the quest for moral and spiritual truth. Our own sincerity and honesty about these matters, our own integrity and willingness to explore difficult questions with them, rather than to give them 'flip' answers, may be more helpful and comforting that trying to give the appearance of having solved life's problems. As G.K. Chesterton said of the suffering of Job: 'Job found more comfort in the puzzles of God than the answers of men' (Chesterton 2000).

The inescapability of the questions concerning the meaning of being for us all, and for nurses in particular, relates to the fact that not only patients have to confront the question of the meaning of suffering, or how we cope with it. Given the nature of their intimate involvement with pain and suffering, death and bereavement, nurses, perhaps more than any other group of professionals, confront and have to wrestle with these questions themselves. Because we all, nurses included, are potentially vulnerable, may be well one day and critically ill the next, we do well to note the counsel of the poet:

> No man is an Island, entire of itself; every man is a piece of the Continent, a part of the main. Any man's death diminishes me, because I am involved in Mankind; … and therefore never send to know for whom the bell tolls; it tolls for thee. (John Donne (1572–1631): *Devotions* XVII)

QUEST FOR THE FOUNDATIONS OF ETHICS

For some people, the quest for the foundations of ethics and morality leads back to belief in a transcendent God who is the source of universal norms, or to metaphysical beliefs about the ultimate meaning of human being-in-the-world. Historically, most systems of social morality have evolved from metaphysical and religious beliefs, so it is always interesting, and often instructive, to trace their pedigree. However, it can be argued that ethics can, or should be, able to stand without the supports of religion and metaphysics, that it should be grounded on rational criteria based on reflection on the given structures and dynamics of human being-in-the-world, and what conditions are necessary for us to fulfil our potential 'species nature' as human beings.

For many people on the other hand, those who are less bothered by sceptical doubts, the matter is more pragmatic – how to reconcile their moral beliefs with those of other people in such a way that conflict can be avoided or reduced and cooperation made possible (Mitchell 1970, Davies 2000, Pt VI).

If we are to avoid giving unnecessary offence, or injuring other people's moral sensibilities, we need to develop tolerance and understanding, even respect, for moral standpoints that differ from our own. This is not easy. We are born into particular families and societies, with their own unique traditions and values. Commitment to these values and willingness to live by them, fight for them, and in some cases to die for them, is a vital source of cohesion and solidarity in families and communities. Also, such values serve to define our identity as members of such social groups. For children born of parents of widely different cultural and religious views or ethnic origin, the conflict of values can be both painful and a source of enrichment. For people working in the caring professions, awareness of cultural and religious differences is not only important for dealing with their own confusion or disagreements with colleagues of a moral nature, but may be vital in understanding what factors (dress, diet, genetic differences, customs relating to birth, reproduction and death) are directly relevant to the sense of dignity and identity, physical and mental health of their patients or clients. Charles Taylor points out that there are many factors that enter into our definition of personal identity, cultural, philosophical, religious and moral (Taylor 2002).

At a broader level, Christianity, Marxism and Islam, as three great 'religions', have sent out missionaries to spread their respective 'gospels' and to make converts. In the course of their endeavours they have often treated with contempt the traditional religion and customs of the societies they have penetrated. At best, they have been guilty of a kind of cultural imperialism – the arrogant and often self-righteous claim to proprietorship of the truth or of privileged access to moral wisdom. At worst, they have been guilty of forced conversions, witch-hunts, massacres, persecution and suppression of religious practices other than their own. Against this, the painstaking studies of anthropologists and sociologists and the cross-cultural comparisons made on the basis of more objective and scientific analyses have not only brought to light the diversity and relativity of social customs and mores, but also the many common features shared by different cultures. They have helped us to become more tolerant, and to gain insight into the rich wisdom and dignity of many cultures we might be tempted to call primitive.

SHARED AND CHANGING VALUES

In what has been written so far, moral values have been discussed mainly in terms of the values of individuals and how these may differ from those in both their own and other cultures. But values, of course, are something we share with others. This can be seen in the fact that morals and politics are not distinct activities but are part of a continuum. People, it is true, sometimes talk about politics as if it were only a matter of power for power's sake. However, while power is clearly of importance in politics generally, and to some politicians in particular, politics is also concerned with ideals and social goals. Values too play an important part in political as well as moral decision-making. Some of the earliest moral philosophers, Aristotle, for example, in the 4th century BC, considered that the study of ethics was part of the study of politics; and clearly enough the purposes, values and principles we have as individuals cannot be properly studied in isolation from those of the society and culture which have made us what we are (Thomson 1976).

The fact that we have both shared and individual values is of obvious importance in considering practical moral issues in nursing and the ethics of nursing care in general. In the broader context of everyday moral choice, however, it may be worth asking how our shared values have been changing, and what effect this may be having on our contemporary moral decision-making. In doing so it is necessary to distinguish between attitudes, beliefs and values (Box 1.1).

One of the major changes that seems to have taken place in our society during the last century is a shift from general public agreement about moral values to a much greater variety of expressed moral opinion and tolerance of diversity. Not everyone 100 years ago, of course, agreed about what was morally right and wrong, nor today is society without consensus on some moral issues. The variety of moral viewpoints, which it is acceptable to express and possible to justify in public today, does seem to have become greater. This situation of moral pluralism may well be one reason why we are particularly aware today of moral conflicts and dilemmas. How we view this situation will depend on our moral presuppositions: some of us will see it as symptomatic of moral liberation, others of moral decay. The truth is probably, as usual, more complex and, because we are living through it, largely hidden from us. On the basis of what has happened to societies in the past, one way of interpreting what is happening now may be by comparing it with the transition from childhood to adolescence.

> ### Box 1.1 Attitudes, beliefs and values
>
> ATTITUDE (Latin: *aptus*, fitting): An uncritical, or unexamined position one adopts about something, a conditioned way of regarding or behaving towards someone, towards ideas or things, positive or negative feelings, dispositions, or reactions towards someone or something.
>
> BELIEF (OF: *beleafe*: trusted, dear): Beliefs form a subset of acquired opinions and attitudes to which we give personal assent and for which we are prepared to make truth-claims, that is, we make judgements based on our beliefs that are open to testing by others.
>
> VALUE (Latin: *valere*, to be strong, worthy): The basis from which we assess the importance or worth of something, estimate the relative salience of various things or actions, for the achievement of our life goals, or the well-being of others/society. Values are beliefs, which we often share with others, to which we are personally committed and on which we are prepared to act – to stake our decisions and our futures.
>
> *Adapted from Oxford Reference Dictionary (Hawkins 1986).*

An obvious aspect of this comparison is the way in which many people today look back nostalgically to the lost moral certainties of the past. This nostalgia is reminiscent of what, in retrospect, seems so attractive about childhood – its security and particularly the certainty of childhood ideas. Grandmother is a saint, father can do anything, our family's ways are the best ways, the others' are rather odd. The pain, but also the excitement, of adolescence lies in discovering that things are really much more complicated and often not what they had seemed. Grandmother can be an emotional tyrant, father has not conquered the world, other families' ways and moral standards may be as good as, if not better than, ours. The change experienced in adolescence, in other words, is from a world in which things are morally black or white to one in which we discover an infinite variety of moral shades of grey. In this situation we are faced with two major temptations. One is to deny that the shades of grey exist, possibly by adopting a new black and white morality supplied by some dogmatic moral, religious or political ideology. The dangers of this are those of moral short-sightedness about the complexity of real-life decision-making, and moral insensitivity towards those with different convictions. The other temptation is to accept the infinite variety of moral shades of grey and to say that they are all the same. The dangers here are those of moral indifference and moral indecisiveness.

One way of understanding what has been happening to morality in our society, then, is to compare it with this transition from the moral certainties of childhood to the uncertainties, temptations and dangers of adolescence. Similar changes have taken place in the past, when individuals or societies have experienced the transition from tribal or village life to the life of large cosmopolitan cities. In the tribe or village, morality was a matter of shared fixed conventions, which gave people considerable security – but at the price, often, of hypocrisy, guilt, and even open cruelty towards those who deviated from the moral norm. The shift to city life, where people from different origins with different moral views lived together, made it difficult to maintain the old black and white certainties, revealed the moral shades of grey and exposed individuals and society to the adolescent's temptation to question all values or take refuge in dogmatism. In our time, something of the same kind seems to have been happening to society generally through experiences of war, the growth of travel, international communications, the mass media and public education. These changes have made more people aware than ever before of the variety of moral viewpoints which it is possible to hold, and consequently of the difficulty, in the face of this, of maintaining that any one traditional moral viewpoint is right or the best. Here we face the same risks, of moral dogmatism – the uncritical acceptance of a particular moral position as infallible – or moral relativism – the view that any moral position is as good as another.

Against this background, one particular value, which has fallen in public esteem, is that of paternalism and the principle that 'father knows best'. This shift is associated with greater respect for the value of self-determination (or autonomy) and the related ideal of human rights – especially the rights of women and of minorities. Involved in this change also is an emphasis on the individual, which favours such values as self-expression rather than self-sacrifice, tolerance rather than conformity, and flexibility rather than strict obedience to moral rules. Changes of this kind seem to be reflected today in changing attitudes within nursing, traditionally a female, obedient, self-sacrificing and sometimes rigid profession. These changing attitudes focus on questions about the authority of the traditionally male profession of medicine, the separate identity of nursing as a profession in its own right and the need for more flexible ways of providing care. Changing values also seem to be reflected in contemporary concern for such things as the patient's right to know and the right to choice and self-determination in healthcare.

CULTURAL DIVERSITY AND COMMON ETHICAL PRINCIPLES

In the study of ethics we set out to study the underlying principles common to all types of personal and social morality. But are we justified in assuming that there are common underlying principles? And, what do we mean by 'principles'?

Many people think of *principles* as dogmatic beliefs, statements of absolute or infallible truths. This is unhelpful to ethics, for it removes the making of moral judgements from the domain of what can be debated on rational terms. Ethics from this standpoint becomes either an appeal to subjective intuition or a slanging match between competing fundamentalisms. We wish to use the term in its classical meaning, where the original meaning of the word 'principle' is a 'beginning', or 'starting point' for reasoning. Thus 'principles' refer to where you start, not where you end up, and refer to the basic questions you must ask, rather than providing you with ready-made answers. Unfortunately for those who believe in absolute moral truths, being able to recite a list of moral principles does not help you decide which principle is applicable in a given situation, nor how to apply it, nor how to resolve conflicts between principles when these arise. Principles help give us direction; they point the way, but do not tell us where we will end up, or what will happen along the way (Box 1.2).

We often hear it said, 'When it comes to morality everyone seems to have different views of what is right and wrong.' And 'Who are we to say that one person is right and another wrong?' In an increasingly multicultural Britain and in other European countries with a colonial past, colonialism brought European 'Christian' culture into contact, and sometimes

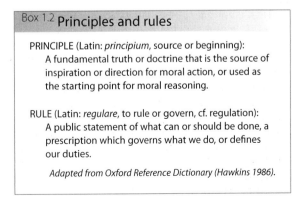

Box 1.2 **Principles and rules**

PRINCIPLE (Latin: *principium*, source or beginning):
A fundamental truth or doctrine that is the source of inspiration or direction for moral action, or used as the starting point for moral reasoning.

RULE (Latin: *regulare*, to rule or govern, cf. regulation):
A public statement of what can or should be done, a prescription which governs what we do, or defines our duties.

Adapted from Oxford Reference Dictionary (Hawkins 1986).

conflict, with other cultural and religious traditions. The massive social upheavals resulting from wars and revolutions in the 20th century – causing the dislocation of millions of people, and creating refugee populations on a scale unseen before – have also brought people into contact with migrants from all over the world. These changes, coupled with global trade, travel, emigration and immigration, have left few cultures unchallenged by interaction with others. We are thus confronted with a rich variety of different religions and philosophies competing for our allegiance – i.e. besides Christianity – Judaism, Islam, Hinduism, Buddhism and Taoism as well as secular ideologies such as Marxism and Humanism – offering us different systems of values to live by and different means of salvation.

The reality is that few of us live any longer in isolated or culturally homogeneous societies. Britain itself has become a multicultural society (and perhaps always has been), and it is increasingly a multi-ethnic society too. The UK National Health Service not only has to deal with patients from an incredible variety of religious, political and cultural backgrounds, but its healthcare staff represent the same variety and diversity too.

On the one hand, this diversity and confusing variety of traditions of religious and social morality seems to make the talk of common principles appear naive and moral consensus an unrealistic dream. On the other hand, if we are not overwhelmed by the relativities and driven to moral scepticism, we can only wonder at the richness and variety of forms in which human beings have sought to express what they believe it means to be human and what values they see to be necessary to make possible a full life (Downie 1987, Veatch 1981). Moral relativism and scepticism are also useful challenges to thinking about ethics. As the German philosopher Kant pointed out in the 18th century, when we say that something is right or wrong we are making an implicit or explicit claim that this is, or should be, true for everybody (Paton 1969).

This claim to universal validity, implicit in our ordinary moral judgements, is challenged by the evidence of moral disagreements between individuals and the diversity of moral rules in different systems of social morality. This may lead us to make dogmatic claims for the universal applicability of our own moral values and traditions; or lead us to sceptical relativism. In the face of scepticism based on moral relativism, namely that all moral beliefs are relative either to each individual or to their culture, we can either take refuge in cynicism, or we are driven to find more fundamental principles which underlie these apparent individual and cultural differences.

The challenge represented by moral scepticism is to provide some kind of rational justification for these fundamental principles, once we have found them. The rational debate about the foundations of ethics as such takes us into the sphere of moral theory – a subject we will return to in the final chapter. We can pursue the demand for rational justification for moral principles only so far as is reasonable. If nothing will satisfy us but absolute certainty, then perhaps nothing will satisfy us, and we are left with paralysing scepticism or apathy. In practice, we do manage to get along more or less well with people of other religious and cultural traditions and we share enough common ground to do business with one another, intermarry, and even vote for the same political parties. Moral scepticism has to make sense of this creative interaction between widely different human cultures, or it simply leads to a kind of cul-de-sac of thought and action.

Moral relativism has therefore helped to challenge cultural imperialism, religious and moral dogmatism, intolerance and arrogance. However, it must also be pointed out that there have been thinkers and leaders among Christians, Marxists and Muslims who have also criticised religious intolerance among their co-religionists or party supporters. For Christians it has been in the name of a god who transcends and judges all human institutions. For some Marxists it has been in the name of a science which is experimental and tentative, not dogmatic, and recognition of the need for ongoing reform even after the Russian Revolution! For the great philosophers of Islam, it has been in the name of an uncompromising ethical monotheism, and a belief in universal human values. The recognition of some kind of transcendent ideal itself may be grounds for a kind of moral relativism – the humility to recognise the limited and fallible nature of our own moral systems or personal insights. This view was given a somewhat paradoxical expression in the posthumous writings of Ludwig Wittgenstein, whose mystical philosophy of religion was as much a response to religious and moral relativism as to deeper personal considerations (Kerr 1997).

The argument based on moral relativism can, however, be so exaggerated as to make nonsense of moral argument and the reality of human intercultural cooperation. If there were no common ground between the moral beliefs of different individuals or different peoples, then no rational debate and intelligent disagreement about ethical and political concerns would be possible. The reality is that even people with the most widely divergent views continue to debate moral principles and values in a way that they do not do about mere matters of taste (*de gustibus non est disputandum* – concerning matters of taste there can be no dispute). This suggests that there is sufficient common ground for each disputant to at least understand (or partially understand) what the other is saying, and thus attempt to marshal arguments, feelings and evidence in the effort to persuade the other.

The reality is that throughout history diverse nations and cultures have been able to form pacts and alliances, cooperate in peace and war, and even develop the basis of public and international law. The United Nations Universal Declaration of Human Rights (UNO 1948), despite not being signed by the USSR and South Africa in 1947, was signed by the official representatives of all other member states. The further elaboration of this Bill of Rights and the growing body of international law, together with the enhanced authority of the International Court of Human Rights, suggest that there is in fact more agreement about fundamental principles and human rights than might at first sight be apparent. The seemingly interminable wrangles in public debate and in forums such as the European Parliament or the United Nations General Assembly (Eide 1992) do not gainsay the achievement of international agreement over the UN Universal Declaration of Human Rights (UNO 1948) or European Convention on Human Rights (Council of Europe 1950) or even the UK Human Rights Act 1998.

This should not altogether surprise us, for, despite the seemingly infinite variety of individual human beings and their forms of social, cultural and political organisation, some things are universally common to all members of our species. For example, in all human societies babies are born through the fertilisation of sperm and ovum from parents of different sex; children are initially very small and vulnerable – needing to be fed, nurtured and protected. With luck, good management and effective healthcare they may survive the infections and traumas of childhood; may reach maturity, reproduce themselves, decline into old age and sooner or later all will die. These universal features of human life suggest that there are bound to be features of all systems of social morality that are similar. If certain general conditions must be satisfied before human life can develop and flourish, then the principles of morality will seek to protect vulnerable human life and promote the conditions necessary for human flourishing (Maritain 1944, Finnis 1999).

This question can be approached in two different ways: either by attempting to clarify the fundamental values by which we seek to direct human action and social organisation to protect human beings and to promote human flourishing, which leads to the formulation of *fundamental principles*, or by attempting to define the essential conditions that must be satisfied if human life is to be human, which leads to the formulation of *fundamental human rights*. We will discuss the first of these options in this chapter; the question of fundamental human rights will be examined in more detail in Chapter 7.

CONSTITUTIVE AND REGULATIVE PRINCIPLES IN ETHICS

In his 1785 *Groundwork of the Metaphysic of Morals*, the German philosopher Immanuel Kant set out to clarify what he called the principles presupposed in and necessary to ethics as such (Paton 1969). He distinguished between two kinds of rules or principles that apply to moral behaviour, and for that matter to all rule-governed human activity: namely those rules that are *constitutive* of a universe of discourse or activity, and those rules that are *regulative* for operations within that universe of discourse or activity. Like the rules of football, the *constitutive rules* are those that relate to the size of the pitch, the number of players, the shape of the ball etc.; they *constitute*, that is, set up the game; whereas the *regulative rules* are those that relate to scoring, penalties, throw-ins and being off-side, and these rules are *regulative* of the game itself. Wittgenstein, in his *Philosophical Investigations*, suggests the analogy of games to explain a variety of different types of rule-governed human activity, including logic and ordinary language, in which we can lay down a variety of rules in different universes of discourse, and then play the game according to the rules. In all cases *constitutive rules* define the domain and boundaries of the game activity, the *regulative rules* the permissible rules of play (Wittgenstein 1958).

Kant argued that the concept of 'person', or 'person-hood', is fundamental to ethics, and is a formative or *constitutive principle* of ethics (Paton 1969). Without the concept of a person – defined as an individual who is a bearer of rights and responsibilities – ethics cannot get started. Such individual persons must always be treated as ends in themselves and never simply as instrumental means to an end or we contradict ourselves, and the nature of ethics itself. The concept of a 'person' defined as 'a bearer of rights and duties' also serves to define the membership and boundaries of the 'moral community'. 'Respect for persons' thus functions as a *regulative principle* for our ethical conduct by requiring us to respect the rights of others, and to avoid the exploitation or abuse of persons in our everyday practice.

The concept of a person, as a bearer of rights and responsibilities, implies an individual who is able to exercise some degree of self-determination, can understand the requirements of membership of the moral community to which they belong, and who is free and able to act, to exercise their rights and to recognise their duties to others. Kant points out that this freedom and moral independence is necessary for any moral agent to qualify as a moral agent, or to be held responsible for their actions. However, in order to exercise one's power of self-determination and choice, one must not be subject to oppression or imposed constraints and must be able to adopt one's own moral values. Kant calls this kind of moral independence 'autonomy'. He contrasts it with 'heteronomy', that is, subjection to or forced submission to externally imposed authority. Thus, he argues that the *principle of autonomy* is a necessary theoretical and a practical presupposition for any functioning system of ethics or law. Responsibility and accountability, rights and duties do not make sense unless we can assume people are capable of self-determination and of making a personal commitment to a set of values. Respect for persons also requires that we respect this autonomy in others.

However, the concept of a person, or even a derived list of personal rights, would not alone be sufficient to establish a coherent system of ethics, let alone ensure its effective operation. Personal rights alone would not provide an adequate basis for a system of social ethics unless these rights could be justified, promoted and protected as rights for all. This demand for universal human rights, or the universal applicability of moral principles, requires a second kind of constitutive principle – namely the *principle or criterion of universalisability*, as Kant called it. The principle of universalisability in ethics seeks to ensure that as individuals we act consistently and that the rights we claim for ourselves are applied to all without discrimination. This demand for equity or universal fairness is a demand of the regulative ethical principle of justice.

Justice and respect for persons together would make for a reasonably satisfactory combination of pillars for any system of ethics but for the fact of given inequalities – the fact that there are wide discrepancies of size and age, wealth and power, intelligence and skill, health and strength among human beings. To ensure a workable system of ethics we require another constitutive principle, which we might call the *principle of reciprocity* (do unto others as you would have them do unto you). This principle or criterion is necessary because at certain times in our lives we all experience extreme vulnerability – when we are infants, sick, injured, mentally disordered, senile or dying. Unless we build in a principle of reciprocity – the recognition of a reciprocal duty to care for one another – we cannot ground the social obligation to care for or protect the interests of the weak. The regulative moral principle of beneficence (the duty to care, or to do good) or its negative form, the principle of non-maleficence (the duty to do no harm), serve to complement respect for personal rights and justice, and thus complete the minimum basic requirements for a coherent system of ethics.

CONFLICT, CHANGE AND STABILITY IN HUMAN LIFE AND VALUES

In this chapter we have pointed out that there are features of our life that are changing and others that remain constant. Human life is being impacted on dramatically by rapid cultural change, especially in the area of scientific and technical advance, in medical science and understanding of our genetic and psychological make-up. On the other hand, there are universal features of the human condition that remain constant, and invariable in time across human cultures:

> Birth, copulation and death.
> That's all the facts, when you come to brass tacks.
> *Sweeney Agonistes* (Eliot 1969)

We are all subject to the processes of growth, maturation, the expression of our sexual and reproductive potentialities, and we will all eventually have to face suffering, death and bereavement. As St Augustine remarked: 'When a man is born, you might as well say his condition is fatal. He will not survive!' (Augustine (Tasker, ed) 1967, 13.9–11).

We have argued in this chapter that certain values are common to all moral communities, and necessary for their functioning and survival, namely the values of beneficence, justice and respect for the dignity and rights of others. These values underlie and shape the way we prioritise other more personal values and our individual and communal life goals. As the relative importance of these values may change in family life, from a preponderant emphasis on the duty of protective beneficence of parents towards their children, to a struggle with parents for justice and equal treatment by adolescents, to a mature mutual respect for one another in adult life, so the priority we give to different values will change with changes in our economic and social circumstances, and with wider changes in society.

The account we have given of changing attitudes and moral values in our society is merely one impression of what has been happening. It can be immediately conceded that the changes suggested are far from universal However, these social changes contribute to the unpredictability of what values will be held by other people, contributing to the difficulty of moral decision-making today. Frequently, it is not possible when making difficult moral choices to rely on an appeal to values which, in the past, might have been expected to command general support. In nursing, for example, there is still considerable reluctance to go on strike. But this reluctance cannot be relied upon as much as in the past and it is likely to be defended only in some cases by an appeal to the traditional values of duty and obedience. In other cases the defence is more likely to be in terms of the value of care or concern for patients, or even of the profession's self-interest where strikes are thought to be counterproductive.

As this example suggests, the variety of moral values that people hold today is a matter of practical concern as well as of theoretical interest. Conflict between moral values exists not only on either side of the moral dilemmas confronting individuals, but also within society and between different societies. The great divisions in today's world are not only about material issues of power, wealth and poverty, but also about which moral values should have priority in the ordering of society. Should liberty be put first, as we attempt to do in Western societies, or should it be equality as in socialism, or obedience to the law of God as in resurgent Islam? Moral conflicts of this kind, clearly, can spill over into social, economic and even physical conflict within societies as well as between them. While political bargaining can play some part in the attempt to reconcile different interests, the purposes, ideas and values which move individuals and societies to action must also be taken into account, in our decision-making, if the harmful consequences of conflict are to be avoided.

In seeking to avoid these harmful consequences, it is important to remember that moral conflict in itself is not bad. Indeed it is only through moral conflict that society can resist tyranny or individual moral dogmatism and moral relativism, and thus remain responsive to the variety of moral values in personal and communal life which makes life fully human. To resist these temptations and at the same time avoid the harmful consequences of conflict is not easy, and not even possible, unless individuals and societies have some way of communicating with one another which helps each to understand the importance of the other's moral values without thereby diminishing the importance of their own. In human life there are many ways of establishing such communication, ranging from marriage, negotiation and industrial bargaining, to international diplomacy. But one useful way, we would suggest, is through the kind of informed and reasoned public debate about moral issues which we undertake in the study of ethics. Such debate provides a framework within which people can communicate with one another about the values and principles that move them to action. Ethics provides a framework within which we can give one another reasons why we believe these values and principles to be important, can offer and listen to reasonable criticism and can, on occasion, find ways of establishing public consensus about the rights and wrongs of particular conflicts. In an area such as healthcare, at a time of increasing recourse to the courts and to political bargaining, ethics would seem to have a particularly useful contribution to make.

Of course, this is not to suggest that we all need to become philosophers any more than we are all able to be saints. Nor is it to suggest that someone who has mastered the technical language of ethics is necessarily thereby a better person or even someone better able to resolve moral difficulties in practice – indeed the opposite is sometimes the case. But it does suggest that to make ourselves vulnerable to, and critical of, the ethical arguments and moral sentiments of others is a more creative and constructive way of responding to the moral complexity and conflicts of our time than by retreating either into moral dogmatism or into moral relativism.

Vulnerability is probably the key word here. Moral dogmatism and moral relativism are each in their own way attempts to be invulnerable to moral conflict, by pretending either to have no doubts or that none of it matters. The point we have been trying to make in this chapter and which, we hope, will be apparent in the following chapters is that moral conflict does matter and that, in practice, we can rarely be entirely sure that our actions have always been right or for the best as even the most prudent and informed moral judgements are necessarily fallible. This is particularly true in the field of healthcare, where professionals are frequently required to act quickly and decisively in matters affecting the vital interests of patients. To ask such professionals also to be vulnerable to such knowledge, and thus open to the pain and guilt it may involve, is no doubt hard. But it is only in accepting such vulnerability, perhaps, that any of us has the courage to be ourselves and to escape from moral adolescence into precarious adulthood.

further reading

Davies B 2000 Philosophy of religion. Oxford University Press, Oxford

Finnis J M 1999 Natural law and natural rights. Clarendon Press, Oxford

Freidson E 2001 Professionalism: the third logic. Polity Press, London

O'Neill O 2002 Autonomy and trust in bioethics. Cambridge University Press, Cambridge

Stevenson L, Haberman D L 1998 Ten theories of human nature, 3rd edn. Oxford University Press, Oxford

Taylor C 2004 Modern social imaginaries. Duke University Press, Durham

Nursing ethics – what do we mean by 'ethics'?

2

AIMS

This chapter has the following aims:

1. To clarify what we mean by ethics and some of the basic concepts like 'right', 'wrong', 'good' and 'bad', 'virtue' and 'vice' that we use in our everyday ethical life and discussion

2. To clarify the important connection between power and responsibility in the moral life

3. To distinguish between ethical problems and ethical dilemmas, and personal and shared social values

4. To examine the foundations of common ethical principles and how we deal with cultural and personal differences

5. To explore some of the connections between religion and morality and how ethics can be distinguished from religion.

LEARNING OUTCOMES

When you have read and worked through this chapter, you should be able to:

- Give a critical account of the nature of ethics, and how it is distinguished from social convention, customs and etiquette

- Illustrate how the relationships of power and dependency, responsibility and accountability link with the exercise of ethical practice in professional life, especially in nursing and healthcare

- Distinguish between the different types of discourse in which we judge things to be 'right or wrong' and that in which we judge things or actions to be 'good or bad', 'virtuous' and 'vicious'

- Give examples and explain the difference between an ethical 'dilemma' and an ethical 'problem', and how we attempt to deal with them

- Explain in what sense justice, respect for persons and protective beneficence, are fundamental and universal principles

- Discuss the nature of 'ethical relativism' and give examples to explain the value and limitations of relativism in ethics

- Give a critical account of the relations between ethics and religion.

Part A Ethics – issues of power and responsibility

ETHICS AND THE ETHOS OF A COMMUNITY

Public interest in and debate about ethics may appear to have increased over the past century, with our constant exposure to both sensible and sensationalised discussion in the mass media of controversial cases of 'unethical conduct' or 'moral dilemmas'. However, concern with ethics is not new, and the roots of ethics run deep into the past histories of our different cultures and communities. So, we cannot do justice to the subject by simply taking at face value the pronouncements of so-called experts in televised discussion on ethical issues today. We must probe some of the historical and cultural origins of ethical concepts and of ethics itself.

While every known society has developed its own customs and rules of moral conduct, historically the discipline of moral philosophy, or ethics, evolved in Europe. This does not mean that Europeans have a monopoly of wisdom in ethical matters or that we do not need to be aware of the rich diversity of moral traditions in other cultures. On the contrary, as our societies become increasingly multicultural, it is all the more important to understand the distinctive emphases and moral priorities of other people. However, the seminal work of ancient Greek philosophers, over 2000 years ago, created the vocabulary and conceptual distinctions that we still use in ethics today. Their contribution to the critical analysis of both the individual and social dimensions of moral responsibility and the regulation of human conduct has been definitive in shaping the course of ethics ever since.

The Oxford Reference Dictionary (Hawkins 1986), for example, relates the term 'ethics' to the root meaning of the Greek word 'ethos', which it defines as 'the characteristic spirit or attitudes of a community'. This connection between the ethos of a society and the form of its ethics serves to remind us that *ethics is essentially concerned with our life as members of a community, and how we behave and function in society*. This is true at a number of different levels, for we are members of various interconnected and overlapping communities within our broader society, and within the international community. A nurse, for example, will belong to some kind of family, may be a member of a church or political party, play for a sports club, be a staff nurse on a hospital ward or manager of a team of nurses, a member of a professional association or trade union, and a concerned voter and taxpayer. In each case, the nurse is a member of a different kind of *moral community*, each with its own rules, rights and responsibilities for members.

INDIVIDUAL AND SOCIAL DIMENSIONS OF ETHICAL RESPONSIBILITY

There have been two major sources of inspiration for ethics in the European tradition, the first coming from Greek and Roman culture and the other from Judaeo-Christian culture. We will discuss each of these briefly in turn to identify some of their distinctive emphases.

For the Greek philosophers, notably Plato and Aristotle, ethics and politics are inseparable, because they see the individual as belonging to a city-state (*polis*) and human beings as essentially social beings. While ethics may be concerned more with the individual, and politics with life as a member of society, ethics and politics actually represent different poles of the same continuum of communal life. There is little emphasis on *moral rules* in Greek ethics, and the ultimate goal of both individual and political life is seen to be rather the achievement of the good life, a healthy and balanced life that contributes to our *personal fulfilment and happiness* and *to social harmony and the well-being of others*. The cultivation of the virtues (or the moral potentialities and competencies of the individual) is seen to be essential both to achieve personal happiness, and for the proper exercise of our social and political responsibilities.

With both the traditional focus in nurse training on the cultivation of personal integrity, a healthy lifestyle and habits of good practice, and the modern emphasis on competency-based training and continuous improvement, this classical Greek view of ethics will be seen to have considerable relevance for nurses individually and for nursing practice.

For the later Stoic philosophers, like the Roman senator Cicero or Emperor Marcus Aurelius, ethics is concerned with living a well-ordered, healthy and noble life, in accordance with Nature, and *regulated by rational moral laws*. The famous saying *mens sana in sano corpore* (Juvenal (Braund, tr) 1996) summed up the Stoic belief that a sound mind requires a healthy body and that ethics is concerned with promoting both our physical health and mental well-being. The Stoics believed that Roman law should be both rational and moral, not based on the arbitrary edicts of tyrants. They believed that by rigorous intellectual debate we can arrive at laws which conform to 'natural law' –

'natural law' being the implicit and universal moral demands which we must obey if we are to lead healthy lives, realise our true nature as rational beings, and be effective members of human society.

In this context, nurses as health professionals are concerned not only with care of the sick and the dying, but with prevention of disease, health education, health protection and health promotion. Nursing ethics should thus encompass more than a narrow moralistic view of ethics and take on board the Stoic commitment to a wider view of how ethics and law can contribute to the health and well-being of individuals and society.

Judaeo-Christian (and Islamic) ethics, by contrast, has placed greater emphasis on moral commandments and obligations, and on rules. The moral command-ments are claimed to have a Divine origin and endorsement. They bind us into a community of reciprocal covenants and promises with God and other people that are seen to be necessary for the health and well-being of individuals and society. The biblical emphasis on salvation – the need to be healed and made whole – means that obedience to the law is not simply a matter of subordination to authority, but rather a recognition that the law serves to protect us from harming ourselves or others. While the Judaeo-Christian and Islamic traditions have sought to emphasise that authentic moral conduct cannot be merely a matter of external observance of the law, they have given prominence to the idea that ethics is concerned with the regulation of human conduct by rules and laws. Historically in the Western Church and in Christian societies this emphasis on prescriptive moral rules and laws has been reinforced by associa-tion with the tradition of Roman law and governance. However, Judaeo-Christian ethics has also emphasised that in seeking to observe the spirit, and not just the letter of the law, the motives and intentions of the moral agent are important to factor into the equation. It is not just what we do, or whether we act in conformity to the rules, but what we think and how we feel in our hearts when we act, that is important for understanding whether actions are genuinely moral or not. This emphasis on inner motives and intentions serves to focus on personal responsibility for moral action in a new way, giving moral duty and obligation a deeper personal meaning.

The emphasis in nursing, as in other professions, on regulatory Codes of Conduct or Codes of Ethics, mirrors this recognition that rules play an important part in ethics in defining right and wrong conduct, or, in this case, the responsibilities of nurses towards those dependent on them for care and treatment. However, these rules are grounded in recognition of more fundamental values relating to what it means to be human and how we protect and promote what we regard as most precious about being human.

What the two Western traditions have in common is an emphasis on the *centrality of the concept of justice* in our understanding of both ethics and politics, and in our exercise of personal and social responsibility as members of a variety of different kinds of community. Justice is essentially an *interpersonal* virtue, concerned with both fairness to ourselves and to others, and it is grounded in responsible sharing of power and resources with others. For Plato, justice (or *dikaiosune*) is the principle of order in human life that preserves the proper balance between all our human gifts and potentialities, and it is the principle of order or harmony that keeps the individual, political and cosmic orders in balance and harmony with one another. For Jewish thought, too, justice is central to the achievement of *shalom*, peace or social harmony based on right order. The key term in Hebrew (translated as *righteousness*) combines both the concept of justice as fairness and the principle of order in personal and social life. Righteousness means living in accordance with the demands of fidelity to one another and to a God of covenant love. Finally, Christian ethics has sought to emphasise the insepar-able connection between justice, love and power, and of reciprocal care and responsibility for one another. The central challenge of Christian ethics to secular ethics is perhaps how a love ethic is to be harmonised with the sometimes harsh demands of justice, or how an ethic of caring is to be translated into public service in rule-governed institutions (Boman 1960).

Nurses, as members of one of the 'caring professions', with a particular 'duty of care' towards vulnerable patients, are faced with the constant tension between the demands of providing a fair and equitable service to all their patients, and the respons-ibility to care for the particular needs of individuals.

What the European tradition has emphasised is that individual ethics and social ethics, individual responsibility and corporate or social responsibility, cannot be separated from one another without significant loss of balance in our understanding of the nature of human society. We do not exist in god-like isolation, we are part of one another, interact with one another, are dependent on one another. Ethics therefore has to do with our reciprocal responsibility to one another as well as responsibility for our own lives, decisions and actions. We are held accountable to the moral communities in which we live and work, through formal and informal scrutiny, and review of our performance and conduct, both as individuals and professionals.

CHANGING PERCEPTIONS OF THE RELATIONSHIP OF THE INDIVIDUAL AND COMMUNITY

In the first chapter we explored some of the historical factors that have contributed to the development of professions in the contemporary world, and drew attention to the changing 'social imaginaries' or belief and value systems that provide the context for the definition of the roles of nursing and other professions. One of the key cultural changes has been in perceptions of the role of individuals in relation to society.

Tensions between individualism and collectivism have been present in most societies from the most traditional to modern. The Greek tragedies of Aeschylus, Sophocles and Euripides are concerned with the struggles of individuals against fate and the oppressive forces of traditional society or tyranny. The biblical prophets protest in the name of a faith that is both personal and based on inner righteousness against a religion of external obedience and conformity to the law and ritual of the Jewish religious establishment. The European Renaissance and Protestant Reformation gave a new emphasis to personal moral responsibility (before God) on the authority of individual reason and conscience, and on individual rights and dignity, against what was seen to be the overbearing authoritarianism of the Roman Catholic Church. The rise of European nationalism in the 18th and 19th centuries (and in the rest of the world in the 20th century) can also be seen as the result of new movements of peoples to define their individual identity in relation to their ethnic and cultural origins.

The 20th century, however, marked perhaps the most extreme expressions of and conflicts between collectivist and individualist ideologies, e.g. between communism and fascism on the one hand and liberal democracy and free-market capitalism on the other. Conflict between these collectivist and individualist ideologies was expressed at many different levels.

At the cultural and political level it took the form of a struggle to win the hearts and minds of people by all available means, including the use of the newly invented and powerful mass media of radio, film and television. At the economic level it was expressed by increasingly aggressive national and industrial competition to win global markets and access to natural resources through conquest and colonisation. Industrialised colonial powers penetrated more traditional societies in the name of 'modernisation', and subverted their cultures and communitarian values by promoting individualism and commercial competition. At the international level this led inevitably to a century of wars and global conflicts of unprecedented ferocity.

But what has this to do with ethics? In a sense it has everything to do with ethics, for the tension between individual and society, personal and political responsibility, is at the heart of ethics. However, there is another sense in which the conflicts of the 20th century have also profoundly influenced and set the agenda for ethics in the 21st century. Ethics acquired a new prominence on the world stage, and in public debate, as a result of the appalling human rights abuses associated with the wars and conflicts of the 20th century.

For example, in marking the 60th anniversary of the liberation of Auschwitz, we remember the six million Jews, Poles, Gypsies, homosexuals, and mentally or physically disabled people who were exterminated in Nazi concentration camps, and are reminded of the so-called medical experiments performed on captive men, women and children in these camps. As a result of worldwide outrage at these atrocities, public pressure led to a fundamental review of human rights and ethics in public and professional life. In particular, it led to a review of medical ethics by the World Medical Association and a new level of public interest in biomedical ethics and the ethics of research. This in turn led nurses and other professions to develop codes of ethics and practical means for the regulation of professional conduct and practice. The establishment of the United Nations Organization after World War II represented first an attempt to secure world peace and prevent further global conflict by setting up a framework for world government. However, it also led to the formulation of UNO's *Universal Declaration of Human Rights*, (1948) and this has been followed by a variety of other declarations and international conventions, for example the *European Convention on Human Rights* (UNO 1950) and the *Declaration on the Rights of the Child* (UNO 1959).

As we shall see, when we come to discuss human rights later, *we acquire rights as a result of being members of a moral community, to which we also owe duties and obligations*. While traditional societies have tended to emphasise the priority of our social obligations and civic duties over individual rights and liberties, the focus has shifted recently towards an emphasis on individual rights often divorced from consideration of our correlative social duties. Exploring the relationship between rights and duties, personal liberty and social obligation, is the very stuff of ethical debate. These questions are often at the heart of what we experience as ethical problems or dilemmas, both in personal life and in our professional work with clients and patients. Fundamental to this debate, as the Greek philosopher Aristotle (384–322 BC) recognised, is the question of how we share power and responsibility, in individual and political life, how we put checks on the abuse of power and how we educate people for the exercise of moral and political responsibility.

ETHICS AND POLITICS – QUESTIONS OF POWER AND QUESTIONS OF PRINCIPLE

Plato introduces Book 3 of his *Republic* with a spirited debate between Thrasymachus and Socrates on the nature of justice in individual life and society (Plato (Cornford, tr) 1961). Thrasymachus attempts to defend the view that 'might is right', that it is the powerful, those who exercise control in society, who define what is right or wrong, and concludes that 'justice' is 'but the rule of the stronger'. Socrates questions this popular view, by criticising both what Thrasymachus says and how and why he says it. He questions Thrasymachus' cynicism and the aggressiveness with which he defends his position in the face of rational criticism. He questions, too, his ulterior motives in rejecting the idea that there can be a principled basis for believing in justice as an ideal or as a critical norm for individual and social life.

Plato is sufficient of a political realist to recognise that the apparent choice between power and principle is not a real choice. In the real world human appetites and desires, the lust for power and wealth, are forces to be reckoned with, both in individual and corporate life and in society. To achieve order and harmony in our own lives these powerful forces need to be subject to rational direction and discipline or we can destroy ourselves. In the state, which has greater power than the individual because it is built on the collective power of the people, power needs to be accountable, to be subject to rational ordering and direction if it is not to lead to the abuse of power, and to disorder, conflict and anarchy.

In the *Republic*, Plato describes justice both as the individual virtue or competence required to balance our appetites, desires and ambitions with the need for rational order in our lives, and also as the rational basis for the organisation of society for the common good. How this is to be achieved in practice is a matter of debate – whether rational direction of the state should be by one powerful man (autocracy), by a small powerful and rich elite (oligarchy or timocracy), by noble people of recognised moral competence and political wisdom (aristocracy), or rule by the mob (anarchy) (Plato (Cornford, tr) 1961, Bks VIII and IX). Plato himself was disillusioned with Athenian so-called 'democracy', because it had put to death his revered teacher, Socrates. As he saw it, democracy too

easily degenerates into mob rule, through the cynical manipulation of public opinion by demagogues (or 'spin-doctors') employed by those with vested interests. Recognising the reality of power, and the need for the exercise of power to be subject to rational and moral control, he believed that those elected to rule should be noble, not in terms of birth or wealth, but because of their recognised wisdom, experience and moral integrity. In a just society he believed proper respect would be given to the contributions of workers and producers, traders and administrators, soldiers and guardians, and those who ruled would ideally be lovers of wisdom.

While Plato thus favoured a form of 'aristocracy' – rule by the best, most virtuous and wisest of men – Aristotle, a contemporary disciple and critic of Plato, favoured a form of rational democracy in which those who rule are accountable to the people and where restraints and balances can be built in to the structure of the state, to prevent the abuse of power by individuals or groups with vested interests (Ross 1952, Vol. X, Bks IV and V).

However, one might ask what is the point of discussing these historical matters, interesting though they may be, in a textbook on nursing ethics? Well, this is because we may see that there are parallels between the classic forms of government and different types of management in institutions and professional bodies. Nurses and other health professionals do not function in isolation, but within an organised profession, and in hospitals, health centres and other institutions that require leadership and structures of governance to operate effectively. Health visitors or district nurses do not function on their own but as members of a team. They are responsible to the primary care team, as they are also responsible to their managers and to society, for the quality of care they provide to clients.

Patterns of management in hospitals and institutions can also be autocratic, run by a board or management team, based on a hierarchy of seniority based on expertise, or they may be more democratic, with staff representation in formulating policy and organisational decision-making. The form of management adopted will depend on the way power and responsibility is shared and on the pattern of organisation required.

'Line management' is commonly the type of management adopted in large institutions that require a hierarchical form of organisation and division of power or responsibility. Many examples may be found in the way hospitals and most public sector departments are organised.

'Partnership', a model adopted from business and industry, has recently become a popular model in the public sector in the UK. This model is being recommended in areas where inter-agency collaboration is necessary, as in children's services. Ideally 'partners' should share staff and resources in 'joined-up' services and share collective responsibility for outcomes. However, 'partnership' is often more a matter of rhetoric than genuinely shared values, or investment of capital, shared management or real collaboration.

Teamwork or co-responsibility are models more commonly adopted in the organisation of inter-professional work in primary care, community psychiatry and social work, and in some types of collaborative sharing of decision-making and responsibility on ward teams.

The specific ethical issues that confront us as individual professionals in dealing with patients or clients, or as members or managers of organisations, may be different in some ways from those faced by the ancient Greeks, but they are similar – for in professional life, we make decisions within the context of organisations where we are accountable in different ways at different levels.

DIFFERENT LEVELS OR SPHERES OF RESPONSIBILITY

The exercise of moral responsibility in public life and in the exercise of one's duty as a professional is many layered. In order to get away from the simplistic and narrow individualistic view of ethics that has dominated thinking and discussion of the subject in the past century, we need to adopt a more complex model that does justice to the interconnections between individual, team, organisational and inter-agency levels of responsibility. It means recognising that nurses and health professionals do not work in isolation, or teams in a vacuum – but in complexly structured organisations with many kinds of connections within them and to other agencies and to society.

To understand better the multilevel nature of ethical responsibility, we might again take a cue from Plato and the Greek philosophers, who saw social life as operating at three different levels: that of the individual (the *micro-cosmic* order), at the level of

society and the state (the *meso-cosmic* order), and in relation to the wider world (the *macro-cosmic* order). Adapting this model we can apply it to the various levels at which we exercise moral responsibility and accountability. Thus we might apply the terms 'micro' to the individual level, 'macho' to team leadership (because who leads the team can be a contentious issue), 'meso' to organisational management, and 'macro' to the politics of inter-agency relationships, and relationships with government.

All moral action takes place as it were within a series of interconnected and concentric spheres of social responsibility. At the centre we stand on our own, sometimes having to make individual decisions and difficult personal moral choices. This sphere, however, is encompassed within the wider sphere of responsibility we have to family or professional peers and to managers to whom we are immediately accountable, and from whom we can also draw advice and support. Around this sphere is the sphere of the wider organisation in which we work, which gives us enhanced power and an official status. Beyond that, there may be further spheres of responsibility relevant to our own exercise of responsibility, e.g. our duty to act with integrity towards people in other organisations with which ours has to cooperate, or who supply us with services.

Given this complexity and many-layered nature of moral responsibility, it is important in discussing the subject of ethical responsibility to recognise these various levels. Working with others in large organisations involves possibilities for both cooperation and conflict over resources and dominance. Outside the institutions in which we work are other organisations, businesses and voluntary agencies with which we have to cooperate or compete, and then there are the structures of the state on whom we depend for resources, and public authorities to which we are accountable, e.g. our health authority, local and state government.

One way of distinguishing the 'micro', 'macho', 'meso' and 'macro' levels might be called the *'Russian dolls' model* of organisational ethics, because each level is contained in a wider, more embracing structure.

Box 2.1 Levels of responsibility in organisations		
Macro level	External stakeholder level	Ethics in strategic planning and inter-agency relations
Meso level	Internal stakeholder level	Ethics in corporate management of human and financial resources
Macho level	Team leadership level	Ethics in interdisciplinary cooperation and teamwork.
Micro level	Individual level	Ethics in personal decision-making and employee development

It serves to illustrate that the exercise of ethical responsibility, and taking ethical decisions, means different things in different contexts – at individual, professional, management and inter-agency and political levels. The various encompassing levels of ethics in professional and organisational life and levels of moral action and responsibility can be illustrated hierarchically as in Box 2.1.

Alternatively the various overlapping spheres of individual responsibility (micro), team leadership (macho), organisational management (meso), and inter-agency collaboration (macro) can be illustrated by a kind of 'spider's web' (Fig. 2.1) – an image that emphasises the interconnections between the various spheres of action and operation.

Recognising that we exercise responsibility and make ethical decisions within a context where our actions have implications at a number of different levels helps to remind us of the complex ramifications of what we do, and of the necessary complexity of ethical decision-making in professional life. It should also help us to clarify the different kinds of responsibility that we exercise at these different levels. Instead of being overwhelmed by the many kinds of demands we have to satisfy in institutional life, we can begin to address these separately and thus deal with them in a more rational way.

Traditionally the teaching of ethics in the professions has tended to focus attention on codes of conduct, or to approach ethics from a very individualistic perspective emphasising personal responsibility for decision-making. In organisational life most decisions are made in teams or committees or by higher management. Little attention has been given to the way these groups make decisions or to training people to play an effective part in group decision-making on ethical policy or in dealing with specific ethical problems. Adopting a comprehensive and corporate approach to ethics helps us to understand that making ethical decisions as a professional, or employee, cannot be separated from one's role or function in the organisation and one's accountability to the whole moral community which that organisation comprises. *Thus ethics is not simply a private matter but one which applies to the life of the whole organisation* (Kitson & Campbell 1996, Barrett 1998, Sternberg 2004).

A corporate approach to ethics requires that ethics is integrated into all aspects of our work, viz:

- achieving standards of excellence in the performance of our work, in serving our clients
- good leadership and effective teamwork,
- sound, fair and efficient management, and
- responsible dealings with other agencies and government.

Ultimately, the demands for strategic planning, performance management and evidence-based practice arise from outside as demands for publicly accountable services, and from within as demands from the profession for responsible ethical practice. When corporate management integrates ethics into its strategic planning, recognises the multilevel nature of its ethical responsibilities, and negotiates ethical policy with all stakeholders, this helps to ensure that an institution is an ethical organisation, not just a collection of ethical individuals:

- Instead of ethics being seen as a purely private matter, ethics is recognised to be at the heart of what it means to be a responsible and publicly accountable professional, who, as a responsible employee of an organisation, is a member of a specific moral community.
- Instead of ethics being seen as merely necessary for dealing with malpractice or corruption, it is the basis for the ethos, mission, value base and strategic planning of an organisation.
- Systems, procedures and training programmes are set up in such a way that ethical policy directs the way the whole organisation does its business, for the benefit of its clients, while also contributing to the well-being of the institution, its planning for growth, organisational change and staff development.
- Sound ethical policy is seen to contribute to both corporate and individual well-being, and collective commitment to the new ethos of 'ethical management and practice' is seen to be advantageous to all, and to be secured by negotiation rather than edict from above.

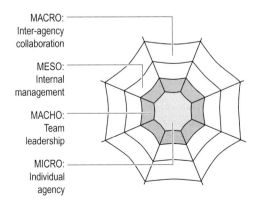

Figure 2.1 Overlapping spheres of responsibility.

- Quality assurance, standards setting, and peer review are seen to be a normal part of ethical management – encouraging development of skills and confidence in self-audit or monitoring, thus reducing dependency on legalistic, authoritarian and merely 'disciplinary' approaches.

What is outlined above may be open to the criticism of being unlikely to translate into practice due to the vested interests of different stakeholders and that not everyone will give the same priority to ethics in practice. However, there is good evidence from research on both private and public sector organisations that sound strategic ethical management does contribute to the improvement of standards of performance, staff morale (as well as morals!) and the general well-being of the organisation, including its efficiency and effectiveness (American Accounting Association 1975, Bruce 1994, Bruyn 1987, Markowitz 1992, Robertson & Schlegelmilch 1993).

Part B Ethics – some basic conceptual distinctions

WHAT DO WE MEAN BY 'ETHICS' AND/OR 'MORALS'?

Nursing is only one area of life in which we face moral choices, and while it has many special features which we will consider later, it also has much in common with the rest of our moral experience. By way of introduction, therefore, we will begin by defining some terms and discussing what we mean by them in the context of this book, namely: 'ethics' and 'morals', 'moral problems' and 'moral dilemmas', 'moral choice', and 'moral values'. We will discuss these first in the context of ordinary life, noting how perceptions of moral issues and choices are related to the ways in which moral values may change over time.

What, in the first place, do we mean by *ethics* and *morals*? These terms originally meant much the same thing, 'ethics' coming from Greek and 'morals' from its Latin equivalent. Both words referred to social customs and etiquette regarding what is 'right' and 'wrong', in theory and social practice. In everyday usage the terms 'moral' and 'ethical' can still be used more or less interchangeably, but a distinction has grown up between the two terms in more formal usage. Morals (and also morality) now tends to refer to the standards of behaviour actually held or followed by individuals and groups, while ethics refers to the science or study of morals – an activity, in the academic context, also often called moral philosophy.

This distinction, however, is complicated by three popular ways of using the words. 'An ethic' can also be used to refer to the moral standpoint of certain groups, e.g. 'a nursing ethic' or 'legal ethic'. It is sometimes applied to the moral beliefs of individuals, e.g. 'her personal ethic'. The implication behind this usage is that the group or individual moral convictions involved have been codified or carefully worked out, or that they are in some sense high-minded. Associated with this kind of high-mindedness is the second popular use, where 'moral' and 'ethical' are used as terms of approval, and their opposites are 'immoral' or 'unethical'. The more formal use derives from the idea of ethics as the impartial study of moral systems or science of morals. In formal discourse 'ethics' and 'ethical' seem to be preferred to 'morals' and 'morality' because of the common association of 'morals' with personal conduct. Another critical use of 'morals' is when it is linked to personal prejudice or religious dogmatism. 'Ethics' and 'ethical', by contrast, are thought of as involving something more academic or objective. There is no substantial reason for these associations of ideas, which are largely a matter of convention or preference (Audi 1995). However, we do need to adopt some distinctions and definitions in order to clarify our discourse and to avoid confusion and ambiguity.

Some distinctions and definitions with which we might begin are taken from common usage (Box 2.2).

CONSIDERING WHAT ETHICS IS AND IS NOT

Our everyday ethical life and discourse has three distinct but interconnected aspects, expressed by the universal distinctions between three pairs of interrelated terms, namely: *right* and *wrong*, *good* and *bad*, *virtue* and *vice*. Understanding the meanings of these terms and how they relate to one another is a useful way to begin the exploration of ethical discourse and the emphasis given to these different terms in different ethical traditions as well as different moral theories. In general these pairs of terms serve to emphasise different things.

We decide with reference to *rules and principles* whether our actions are *right or wrong*. The terms *virtue and vice* relate to our assessment of *moral character* and whether our actions are morally competent or incompetent. *Good and bad (or evil)* are terms that we apply to assessment of whether our actions *promote*

Box 2.2 Defining etiquette, morals, ethics and meta-ethics

ETIQUETTE – (French: ticket) refers to the written or unwritten rules of a society relating to:
- conventional manners or rules of behaviour in public
- social customs relating to gender roles, dress and to people of different status
- court ceremonial, rules for 'professional' conduct.

MORALS and MORALITY – (Latin: mores = custom or convention) – generally refer to:
- the domain of personal values and rules of behaviour
- conventional rules of conduct regulating our social interactions
- culture-specific mores, customs grounded in religious and ideological beliefs.

ETHICS – (Greek: ethos = the spirit of a community; its custom or conventions)
- 'An ethic' refers to the collective belief-and-value system of any moral community, or professional group.
- 'Ethics', meaning the 'science of morals' studies:
    how we determine what is good or bad for the flourishing of society
    what rules are required to prevent people being harmed
    what form of education or training is necessary for moral competence (virtue).

META-ETHICS or MORAL PHILOSOPHY
Moral philosophy is the systematic and critical study of the different kinds of theories that we invoke, or fall back on, when challenged to justify the ethical policies on which we base our moral lives and decisions. This higher-level kind of study of the foundations of our belief-and-value systems is sometimes called 'meta-ethics' because it represents a 'second-order' reflection on our 'first-order' moral experience, principles and rules.

Adapted from the Oxford Reference Dictionary (Hawkins 1996).

by fiat or by relying on people to just 'follow their individual consciences'. Provision must be made for time and opportunity to build up trust and understanding among all staff and stakeholders, so that a workable moral consensus can be built.

In broad terms any adequate account of ethics must comprehend all three types of distinction, namely right/wrong, good/bad and virtue/vice, and give meaning to these in practice, because:

- *Ethics is concerned with what is good or bad for human beings,* that is, with the pursuit of values that will ensure the flourishing of human societies, and the avoidance of what will cause harm. Ethics is concerned with specifying the requirements for the general well-being, health and happiness of people, and what kind of things prevent this happening.
- *Ethics is also concerned with defining what is right or wrong,* that is, with such regulation of human society as is necessary to foster an environment in which individuals and communities can flourish, and with what means are necessary to protect people from those who would harm them. Protective rules or regulations defining what is right or wrong, legal or illegal must be value-based and promote personal and social well-being if they are to be fair and ethical.
- *Ethics is concerned with how we cultivate a virtuous character and avoid moral incompetence or vice.* That is, ethics is practically concerned with striving for excellence, with how we should develop our human potentialities, both our intellectual and moral competencies, in order to flourish as individuals and contribute more effectively to society. It must address the issues of defective will, bad habits and moral weakness, as well as social evils.

In practice, who defines these will serve to characterise the kind of organisation in which we find ourselves, and its style of management. If ethical policy is defined by prescription from above it may be ignored, or not taken seriously by subordinate managers and employees. If trade unions assume that they have a monopoly of wisdom in ethical matters and seek to dictate ethical policy from below, this may encourage a cynical and amoral attitude on the part of management. If ethical policy development involves genuinely participative methods in which all stakeholders have a part in shaping ethical policy, then there is some hope that it will be 'owned' and respected by all who shape the policy and accept responsibility for its implementation.

Having attempted above to distinguish between what ethics is and what ethics is not, and having

human flourishing, and whether our actions have *beneficial or detrimental outcomes or consequences.*

It should be noted that as pretty well everything in ethics is contestable, there will be argument about what we mean in practice by each of these concepts: 'moral character', 'human flourishing' and 'beneficial or detrimental consequences'. This is the stuff of moral debate. However, we can only cooperate with others if we can reach some consensus about what we mean when we use these terms. A sound moral community in business or professional life cannot be created clarified the function of the terms good/bad, right/wrong, virtue/vice in moral discourse, we suggest the following summary definition of ethics as a starting point for our discussion:

> Ethics is that universe of discourse in which we are concerned with the appraisal of human conduct, from the point of view of:
> - whether it promotes the well-being of the individual and society
> - whether it conforms to the moral rules and laws formulated by the moral community in which the individual lives and works
> - whether it is conducive to building sound moral character and community life.

We may summarise the main points we have made above as in Box 2.3, distinguishing common misunderstandings of what ethics is, from a philosophical understanding of ethics.

THE RELATIONS BETWEEN RIGHT AND WRONG, GOOD AND BAD, VIRTUE AND VICE

(Note: For some classical works on these topics, see: Ross 1930 (*The Right and the Good*), Murdoch 1970 (*The Sovereignty of Good*), Macintyre 1985 (*After Virtue*).)

Right and wrong

We are all born into a morally structured world, and encounter rules and regulations whichever way we turn. Our parents lay down rules for us to obey, the church and religious communities and professional bodies seek to lay all kinds of rules on us. Schools seem to be rule factories. Society is governed by rules, laws and regulations. Not surprisingly some say: 'In the beginning was the Rule!' However, this legalistic perspective tends to focus on regulation, 'black letter'

law, and to devalue the virtues of informed and prudent moral judgement (Solomon 1994, Ch. 4).

Rules are not absolute, we may always question whether a rule is a *good* rule or not. As adolescents, we challenge family rules in this way, and will not 'own' a rule unless we feel that the rule benefits us as well as others. In this sense, judgements of value have to be made about rules, as to whether they are fair, respect the rights of all parties, and protect those who cannot defend their rights. Value judgements are therefore more fundamental than rules. Like the law, sound statutory law must be based on and be consistent with common law and the principles of natural justice. Legislation alone does not make a law just or fair. It must also serve to promote human well-being and prevent harm to people.

To be a mature and responsible moral agent means that we do not simply do our duty because we are ordered to do so by some authority, or because the law says we must. We have to make our own commitment to the law (or conscientiously object to unjust laws) and we have to take full responsibility for our actions. To make conscientious moral choices means that we must have internalised the moral law, and made it our own.

Good and bad

Deciding what things are good or bad for us is not something other people can do for us. Parents and other people may well try to tell us that smoking or lazing about on the beach is 'bad' for us. We are not convinced until we have examined the facts or tried these things for ourselves. We may learn from bitter experience to avoid certain things that hurt us and to strive for others that bring us greater pleasure or fulfilment.

Box 2.3 What ethics is and is not

What ethics is not	What ethics is
ETHICS IS NOT simply about matters of a private nature or about personal feelings, attitudes and values.	ETHICS IS a community enterprise, based on universal principles and reasoned public debate.
ETHICS IS NOT about mysterious occult processes, feelings in the gut, or privileged access to moral truth.	ETHICS IS about real power relations between people and the basis of power-sharing between them.
ETHICS IS NOT a business for experts, for religious authorities, lawyers, philosophers or gurus.	ETHICS IS about participation in a moral community and ownership of the policies it develops.
ETHICS IS NOT about endless disputes, disagreements and dilemmas, nor about grandstanding our opinions.	ETHICS IS a problem-solving activity based on knowledge of principles and skills in their application.
ETHICS IS NOT a matter of innate knowledge, special powers of intuition or supernatural revelation.	ETHICS IS an educational process in which we can discover what it means to be responsible moral agents.

Although the attempts to make the pursuit of pleasure and avoidance of pain the basis for ethics are as ancient as Plato and Aristotle in the 4th century BC and Epicurus in the 3rd century BC, it was the utilitarian philosophers Jeremy Bentham and John Stuart Mill in the 19th century who gave particular prominence to the pleasure principle as a basis for ethics. We can only be said to be free moral agents when we can challenge our inherited attitudes and test these by the light of reason and experience. In this way we come to adopt beliefs as our own. In the light of tested beliefs about ourselves, and the world around us, we may come to change our attitudes to many things, to challenge the prejudices of our parents or teachers, and may begin to react differently to people. It is in this way that we develop our own set of values.

We cannot inherit values from other people, nor have them imposed on us, as is the case with attitudes and unquestioned beliefs. Values must be of our own choosing, or they are not values. Values determine our choice of means to achieve our life goals. While we make testable truth claims for our beliefs, we need not act on them. Value judgements embody commitments we make, lifestyle choices, things on which we stake our decisions, and sometimes our lives.

Virtue and vice

'Virtue' literally means 'strength' or 'power'. It is important to emphasise that virtue does not have a narrow pious or religious meaning, but relates directly to the development of our personal character, our mental, physical, emotional and social potentialities and skills. In striving to improve our health and strength, knowledge and expertise, our powers of self-discipline and ability to control our feelings and appetites, and to develop our social skills and ability to communicate effectively with other people – in all these activities we are cultivating our personal identity and integrity of moral character. Virtue is a matter of moral competence.

'Vice' is a word that has gone out of currency, but it comprehends at least three forms of deficient character for which we can be held responsible: first, incompetence, due to the failure to develop our potentialities; second, dysfunctional forms of behaviour or bad habits that frustrate our attempts to achieve our own or society's goals; and, third, corrupt or destructive actions which damage ourselves, or our friends and families, or our work and professional colleagues – and may lead us into crime.

What this means is that we are not simply born good or evil, but these dispositions are learned and hardened into habits, for good or ill, through the pattern of our practice. To become skilled in driving a motor car, or playing a musical instrument, requires a complex process of learning, effort and practice. In the same way the achievement of a state of realised moral integrity and virtuous character is the result of growing knowledge and life skills, self-insight and self-mastery through discipline and practice. Virtue is a developmental concept and is linked to our striving to improve our personal competencies, our striving for excellence. So too, unfortunately, is vice learned and, as we all know, bad habits are often difficult to unlearn. In this connection, the work environment in which we are employed may encourage sound moral practice and development of practical competencies in applied ethics, or the organisational context may inhibit and even discourage sound ethical practice. Like all our human potentialities moral virtues need nurturing and support, and the right kind of environment in which to flourish. However, some exceptional individuals may display heroic virtue under very difficult circumstances.

THE STRUCTURE OF MORAL ACTION AND MORAL THEORY

Aristotle, in his attempt to characterise practical wisdom, and in analysing the nature of human action and the structure of moral judgements, suggests that all human acts have the same basic structure. He describes this structure as one in which we have to take account in turn of what he calls: *causes*, *means* and *ends* (Thomson 1976, Bk VI).

- '*Causes*' here refer to the forces operating in a situation, the principles and rules that apply in the given circumstances and which provide the context and impetus to act.
- '*Means*' refer to the human and material resources, skills and expertise required to act effectively in the situation to address a given problem.
- '*Ends*' refer to both the specific aims and objectives of a plan of action, and to the long-term goal/s of individual or corporate actions.

The key pairs of terms we have discussed above, namely right and wrong, virtue and vice, good and bad, relate directly to different aspects of the above structure.

- '*Right*' and '*wrong*' relate to the practical and moral principles that underlie the laws and rules which define our duties, and responsibilities to others; we judge actions to be 'right' or 'wrong' depending on whether we have applied these principles correctly or incorrectly.

- *'Virtue' and 'vice'* relate to whether or not we have the competence to choose not only the right course of action, but also appropriate and effective means and methods to achieve our objectives. The classical virtues relate to fundamental values, to standards of moral excellence and practical moral competence, which are essential for effective and efficient moral action.
- *'Good' and 'bad'* relate to both our anticipation and assessment of the outcomes of our actions. In relation to short-term objectives, we are concerned to establish whether or not the consequences of our actions are beneficial or detrimental to solving our problem. In relation to our long-term life goals we are concerned with whether our actions collectively contribute to our well-being and the good of society.

On this basis it is logical to suggest that in planning a course of action, in making a rational decision, or acting in a purposeful and responsible way, we should:

- review the prevailing circumstances and the facts of the specific situation, including what principles and rules apply to the particular 'ball-game' in which we find ourselves
- consider what practical options are available to us, what expertise, assistance or resources we will require, and what means or methods we need to solve a pressing problem
- anticipate the likely outcomes of each option, ensure we have specific goals and realistic objectives so that it is possible for us to evaluate whether our action is successful or not.

These steps are all involved in any action that is intelligently planned, but we may not consider them in the given order, and may in reality move backwards and forwards between these three levels until we have clarified how we decide to act. Further, in situations of crisis we may not have time to reflect and either skip steps, or rely on well-tried courses of action used before.

The three complementary features of our moral experience set out above also relate to the three classical types of moral theory, namely: *deontological*, *axiological* and *teleological* (from the Greek words 'deon' for duty, 'axios' for virtue or value, and 'telos' for goal or end.

Deontological ethical theory focuses attention on the 'prior conditions' or *'causes'* which set the boundaries of the situation in which we act. For Aristotle these pre-existing conditions include not only the objective context and what critical event/s make it necessary for us to act, but also the framework of principles and rules that serve to define our duties.

Axiological ethical theory focuses on the *'means'* needed to achieve effective action, and these include moral knowledge and practical moral competence. The cardinal moral virtues, namely, temperance, courage, justice and prudence, relate to the key values of self-mastery, emotional balance and maturity, consistent fairness and practical wisdom respectively. Axiology is therefore concerned with the mastery of the virtues that are necessary to act effectively.

Teleological ethics focuses attention on both the short- and long-term goals or *'ends'* of action. Since our actions cannot be rational unless they are planned and have clear objectives, our first task in acting responsibly is to clarify our intended goals for acting. Only if we have clear objectives can we evaluate whether or not our actions succeed in achieving the outcomes we desire. ('Consequentialism' and 'utilitarianism' are specific forms of teleological ethics that direct our attention to the outcomes of our actions.)

We can tabulate the points we have been making about these three interconnected aspects of moral experience and the various aspects of moral practice which they help us to evaluate. In Box 2.4 we set these out schematically.

Aristotle considers that the key form of moral competence that we require to make morally sound and effective decisions is the virtue of practical wisdom or prudence. We may paraphrase Aristotle's definition of prudence or practical wisdom in the following terms: *Prudence is the ability to apply universal practical and moral principles to the demands of particular situations, using our knowledge and past experience to make sound judgements about the best available means to achieve a good result or outcome for ourselves and others.*

Following Aristotle, we believe that sound moral judgements involve consideration of all three aspects of human actions, namely *causes → means → ends*, and review of moral situations in terms of all three types of moral criteria (deontological, axiological and teleological). The appraisal of moral judgements and actions requires determination of whether they are right, likely to be effective and whether they produce good outcomes. We can also justify our moral judgements and actions if we have circumspectly considered: relevant principles, rights and duties, the kinds of moral competence and resources needed, and whether the desired ends are good and actual outcomes are beneficial rather than harmful. Given Aristotle's insight into these elements in human actions, it is not surprising that he regards prudence as the keystone which holds together and gives strength to the arch of human theoretical and practical virtues.

Box 2.4 Interrelated key concepts in ethics

Right and wrong	Virtue and vice	Good and bad
'Right' and 'wrong' are terms that relate to and presuppose a system of *formal rules*, laws and regulations	'Virtue' and 'vice' are terms used in appraising *competence/incompetence in ourselves or others as moral agents* and the effectiveness of actions	'Good' and 'bad' are terms that relate to *value judgements* about what does/does not promote our well-being or that of others
'Right' and 'wrong' belong to a *binary system* where things must be *either* 'right' *or* 'wrong'. They are mutually exclusive and collectively exhaustive terms	'Virtue' and 'vice' are antithetical *states of being or character* of a person, and/or the developed or under-developed nature of their personal potentialities	'Good' and 'bad' are *polar terms in a continuum* (like 'health' and 'disease'); they are not mutually exclusive opposites, but admit of degrees of comparison
'Right' and 'wrong' only *appear 'absolute' and 'objective'* so long as one does not question the system of rules in question	'Virtue' and 'vice' relate to the *personal attributes we value and cultivate*, in ourselves or others, as expressing our nature as human beings	'Good' and 'bad' may *appear 'relative' and 'subjective'* because we have to make personal appraisals of things, events or experiences
Justification of judgements that things are 'right' or 'wrong' is based on *appeal to authority* – the authority of the rule or rule-giver	We seek to justify claims that people are virtuous or vicious (evil) by evidence of the *good or harm they do to themselves or others*	Judgements that things are 'good' or 'bad' have to be based on *appeal to evidence, facts and experience* (not authority or rules)
A system of rules defining what is to be regarded as 'right' or 'wrong' also serves to define our *rights and obligations* within that system	'Virtue' and 'vice' are *axiological terms*, by which we assess whether the way a person develops helps or hinders them in achieving their life goals	'Good'/'Bad' are *normative terms*, by which we judge the degree things approximate to or deviate from a given norm or ideal standard
'Right'/'Wrong' thinking *seems to offer moral certainty* and security and is often associated with authoritarian dogmatism	'Virtue' and 'vice' *are states of being or fixed dispositions*, in which we gain possession of moral knowledge in the course of our life and experience	Judgements that things are 'good' or 'bad' involve making *our own riskful decisions* about things based on personal experience
***Deontological moral theory* focuses on 'right/wrong', rule or duty-based thinking**	***Axiological moral theory* focuses on 'virtue and vice', and prudential value-judgements**	***Teleological or utilitarian theory* focuses on whether goals and outcomes are 'good or bad', beneficial or detrimental**

Understanding of the relevance of this *causes →* *means → ends* structure of intentional acts to the logic of sound problem-solving has been common to many approaches to ethical decision-making in the past, and is employed both in this text and by other modern authors (ICAA 1997, Grace & Cohen 1998, Appendix 1, Seedhouse 2001, Pt 3 Moral Reasoning).

MORAL PROBLEMS AND MORAL DILEMMAS

Given this background of different usage of ethical terms, what do we mean by 'moral problems' and 'moral dilemmas'? Both terms confront us with choices that involve our beliefs and feelings about what we fundamentally regard as good, virtuous or right – our moral values, standards of conduct, or moral principles. We must distinguish between moral problems and moral dilemmas because there is a tendency in popular discussion in the media, and the

nursing press, to refer indiscriminately to all difficult situations requiring moral decisions as 'dilemmas'. There is also a risk that people, confronted with a situation which they see as a 'dilemma', will avoid taking responsibility for making hard decisions – either regarding the 'dilemma' as insoluble, or simply a matter of personal opinion or preference. We argue that if the issue can be reframed as a 'problem' there may be things that can be done, provided someone is prepared to take responsibility to find a practical solution that meets the needs of the situation. (Box 2.5 gives definitions of 'problem', 'dilemma' and 'quandary'.)

In everyday life we often deal with *problems* which require us to make moral decisions. These may involve completely new and unfamiliar situations, but more often we are dealing with day-to-day problems which tend to recur. Past experience of similar situations equips us to face specific problems with some

> Box 2.5 **Problems, dilemmas and quandaries**
>
> *Problem* (Greek: *problema* from *pro-ballo*, throw at or towards). A doubtful or difficult matter requiring solution, 'thrown up' by life or experience, something hard to understand or to deal with, an exercise, test or challenge set for us, but something soluble in principle, with appropriate effort.
>
> *Dilemma* (Greek: *di-lemma*, double argument with conflicting assumptions). A specific situation in which a choice has to be made between alternatives that are both undesirable, or, in ethics, a situation involving a real or apparently irresolvable clash of principles or duties, where there are no rules or precedents to follow.
>
> *Quandary* (origin unknown). A perplexed state, a state of practical uncertainty or puzzlement over alternative choices, sometimes loosely called a dilemma.

confidence because we have knowledge of how to deal with them, however painful or difficult they may be. Because 'problems', clearly defined and understood, usually have solutions, or possible solutions, they are not of the same kind as moral 'dilemmas', although we may also need courage to tackle them.

A *dilemma*, on the other hand, is a choice, of whatever kind, between two equally unsatisfactory alternatives. Not all dilemmas are moral dilemmas; some 'dilemmas' or 'quandaries' are the result of not knowing the best means, in theory or practice, to an agreed end. Nor are all moral choices moral dilemmas, since in many cases we may well know what we ought to do and the real question is whether or not we are willing fulfil our obligations. Classically a moral dilemma involves a conflict of duties. What makes the choice a *moral* dilemma is the fact that it involves conflict between competing moral principles or values, which are both applicable to the situation – what we believe we ought to do, or what we believe to be fundamentally good or important. We feel, in other words, that certain moral values or principles would make us adopt the one alternative, whereas consideration of other factors would make us adopt the other alternative; but the point about a dilemma is that we cannot adopt both. Choosing the one alternative means not only not choosing the other, but actually going against what the value or principle it represents would require us to do in the circumstances.

If situations demanding a decision present as 'dilemmas', we may be able to reframe these as *problems* and then apply suitable *problem-solving strategies* to them. Regularly applying problem-solving strategies to moral problems may then enable us to

develop standardised approaches to ones that recur. In practice this facilitates decision-making, and training, because there are rules and precedents that can be applied and routines and policies established to deal with recurring types of moral problems.

However, genuine moral dilemmas do arise, and while these are not nearly so common as the popular media would suggest, they do confront us with the need to adopt different strategies. To act responsibly, one would have to demonstrate that one had rehearsed the standard processes for dealing with recurrent problems, and that in doing so had failed to resolve the dilemma. Then one is faced with a number of choices. One might seek to abrogate responsibility for the decision by 'passing the buck' to someone else. One could do nothing in the hope the dilemma would go away, but action through inaction has its own consequences for which we would have to accept responsibility. Finally, one might have to accept the risk of being wrong, and then take what one believes to be the best course of action in the circumstances, being willing to accept personal responsibility for the outcome/s, whether good or bad.

Moral dilemmas arise from time to time in the lives of most people. Consider Case Study 2.1, for example.

These experiences present as moral dilemmas because a choice between conflicting moral values

case study 2.1

Some everyday dilemmas

A student has promised her classmates that she will write up their group project, which must be handed in to their tutor the next morning. Just after she has started to write, her closest friend telephones in great distress, demanding to see her right away because her fiancé has just broken off their engagement. A few days later the student is approached on a bitterly cold morning by a beggar who asks her for the price of a cup of tea. The student can easily afford to give him this, but the beggar clearly has alcohol on his breath and it is only 10 o'clock in the morning. Later in the day the student meets her married sister who is worried about her 14-year-old daughter. The daughter has asked if she can go to the next town tomorrow with a girlfriend to see a new film and come back on the late train. She says that the other girl's parents have agreed, but her mother is unable to contact them and is not sure that her daughter has told her the whole story.

or principles seems to be involved in each case. The first experience involves, on the one hand, the moral principle that we should keep our promises: on this side of the dilemma there is also the moral value of being a good or dutiful student. On the other side there is the moral value of being a good friend; there is also the moral principle that we should help others in need. The conflict here is not between different things the student *wants* to do (her best friend or the group project may each in their own way be tiresome and the alternative a welcome excuse) but between different things which she feels she *ought* to do.

Meeting the beggar, the student may want to give him the money – perhaps to get him out of the way, perhaps to make herself feel virtuous – but she may also feel that she ought not to, because it would not be in his interest to continue drinking himself to death. On the other hand, she may not want to give him the money in the first place – perhaps because she is afraid the beggar may recognise her and pester her again. She may also feel that she ought to give it, because as another adult the beggar has a right to decide what is best for himself – and because one ought to help others in need.

The sister's dilemma, too, involves the right of other people to decide what is best for themselves, but in this case it is complicated because the other person is a child. If teenagers are to become responsible adults, parents have to learn to trust them to be responsible, even if this means letting them make their own mistakes. On the other hand, some mistakes can have serious consequences, and parents also have a responsibility to protect their children. If the mother values responsibility, that value will exert considerable moral force on both sides of her dilemma.

The above examples all seem to be genuine irresolvable moral dilemmas. But certain facts may emerge that could question this. The student might have failed to read a notice from the tutor postponing the project deadline for a week. The beggar might have been at a crucial stage in voluntary psychiatric treatment for alcoholism. The other girl's parents might have agreed to her going to the cinema on the condition that one set of parents collected the two girls by car. In each case this vital information, if it had come to light, might well have resolved – or dissolved – the respective dilemmas. In the case of the project this would be for obvious reasons. In the case of the beggar, the student might be able to argue that because his psychiatric treatment was voluntary her refusal of money was supporting his own prior decision about what was best for himself. As far as the girls were concerned, the information might allow the mother to negotiate an agreed compromise with her daughter

about the degree of responsibility appropriate to the circumstances.

Possibilities of this kind illustrate the importance of good communication and adequate information about the circumstances, when facing moral quandaries in everyday life. Quite often, what appears to be a moral dilemma is the result of a breakdown in communication, or the absence of relevant communication between different people. This is certainly true of some areas of interprofessional and professional–patient communication, where the absence of clear procedures may give rise to 'dilemmas' that have more to do with poor professional practice than ethics in the narrower sense. If a nurse does not know what a doctor has told a dying patient, she may be left in a quandary about what to say if the patient asks her directly what is happening to them. When the bed of a patient awaiting discharge is urgently needed for another patient, and the nursing staff fail to discover, for example, that a relative has just arrived at home to look after the first patient, the misconception that this patient has nowhere to go could create an avoidable moral dilemma about priorities. So when the same kind of difficult moral choices recur, rather than agonising over each 'dilemma', it may be worth asking whether institutional or personal networks of communication cannot be improved in some appropriate way, either by some organisational means or by those involved cultivating a greater degree of tact or ingenuity.

Access to the 'bigger picture' that students acquire as they become more senior may reduce some apparent 'dilemmas' but increase others, as the more knowledge and experience they have, the more they may become aware of the complexity of ethical decision-making. It has been well said by a student that 'education and training in ethics is as much as anything about learning to tolerate complexity and not think there is a simple solution to every moral problem'.

MAKING ETHICAL DECISIONS WE CAN JUSTIFY

Improvements in communication clearly have a part to play in avoiding certain unnecessary moral dilemmas. On the other hand, there may be a temptation, particularly among practically minded people, to overestimate what can be achieved in this way. The student's difficulty, we might say, could have been avoided either if the college had had a better system of informing students, or if the student herself had cultivated the habit of checking notice boards more carefully. Her sister's problem, too, might have been avoided had she worked harder, over a longer period of time, at communicating with her daughter. Even the moral quandary involving the beggar might have been avoided if the student, on meeting him, had talked to him and elicited the vital information. A way round the apparent moral dilemma can be found in each of these situations, just as, often enough, it can be found in everyday life. On the other hand, there are many situations in everyday life when no such way exists; and even when it does, difficult moral choices and moral conflicts may remain.

To illustrate this fact, consider the examples again. Meeting the beggar, the student might have started to talk with him and he might just possibly have given her the vital information. But in thus delaying any decision about whether to give him the money until she had more information, the student was already acting in a way which – at that time, with the information she had – went against what on one side of her 'dilemma' she felt she ought to do; on the other side it went against another adult's right to decide what was best for him. Her decision to seek more information in this case was not a neutral matter: she had come down on one side of the dilemma and made a moral choice.

Prior moral choice might equally have been involved in any means by which the other two apparent dilemmas could have been avoided. A better system of informing students might have been possible for the college only at the cost of choosing not to spend its limited resources on, say, library facilities or student amenities. Again, in cultivating the habit of checking notice boards more regularly the student might have been opting for a general style of living which gave greater priority to the demands of work than to the demands of friendship. Here, too, moral choices would have been involved, as they would have been in the sister's decision to spend more time with her daughter – which might well have been at the expense of time spent on her own work or with her husband.

Even when ways exist of avoiding painful conflicts between moral principles, then, this does not mean that moral choices are not being made. Such choices may have been made over a long period of time, as the characters of individuals, relationships or institutions were being formed. But the succession of small choices made every day by everyone, or collectively, is no less significant than the large choice with which an acute moral dilemma confronts us. In this sense, every purposeful moral choice we make, in principle at least, is the result of some earlier moral choice we have made as individuals or as part of present or past society.

What all this suggests is that moral problems and even dilemmas, which we may reasonably wish to avoid in everyday life, can nevertheless play a useful part in our understanding of the moral dimension of our experience. The point about moral dilemmas, in particular, because they appear to confront us with irresolvable conflicts of duties, is that they demonstrate, more dramatically than anything else the complexity of moral experience, and the inescapability of moral choice in life.

A moral dilemma brings into sharper focus the moral values and principles which matter to us even when they conflict with one another – because of our previous moral choices. Many of these will have been everyday choices and relatively unconsidered but which, cumulatively, have gone to make up what we may call our moral character. Confronted by a genuine moral dilemma, the fact that we recognise it as such challenges us also to recognise the strength of our conflicting values, and in making – or not making – a moral choice, to adopt, change or reinforce the nature of our moral character. In studying moral issues, then, while it is reasonable enough to look – as we would in everyday life – for ways round or out of the dilemma, it is also useful to consider the dilemma on the assumption that there are no such ways, and to ask, if that is the case, which option we would choose and how we would defend our choice in the light of the values involved. When we have begun to do that, we have begun in practical terms to explore the nature of ethics.

Most people in the course of their lives learn to make ethical decisions, mainly by imitating others, or by a process of trial and error rather than by learning systematic ways of doing so. As a result, people tend to believe it is 'all a matter of common sense' or 'intuition'. Alternatively people say that when making moral decisions they go by 'gut feelings' or are guided by 'the voice of conscience'. Is this satisfactory? Without wanting to belittle these claims of people about how they take decisions, one can hardly say that they are convincing explanations, nor do they comprise adequate justifications for their actions. They are not the kind of explanations that would stand up in court, for instance, as explanations of why someone did something that caused harm to another person (e.g. 'I shot the man because I had a gut feeling that he would attack me', or 'My conscience told me to inform my boss of his secretary's dishonesty, despite having heard this second-hand') (Thompson & Harries 1997).

To treat every moral quandary as a 'dilemma' that necessarily leads to endless disputes and disagreement, or to treat all moral judgements as subjective, arbitrary or capricious, is a 'cop out'. It is a refusal to take responsibility for making sound ethical decisions. Such talk leads all too easily to cynicism about ethics, or to scepticism about finding any rational basis for our moral choices. If every moral quandary is a dilemma, in the sense that it involves an irresolvable conflict of duties, then the study of ethics would be pointless. If it is possible, as we said earlier, to reframe an apparent dilemma as a problem, then we can begin to think of applying problem-solving methods to it, and may possibly find a 'solution' to the difficulty confronting us (Thompson & Harries).

Ethical decision-making is not some kind of occult process, but is just one kind of problem-solving process among many others. There is no mystery about applying common-sense methods of problem-solving to *ethical* problems. Traditionally, nurses have not given the same time and effort to learning skills in ethical decision-making that they do to learning the application of problem-solving methods to the technical aspects of their professional work. It is for this reason that the Nursing and Midwifery Council (NMC) identified awareness of ethics and responsiveness to moral issues as one of the competencies which students *must* achieve. This is now clearly explicit in all approved nursing curricula in the UK, and nurses expect to be assessed during the programme in a variety of ways. In addition to theoretical assignment(s) there are practice assessments during their placements with a focus on ethical competence. Students are required to prepare a portfolio in which they focus on an ethical/moral issue that they identify in their practice placement and then must discuss the various possible ways in which this might be addressed.

Problem-solving demands careful appraisal of all relevant evidence. It involves reflection on alternative courses of action and their possible outcomes, and what kinds of reasons can be given in justification for a course of action chosen. A problem-solving methodology also builds the 'feedback loop' into the learning process. The value of using systematic and standard methods of decision-making is that it helps us deal with immediate problems. However, it also equips us to deal more effectively with future problems because we can repeat the process, learning from the results of past decisions and actions. This knowledge enables us to some extent to predict what will happen in future situations of the same kind, and helps to guide our future actions. Carol Gilligan, in her classic book *In a Different Voice: Psychological Theory and Women's Development* (Gilligan 1977, 1993), sums up the findings of her research by an analysis of the different kinds of narrative in which women and men explain or justify their moral judgements. Briefly

stated she claims that men tend to adopt a justice perspective and women a greater emphasis on care for others, that women are less inclined than men to adopt purely formal and rational models of problem-solving, and that women tend to take greater account than men do of the emotional impact of ethical decisions on personal relationships and interpersonal trust.

Gilligan did not focus her research solely on women. One study was of college students of both sexes and this indicated that, although there were substantive differences between men and women, both sexes moved from adherence to moral absolutes over a period of 5 years (between initial and last interview) to an increasing awareness of the complexity of ethical situations. The upshot is that in making ethical decisions we must take account of a variety of perspectives on 'the truth' that render moral judgements contextually relative and demand practical wisdom in reaching sound conclusions. In this context we cannot afford to overlook those different dimensions of ethical decision-making that she maintains are important to women and men. However, whether or not we agree with Gilligan that men and women tackle ethical decision-making in different ways, both men and women can benefit from adopting a systematic approach to the process of ethical decision-making, based on the requirements set out below.

In many different types of situations in life people learn to apply systematic ways of dealing with problems. For example, part of our fascination with detective thrillers, lies in being drawn into the problem-solving process and methods of the detective hero. Conan Doyle has his famous detective hero, Sherlock Holmes, reflect with Dr Watson on the logic of 'deducing' the right conclusions from the evidence. Whether detective, lawyer, scientist, doctor, counsellor, nurse, accountant or public servant, we tend to follow the same steps in problem-solving, viz:

- collect and assess the evidence and define the problem
- consider what principles and values apply to the case
- review the options and choices available in the situation
- devise an action plan, with clear objectives
- act effectively to implement the plan and observe and monitor the process
- analyse the results, and feed back what you learn into the next problem you face.

What this process does is to get away from simplistic binary, 'right or wrong' answers to every situation. Even in those areas where rules, regulations or laws apply, most of the time and effort involved in dealing with moral problems or dilemmas has to do with the appraisal of evidence for and against a case, not automatic application of a rule. In fact the first issue to be decided in a public trial in court is whether, in the light of the evidence led by the prosecution and defence, the case actually falls under the rule or not. Once that issue is settled the court can proceed to engage in a process of deliberation that takes account of a number of factors: the appropriateness of the indictment (or charges made against the accused), the evidence led by the prosecution and defence, the relevant principles (or laws) that apply, issues of the competence of the accused to face trial, questions relating to motive, intention and means employed, and finally a review of the actual consequences or outcomes. Before passing judgement, lawyers on both sides will be allowed to offer evidence based on the past record of the accused, or pleas in mitigation of sentence.

In approaching ethical decision-making, especially in relation to weighty matters, we could do worse than follow the example of courts in systematically reviewing the kinds of factors described above. Both the criminal and civil courts exist to assist us to resolve matters of conflict, or compensation for injury, loss or damage to property. We have recourse to the courts when the ordinary processes for conflict resolution in families and society break down. Ethics is concerned not only with the promotion of human well-being or flourishing, but also with the resolution of conflict that can harm us. Applying systematic processes to ethical judgement in community settings can be a powerful way of resolving differences, clarifying different perspectives on situations, and building trust and cooperation in society, but this requires wisdom and skill based on routine practice.

✳ FUNDAMENTAL ETHICAL PRINCIPLES

If ethics is to have any credibility it must be based not only on our shared and changing values, (as discussed in Chapter 1), but on principles that are universally acknowledged and respected. Here, as we have already indicated, we seem to be up against an immediate difficulty. The popular view of ethics is that everyone has different ethical principles. Everything is relative and no agreement is possible in ethics. Is this really true, or is this just a 'cop out'?

In a liberal society tolerance of religious, moral and cultural diversity is encouraged. Living in 'multicultural societies' we are taught that

- everyone is entitled to their own opinions about matters of ethics and politics

- people should not be prevented from expressing these views, and
- people should not be discriminated against because of the views they hold.

Now, this seems to imply that all points of view have equal validity, or that all moral points of view are relative. If all moral beliefs are just that (points of view), then it would not seem to be possible to talk of moral truth or of universal moral principles.

However, arguing that we *ought* to allow everyone the right to express their views on ethical and political matters is based on an unstated ethical principle, namely, that of *respect for persons and their rights.*

Emphasis on freedom of conscience and expression for individuals and respect for others' personal rights gained prominence in the struggles for religious and political freedom in Europe, following the Protestant Reformation and in the 18th century Enlightenment. Great philosophers of this period who championed individual rights were: John Locke, Jean Jacques Rousseau, Immanuel Kant and John Stuart Mill. Kant, in particular, built his whole system of ethics on the principle of respect for persons as fundamental to the ethics of any moral community.

This principle informs the whole of the ICN Code for Nurses (ICN 2000) (and many others) and is specifically expressed in the preamble namely:

> Inherent in nursing is respect for life, dignity and the rights of man.

To argue that we *ought not* to discriminate against people with moral, political or religious views different from our own beliefs is based on appeal to the *principle of justice* (Rawls 1971). Again, this principle of justice, or universal fairness and non-discrimination, is manifested in the statement in the ICN Code:

> [Nursing] is unrestricted by considerations of nationality, race, creed, colour, age, sex, politics or social status.

Other elements in the Code which arise out of the demands of justice are such obligations as the requirement that nurses accept responsibility to maintain their level of competence, that they share with other citizens the responsibility to 'initiate and support action to meet the health and social needs of the public', and play 'a major role in determining and implementing desirable standards of nursing practice and nursing education', and participate 'in establishing and maintaining equitable social and economic working conditions in nursing'.

Historically, the liberal tradition has used relativist arguments both to attack religious and political bigotry on the one hand, and to defend civil liberties like freedom of speech and association on the other hand. However, underlying the liberal defence of personal rights and freedoms is an appeal to the more fundamental and universal principles of justice and respect for persons.

Linked to these arguments are similar arguments about our duty to defend the rights of those who are too young or too weak to defend their own interests, including ethnic and religious minorities. Here appeal is being made to the underlying *principle of beneficence* or the protective duty of care the strong owe to the weak. The basis for this moral demand for reciprocity in mutual care and protection is the need to recognise that we are all weak and vulnerable at different times of our lives, and need others to care and advocate for us, classically expressed in the *Golden Rule*: 'Treat other people as you would like them to treat you', 'Do as you would be done by', etc. This so-called 'Golden Rule' occurs in one form or another in the ethical traditions of many ancient cultures, e.g. the ancient Babylonian Code of Hammurabi, in the *Analects* of Confucius, the Bible (Matthew 7: 12), and is the basis of Kant's principle of reciprocity in his *Groundwork to the Metaphysic of Morals*. For wider discussion of the principle and defence of its importance in healthcare, see Beauchamp & Childress (2004) and Veatch (1981).

Nurses usually encounter people when they are sick, at their most vulnerable, injured or mentally ill, and when they, as nurses, are in an inherently more powerful position – based on their supposed knowledge, expertise and professional skills. Thus, nurses are said, in both law and ethics, to have a *fiduciary responsibility* not only to care for and to advise patients, but also to act on behalf of and advocate for those who are less well-informed or actually incompetent. The nurse has a fundamental duty of care to protect the interests of patients, and not to take advantage of their naivety, ignorance or vulnerability.

The *principle of beneficence* – to do good – and the corresponding negative form of the same principle, *non-maleficence* – not to do harm – are fundamental to all moral communities. Parents have a basic duty of care, of protective beneficence towards their children (as also to elderly and dependent relatives). Teachers exercise a legal duty of care *in loco parentis* (in place of the parent) towards the children in their care. Doctors and nurses, social workers and counsellors and all members of the caring or consulting professions (including lawyers and accountants) have to exercise a similar duty of care or protective beneficence towards their clients. This is in virtue of the *relationship of trust* or fiduciary responsibility in which they stand relative to their patients or clients.

The fact that the principle of reciprocity, or 'Golden Rule', crops up in virtually every known system of community morality is because it is universally true that while we are strong today we may be vulnerable tomorrow, we may be nurses today and patients tomorrow. As such, the requirement that we should do good and not harm to one another, the principle of protective beneficence and/or non-maleficence, is the necessary foundation for membership of any moral community. Without this principle no society could survive or function very well.

FUNDAMENTAL ETHICAL PRINCIPLES IN THE CONTEXT OF HEALTHCARE

The principle of respect for persons

In the context of healthcare, respect for persons basically means treating patients as persons with rights. It means further respecting the autonomy of individuals and protecting those who suffer loss of autonomy through illness, injury or mental disorder, and working to restore autonomy to those who have lost it. It means recognising that patients have such basic human rights as: the right to know, the right to privacy and the right to receive care and treatment. Clearly, there may be a tension between the patient's rights and the helper's duty to care, just as there may be practical difficulties in determining adequately informed and voluntary consent to treatment; or in setting sensible limits to confidentiality, or physical privacy, in institutions where care may be shared by a team of nurses, paramedics, social workers and doctors; and distinguishing between 'care' and 'treatment' (or the choice of therapies). Paul Ramsey, in his classic book *The Patient as Person*, pointed out that for the carers, respect for persons in their care means working to maintain the optimum degree of independence for the patient, and sharing knowledge, care and skills in such a way as to empower the patient and avoid creating and perpetuating dependency (Ramsey 1970). Following in this tradition, the British Royal College of Nursing stressed in its first draft Code of Ethics (RCN 1979) – the lineal ancestor of the NMC 2004 Code – that the primary duty of the nurse is to work to restore the optimum degree of autonomy to the patient that is compatible with what they have lost as a result of disease, injury or me͏· ͏ ·͏ ͏rder.

The principle of justice

Justice, or the demand for universal
a relationship of tension with respe

individual persons. The exercise of our individual rights (such as freedom of movement or association) may have to be curtailed in times of crisis, in the interests of the common good – for the sake of public order in war or emergencies, or where public health measures have to be introduced to control epidemics. Action is taken here in the interests of distributive (not retributive) justice, but the restriction of their individual liberties may be perceived to be punitive by infected individuals – e.g. the way people with AIDS have been segregated or incarcerated in some societies is reminiscent of past treatment of lepers or the mentally ill. When we consider the social controls imposed on mentally disordered people and the loss of rights of people in institutional care generally, or the policing role which nurses and other healthcare workers may have to perform, the analogy with retributive justice seems close (as the sociological analysis of sickness behaviour as a kind of deviance illustrates) (Freidson 1970, 1994). However justified public health measures may be, we must not lose sight of the rights of individuals. Justice to individuals also means non-discrimination on the basis of sex, race, religion (or because of youth, old age, having a contagious disease, mental handicap or mental illness). It means equal opportunity to benefit from, or have access to, preventive medicine and treatment services and to the benefits of medical research.

Justice also means equality of outcomes for groups. This raises questions of the broader 'political' duty of health professionals to contribute through research to informed debate on justice in healthcare, and to contribute to fairer distribution of and access to health resources, by sound social and economic research and policy development. The well-documented evidence by health researchers of inequalities in health status of people in Britain during the so-called Thatcher 'boom years' (Townsend & Davidson 1982) and the growing health divide between rich and poor (Whitehead 1987) showed that to ensure justice in healthcare, political action was required to get the state to shift greater resources to deprived areas, even at the expense of more privileged sectors. Campaigning for resources to improve services or to defend standards of care are both demanded of health professionals committed to the principles of justice and equity. This has been the theme of major international reports in the past, e.g. the WHO Report: *The Health Burden of Social Inequalities* (Illsley & Svensson 1984), and the *World Development Report – Investing in Health* (World Bank 1993).

More recent research has been focused on trying understand what factors related to poverty are

particularly linked with poor health. Kendall (1998) and Graham (2000) have observed that health inequalities can be exaggerated if we fail to take account of changes in demographic and socio-economic change; e.g. between 1931 and 1981, social class V shrank by 55% while social class I grew by 217%. These and other researchers have emphasised that there is no simple relationship or equation between poverty and ill-health. They have emphasised the multifactorial nature of the causal factors linking health and social deprivation. For example, Graham (1993) focused on the predicament of women affected by poverty and unemployment, while Donkin et al (2002) and Chandola et al (2003) established that social selection plays a role in producing health inequalities, and studies by James et al (1997) and MAFF (1998) have looked at the association of lifestyle, and how factors such as smoking, excessive drinking and obesity contribute to ill-health among those of lower income. Perhaps not surprisingly, Benzeval et al (2001) established that lack of income appeared to have a greater impact on inequalities in health than did either occupation or educational attainment.

The principle of beneficence

Beneficence has had a bad press recently. Attacks on paternalism in medicine and nursing, lay resentment of the medicalisation of life, the emphasis on patients' rights by militant pressure groups, as well as action by politicians concerned with social justice and the political economy of healthcare, have resulted in health professionals becoming defensive about beneficence. Certainly, beneficence, or the duty of care, may be exercised in a way that 'infantilises' people and creates dependence, but it need not do so. In fact, it has been argued that patient advocacy, defending the rights of the vulnerable patient, or acting on behalf of those unable to assert their rights, is a requirement of beneficence. Beneficence is indispensable wherever there are dependent, severely disabled or helpless people in need of support or urgent care and attention. The reciprocity in our duty to care for one another should make us realise that we all need others to speak for us, to do things for us, or to defend our rights, when we are too weak to do so for ourselves. But if knowledge is power, true carers will aim to share their knowledge and skills with vulnerable individuals so as to empower them to reassert control over their own lives, if this is humanly possible (May 1983, Campbell 1984a, Chs 2 and 3).

Constitutive and regulative ethical principles discussed above are summarised in Box 2.6.

Box 2.6 Fundamental ethical principles

The principle of respect for persons

- The duty to respect the rights, autonomy and dignity of other people.
- The duty to promote their well-being and autonomy.
- The duty of truthfulness, honesty and sincerity (honour = respect), for deceit dishonours a person.

(The concept of a 'person' (as a bearer of rights and duties), and the principle of autonomy (that one should be free to determine one's own choices) are here both constitutive principles essential to legal, ethical and political discourse.)

The principle of justice

- The duty of universal fairness (equal opportunity for individuals) and equity (equality of outcomes for groups).
- The duty to treat people as ends in themselves, never simply as means to an end (i.e. not to exploit them).
- The duty to avoid discrimination or abuse of people on grounds of race, age, sex, class, gender or religion.

(The principle of justice requires of us that any personal rule of action we use, should, in principle, be capable of being universalised for all people. For this reason it is sometimes described as the constitutive principle of universalisability.)

The principle of beneficence (or non-maleficence)

- The duty to do good and to avoid doing harm to others.
- The duty of care, to protect the weak and vulnerable.
- The duty of advocacy, defending the rights of those incompetent or temporarily unable to defend their own.

(Like the Golden Rule (do unto others as you would have them do unto you), this principle is sometimes referred to as the constitutive principle of reciprocity, and is a necessary condition for any moral community to survive or function.)

CONFRONTING THREE TYPES OF MORAL RELATIVISM

The claim we make here is that all moral communities share at least these three fundamental ethical principles, as the basis for coexistence and cooperation. This runs counter to the popular relativist argument that 'everyone has different values' and 'ethics is a personal matter and just a matter of taste'. The view that all ethical values and judgements are relative to the individual, or to the societies within which they operate, is so widely held that it deserves further comment (Thompson 1987b, Beauchamp & Childress 2004).

First of all, it must be said that the opposite to moral relativism is not moral absolutism, or fanatical fundamentalism – of either the religious or moral variety. The movements associated with the self-styled 'moral majority' often but thinly mask new types of moral bigotry of the right, while arguments about what is or is not 'morally or politically correct' are often driven by ideologues of the left.

Against these forms of authoritarian thinking, ethical relativism and sceptical realism is a refreshing antidote. In the past, and in opposition to European cultural imperialism of the past, social scientists, historians and psychologists have rejoiced to point out the variations between the beliefs and values which form the foundations of different societies, and the lifestyles of individuals. There are indeed interesting and often profound differences in the way various cultures (e.g. Anglo-Saxon, Asian, American or African) articulate themselves as moral communities, and how they come up with different social customs and conventions for behaviour in various circumstances. 'Ethical relativism' in one sense can be a safeguard against ethnic chauvinism, religious intolerance and cultural arrogance. However, maintaining that certain ethical principles are universal, and applicable to all moral communities on this planet, is not incompatible with a sincere recognition of this cultural diversity or the individual differences in moral beliefs and values which exist.

It is of the nature of principles that they are just that, namely, starting points, from which we have to derive duties and rights and specific moral rules. It is part of the interest of comparative ethics that we can study the incredible variety of forms and practices in which different human societies have expressed their intuitions of beneficence, justice and respect for persons.

However, ethical relativism can lead to ethical scepticism and cynicism about the possibility of moral agreement, and the applicability of universal rights or moral duties. For this reason, we need to address three types of ethical relativism:

Interpersonal relativism emphasises that different people (even within the same family) may base their lives on different values and belief systems. Does this disprove the universal nature of moral principles? Of course not. A brother and sister may be brought up in the same family traditions and one become a priest and another an atheist Marxist, but this does not mean that they abandon faith in universal ethical principles. Instead, what happens is that each of the positions they adopt results in different emphasis or priority being given to justice or beneficence, or respect for persons as human values, or for their primary life goals in different belief systems. Like navigation instruments, principles help us orient ourselves. They do not provide us with a map, nor dictate a particular course to us. We have to choose our own destinations and routes for getting there. The articulation and adoption of our own moral beliefs, values and ethical rules is necessary to enable us to chart a personal course through life, and to achieve our life goals.

Cultural relativism is a healthy alternative to dogmatic fundamentalism, smug parochialism, gender-based sexism or chauvinistic nationalism. As we have seen earlier, the basis for the moral demand that we show tolerance and respect for cultural differences involves an implicit appeal to underlying universal moral principles. These principles each express different modalities of power and power relations that are common to our relations with people in any and every kind of society. For these fundamental ethical principles deal with the different ways that power can be expressed or shared in relations between people. For example, the basis of the *principle of justice* is *equitable power-sharing* between people. *Beneficence* has to do with the *responsibility of the powerful to protect the weak* and vulnerable. *Respect for persons* expresses our duty, as members of a moral community, to *empower others to achieve their full potential*, to claim and exercise their rights.

Philosophical relativism is the argument that there cannot be agreement between people who hold different moral theories such as a utilitarian or duty-based theory, or one that emphasises personal virtue or integrity. We pointed out earlier that there are some significant differences between thinking about ethics in terms of right and wrong – of principles and rules, rights and duties, and thinking about ethics in terms of good and bad – where we are more concerned with values and goals, costs and benefits. While some philosophers ('deontologists') have attempted to develop a complete account of ethics in terms of the former, other philosophers ('teleologists') have been exclusively concerned with the latter. Recently some philosophers have reaffirmed 'virtue ethics' as a third type of ethical theory which focuses on the moral agent as having to mediate in reality between principles and outcomes. These three types of moral theory are briefly defined in Box 2.7.

Box 2.7 Three main types of ethical theory

Deontological ethics (duty-based ethics)
The *deontologist* (from the Greek *deon* = duty) argues that what makes actions right or wrong is their consistency with unconditional moral principles, or rules, and that these alone are the necessary foundation for a responsible ethics. The deontologist develops a system in which our moral duties and rights are clearly defined by rules. Sometimes referred to as 'principle-ism', deontology emphasises the priority of principles and rules, rights and duties.

Teleological ethics (consequentialism or utilitarianism)
The *teleologist* (from the Greek *telos* = goal or purpose) stresses that what makes an action good or bad (rather than right or wrong) is not the principle someone professes but the actual consequences, benefits or costs of their action. Teleologists are hence often called 'consequentialists' or 'utilitarians', as they consider what is morally important is the usefulness of the consequences in achieving good results.

Axiological ethics (prudential or virtue ethics)
However, *axiology or virtue ethics* is another tradition which has ancient roots and has recently gained more attention, namely, the tradition which attaches crucial importance to the integrity and competence of the moral agent who has to decide how to act in a specific situation in the light of principles to achieve good ends. 'Virtue ethics', or 'prudential ethics' focuses on the crucial role of competence and integrity in the agent making value judgements.

We have argued that moral relativism in its inter-personal, cultural and philosophical forms can play an important role in challenging moral dogmatism and uncritical moral prejudices, and as such needs to be taken seriously. Awareness of the diversity of moral viewpoints and people's personal perspectives on morality may help to make us more understanding and tolerant of the way other people act and of the things they say. Sensitivity to ethnic, religious and cultural differences, and the moral relativities involved with different customs and practices, may help us to avoid misunderstanding of other people's ways of life, and racial prejudice. Awareness of the fact that philosophers may use different theoretical justifications for the type of ethics they adopt may help us to understand the different emphases in their ethical systems, and that different kinds of meta-ethical defence of ethics are possible but serve different functions.

As we shall see in the final chapter, these different moral theories do not necessarily contradict one another, unless they are interpreted absolutely, that is, when viewed as the only possible way of determining whether or not our actions are ethical.

In Chapter 13 we argue that an adequate account of any moral judgement must take account of prior conditions and basic moral principles, choose the best means and methods to achieve our goal, and assess the likely consequences, costs and benefits of our action. 'Deontological' moral theories tend to emphasise prior conditions and principles as of paramount importance. 'Pragmatism' emphasises the efficacy of the method used and 'virtue' ethics emphasises virtue as an essential means to achieve a moral outcome. 'Teleological', 'consequentialist' and/or 'utilitarian' theories focus attention on ends or goals and out-comes. In reality we need to take account of all three aspects to give an adequate account of moral acts.

We will argue that they each emphasise complementary aspects of human acts and relate to different aspects of our moral experience. If we wish to give a complete or comprehensive account of moral action, then we must pay attention to each of these different dimensions of moral action. These ethical theories each seek to justify our moral beliefs and ethical policies by reference either to principles, or to means or consequences. In this book we argue that ethics can be defended as the rational study or 'science' of morals and that each type of moral theory has its own value within a broader theory of the nature of moral action – that the classical ethical theories are complementary and not neces-sarily mutually exclusive or incompatible with one another.

 ## further reading

The meaning and scope of ethics

Frankena W K 1973 Ethics, 2nd edn. Prentice-Hall, Englewood Cliffs, NJ

Macintyre A 1993 A short history of ethics. Routledge Paperback, London

The nature of ethical decision-making

Holm S 1997 Ethical problems in clinical practice: the ethical reasoning of healthcare professionals. Manchester University Press, Manchester

Josephson Institute of Ethics 2005 Making ethical decisions. Josephson Institute of Ethics, Los Angeles, CA. Online. Available: www.josephsoninstitute.org

Fundamental principles and ethical relativism

Beauchamp T L, Childress J F 2004 Principles of biomedical ethics, 5th rev edn. OUP, London

Holloway R 1999 Godless morality: keeping religion out of ethics. Canongate, Edinburgh

PART 2

Socialisation, professionalisation and nursing values

Becoming a nurse and member of the profession

3

Chapter contents

AIMS

This chapter has the following aims:

1. To describe some of the sociological perspectives that are relevant to healthcare
2. To explore the effect of the media on public perceptions of health and healthcare
3. To discuss the processes by means of which nurses are socialised into their professional roles.

LEARNING OUTCOMES

When you have read and worked through this chapter, you should be able to:

- Reflect upon your own socialisation into nursing
- Examine your current nursing practice in the light of sociological theory
- Discuss the role of the media in forming perceptions of health and healthcare
- Explore the impact on patient care of the issues addressed in the chapter.

SOCIOLOGICAL PERSPECTIVES ON NURSING AND ETHICS

In this chapter we shall discuss some aspects of what it means to 'become' a nurse and consider both the practical and ethical aspects of this process. The focus will be on undergraduate students. In Chapter 5 we will focus on registered practitioners. A sociological approach is adopted throughout in order to set the individual nurse who makes moral decisions within the social and organisational context that shapes and influences these decisions. As ethics is not merely an individual matter, but concerns our participation in a variety of social contexts or moral communities, sociology can help to throw light on ethical issues and decision-making in nursing practice. The sociological outlook, which sees the world in terms of roles, processes of socialisation, social organisation and social structure, contributes to understanding the perspective of others and the social factors that may facilitate, or constrain, their actions.

There are many sociological traditions. One line of theory has focused on the structures (e.g. social, economic, political and organisational) within which individuals live, and the extent to which these structures facilitate or constrain the actions of those individuals. Other theories take a more individualistic approach, placing emphasis on the individual and their capacity to be active and autonomous agents within their environment. More recently, however, sociology has focused to a greater extent on a synthesis of different approaches, i.e. those that acknowledge the influence of structures on an individual's capacity to act, but at the same time accord importance to the ability of individual 'agency' to influence structures and even to modify or overthrow these structures.

In order for individuals to influence the structures within which they operate they need to be able to reflect upon these structures, and upon their own role and the roles of others in relation to these structures. The emphasis upon reflective practice in nursing in recent years (e.g. Ghaye & Lillyman 2000, Johns 2000, Rolfe, Freshwater & Jasper 2001, Bulman & Schutz 2004) links with the concept of reflexivity, whereby an individual identifies, reflects upon, and challenges the prior assumptions held by themselves and others about the nature of the world and the structures within which they operate. Here both philosophy and sociology can be of help, as they are essentially reflective disciplines. Philosophy is concerned with critical examination of the patterns and structures of thought – e.g. in relation to theory of knowledge, ethics, aesthetics, metaphysics, logic and philosophy of science. Sociology, on the other hand, is concerned with the nature and structures of human societies and patterns and regularities of human social behaviour. In this book we attempt to combine both these reflective approaches to help illuminate the scope and nature of nursing ethics.

The nature of nursing requires nurses to have a knowledge of micro-social theories (e.g. those of Mead (1934) and Goffman (1969)) because these deal with the interactions that people have with one another on an individual level (interactionism), but nurses also need knowledge of macro-social perspectives that deal with the formation and maintenance of social structures, such as health services and regulatory bodies (structuralism). Giddens's (1984) theory of structuration proposes that neither interactionism nor structuralism is adequate by itself, and that a more comprehensive sociological explanation of human behaviour should combine elements of both. 'Structure' and 'agency', in Giddens's view, are two sides of one coin, but he does appear to place greater emphasis on individual agency than upon the social structures within which individuals operate. This means that he considers individuals to have the freedom to act autonomously even within relatively rigid social structures. Students and registered nurses, however, arrive in healthcare settings in which structures are

case study 3.1

Structure and agency

A student nurse, who is undertaking her first practice placement, feels unhappy about some aspects of the care provided for frail older people who have dementia. These people are not physically abused, but they are shouted at by some of the care assistants if they do not eat their food, or if they decline to have a bath or are incontinent.

Activities

Either on your own, or with someone else, identify the different factors that you think that the student would take into account in this situation.

Try to identify which factors are related to 'structures' and which factors relate to the individual 'agency' of the student.

Try to determine which factors you consider would be the most influential in the student's decision-making and provide the reasons for your answer.

already in place and these are likely to be resistant to change by any one practitioner or student!

For a practical example of the possible tensions that may exist between structure and agency, please read Case Study 3.1 and carry out the suggested activities.

Case Study 3.1 – discussion

New situations may create insecurity about one's own competency and one's ability to judge the practice of others. Students' own values may indicate that treating people with respect, and as individuals, with active acknowledgement of their preferences, is important. Students may also consider that people who are frail, vulnerable and dependent should be afforded protection from emotional as well as physical abuse. However, in this situation students may also feel some degree of doubt, due to their own inexperience, as to whether the practices that they witness are acceptable or unacceptable. The expectation would be that healthcare assistants provide a high quality of care. If the placement culture (i.e. the apparent attitudes and behaviours of the permanent members of staff) indicates that shouting at patients is in some circumstances acceptable, then students may consider that they are not in a position to contest this, due to their lack of experience. Students may also not wish to jeopardise their prospects of gaining good placement assessments by raising concerns and possibly making themselves unpopular. Further, having to work alongside people, the adequacy of whose care provision they have questioned, may be a daunting prospect. Finally, students may feel that the placement manager and/or the university staff will not believe them and/or be unsupportive of their claims.

It can be seen that, in situations that are unfamiliar, students may experience insecurity and doubt. The extent to which the structures within which they have to operate (practice placements and university) provide them with support may appear unclear. A student's individual ability to take action may be very limited.

Questions of power and authority, consensus and conflict are addressed by sociology, both at the personal and social (including structural) levels of nursing, and these issues are directly relevant to debates in nursing ethics. Here we examine the moral aspects of nursing, both from the standpoint of the individual nurse, and also in the actual context of nurses' relationships with colleagues and patients within health service structures. In doing so we aim to strike a balance between emphasis on corporate and individual responsibility. At an individual level, it might seem that nurses are motivated to a great extent by an ethic of caring. However, when we look at the way in which nursing care is organised and delivered in health services, it becomes clear that professional nursing has to be operated on principles which are less individualistic than the notion of personal care for individual patients. Because nurses exercise moral responsibility not only as individuals, but also as members of teams and as employees in hospitals and other institutions, this means that understanding of both nursing care and nursing ethics requires a sound knowledge of the social and behavioural sciences and concepts of justice and respect for people's rights.

NURSING: INFORMAL AND PROFESSIONAL

It is important to differentiate between two forms of caring that are well recognised within our society. The first is 'informal' care that is provided by lay people who are usually related to, or friends of, the individual who requires care. These carers have received no formal preparation for practice and are unlikely to receive financial recompense for providing care. We have all experienced, and probably have also provided, this form of care.

Healthcare may also be provided by 'formal' carers, i.e. those who have received some form of preparation for their practice and who receive financial remuneration for this. Formal care may be provided by healthcare assistants in the UK and/or by professional nurses, who undergo a selection process prior to acceptance as undergraduate students. Students subsequently receive a formalised preparation and training, the successful completion of which results in registration with a regulatory body (in the UK, this is the Nursing and Midwifery Council (NMC)). Registration is a prerequisite for subsequent qualified practice. The UK *Code of Professional Conduct* (NMC 2004) sets out the expectations which the NMC has of registered practitioners, and post-registration education and practice (PREP) requires all registered practitioners to provide evidence of having undergone updating education and practice at regular intervals, in order to remain on the register (NMC 2005b). The implications for registered nurses will be discussed in detail in Chapter 5.

Nursing students are not *professionally* accountable during their preparation for practice (NMC 2002a), but are nonetheless *responsible* for their actions and omissions. (Students' responsibility for their practice is discussed further in Chapter 5.) Professional accountability for practice lies with the registered practitioners with whom students work. Registered nurses (RNs) who supervise students' practice during their placements are usually referred to as mentors or preceptors. Mentors will have undergone some preparation for practice in relation to this role. The expectations of students of nursing within the UK are set out by the NMC (2002a). Whilst students do not have *professional* accountability they may be called to account for the consequences of their actions and omissions by their higher education establishment and/or by the law where a criminal offence is alleged to have been committed.

Students and registered nurses undertake their work not solely on the basis of duty, altruism or necessity, but on a contractual basis. Professional nurses look after patients in return for payment and students do so in order to gain the qualifications that are required for their subsequent practice as registered nurses. The differences between informal care and professional care are important both in relation to the public's perception of nursing care and also in relation to the different kinds of ethical responsibility that may arise in nurses' relationships with other members of the healthcare team, with patients and with the public.

Nursing work often requires nurses to take responsibility for difficult ethical decisions which may call into question the nurse's own personal convictions and values. However, it is important to remember that ethical decisions in nursing are not necessarily of the 'life and death' variety, as tends to be the case in the world of TV soap operas. The public's perception of nursing does involve some appreciation of the difficulties and conflicts faced by health professionals, based on discussion in newspapers and on television, and the internet. All these media have served to enhance public awareness of ethical issues in healthcare, but they can also distort people's perception of the frequency with which 'dilemmas' arise. While the media can contribute greatly to raising public awareness of health issues, it is also true that the greater the volume of health information available 'online', the greater the potential disadvantage for those to whom internet access is unavailable. Lack of access to these information resources may increase current health inequalities in society, or between developed and developing societies, as those who lack internet access may be those already disadvantaged by other socio-economic factors, or by disability.

THE ROLE OF THE MEDIA

The public's perception of health, healthcare and nursing is shaped by a variety of media. These media do not, however, always present a neutral perspective on these matters. Media proprietors, producers, directors and special interest groups do influence presentation in a number of ways and with a variety of motives. It is important to emphasise that all the media, irrespective of their specific purpose and format, have to compete for customers or subscribers and 'sell' their programmes to the public. To raise their circulations, or viewing figures, they have to present eye-catching images and unusual or sensational story-lines, accompanied by short and easily-assimilated explanatory accounts of the issues involved. The result is that in the presentation of scientific and medical material, for example, issues are often misleadingly over-simplified and alternatives presented in an adversarial manner, in order to make an impact.

In relation to the sociological concepts of 'agency' and 'structure', the media, despite their substantively disparate interests and foci, provide collectively an example of a social structure that exerts powerful influences over the ways in which human beings view themselves and others. The depiction by the media of healthcare is influential in forming the expectations of both healthcare providers and recipients.

Seale (2002) argues that health research has not fully acknowledged the role of the popular media in shaping people's views and experiences of illness and their expectations of the healthcare system. One exception to this lack of research has been in the evaluation of health education and health promotion campaigns in the UK. Naidoo & Wills (2000) found that, whilst health education may raise people's consciousness of issues at a relatively superficial level, it is less effective in addressing the complexities of individuals' enduring beliefs or the psychosocial factors that may affect their initiation into and maintenance of lifestyle changes. Indeed, one of the problems Naidoo & Wills (2000) identified is that lifestyle change is often assumed to be unproblematic, e.g. that if information is given by a 'credible' authority individuals will act on it, and that behavioural change is achievable by individual agency rather than requiring changes in social conditions or social structures. The study by Graham (1993) of the smoking habits of young single mothers found, not that they lacked information about the dangers of cigarette smoking, but that they used cigarettes as a means, often their only means, of coping with the stress and poverty with which they had to contend as single parents.

In more general terms Seale (2002) argues that policy-makers and professionals often assume that once information is established as factually 'correct' its transmission to, and internalisation by, the public will be unproblematic. Reports by the media of 'exciting new scientific discoveries' tend, however, to be over-simplified and presented under eye-catching headlines that frequently minimise or ignore any dubiety about the results of the research quoted. For example, 'research' which suggests that drinking alcohol may have health benefits receives intensive coverage of a frequently misleading nature. The media tend not to give the same prominence to reports of the individual and social pathology associated with alcohol misuse.

Coverage given in the media to health risks, or threats to human life and welfare, is frequently inversely related to the statistical likelihood of the threat in question. Much of the coverage, for example, of the alleged link between the mumps, measles and rubella (MMR) vaccine and autism has been misleading. Statistically the risk of death as a consequence of cigarette smoking, road usage or alcohol abuse is many times higher than death by most causes highlighted by the media.

By a similar process, aspects of life such as sadness or anxiety (previously regarded as integral to the human experience) may be medicalised by the media, so that their presence becomes equated with the possibility of cure. This then contributes to a demand for 'treatments', frequently in the form of prescription medication. Please read the short scenario in Case Study 3.2 and, either on your own or with others, consider the options open to the general practitioner (GP) in this situation.

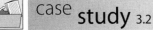

case study 3.2

Stress in the workplace

During a consultation with his GP, a young man speaks of his current unhappiness with his job, which he finds stressful. He explains that he feels anxious all the time and has difficulty in sleeping. This anxiety has had an adverse impact on his relationships with his partner and his friends. He asks the GP if he may have medication to reduce his symptoms.

Activities

- Identify the factors that you think that the GP would take into account in this situation.
- Which of these factors could be attributed to structures?
- Which of these factors could be attributed to the individual 'agency' of the patient or GP?
- What action do you think should be taken? Please provide the rationale for your answer.

Case Study 3.2 – discussion

General practitioners may come under pressure, from patients and because of the limited consultation time allocated to each patient, to collude with the patient in provision of a speedy 'remedy', even though the GP might wish to spend time in exploration of the individual's specific problems in order to identify the most appropriate course of action.

The structures, in the situation in Case Study 3.2, consist of both the healthcare system within which the GP works and the structures of the patient's work situation. A relatively short period of time (usually 7–10 minutes) is allocated for each patient consultation and the lengthening of one consultation will impact on the waiting times of other patients. There is no guarantee that the queuing patients do not also have problems that merit discussion exceeding their allotted time. Extension of the surgery hours will subsequently impact on other aspects of the GP's day, for example, the ability to conduct home visits. Another structure that may be influential in this case is the mass media, which may foster in patients unrealistic expectations of the efficacy of prescription medication. In addition, the way GPs and nurses are represented in television dramas frequently indicates that they have limitless time, both at work and at home, to focus on patients' problems, emotional as well as physical.

The scope for 'agency' in this case, i.e. the ability of the GP to act autonomously, might result in her deciding to devote extra time to that patient's consultation, in order to explore his problems and the most appropriate course of action, regardless of the impact this may have on other patients and on her own work schedule for the day. The GP may consider that her major responsibility is to patients as individuals, rather than being constrained by the health services' structures. These structures result in patients being treated as 'units', a certain number of whom should be 'processed' within each surgery time. Alternatively, the GP may shift the responsibility back on to the patient, by encouraging him to do something to change his work situation or lifestyle.

Intensive and extreme forms of medical intervention receive a disproportionate amount of attention from the media, usually with a specific focus on either the positive or the negative effect(s) of these interventions. Saving the lives of very premature babies is usually depicted as desirable. There is seldom a serious discussion of the long-term and frequently severe consequences for the baby's future physical and mental development. The care responsibilities that are imposed upon the parent(s) and the cost in social and financial terms to society are not usually addressed.

Television 'soap operas' attract large audiences. A study by Crayford, Hooper & Evans (1997) found that few of the leading characters die 'naturally', the majority meeting statistically rare violent and unexpected deaths. The central characters are seldom overweight, let alone obese. They frequently have several sexual partners but do not contract sexually-transmitted disease and they drink large quantities of alcohol over many years without experiencing apparent long-term health problems!

Healthcare dramas

The distorted and atypical picture of healthcare created by media fiction has implications for what the public perceive to be nursing practice and typical ethical issues and dilemmas in healthcare. For example, in hospital dramas cardiopulmonary resuscitation (CPR) success rates are unrealistically high. The focus tends to be on young people and trauma, older adults and enduring conditions being under-represented in relation to their actual incidence and prevalence within society. The emphasis in medical dramas is on the initial crisis situation, and seldom on the long-term process of recovery and rehabilitation. This distorts reality in terms of where the bulk of nursing work is carried out. Generally, portrayal in the media of individuals who have mental health problems is rarely positive. They are frequently shown as having disturbing, and frequently violent, behaviours. The media tend to highlight cases in which an individual with a history of mental health problems carries out a violent assault or murder. However, *absence* of mental health problems in the perpetrator of crime is seldom reported. Different occupational groups within the healthcare system are accorded the type of treatment in the media that tends to reinforce traditional stereotypes. Hospital managers, for example, are almost invariably portrayed negatively. They are portrayed as officious, heartless bureaucrats attempting to thwart the valiant attempts of medical and nursing staff to provide optimum patient care – despite the imposition of savage cost-cutting and endless paperwork by management! Demonstration of responsible care for groups of patients and management of limited resources for the common good is not awarded the same endorsement as care focused solely on individual patients.

Representation of medical staff and nurses in the media has altered over time, more emphasis being placed today on 'human' qualities and private lives.

There is usually a less idealised view than was promoted in the past by television series such as *Dr Kildare* and *Angels*. There is acknowledgement that mistakes can, and do, happen, usually as a result of practitioner fallibility, or negligence. Highly successful dramas such as *ER* portray characters that have complex lives and who do not always possess altruistic dedication to their work in the face of distraction by personal affairs. However, the significance and complexity of the role that nurses play in relation to patients' long-term rehabilitation, recovery and care seldom receives recognition.

Health 'consumers'

The increasing emphasis on patients' rights and 'consumer focus' in healthcare means that medical experts are subject to scrutiny by, and are expected to be accountable to, the public. Patients are presented as active and valiant service 'users' or 'consumers', rather than as passive (and grateful) recipients of care. Successful and influential television shows, such as *Oprah*, extol the value of people's everyday life experience as opposed to the expertise of a professional elite. Society within the UK has arguably changed over recent decades and the structures of the establishment (e.g. the Church, medicine, law, government, police) have become less revered and more open to question. Establishment structures are less frequently perceived as unequivocally benign forces. Ambiguity in their functions is actively acknowledged and commonly used as a rationale for changes in their status. This includes demands for greater transparency of decision-making and accountability to the public.

High profile cases where healthcare professionals have demonstrated negligent and sometimes criminal behaviours have dented public confidence. The most sensational example is that of Harold Shipman, a GP who murdered an unknown number of his patients, but probably in excess of 250. It may be argued that Shipman was a highly unusual case, being a serial killer and quite unrepresentative of the medical profession. However, the fact that he was able to escape prosecution for decades, despite the disquiet of some colleagues, has identified shortcomings in the regulatory framework that governs medical practitioners. It has also highlighted the power that individual medical practitioners possess. The Shipman Inquiry (HM Government 2005a) expressed concern that the UK General Medical Council (GMC) has been preoccupied with maintaining the medical profession's power and status, rather than fulfilling its remit, namely, protection of the public. Several recent inquiries (e.g. the Bristol Royal Infirmary Inquiry (HM Government 2001b), the Royal Liverpool Children's Inquiry Report (HM Government 2001a)) have led to public demand for greater public accountability and transparency on the part of the medical profession, and for root and branch reform.

Public perceptions of healthcare are thus greatly influenced by the media. The media are also of importance in forming the perspectives of entrants to nursing. They influence the perceptions and expectations of those who access healthcare for themselves or who have relatives or friends who do so. Thus, the media collectively form a societal structure that will both facilitate and inhibit the socialisation of entrants into nursing – by virtue of its influence on nursing students' pre-existing perceptions of healthcare and nursing practice. This in turn will impact on the extent to which students are subsequently able to assimilate and internalise the actual requirements of nursing work. The slant adopted by the media on moral and ethical issues in healthcare, and the controversial cases that are selected for coverage, have a considerable impact on perceptions of nursing ethics both by providers and by recipients of healthcare.

CONCEPTIONS OF CARE

Historically, care has been associated in many societies with low-status work requiring little, or no, formal preparation for its practice and the care provider's receipt of little, or no, financial reward for its delivery. Therapeutic intervention or 'cure', in marked contrast to 'care', has been traditionally associated with power, status and being in control.

Davies (1995) differentiated between three types of care:

- *caregiving work*, which refers to caring carried out on an unpaid basis within networks of family and friends
- *care work*, which refers to a variety of paid jobs within the health and social services (e.g. by home helps and healthcare assistants)
- *professional care*, which refers to caring work carried out within the public sphere and for which the carers have received systematic and formal preparation for practice.

Whilst it is clearly professional care that is the focus of this book, the historical association of care provision with domestic work and 'women's work' is significant. Although professional carers receive a formalised preparation, a qualification and financial rewards their role may continue to be undervalued.

Sourial (1997) agrees that caring has numerous interpretations and this view is supported by Webb (1996, p. 962), who identified from nursing literature more than thirty words associated with care. This serves to highlight the confusion and ambiguity attendant on attempts to find one definitive explanation of the concept. The concept of care as it relates to nursing work has been the subject of much theorising, study and polemic but no definitive conceptualisation has yet been agreed upon. It may be suggested that the reason for this relates to the complexity of care rather than a lack of time spent in conceptualising it.

The claim that a capacity for caring is an inherent human trait has been proposed by influential writers such as Benner & Wrubel (1989), Leininger (1988), Roach (1992) and Watson (1988, 1990). Morse et al (1990) make the point that these authors minimise, or ignore, the effect(s) of organisational frameworks upon the ability of individual carers to provide it. Cultural and organisational frameworks within which care takes place help maximise, or constrain, the range of interactions available to individuals. (This analysis again links to the ideas of agency versus structure, discussed earlier.)

Watson's work (1990) inspired some nurses by advocating that good nursing care requires altruism and spiritual connection, in addition to a knowledge base and clinical competence. Her ideas can prove problematic, however, in the realities of nursing practice. Sourial (1997) suggested that, within existing organisational frameworks, instrumental (i.e. technical) care is easier to provide than affective (i.e. emotional) care. This is due to the necessity for any organisational structure to adopt a wider, more utilitarian perspective, i.e. to go beyond care for the needs of individuals to ensure equitable provision for all who are their responsibility. This may result in conflicts between the individualistic philosophy of care espoused by many nurses and the more impersonal concern with the common good demanded by organisations.

Aside from the views of individual nurses as to whether the level of care proposed by Watson is desirable, or indeed appropriate within nursing practice, there is the practical problem that, in most care settings, the depth of interpersonal interaction required would be impossible to achieve. Indeed, allocation of the quantity and quality of attention which Watson proposes would be unachievable in most care settings, and/or necessitate neglect of some clients at the expense of others. This might create feelings of frustration, failure and guilt in nurses. For a practical example, please read Case Study 3.3.

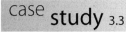

case study 3.3

Who gets priority?

A community psychiatric nurse (CPN) had a large and varied caseload of clients, the majority of whom had economic and social difficulties in addition to their specific mental health problems.

On one particular Friday, the CPN's last client was tearful and said that she was having increasing arguments with her partner in whose house she lived. She was afraid that if the situation continued to deteriorate she would become homeless. The client had a previous history of intravenous heroin use but had undergone a rehabilitation support programme. Following this she had remained heroin-free. The client indicated to the CPN that a return to her previous drug habit was imminent as she felt unable to cope with everything that was going wrong in her life.

Activity
Either on your own, or with someone else, identify what you consider to be the CPN's responsibilities to her client in this situation.

Case Study 3.3 – discussion

It would seem that, in this situation, the community psychiatric nurse (CPN) has a responsibility to attend to the client's mental health problems. However, these are to some extent inseparable from the client's social and economic difficulties (which she may be able to do little to change). The level of attention that the CPN can devote to one client is limited by her total work-load, the competing needs of other clients, and the CPN's own social and domestic commitments. Attempting to achieve the level of care proposed by Watson (1990) may appear to be unrealistic and unattainable. If nurses do strive to live up to this ethos then they may become disillusioned by their inability to maintain the standards that they have set themselves. These issues may be addressed by development of guidelines that clarify, for both nurses and their clients, the boundaries of the nurse's role. Of course, whilst guidelines may assist in minimising the risk of unrealistic demands being made of the nurse, they may be easier to formulate than they are to implement, given the complexities of situations in which nursing care may be required.

Changes in health services' provision

The move within the UK to provide care in the community, rather than in institutional settings (formalised by the Community Care Act (HM Government 1990)), has provided an impetus to ensuring that care takes place, wherever possible, in the community rather than large institutions. This shift to care in the community applies not only to individuals who have mental health problems and learning difficulties, but also to adults with acute physical health problems. Treatment for these patients is now frequently provided in primary care settings. Patients who require hospitalisation are discharged more speedily than in the past. However, this rapid discharge has had two effects. The first is in primary care, where there is now much pressure on district nurses and home helps to provide a greater quantity and quality of technical care than previously, as well as fundamental care related to patients' activities of daily living. The other effect is within hospitals, where a much higher proportion of patients tend to be acutely ill and highly dependent than was the case in the past (when most wards and units comprised a mixture of highly dependent and relatively self-caring patients who were progressing towards discharge).

In the next section some specific changes that have taken place in nursing education will be discussed. These cannot be viewed in isolation from the changes that are taking place within society. These are changes that have impacted upon expectations of the public in relation to nursing, and changes in nursing practices that have influenced society.

Entrants to nursing

Within the UK, the demographic profile of entrants to nursing has changed considerably over the past twenty years. There is greater heterogeneity in the intake, in relation to age, gender, and prior life and work experience than previously. Nurses' preparation for practice has undergone radical change with the preparation for practice programmes initiated by the United Kingdom Central Council (UKCC) for Nurses, Midwives and Health Visitors (*Project 2000*: UKCC 1986). Most UK nursing programmes now offer a choice between a bachelor degree or diploma as the registration point for students. Additionally, there has been a burgeoning of postgraduate Bachelors, Masters and Doctoral level programmes aimed at registered practitioners. Post-registration nursing degrees, particularly in relation to specialised practitioner status, link conveniently with the pragmatic desire of the medical profession to devolve some aspects of its work to registered nurses. Students of nursing operate within two different structural frameworks, those of education and of practice. Both of these may challenge the students' previously held attitudes, beliefs and values. The requirement to undertake academic work to diploma or degree level may create difficulties for some students, as may the need to obtain satisfactory assessments in practice placements. Students within the UK are now supernumerary to the staff quotas in practice settings, and receive a bursary rather than a health service funded salary. They undertake practice placements, during which they work within the organisational framework provided by health services, rather than by higher education. These two different structures have the potential to facilitate, but also to constrict, students' individual agency (i.e. ability to act autonomously) and both types of structures exert a powerful influence upon students.

During the transition from matriculation to quali-fication, the socialisation process means that students learn, and adopt the approach of registered nurses, by acquiring knowledge and practical skills which may change their existing attitudes, beliefs and values. The regulatory bodies in each country stipulate the academic and nursing practice competencies that must be achieved. In the UK, these are the Nursing and Midwifery Council (NMC) and, because health is a devolved issue, country-specific non-governmental organisations (NGOs) within the UK. Within England the quality assurance framework is delivered by 'Visitors', who represent the NMC and monitor the quality of education programmes. The organisations contracted to carry out this function within the other UK countries are:

- NHS Education Scotland (NES)
- Health Professions Wales (HPW)
- The Northern Ireland Practice and Education Council for Nursing and Midwifery (NIPEC).

Registered practitioners in the UK are accountable to both their employer and the NMC as their regu-latory body. In addition to these separate structural frameworks, which may impose potentially conflict-ing obligations on nurses, practitioners bring indi-vidual attitudes, beliefs, values and personal commitments to their work. These may agree with those of the structures within which they are required to operate on most occasions, but may sometimes collide.

University lecturers

For most lecturers within the UK who provide the preparation for practice for both undergraduate and postgraduate nurses, the move to establishments of higher education, discrete from health services' provision, has taken place within the past 10–15 years. The majority of lecturers are registered nurses and must provide evidence of clinical competence, as well as educational development, in order to maintain their registration. However, the extent to which clinical commitments are maintained is widely variable. Lecturers have become more vulnerable than previously to the charge of working within an 'ivory tower', removed from the realities of nursing practice. The decision to maintain clinical contacts may not be a matter of individual choice, but of organisational constraints imposed on lecturers by higher education institutions. This is an example of the tension that may exist between structure and agency for lecturers in nursing. In addition, universities expect lecturers to participate actively in income-generating research. These tensions invariably impact on students' experiences, within the organisational frameworks of the university and those of the health services.

Relationships with patients

As was highlighted earlier, public perceptions of nursing may prevent appreciation of the level of knowledge, skill and complex responsibilities that nursing work entails, and misunderstanding of the nature of the moral conflicts that nurses actually encounter in their daily practice.

In order to appreciate these responsibilities, complexities and conflicts, it is necessary to examine further the similarities and differences between 'informal' (or 'lay') care and 'professional nursing'. When assisting patients with activities of living there may be little difference between an informal carer, a home help, a care assistant, a nursing student and a registered nurse. There are differences, however, in the preparation for practice that each carer receives, and in the purpose of that preparation. With the exception of informal carers, all receive some form of financial remuneration for their efforts. (Informal carers may, however, qualify for state benefits if they fulfil specified criteria in relation to their care commit-ments.) Paid nurses, unlike informal carers, do not usually have prior knowledge of the person for whom they provide care. Contact between the care provider and care recipient is usually restricted to the situation in which care is provided and received. Indeed relationships above and beyond this boundary are usually regarded as undesirable, if not actively forbidden. Many healthcare providers, and regulatory bodies such as the NMC, provide specific policies and guidelines which seek to regulate patient/client relationships. Care providers are usually in positions of relative power compared to care recipients, and setting clear boundaries helps ensure that the potential for abuse of this power is minimised.

SOCIALISATION: CARE SETTINGS

The processes involved in becoming first a nursing student and second a registered and qualified practitioner are rather different. Some entrants to nursing have prior experience of providing paid care, in either community or institutional settings. They have therefore undergone a partial socialisation into one aspect of paid care work. This may make their transition to the role of student nurse more, rather than less, difficult.

The expectations that registered nurses have of care assistants and students are different. Care assistants are expected to provide fundamental care as and when required, in fulfilment of their employment contract. Whilst care assistants may acquire practice-based vocational qualifications the focus is on the practicalities of care provision. The focus in students' education is on acquisition of knowledge and competence in a wide range of technical and psychosocial skills. The aim is to produce competent registered practitioners who have the ability to direct as well as implement care.

The financial constraints of having a bursary rather than a salary mean that some students have to work part-time in addition to undertaking their nursing programme. This work may be as a care assistant. The student may experience tension or conflict between the roles of student and care assistant although some find the additional perspective helpful. Some students may have experience of having been a patient, or may have relatives or friends who have been patients. All of these experiences will affect students' perceptions of their current role and their future role as registered nurses.

Labelling patients

The theory of labelling originated within sociological perspectives of deviance (Lemert 1951, Becker 1963) and refers to attitudes towards people who have attributes that society considers abnormal. These attributes may relate, for example, to an individual's physical or mental health problems, their physical appearance, personality type or sexual orientation. It is important to bear in mind that labelling may have advantages for both professional and patient. For the professional it means using a standard vocabulary when referring to specific disorders. For the patient the diagnosis of a specific illness will legitimise their access to appropriate services, including medical and nursing care or state benefits. Acceptance of a label not only brings rights but may also impose obligations on the patient, for example to cooperate with prescribed forms of treatment. However, medical labels, like personal ones, may potentially stigmatise individuals (e.g. 'alcoholic', 'depressed' or 'feckless'). Understanding the implications of labelling and stereotyping of patients by nurses is important in nurse–patient relationships, as discussed by Bond & Bond (1994), for example.

Please read the outline provided in Case Study 3.4 (which relates to the situation described earlier in Case Study 3.1) and carry out the activities associated with this.

case study 3.4

Personal labelling

(This follows on from the scenario in Case Study 3.1.)

The student noted that the staff treated patients differently, treating some with respect and shouting at others. One of the patients was treated with affection and was 'allowed' to make decisions about her care. She was referred to in good-humoured terms by staff at the handover report. This was in marked contrast to the staff's attitude to one of the other patients whom they seemed to dislike and whom they referred to amongst themselves (but within earshot of the student) as 'that awkward so-and-so'.

Activity
Either on your own, or with others, identify the ways in which the situation described relates to the concept of labelling.

Case Study 3.4 – discussion

When nurses use the technique of personal labelling of a patient, it may serve to legitimise the feelings (positive or negative) that individual nurses have towards a patient. It also enables staff to think that their own impatience with a patient is the result of the patient's negative characteristics rather than the staff's own behaviour. In the label given, the adjective 'awkward' does not identify one single behaviour, but conjures up a variety of 'non-compliant' patient behaviours that interfere with the smooth running of the routine.

To some extent labelling and stereotyping are a common part of social interaction, as they help us to make sense of the world by reducing challenging complexities to simpler and more manageable categories. However, the vulnerability of patients, and their dependence on nursing staff for understanding and support, means that labelling in a ward situation can have further reaching effects than in everyday social interaction. Unpopular patients may be at some risk of having their psychological and physical needs ignored or neglected. The principles of beneficence and justice are of equal importance here. If patients are in danger of having their rights to appropriate physical and psychological treatment compromised, then nurses are failing in their duty of care. Another example of labelling occurs when patients do not adhere to prescribed treatments (see Case Study 3.5).

case study 3.5

Non-adherence to treatment

During a placement in a respiratory unit, a student was involved in the care of a young woman who was admitted with severe acute asthma, a life-threatening condition. The patient required emergency treatment, following which she made a successful recovery. It was subsequently discovered that the patient had not been taking her prescribed steroid inhaler for some time, and that she had become increasingly breathless and wheezy for several days before the severe acute attack. The student overheard the patient being referred to by staff as being 'non-compliant'.

Activity
Either on your own, or with someone else, consider the meaning and implications of the phrase 'non-compliant'.

Case Study 3.5 – discussion

The phrase 'non-compliance', or its more recent successor, 'non-adherence', does seem to imply that the treatment deemed appropriate by healthcare staff is the yardstick by which patient behaviours are judged. It seems unlikely that the young woman in the situation outlined in Case Study 3.5 chose to develop a life-threatening condition by neglecting to follow the health advice that she had been given. Rather than labelling the woman as 'non-compliant' or 'non-adherent', it might have been more useful to explore with the patient the reasons for her behaviour. This approach would encourage better understanding between healthcare staff and patients in relation to the reasons for treatment and the reasons for non-compliance.

Group labelling

Another type of labelling occurs when *groups* of individuals are perceived as being homogeneous. The public's perception of schizophrenia, for example, is that it is associated with incomprehensible, unpredictable and possibly dangerous behaviour. We have already seen that the media frequently depicts people with mental health problems in a negative light and plays a powerful role in public attitude formation. People who have schizophrenia may be labelled as a *group* who have similar attributes, rather than being seen as individuals. Negative labelling may also apply, for example, to people who have HIV, or who are admitted to care settings because of alcohol abuse, attempted suicide or self-harm. This form of labelling may lead to discrimination against *groups* of individuals. It may ultimately have a more extensive effect than personal labelling because the discrimination may become enshrined in policy or law. For an example of group labelling, see Case Study 3.6.

case study 3.6

Self-harm

A 16-year-old girl was admitted to the accident and emergency department, having taken a deliberate overdose of shop-bought analgesia. After initial treatment she was transferred to a ward for observation. The student noted that whilst the staff provided necessary physical care, their comments about the patient at the handover report were derogatory. One of the registered nurses referred to the patient as 'another of those time-wasting self-harmers'.

Activity
Either on your own, or with someone else, identify why the staff may have this attitude.
   What are the effects of labelling individual patients in this way?
   You may also wish to identify and discuss your own attitudes and beliefs about individuals who self-harm.

Case Study 3.6 – discussion

Staff may consider that people whose illness is perceived as being 'self-inflicted' are less worthy of care than others. Such patients may be seen as using resources that could be better employed elsewhere. Staff may feel that their own expertise should be used to care for people whose problems are viewed as 'legitimate'. These attitudes may mean that individuals who deliberately self-harm, or whose illness is perceived as 'self-inflicted', are seen as a *group* whose behaviour is unacceptable and who are consequently stigmatised. Even though, in this situation, the staff provided physical care, their negative attitudes may be detrimental to the patient's psychological well-being.

Attitudes, beliefs and values

We noted earlier that student nurses enter their undergraduate programme with pre-existing attitudes, beliefs and values. This 'moral baggage', including unexamined moral assumptions which they bring to their work, affects the way nurses relate to people in their care. Nurses may be uneasy or judgemental about the lifestyles, past and/or current, of some patients. However, the practical nature of nursing work undertaken by students on practice placements means that they may experience these conflicts at first hand. For example, if nurses hold strong views about alcohol abuse or tobacco use then these may impact negatively on their perceptions of patients who present with problems associated with these behaviours. The NMC's (2004) expectation of nurses is that they should not allow their personal health beliefs or moral attitudes to prejudice their approach to any person and these should not impact negatively on the physical or psychological care that they provide for patients.

One situation in which UK nurses have the option to refuse to participate in treatment is when a patient is undergoing a planned termination of pregnancy or abortion. (The clinical use of the term 'abortion' denotes removal of a fetus from the uterus by either deliberate or accidental means. The lay term for the latter occurrence is usually 'miscarriage'.)

Refusal to participate is often less clear-cut than may appear at first. The option to refuse applies only to participation in the termination procedure, and nurses retain a legal and moral duty of care to the patient before and following the event. When terminations are carried out in operating theatres then the procedure is clearly located and time limited. Terminations may, however, be carried out within ward settings, by means of abortifacient drugs that induce uterine contractions and expulsion of the fetus. While nurses may refuse to participate in the administration of such drugs, they may be required to assist patients (e.g. if vomiting) during the time that the medication is having effect. It is not clear that nurses have the right to refuse to provide assistance in those circumstances.

Reporting inappropriate practice ('whistle-blowing')

Earlier we discussed situations where students may feel uneasy when they witness, or are asked to

participate in, forms of care that they consider inappropriate. In the UK, the Public Disclosure at Work Act (HM Government 1998b) provides legal protection for employees who divulge unacceptable work practices. Although students are not employees, they are subject to the regulations of their higher education establishment and liable to censure by their college for misconduct or incompetence. (Registered nurses who are employees with organisations may have professional indemnity, but this does not protect them from censure by colleagues for unacceptable practice, or disclosure to the employing authority of incompetence or unprofessional conduct.) For students who witness what they consider to be inappropriate or unacceptable practices in placement settings, there are several kinds of action they can take. However, their ability to take action may be constrained by the structures of power and authority within the organisation where they are working. This again illustrates the tension between the placement and university 'structures', and the limitations they place on the individual agency of a student on a placement.

In the situation in Case Study 3.1, the student might raise her concerns with the care staff involved at the time, but as indicated earlier this might present difficulties for her. It is recommended that students in placements should be allocated a mentor, who is a registered nurse. In this way it is possible for students to voice concerns either to their mentor or to the charge nurse. In practice this may prove to be difficult if the student wishes to avoid the possibility of being viewed as a troublemaker, or if the care assistants and registered nurses have befriended them, or if the registered nurses already appear to be aware of the questionable practice. In such situations, students should seek advice from their academic supervisor, either a lecturer who has a formalised link with the placement area, or another within their education programme. The student's concerns may then be conveyed by university staff to staff in the placement organisation.

There have been instances in the past, however, where student concerns have been reported or documented but ignored. In 1996 students working within Lakeland Trust in the north of England reported concerns about the treatment of patients to their higher education establishment and wrote to the Trust, detailing these. They reported emotional and verbal abuse of patients, and unacceptable practices (e.g. tying patients to commodes whilst the staff ate their breakfast). An investigation was carried out, but no disciplinary action was taken by the Trust. It was not until further complaints were made two years later, by registered nurses working temporarily in the unit, that a full investigation was carried out (Commission for Health Improvement (CHI) 2000). This case is an instance where complaints about unacceptable practices have given rise to public concern in recent years, and brought about demands for greater accountability by healthcare professionals to the public.

REFLECTION ON PRACTICE

Reflection on practice may take place informally (when initiated by students with their peers), or occur formally, as a preplanned and regular event within university and/or placement settings. These 'debriefings' may assist students to adapt better to their new environment and its responsibilities and challenges. A formalised process of reflecting on practice situations, in company with fellow students and experienced staff, may assist students to come to terms with anxiety-provoking or distressing events. Reflection may also develop the students' skills of analytical and critical thinking. (Note: 'reflection on practice' implies reflection on both the positive and negative aspects of practice.) A number of models may be used as a framework for reflecting on practice (e.g. Johns 2000, Atkins & Murphy 1994). The *DECIDE model* that we describe in Chapter 12 provides a framework for reflection on moral decisions and planning of future action.

For one example of reflection on practice, see Case Study 3.7.

case study 3.7

Use of reflection – nurses and dying patients

A group of students were in university for a study day, at the end of the second year of their programme, having completed two weeks of their current practice placement.

During small group discussion students, with a lecturer as group facilitator, reflected on their experiences. One student spoke about how upset he was when a patient died suddenly and unexpectedly. The patient had been in the unit since the student's arrival and appeared to be making a good recovery following serious illness.

Activity
Either on your own, or with someone else, identify the ways in which you think that reflecting on this situation in a group might be helpful to the student who was distressed and also to the other students in the group.

Case Study 3.7 – discussion

The death of patients is likely to have a powerful effect on both nursing students and registered nurses. Reflection within a small group on their different attitudes, beliefs and values relating to death may be helpful for students and for registered nurses. This may help them to identify the positive and negative aspects of the situation that is described and to address these within their own setting in a way that helps provide one another with support. At least some of the other group members are likely to have experienced similar, although obviously not identical, situations involving the death of a patient. Group members may then be able to compare and discuss their feelings about, and responses to, these situations. This discussion may provide helpful insight (and opportunity for input from the lecturer) that will be of value both in that situation and also for their subsequent nursing practice. The discussion may help identify therapeutic approaches to caring for people who are dying, and ways to build on these. The group may need help to understand that the distress experienced by an individual student represents a normal response to loss and this can lead to useful discussion of bereavement and loss, as well as strategies that nurses might employ to help themselves and others to cope with this and other kinds of stressful situation.

Socialisation: academic assessment

The requirement within the UK is that students undertake theory and practice on a 50:50 weighting. The fact that qualifications at registration are now at diploma or degree level makes this balance important. Entry qualifications to nursing have not been raised in keeping with changes to the programme, and entrants may find the academic content challenging. One of the requirements of academic writing is accurate acknowledgement of source material. Sources should be cited within the body of the text, following standard conventions, and listed at the end of the work. There is some evidence that availability of previous students' work for perusal, and the ease of access to written material, predisposes some students to plagiarism.

Please undertake the activity outlined in Box 3.1.

Box 3.1 Plagiarism

Activity
Either on your own, or with someone else, identify the reasons why plagiarism is unacceptable in academic work.

Box 3.1 – discussion

In the discussion of plagiarism in Box 3.1 a number of issues will have been identified, some of which relate solely to the academic setting. These are likely to focus on the question of honesty and respect for the insights gained from other people's work. The principle of justice also applies here, as it is unjust to use other people's ideas without their permission and without proper attribution and due acknowledgement of your debt to them. There is also the point to be made that students who plagiarise may be unfairly advantaged, and students who undertake work honestly may be disadvantaged if they gain lower grades than individuals who plagiarise.

Some discussion of this issue may progress beyond the specific academic issue to the implications of dishonest practices in more general terms. It may be argued, for example, that students who are prepared to be dishonest academically may also be prepared to be dishonest when they are in placements and, subsequently, when they become registered practitioners. Further, that failure to achieve required competencies by cheating might well put patients at risk, by using the wrong procedures in treating patients, just as a driver who had cheated to pass a driving test might put their passengers at risk.

Mixing and interacting with many other students, of disparate ages, cultural beliefs, socio-economic profiles and life experiences may provide stimulation to students, but also challenges of a variety of kinds. For example, many students undertaking nursing programmes do not have a family tradition of university attendance. If a student's social background has not encouraged them to believe that academic achievement at university level is desirable and attainable, then such students may lack confidence in their ability to succeed.

Evidence-based practice

It may appear self-evident that all forms of nursing care should be evaluated and based upon evidence of their effectiveness. For example, the prevention of most pressure sores has been shown to be possible by implementing research findings based on control trials, rather than depending on trial and error and myth. However, an approach to management that focuses on 'evidence-based practice' itself needs to be open to critical evaluation, and to discussion of what would count as relevant evidence of good performance or best practice.

Applied to nursing systems and procedures, evidence-based practice can be helpful in improving the efficiency and cost-effectiveness of some kinds of routine services or treatments. It is debatable whether those uniquely personal aspects of caring for people in distress are susceptible to the same kind of quantitative study and analysis. It is the distinctive personal style, the embodied and affective engagement of the nurse with particular patients, that underpins nursing practice. The move to generalisability may fail to acknowledge this.

The fundamental questions raised by evidence-based practice relate to what we mean by 'evidence' in this context. To answer this, we must consider: the nature and scope of the term 'evidence', and what scientific, performance and value criteria are applied in determining what kinds of information are to count as evidence. Focusing on what can be easily observed, and subjected to quantitative analysis, risks neglect of areas where reliable evidence is difficult to obtain, because it is more qualitative in nature. Qualitative evidence requires the use of alternative forms of data collection (such as personal interviews) and the application of non-quantitative analysis, but these are no less important forms of evidence. Having a sound 'evidence base' for practice does not mean having exclusively quantitative criteria or data, but documented assessment of outcomes of action or treatment plans can be very useful, provided they have preset objectives against which outcomes can be evaluated.

While methods of meta-analysis, such as 'evidence-based practice' and applied epidemiology, allow us to make sense of great volumes of data, by yielding statistically based guidance, they are nevertheless reductionist and represent only a partial view. The particular tends to be lost in the universal, and individuals become ciphers in statistical tables. The question: 'What is to count as "evidence"?' is not unproblematic. The question is based on certain prior assumptions and value judgements concerning what factors are to be considered 'relevant' or 'irrelevant'. From the perspective of individual patients great emphasis may be placed upon what appears to be clinically irrelevant. Systematic reviews, meta-analyses and randomised controlled trials (RCTs) may be recommended as the 'gold standard', without realising that the criteria that determine 'relevant evidence' may be biased or problematic. 'Scientific practice' itself must be open to critical examination and revision in the light of scientific evidence and ethical principles relating to sound methods and just means to achieve set objectives.

Despite the existence of evidence to indicate unequivocally what care interventions will achieve optimum benefit, this evidence may not be fully, or even partially, incorporated into practice. For example, despite the evidence in relation to pressure sore prevention that has been available for almost 30 years (Norton 1975), the implementation of this is not universal.

Tension between theory and practice

Nursing students may experience conflict between the teaching provided in the university setting and the reality of practice placements. According to theories that place emphasis on individual agency, students are free to make their own decisions about their own learning and strategies for dealing with problematic situations. According to theories that place emphasis on structure, the students' abilities to act autonomously are limited by a number of factors, for example their junior status, the need for competent staff to undertake placement assessments, and/or students' performance in their transitory position on any one placement.

Theories that synthesise elements of structure and agency consider that, on the one hand, individuals can provide responses based on their personal inclinations, but on the other hand, decisions are reached on the basis of a need to 'fit in' with colleagues and to acquire satisfactory assessments. The adequacy of support structures for students, such as student counselling services, may also be important in enhancing or reducing students' abilities to make choices.

Ruth Caleb, Head of Counselling at Brunel University and member of the British Association for Counselling, has commented on the efficacy of counselling for students as follows (Caleb 2005):

At this point there is little research evidence into the effectiveness of the counselling process in universities. Rickinson and Rutherford found that students felt that counselling helped them perceive their difficulties as surmountable rather than overwhelming (Rickinson and Rutherford 1996). This may be of especial importance to those students who find the adjustment to university particularly hard, such as students from communities that do not traditionally study at university. More recently, at the University of Cambridge, a sample of students (both undergraduate and postgraduate) was researched throughout their courses, and three quarters

of the sample that had attended counselling had found it beneficial (Surtees et al 2000).

Caleb also observed:

The efficacy of counselling is acknowledged by the DoH (Department of Health), which supports therapy as an effective means of treating depression ... A further DoH report reviewed the evidence for counselling and psychotherapy, and concluded, 'psychological therapy should be routinely considered as an option' (DoH 2001[e]). The Royal College of Psychiatrists Report, having reviewed the evidence concerning student mental health, states that the university counselling service will normally be the favoured route for students with mental health problems (Royal College of Psychiatrists 2003).

Socialisation into professional practice

We have discussed the socialisation of student nurses into undergraduate programmes and identified factors that impact on students during their transition from matriculation to qualification. Some of these factors inhibit, and others facilitate, students' preparation for qualification and registration.

A second transition occurs following registration, when individuals progress from being students to being qualified and registered practitioners. Registration is likely to bring a sense of achievement but may be accompanied by anxieties about the challenges that lie ahead. Registered nurses are legally and professionally accountable for decisions about what care is provided or omitted, by themselves, by students and by care assistants within the practice area. The Nursing and Midwifery Council (NMC) distinguishes very clearly between the role of students and registered practitioners (NMC 2002a, 2004). While the Council has expectations of the former, in their capacity as future professionals (NMC 2002a), it is registered nurses who are professionally *accountable* for their practice. The feelings of insecurity that may accompany students in their movements from one practice placement to another are also likely to affect newly qualified practitioners. These issues and challenges encountered in nursing practice by registered practitioners will be addressed in some detail in Chapter 5.

further reading

Bond J, Bond S 1994 Sociology and health care: an introduction for nurses and other health care professionals, 2nd edn. Churchill Livingstone, Edinburgh

Bulman C, Schutz S (eds) 2004 Reflective practice in nursing: the growth of the professional practitioner, 3rd edn. Blackwell, Oxford

Collins R 1994 Four sociological traditions. Oxford University Press, Oxford

Hallam J 2000 Nursing the image: media, culture and professional identity. Routledge, London

Jones P 1991 Theory and method in sociology: a guide for the beginner. Collins, London

Naidoo J, Wills J 2000 Health promotion: foundations for practice, 2nd edn. Baillière Tindall, London

Seale C 2002 Media and health. Sage, London

Power and responsibility in nursing practice and management

4

AIMS

This chapter has the following aims:

1. To demystify ethics by demonstrating that ethics is about the relations of power and responsibility rather than subjective attitudes and feelings

2. To explore the different levels of power and responsibility in which we have to act as moral agents: the personal, team, corporate and political levels

3. To introduce two sets of models to clarify the different ethical responsibilities of nurses in the various kinds of situations in which nurses relate to patients, and in different kinds of nurse management.

LEARNING OUTCOMES

When you have read and worked through this chapter, you should be able to:

■ Illustrate the inadequacy of a privatised view of morality by examples of power relations and power-sharing in nursing

■ Discuss what 'virtues' are required if one is to be a competent moral agent, and give examples from nursing practice

■ Demonstrate insight into the different kinds of ethical demands involved in relating to patients in crisis intervention, consultative, supportive and service roles

■ Demonstrate understanding of the various forms in which power and authority are expressed in teams, line-management, community nursing and corporate planning

■ Demonstrate sensitivity to the ways in which gender-role stereotyping can affect both personal attitudes and behaviour and institutional practices in hospitals and community nursing.

POWER AND MORAL RESPONSIBILITY

In the first chapter we discussed the significance of our shared and changing values for our everyday ethical decision-making, and sought to clarify the distinctions between 'feelings', 'attitudes', 'beliefs' and 'values'. We have been at pains throughout to emphasise that ethics is not a private matter nor a purely individual activity, but rather that *ethics is essentially concerned with our life as members of a community, and how we exercise moral responsibility within the various kinds of social structures in which we live and work*. We have also emphasised that different social structures are characterised by different kinds of power relations, and ways in which power is shared or abused. In doing so we have sought to bring ethics back into the public domain where the realities of power have to be addressed, (whether these are in personal relationships, professional/client relationships, or in organisational management), in order to bridge the gap between ethics and politics.

However, in British moral philosophy there has been a strong tendency to psychologise ethics. Empiricist and utilitarian philosophers have sought to ground ethics in our subjective feelings and human psychology. For example, David Hume (1711–1776), the Scottish empiricist philosopher, sought to explain the origin of ethics in feelings of sympathy for others, and the fact that such mutual sympathy is necessary for our survival as social beings. Jeremy Bentham (1748–1832) and John Stuart Mill (1806–1873), English social reformers, suggest that feelings of pleasure and fear of pain, and the desire for happiness, dictate our choice of values and serve to explain the nature of ethics. The self-styled 'logical positivists', like A.J. Ayer (1910–1989), maintained that ethical judgements are nothing but personal expressions of our feelings of approval or disapproval of our own or other people's actions. This tradition provides the background to the widely held view that ethics is essentially 'about our subjective feelings, attitudes and values'.

Against this prevailing tendency to psychologise and privatise ethics, we would like to reaffirm the classical view that ethics is fundamentally about power and responsibility, about the conditions for power-sharing and criteria for the responsible exercise of power in our relations with one another. For nurses, the basic question is how this applies to their dealings with patients. We argue here that while psychology has cast light on many aspects of human experience, including the key role of our feelings in making moral judgements, there are also other equally important ways of looking at our moral experience, e.g. sociological, philosophical and historical. To focus exclusively on the subjective and psychological aspects of our moral experience is to ignore and perhaps misrepresent the structures of power and responsibility within which we act as moral agents. There are many objective factors in the exercise of our professional responsibilities in healthcare that have a bearing on our understanding of nursing ethics. Some of these are: the structures of power and authority in institutional life; the organisation of labour and its management and appraisal; the differentiation of roles, rules, responsibilities and lines of reporting; and the kind of moral and legal accountability that we have in public life. All these issues, which are fundamental to nursing ethics, have to do with the relationships between power and responsibility in our routine work.

Sociological analysis focuses attention on the structure of power relationships in different social settings; for example in consulting relationships, in the home, in institutional settings, and in more public and political contexts. It will analyse the different ways moral values and personal or professional responsibility are interpreted in each situation, because each social setting will be governed by its own set of formal and informal rules. It is also concerned, for example, with critical examination of how gender-role stereotyping affects the public perception of the identity and role of nurses in healthcare, and reinforces what many analysts would regard as the institutional exploitation and oppression of women in an essentially patriarchal health service.

Philosophical analysis focuses in ethics more on the logical relationships between the fundamental ethical concepts and the principles which embody our basic moral values, and on clarifying the practical criteria and processes we use in making moral judgements, i.e. how we apply our principles to the concrete situations which demand decisions from us and what means we choose to achieve our desired ends. From a philosophical point of view, we appeal to fundamental moral principles to legitimate our exercise of power, and to define its scope and responsible use.

Historical analysis examines the evolution of a given society (or societies) through time, and seeks to describe the way values have been articulated in the creation of its institutions and in specialised roles in the division of labour. Thus, for example, historians may study how the development of medical science shapes the traditions of medical practice; or the increasing specialisation of nursing functions from lay, religious and military settings to those exercised in modern hospital and community settings. Historical analysis throws light on the evolution of a largely gender-based division of labour in healthcare; and how ethical codes have evolved in each profession, and their relations to one another, which reflect this. As the emergence of different professions has been marked by the formal differentiation of roles and demarcation of different areas of functional power and responsibility within healthcare, so each has developed its own peculiar set of values.

In the first chapter we examined some of the broad historical trends and ideas that have influenced the development of the professions, and nursing in particular. We recognise that a great deal more could be written, and has been written, about the history of healthcare and the nursing profession (e.g. Allan & Jolley 1982, Maggs 1987, Bullough & Bullough 1984, Dingwall et al 1988), here we will discuss mainly sociological and philosophical models for interpreting moral issues in healthcare, and in nursing ethics in particular. As the sociological and philosophical analyses draw much of their material from the history of ideas and the general history of culture anyway, the historical dimensions of the subject are not being ignored and are implicit in much of what follows. Thus, understanding of historical developments in Western society (as distinct from other societies) influences how we perceive healthcare institutions and the relationships between medical, nursing and allied health professionals, and their dealings with patients or clients. It is also directly relevant to our understanding in different societies of the respective rights and duties of professionals and the values and rules which govern their relationships with one another.

Demystifying ethics

(Note: This section is adapted, with permission, from *Putting Ethics to Work in the Public Sector*, by I.E. Thompson and Maria Harries, Public Sector Standards Commission, Perth, WA.)

It is commonly implied in the popular media that ethics is concerned with our subjective feelings, attitudes and personal preferences. While these private and personal factors are clearly important in life, and in our dealings with people, confusion and difficulty are likely to arise in ethics if we treat these psychological states as the primary subject matter of ethics. In fact, the mystification of ethics begins with the relegation of ethics to this realm of subjective and non-rational experience. When this happens, ethics ceases to be open to public scrutiny or debate, and it is difficult to see how ethical decisions can be judged by any kind of criteria that are intersubjectively valid. This mystification of ethics in English-speaking culture arises because of certain pervasive popular misconceptions of ethics current today. (See Box 2.3: What ethics is and is not.)

The belief that ethics is an intensely private matter, concerned only with one's subjective feelings, attitudes and personal preferences, has not been the prevailing view of ethics in the traditions of either Eastern or Western moral philosophy. It has been taken for granted in both traditions that ethics is a public and community enterprise and that the quest for justice and fairness is fundamental to that endeavour. Even the Judaeo-Christian love ethic is not based on how we *feel* about people, but about how we *demonstrate care* for their well-being and fulfilment, *by what we do* for them and with them.

By contrast the modern tendency to privatise ethics, and treat it as a purely subjective matter, makes it into an occult process that is inaccessible to critical investigation. Discerning moral truth becomes a matter of direct intuition, attending to the 'inner voice of conscience', or, in the case of an elect few, privileged access to divine guidance. This privatising of ethics has the consequence of driving a wedge between ethics and law, ethics and politics, ethics and business – the former being seen as belonging to the private sphere and the latter to the public domain. Restating the conviction, as old as Aristotle, that ethics is about power and power-sharing – whether in intimate sexual relationships, in family life, in education, business, professional life, healthcare, politics or international relations – puts ethics back squarely in the public domain.

Our experience of being subjected to the arbitrary moral authority of parents, teachers and religious figures lends credence to the view that ethics, and moral codes, like the Ten Commandments, are handed down from above by God or his self-appointed agents, and that their moral prescriptions are infallible and set in stone. Such an approach tends to be absolutist, authoritarian, and infantilises people by denying them scope for the expression of their own moral autonomy and responsibility. Alternatively, it becomes the domain of experts – philosophers, theologians or gurus – and requires mastery of esoteric knowledge. However, if ethics is about how we articulate, negotiate and agree a set of common principles, and the skills we need to apply them, then ethics must be practical and concerns how we educate people for independence and personal responsibility.

An analogous difficulty arises, as indicated in Chapter 2, if all moral difficulties are treated as 'dilemmas'. In the strict sense, a dilemma has no solution, and arises when we encounter an *irresolvable* conflict of duties. In the face of real ethical dilemmas we can either throw up our hands in despair and abrogate our responsibility for making difficult choices, or treat the matter as one of arbitrary judgement. Real dilemmas obviously do arise, but the overwhelming majority of so-called 'dilemmas', or ethical difficulties that present as dilemmas, prove on careful analysis to be *resolvable problems*. Those that prove intractable demand a particular kind of courage – to act responsibly in the face of painful conflicts of duty, doing the best we can and/or trying to do the least harm. In such circumstances this means accepting moral uncertainty, and being prepared to accept responsibility for the results. If, however, as often proves to be the case, our 'dilemmas' can be reframed as 'problems', then we can and should apply rational problem-solving methods to the resolution of our ethical quandaries and even very complex problems.

Another variant of the privatisation of ethics is the treatment of ethics as a 'skills package' which can be marketed as a 'training product' – skills for improving our public relations, or techniques for 'winning friends and influencing people'. Ethics, from this point of view, becomes just a matter of technique, or manners, or knowing the right rules, possessing the right management competencies – which usually means being masterful in applying techniques to 'control' people. In contrast to this, our ethical tradition is that moral virtue requires effort and growth in the development of personal integrity and practical moral competence. Even the word 'conscience' in the European tradition does not mean capricious or arbitrary judgement, but stands for an educated and disciplined intellectual faculty in which theoretical knowledge of universal principles and practical experience are skilfully combined and applied to real-life problems to achieve the best possible outcome for all concerned.

In Chapter 2 we pointed out the connection between the fundamental principles (of beneficence, justice and respect for persons) and the different modalities of power in human relationships:

The *principle of beneficence*, or the protective duty of responsible care for others, *has to do with the duty the strong owe to the weak and vulnerable* because we are all weak and vulnerable at different times in our lives and need the help of other people, particularly when we are very young or very old, seriously ill, injured or mentally disordered. Doctors and nurses can become ill, injured or mentally disordered, as readily as other individuals, and will thus need others to exercise a duty of care towards them.

The *principle of justice, or universal fairness, is fundamentally about different kinds of power-sharing. Distributive justice* is concerned with how we share power, knowledge, skills and resources with those who lack them – for the good of both individuals and society. *Protective justice* is about how we prevent the abuse of power, by policing observance of the law, and protecting people from violation of their rights, from insult or assault, exploitation, torture, discrimination or oppression. *Retributive justice* is about how we ensure that victims of crime or abuse have equal access to the courts to make complaints, to seek compensation or redress, or the punishment of offenders; and, if accused, have the right to due process, fair and public trial, and to legal representation.

The *principle of respect for persons*, or respect for the dignity and rights of other people, has to do with *mutual empowerment* of one another within both our local and wider moral communities. Respect for the dignity of all persons, as fellow members of the human moral community, and as bearers of rights and responsibilities, is ultimately in our own interests too, for it helps to protect our own dignity and moral autonomy, thus empowering us as moral agents. The abuse of power, which is involved in failure to respect the dignity and rights of other people, contradicts the principle of reciprocity (Do not do to others what you would not have them do to you). Common sense demands that we recognise that while we may be powerful today, we may be very vulnerable tomorrow, and need others to care for us and respect our rights. While there are all too many cases of patients and clients who are neglected or abused, particularly among the 'captive populations' in institutional care, most carers feel diminished themselves when they humiliate another person, or disregard the privacy or dignity of other people – particularly when the person is vulnerable and dependent on them for care and protection – because they are aware of the contradiction involved.

Against the trend to privatise ethics, we wish to assert therefore that in a fundamental sense ethics is concerned with power, power relationships, and power-sharing – with the responsible use (or the abuse) of power in one's personal life, professional work, and in our social institutions. However, we also wish to assert that ethics is concerned with values – with those things that we choose to value because they enable us to achieve our personal goals and fulfilment as human beings. In fact, personal commitment to a set of values gives us the motivation and power to act (Aristotle (Thomson, tr) 1976).

The connection between power and values should be evident in what we have said above about the way fundamental ethical principles function as power principles relating to the different kinds of changing relationships between people. It relates to both our striving for personal fulfilment and our service of other people.

Our personal quest for health, prosperity, fame, and the respect or admiration of others, is ultimately about our quest for power, for fulfilment of our potential powers of being, whether our quest is 'worldly' or 'spiritual'. The literal meaning of the term 'health' in most European languages connects it with two kinds of reality: the quest for fulfilment of our *potential* (power of being) as human beings, and the ideal or value of *the strength of wholeness*. Both are combined in the WHO definition of health: 'Health is complete physical, mental and social well-being, and not simply the absence of disease, or infirmity' (WHO 1947). Taken in isolation this definition has been widely criticised for being unrealistic and Utopian. However, it needs to be seen in the context of the remarkable achievements brought about by the cooperation of international agencies like UNESCO, the Food and Agricultural Organization, the World Bank, the World Development Agency and the World Health Organization, to address the wider social and economic causes of disease. Collectively they have sought to translate into reality the aspirations of the United Nations expressed in the WHO definition of health. Serious efforts have been made to address ignorance, poverty, hunger, lack of fundamental services (such as water and sanitation), and to improve infrastructure such as roads and communications, not just by direct health interventions, but also by promoting economic growth and social development.

For nurses, as well as other healthcare workers, the responsible use of power, to promote their own health and well-being and that of their patients, combines both the need for the responsible exercise of power and its direction by appropriate values – other-regarding values as well as self-regarding ones.

Different levels of power relationships in human affairs

How are the concepts of power and power-sharing, on the one hand, and values or ideals, on the other, related to one another, and what do they mean in more practical terms in nursing ethics?

Let us attempt to unpack what is implied in these concepts, starting with *our* definition of ethics in terms of its relationship to individual potential, power-sharing and responsibility in interpersonal relationships, power structures in social institutions, and power relations between different institutions:

- *Ethics in our personal and professional life as health professionals* is about our responsibility to develop our own human potentialities or 'virtues', both for our own sake and to be able to contribute more

effectively to the service of others. It also means avoiding those things that prevent us realising our full potential as nurses and human beings. Ethics in nursing means dealing with the power of the nurse, and degree of authority, or lack of authority exercised by the individual nurse within the nursing hierarchy – depending on the actual status and seniority of the nurse.

- *Ethics as related to power-sharing in the relations of nurses and their patients or clients* can be expressed in a number of different modes, which we refer to as code, contract, covenant and charter. In analysing these we explore the ethics of the caring role, service role, the supportive role, and the role as accountable public officer (May 1975).

- *Ethics as related to power relationships between different professions in interprofessional teamwork* concerns the way power is shared (or not shared) in the relationships between nurses, doctors, other health workers, social workers and chaplains in hospital and community settings. While nurses have a certain degree of power over patients, they may have limited power to control their work, and even more limited power to decide what treatment or care patients should or should not be given. This has to do with their generally subordinate professional role, even in relation to junior doctors, but is also related to the traditional status of nursing as a mainly female profession within a male-dominated and largely patriarchal health service. Changes in the gender balance of doctors and other professions may well change the power balance and relationships here. However, within nursing, men in powerful positions are disproportionately over-represented in comparison to their numbers within nursing as a whole. In medicine, despite the fact that more than 50% of entrants are women – and have been for many years now – this is not reflected in a corresponding increase in the number of women holding senior posts in medicine (particularly within hospital settings). The ability of women to achieve powerful positions in healthcare (or indeed other occupations) may be inhibited more by the time (and thus opportunity) 'lost' on the career ladder due to maternity leave, the subsequent lack of childcare support and the inflexible working hours of healthcare occupations, rather than by institutionalised discrimination against women.

- *Ethics as it relates to corporate power structures in social institutions*, including hospitals and colleges of nursing, primary care units and community settings, is concerned with management of relations with the internal and external 'stakeholders' of the institution and development of appropriate systems and procedures for this purpose. Structures of power and authority, in principle, are set up to ensure the flourishing of the corporate body, and the well-being of its members and clients. They are also meant to provide a framework for public accountability of healthcare workers. Managers also have to direct policy and public relations with external stakeholders and institutions, including local and national government. To study the range and variety of these relations we will examine four types of models of management in Chapter 9: command management, critical expert, community development and corporate planning.

Personal moral virtues or competencies

It is perhaps obvious that nursing ethics must relate first and foremost to the integrity and competence of individual nurses, and to the responsibility of the nursing profession to ensure nurses receive appropriate education and training to ensure their personal and professional development as nurses. Thus nursing ethics (as emphasised in Chapters 3 and 5) must address the academic and clinical training of nurses, their moral formation, their personal growth, standards of professional competence and nurses' continuing education.

Developing competence as moral agents requires, among other things, critical insight into the 'moral prejudices' and personal moral baggage that we bring with us to our work. We also need to develop sound theoretical knowledge of moral principles, and practical skills in ethical decision-making, clarifying values and goals and skills in setting policy and standards with colleagues. To achieve this requires what Aristotle would call cultivation of the moral and intellectual virtues, specifically as they apply to nurses at all levels in the care and management of other people. This kind of moral development is now identified (within the UK by the Nursing and Midwifery Council (NMC)), as a 'competence' that must be acquired by nursing students during their undergraduate programme. Its attainment must be demonstrated in theory and in practice settings.

Aristotle's discussion of the virtues, and what is called 'virtue ethics', has direct relevance to the professional development of nurses. Unfortunately, the terms 'virtue' and 'vice', in common English usage, tend to conjure up moralistic associations and images of saints and sinners. In order to understand the relevance of the classical notion of 'virtue' and 'vice', it

is useful to compare their meaning to the notion of competence or incompetence, as used in appraisal of staff 'competencies' and in 'competency-based training' in nursing (Aristotle (Thomson, tr) 1976, Bk III).

In his *Nicomachean Ethics*, Aristotle describes the *intellectual virtues* as combining scientific knowledge with acquired practical expertise in the application of scientific method to everyday problems. Prudence or practical wisdom includes knowledge and technical expertise, and combines reflective and intuitive understanding, intelligence, insight and skill in judgement. Regarding the *moral or practical virtues*, he considers the virtues of courage and temperance as necessary for self-control and the exercise of moral responsibility, but the key social virtue is justice or fairness. Other lesser moral virtues or personal competencies that he identifies are: generosity, magnanimity, honour and a sense of style, a good temper, honesty, amiability, communication skills, a sense of humour, and modesty or a realistic assessment of one's own worth. The intellectual and moral virtues represent as it were, the two legs of an arch in which prudence or practical wisdom is the keystone. Prudence, for Aristotle, is the most essential and critical virtue required by the competent and mature moral agent. Prudence is defined as competence based on skilled application of relevant knowledge of moral and practical principles to specific situations, enabling choice of the best means to a good end (Aristotle (Thomson, tr), 1976, Bk VI, i–vii).

Nurse education has always involved both direct and indirect instruction in ethics, but it was previously more of the 'Ten Commandments' variety, i.e. a set of rules to which the nurse should adhere unquestioningly. In recent years there has been more encouragement within the curriculum to develop 'ethical imagination', and this links with the greater emphasis on 'holistic care'. How much this is just a matter of rhetoric and how much internalisation of 'ethical imagination' actually occurs and is translated into more thoughtful practice, is another matter!

However, modern developments require much more thorough integration of practical training in ethics and scope for the moral formation of nurses in nurse education, as well as explicit integration of ethical review in all nursing processes, including nursing management. In Chapter 3, 'Becoming a nurse and member of the profession', and Chapter 5, 'Professional responsibility and accountability in nursing', it is argued that nurses are being exposed to various forms of moral formation, whether consciously or unconsciously, deliberately or inadvertently, through their induction into nursing and working in a variety of healthcare settings. The challenge facing those teaching ethics to nurses is to ensure that the form and content of direct 'education' rather than training in ethics facilitates the development of relevant skills and competencies in ethical decision-making. Appropriate learning environments also need to be created, where the moral and intellectual formation of nurses can be nurtured. This is not easy, as facilities within universities increasingly have to accommodate large groups that make in-depth exploration of topics difficult. Further, within practice placements a variety of standards and levels of student support apply. Besides a capacity for cognitive learning, other competencies relevant to nurses as moral agents include: skills in individual counselling and sharing in groups, ability to provide mentorship and supervision, skilled facilitation of groups, performance appraisal at personal, team and institutional levels, and both fair and competent management of others.

Talk about 'virtue' and 'vice' in professional ethics has been suspect for some time, unless it is in valedictory speeches praising a departing colleague's virtues, or in disciplinary hearings where someone's misconduct or negligence is at issue. However, recent stress on 'competencies', and attempts to define these, involves a return to something like the classical meaning of 'virtue' as 'proficiency or excellence in performance' and 'vice' as 'culpable incompetence'. The value of this form of language is that it gets away from moralising, and focuses on what kinds of education and training could remedy the deficits of the individual/s concerned. It follows therefore that in assessing the 'virtues' (or 'vices') of nurses, we are not attempting to measure their moral temperature, state of sanctity or moral laxity, but rather their practical competencies, or standards of professional performance under normal working conditions. Some of the ethical competencies that we should be able to demonstrate if we are to act confidently and proficiently as moral agents are outlined in Box 4.1.

Furthermore it is important to stress that ethics is not only concerned with how we exercise power and authority over other people, or exercise responsibility in caring for the health and well-being of other people, it is also concerned with striving to fulfil our personal potential as human beings. Ethics is not simply other-related. It is also about our responsibility to develop our own skills and talents, to ensure our own personal development and fulfilment of our life goals. If ethics is about how we share power in human communities, then it is also about how we protect one another's rights and promote one another's good. An egocentric ethics will place the emphasis on my right to fulfil my own powers of being as a person to the exclusion

> ### Box 4.1 Ethical competencies
>
> - Ability to clarify our own personal and professional values and goals, and exhibit insight into the distinction between them, and to show sensitivity to the different values and goals of other people.
>
> - Understanding of fundamental ethical principles demonstrated in ability to apply these with discriminating judgement to specific practical cases in one's working environment.
>
> - Proficiency in the application of relevant problem-solving and decision-making skills in dealing with general or nursing-specific, routine or difficult and problematic, situations.
>
> - Interpersonal, group-work and group leadership skills, relevant to teamwork, negotiation with management and other professional colleagues, and skills in supervision of junior staff.
>
> - Ability to give a reasoned account of one's decisions and actions – to set out clearly the key facts of the case, one's choice of appropriate means, and the principles or rules applied in reaching a decision.

of consideration of the rights of others. An altruistic ethics will tend to sacrifice self-interest (or one's personal rights) in the service of others, so that the other person may fulfil their rights or potential. Clearly both approaches are needed.

In practice, nursing ethics must recognise the need for a balance between both job satisfaction and personal fulfilment in a nursing career, for without adequate emphasis on the needs of the nurse, the quality of patient care is likely to suffer. Frustration and poor staff morale is likely to undermine competence and efficiency in the service. On the other hand, working within an occupation that delivers care and treatment to others, respecting their dignity and value as human beings, provides practitioners with job satisfaction. Mere careerism, or the attitude of 'it's just another job', deprives nursing of professional dignity if these other-regarding values of care are neglected. However, some forms of care can be dependency creating, turning people into perennial 'patients', if nursing care is not directed to empower patients to 'stand on their own feet again', and to restore autonomy, where possible, to people who have lost it as a consequence of illness, injury or mental disorder. This was stressed as a key obligation in the original, 1979, RCN Draft Code of Ethics for Nurses and continues to be emphasised by the Nursing and Midwifery Council (2004). Thus the ethics of nursing, like that of other caring professions, is fundamentally about the sensitive sharing of power with vulnerable people in order to facilitate their recovery of independence (Campbell 1985). However, Davies (1995, p. 29) has argued that undue emphasis on patient autonomy may be unhelpful, because restoration of full independence is sometimes an unrealistic aspiration. Davies suggests that a focus on *inter*dependence and 'providing appropriate support' may be a more productive and realistic aim for some patients.

Responsibility and accountability, power and authority

Ethically, to be designated a 'responsible person' implies a number of things, namely that one is, or can be presumed to be, *a self-conscious rational being who:*

- is capable of acting as an independent moral agent
- is competent to perform the task in hand
- is capable of making a response to other people
- acknowledges a legal or moral obligation of some kind
- has proved that they are reliable and trustworthy
- can give an account of what they have done and why.

In the last-mentioned sense, responsibility is inclusive of accountability, the ability to *give an account* of one's actions, in particular to give a coherent, rational and ethical justification for what one has done. The main difference between responsibility and accountability is perhaps that the former is self-reflexive, namely relating to oneself as a moral agent, whereas accountability relates to one's relationship to other moral agents, in particular to those who have authority over us, although it may also include reference to oneself.

It may be useful in this connection to distinguish between two different kinds of *responsibility to*, and two kinds of *responsibility for*, and to give their more technical names (Box 4.2).

Box 4.2 **Responsibility and accountability**

Responsibility *for* one's own actions	(personal responsibility)
Responsibility *for* the care of someone	(fiduciary responsibility)
Responsibility *to* higher authority	(professional accountability)
Responsibility *to* wider society	(public accountability/ civic duty)

Personal responsibility

Ordinarily one is held responsible for one's own actions and omissions, and praised or blamed for them, provided the following conditions are satisfied:

- that one knows what one is doing
- one has acted freely and voluntarily
- one is capable of performing or avoiding the action
- one can distinguish between right and wrong.

(The last includes awareness of the obligations one is under and one's liability to be praised or blamed depending on how one discharges one's obligations.)

It is this sense of responsibility that is involved when one's own moral actions are under scrutiny, or one has to appear before an investigating inquiry, or one is being tried for negligence in a court. On the other hand, *excusing conditions*, which may be taken into account in determining the degree of guilt and/or possible diminished responsibility involved, relate to the criteria above, and are:

- ignorance of any of the following: the circumstances, the specific nature of the obligations involved, or of the likely consequences of one's action or failure to act
- inability to perform, or to avoid performing, the required action because one lacks the power, skill or authority to act or to desist from action
- acting under threat or duress, or due to compulsion of some kind, including the effect of the stress of the circumstances, shock or grief, or factors beyond one's control
- one's inexperience in the exercise of the relevant kind of responsibility (see also Chapter 11).

Fiduciary responsibility

When someone is entrusted into your care (e.g. a child, or an unconscious or mentally disturbed patient), or when a patient voluntarily *entrusts* themselves into your hands, whether as a nurse or in the context of lay care, you acquire 'fiduciary responsibility' (from Latin *fiducia* = trust). Accepting responsibility for the care and treatment of patients, or for decisions about their individual and collective well-being, is a matter of fiduciary responsibility, and the moral authority or power of nurses to do these things derives from the trust which patients and society place in them.

Professional accountability

The professional responsibility vested in nurses by society is underwritten in Britain by the Nursing and

Midwifery Council (NMC), which, whilst it has a UK-wide remit, devolves some aspects of its responsibilities to individual countries within the UK. These are: Nurse Education Scotland (NES), Health Professions Wales (HPW) and the Northern Ireland Practice and Education Council for Nursing and Midwifery (NIPEC). As a result, nurses have a basic obligation to their colleagues, of *professional accountability*. In practice this duty of accountability means a variety of different things depending on whether it is to justify their actions to their peers, to their superiors, to the NMC, or to society – through the courts if necessary. This general duty of professional accountability follows from the responsibilities delegated and entrusted to registered nurses, by the profession, the healthcare system, and society.

Professional accountability to the Nursing and Midwifery Council – when complaints made to the NMC about a practitioner are investigated – follows a strict procedure. If the complaint has substance then the practitioner is informed and invited to attend a meeting of the Professional Conduct Committee. Following their investigations, if the complaint is upheld, then a variety of options are available to the Committee: e.g. to remove the practitioner's registration or to give 'advice' to the practitioner. This is rather different from a nurse's general legal accountability before the courts, under criminal or civil law, or where there is a breach of contractual duty to one's employer. Only following such investigations would disciplinary action be taken, but this might not relate to actual professional misconduct, but rather to incompetence or a poor work record. The UK National Patient Safety Agency is consulting on a 'Safer practice notice' on 'Being open when patients are harmed'. This outlines a procedure in which the most senior person responsible for the patient's care should 'acknowledge what happened and apologise on behalf of the team and the organisation'. It notes that 'the National Health Service Litigation Authority (NHSLA) circular 02/2002, encouraged healthcare staff to apologise to patients who had been harmed as a result of their healthcare treatment, and explained that an apology is not an admission of liability'. The Medical Defence organisations have been giving similar advice to doctors for some time.

Many nurses will feel both responsible *for* and responsible *to* their patients, and to relatives as well. Because nurses are responsible *for* the well-being of their patients, they may feel guilty if things go wrong and consider that some kind of explanation or apology is due to the patient or relatives. The sentiment might be right, and in some circumstances explanations or apologies might be in order, but it is generally thought inappropriate for the individual nurse to apologise, or to admit being at fault, or to attempt to offer explanations to patients or relatives, as this might also expose the nurse, or the hospital, to prosecution for negligence in cases where the patient has suffered hurt or injury. In that sense, nurses are not accountable to their patients directly (although they may be held accountable *by* their patients, who may prosecute them or take civil action against them through the courts). The current trend towards Charters of Patients' Rights and Quality Assurance means that in some circumstances it may be appropriate for the Health Authority (rather than the individual nurse) to give the patient a personal apology, after investigating a complaint of alleged negligence – if it is clear that quality standards have not been maintained or a mistake has been made.

Registered nurses are personally accountable *for* their practice to their employers and to their profession. In situations in which an error has been made, they should take immediate steps to rectify it and, subsequently, take action to prevent or minimise its future occurrence. As part of this process, the situation would be reported via nursing line management to determine the appropriate course of action, given the specific circumstances.

Public accountability and/or civic duty

Nurses do not act as private citizens, but as individuals who hold public office – whether working in a state or private healthcare setting, or as permanent or temporary members of staff. That is, they are employed as members of a public institution with corporate responsibilities. As such, nurses are held to be publicly accountable, in both a legal and moral sense, for the standard of care given to patients and for responsible use of public resources. As qualified and accredited members of the nursing profession, also as employees within the state healthcare system (or private institutions), nurses also have a duty of public accountability for maintaining the general standards of nursing. Nurses are public officers, even public servants, with both civic and political duties. For example, nurses have both a civic duty and also a professional duty to report, or draw attention to, specific examples of incompetence or negligence, where patients are being abused, or where standards of patient care have become unacceptable. This is made clear in the NMC *Code of Conduct* (NMC 2004). Nurses cannot avoid the 'political' responsibilities they carry as public officers – for example, the duty to change bad practice, to take action to improve standards of care, to prevent waste, to address injustice or discrimination where it arises, and to influence health policy and the allocation of resources – for the benefit of patients in general.

Power and authority

Public discussion of the ethical responsibilities of nurses tends to focus on their use, and possible abuse, of power over patients who are entrusted into their care. However, from the nurse's point of view, some of the most painful practical dilemmas arise because they lack the *authority* to act on their own – to exercise their own judgement and take the initiative, to go against doctors' or senior nurses' orders, e.g. to give information to patients or relatives about the patient's medical diagnosis or prognosis. However, any nurse who believes that the treatment prescribed for a patient is wrong or inappropriate has a duty to inform their line manager. Here even charge nurses can experience some of the classic problems of 'middle management', namely those of having to carry a lot of responsibility for, but lacking the necessary executive authority to do anything about a situation. This is a common predicament of the person in the mediating or intermediate role between someone in authority and a patient or client.

> Relations (of nurses) with patients are closely tied into relations with other members of the institution, and are importantly influenced by the terms of their place in the hierarchy. Nursing care thus occupies an 'in between' position in the organisation of the public response to the patient's need, and is infused with the tensions of sustaining interdependent but differently focused relations with different levels of authority.
> (Bowden 1997, p. 104)

We have emphasised that ethics is about power-sharing and the responsible exercise of power, but we need perhaps to distinguish more clearly between the responsible exercise of *power over others* (whether power over patients or in managing other staff), and executive authority or *power to initiate action*, intervene, to direct policy or to issue orders. To have power over someone else depends on one having the strength or ability to impress the person to submit to your authority over them – whether it be as a leader, expert or professional carer. Or it may be the result of having been authorised to exercise some function, or delegated power by some higher authority. In each case there is an assumption that if executive power is to be effective it must be based on actual strength, knowledge, skill, competence or experience of the kind required to legitimate exercise of that power. 'Power to act' relates to the concept of 'authority', whether that be the power to act on one's own

authority based on one's position or acknowledged power, or on the basis of delegated authority from someone else with more power in the team or in the institution.

'Power' here relates to potential or actual ability to do something; 'authority' relates to the conditions for actual exercise of power. Authority (from the Latin *augere* = to implement or augment) defines the moral conditions under which we exercise power – *to implement* actions or policies that serve to *augment the well-being* of those for whom we are responsible, and over whom we have authority. These functions of implementing the policy in such a way that it is seen to augment the well-being of all within the institution or moral community legitimate the exercise of authority within it. Unless the exercise of authority can be seen to satisfy these conditions, it is without moral legitimacy, and becomes the naked expression of the will to power or domination of others. These moral constraints apply to both established and to delegated authority – where the power to execute orders or to ensure the implementation of the policies is given by higher authority.

When nurses are compelled to weigh their responsibility for individual patients against their institutional responsibilities for groups of patients, they may be faced with a conflict of duties. The actual authority vested in nurses, and reinforced by their regulatory body (in the UK, the NMC), to serve the best interests of patients may contrast with the actual or relative lack of power which nurses have. This will depend, in part, on the position of the individual nurse within the nursing hierarchy and/or their relationships with other professional staff. In reality, the culture of trust or distrust within a ward team may have a great deal to do with how much or how little power or scope nurses have, individually or collectively, to negotiate care provision. In a climate of trust it may well be that experienced registered nurses may be allowed to exercise discretion and independent judgement. Alternatively, nurses may find both formal and informal ways to put pressure on doctors, or to 'guide' inexperienced medical staff as to what 'ought to be done' and thus achieve increased influence over care provision. In the largely 'gendered' social order of hospital nursing (in contrast perhaps to community nursing services), nurses may find themselves having to resort to the stratagems commonly employed by people in subordinate positions of relative powerlessness, or under conditions of oppression, to achieve their ends.

> In keeping with the dominant norms of this (largely patriarchal) order, nursing care is encumbered with much of the social apparatus that operates to undermine

both the value of women's practices in general and the social possibilities of their practitioners. (Bowden 1997, p. 104)

What nurses are entitled to do by law, and what it is or is not permissible for them to do, according to their regulatory body, their union or professional association, may also have a bearing on the matter. We return to some of these dilemmas of responsibility and authority in Chapters 10 and 11.

FOUR MODELS FOR THE ETHICS OF CARER–CLIENT RELATIONSHIPS

Before examining four models for the ethics of carer/client relationships – *code, contract, covenant* and *charter* – we shall briefly consider the kinds of issues that affect the scope of the ethics of healthcare generally, and of nursing ethics in particular. The first point concerns what has been called the 'medicalisation of life'; the second relates to the relevance of different contexts in defining what is meant by ethical responsibility.

Back in 1977 Ivan Illich put forward a wealth of historical evidence, in his book *Medical Nemesis*, to demonstrate that over the previous century and a half, medicine and the medical profession had come to exercise increasing power and control over our lives, from birth to death (Illich 1977). This process of 'medical imperialism', resulting in what he calls the 'medicalisation of life', is reflected in several historical developments:

- the increasing specialisation and professionalisation of medicine, nursing and allied professions
- the 'colonisation' by medical services of areas of human life that have been, traditionally, the domain of lay care (e.g. antenatal care and obstetrics, care of the mentally ill, terminal care and bereavement counselling, dietary advice, sex therapy and assisted reproduction)
- the growing dependence of lay people on medical and/or alternative medicine experts for help, with the corresponding loss of skills and confidence among lay people
- the increasing institutionalisation of healthcare, and consequent hospitalisation of mentally and physically handicapped people, of elderly people and those terminally ill.

Despite recent trends to deinstitutionalise healthcare (particularly in the case of those with mental health problems or learning difficulties), the effects of this medicalisation of life in industrialised countries have been far-reaching. This is especially important if the effect of other general demographic trends is taken into account (such as declining birth rates and an increased proportion of elderly people in the populations of these countries). These developments also have had profound implications for the way we understand the ethics of healthcare and choices about forms of service delivery.

The use of complementary therapies has increased exponentially since earlier editions of this book. It was recently reported in a study by Molassiotis et al (2005) that an average of 35.9% of cancer patients in the 14 EU countries studied use complementary therapies in addition to, or instead of, those offered by conventional medicine. The authors of this study recommend that health professionals explore the use of complementary therapies with cancer patients, educate them about their usefulness and work towards an integrated model of healthcare provision.

With the rise of a more consumer-led approach to healthcare, and people using complementary therapies, there is a risk that these will reduce the efficacy of, or interact adversely with, the standard medical drugs or treatments that patients have been prescribed. As some patients may be reluctant to tell doctors, or nurses, that they are taking complementary therapies, this increases the risk of complications in treatment. With increased questioning of medical 'authority' and the marketing of so-called 'natural' remedies, some people have become suspicious of 'high-tech medicine' and the 'fancy new drugs' being aggressively marketed by the pharmaceutical industry.

These trends raise important questions for nurses about the extent of their clinical and ethical responsibilities to patients in this changing health environment.

Recognition of these world trends has already led in the past 15 years to major new initiatives such as the World Health Organization's *Health for All 2000* programme (WHO 1978, 1979, 1981). National programmes, driven by state-directed health education and health promotion services, have attempted to reverse this medicalisation of every aspect of life, by raising consciousness of health matters by lay people and so encouraging them to take responsibility for their own health. WHO has also sought to influence governments to shift resources from intensive, high-technology, hospital-based care, to primary care and prevention, for the sake of achieving greater equity in healthcare. However, medicalisation of human life and its *rites de passage* is still the dominant reality in most developing countries, where in many cases dependence on institutional healthcare is promoted by a globalised healthcare industry. Even in Europe the vast majority of mothers still have their babies delivered in hospital rather than at home – with increasingly high levels of technical monitoring, intervention and caesarean sections. People depend on specialist and 'self-help' clinics to deal with problems ranging from drug and alcohol abuse, to obesity, family planning, sexual problems and stress management. Finally, the great majority of people die in hospital or in special terminal care units, whereas in previous centuries these life events would have been dealt with at home or in the community. Medicalisation of life and institutionalisation of healthcare have brought their own special complications to the discussion of ethics in healthcare.

There has been a reaction against medicalisation in the UK and elsewhere, e.g. in areas of mental health and learning disability, due to public pressure. In the UK the National Association for Mental Health (MIND) and the Scottish Association for Mental Health have campaigned successfully not only for the reform of mental health legislation, but also for the provision of more adequate community-based accommodation where people with mental health problems can enjoy more independent living. This has led to a reversal of policies for the institutionalisation of patients with mental illness or severe learning difficulties, and to a well-intentioned but not altogether successful attempt to treat these problems in the community. Through lack of adequate resources, 'community care' has often meant that care of these patients becomes a burden on families that are ill-equipped to cope. Instead of liberating and 'valorising' people who have learning difficulties or mental health problems, this sometimes has had a detrimental effect and individuals are recycled into institutions via the criminal justice system.

The countervailing international movement towards 'self help' has perhaps mitigated the effects of medicalisation, encouraged by the proliferation of alternative medicine and private therapies, state-sponsored health promotion and the focus on health in the media and in particular in glossy health magazines. The public are constantly encouraged, usually by government-funded initiatives, to take more responsibility for their own health.

The second point, namely the importance of context in defining ethical responsibility, relates to the fact that *there are subtle and important differences between the ethics of different situations and settings in healthcare*. Professional ethics in primary care or community settings differs in important respects from that which governs relationships in hospitals or other institutions (Freidson 1970, 1994, Bayles 1989, Windt et al 1989).

Different rules and constraints operate in each case. Yet other rules govern hospital management, political roles in the health professions, and the development of health policy, making the ethics of these domains different again. This is not to say that the fundamental ethical principles and values that are applicable are not the same, but rather that the substantive problems and constraints, rules and forms of accountability, vary greatly with the exercise of power and responsibility in each of these different settings.

In this and the preceding discussion we have made use of four key concepts which are derived from sociological analysis of caring relationships, but which are very important and useful in philosophical analysis of ethics too. These concepts are: *situations, roles, rules* and *arbiters* (first suggested by Emmet (1966) and Thompson (1979a)).

It may seem obvious that the nurse meets patients or clients in a variety of different kinds of *situations*, but we do not usually take account of how much these situations differ ethically.

Consider the following situations:

- a district nurse attending a patient in their own home
- a casualty nurse dealing with an unconscious patient in an accident and emergency department
- a hospital nurse attending a distressed patient in bed in an open or private ward
- a psychiatric nurse dealing with a compulsorily detained patient in a locked ward
- a health visitor offering health education at a 'well woman' or 'well man' clinic
- a nurse manager relating to the staff and patients of a whole hospital.

While we may be aware of these different situations, it is not always so obvious that the nurse's *role* in each of these *situations* may be different, that the *rules* of practice defining ethical duties and responsibilities in each context may be different, and nurses will be accountable to different people, who act as *arbiters* of their performance, in each context.

It is the aim of the next section to explore a number of different models for direct care and management relationships, to demonstrate how roles, rules and arbiters change in different professional settings or situations. The significance of these concepts, for analysing the social context of a moral decision, is examined in detail Chapter 12.

Code, contract, covenant and charter

Nurses work in a wide variety of contexts and each of these presents the nurse with different kinds of ethical demands and ethical responsibility. These may be grouped roughly into four types:

1. *Crisis intervention* – e.g. in accident and emergency, intensive care, emergency obstetrics, or acute medical, surgical or psychiatric units.
2. *Consulting role* – e.g. giving advice on family planning, antenatal or postnatal care, interviewing or assessing competent adult patients, and making domiciliary visits in a monitoring, advisory, supportive or clinical capacity.
3. *Continuity of care* – e.g. assisting people with health maintenance or care with enduring conditions. (The first is the situation where the nurse is being proactive, helping people who are well, but whose lifestyles put them at risk. The second may refer to terminal care, but it applies equally to situations of ongoing care of people with severe learning disabilities, enduring mental or physical health problems, or who are frail older adults.)
4. *Competition for service delivery and 'customer focus'* – e.g. where nurses are part of a consortium tendering to supply services, in competition with other service providers, with the emphasis on best value for money. (Here the institution may have to give certain undertakings, relative to its service delivery, to maintain certain standards of performance on the part of its staff, as part of its quality assurance to customers, i.e. to other hospitals, health centres, clinics, general practitioners, or private patients.)

In these four different situations, (a) in crisis intervention, (b) in a consultative role, (c) in providing health maintenance or continuity of care in enduring illness, and, finally, (d) 'customer focused' service delivery, professional ethics tends to be governed by different kinds of ethical models, namely: *code-based, contractual, covenantal,* and *charter-based* ethics respectively. The original distinction between 'code', 'contract' and 'covenant' was suggested by William May in 1975, in his paper 'Code, Covenant, Contract or Philanthropy' in the *Hastings Center Report*, No. 5, but we have adapted and expanded his useful distinctions and have added another, namely 'charter'.

Let us examine these models, identifying the key ethical principle in each (Box 4.3).

By emphasising the key principle that underlies each model we do not wish to suggest that the other principles have no bearing. For example, the application of the code model will raise questions of justice to other parties as well as the duty to care for an individual patient. The contract model presupposes respect for the rights and autonomy of the contracting

Box 4.3 Code, contract, covenant and charter – models for professional ethics

CODE	The duty of advocacy, to care for the patient or client
Paradigm:	Crisis intervention
Client:	Very dependent, vulnerable
Professional:	In total control, acts *parens patriae* as parent for the state
Key principle:	Protective beneficence (or non-maleficence)
CONTRACT	Regard for mutual rights/duties of health professional and patient
Paradigm:	Voluntary request for help
Client:	Independent, competent, ambulant
Professional:	Offers service, acts in client's interest – fiduciary responsibility
Key principle:	Justice and equity (or universal fairness)
COVENANT	Professional seeks to enable and empower the patient
Paradigm:	Befriending, mutual partnership
Client:	Self-directed, seeking support, companionship, partnership
Professional:	Promotes autonomy of client as equal partner, acts *pares inter pares*
Key principle:	Respect for a person's rights (unconditional regard)
CHARTER	Professional gives assurance of quality and standard of service provided
Paradigm:	Customer service and professional/institutional accountability to clients
Client:	Seen as 'customer' or 'purchaser' of service
Professional:	Professional makes themselves professionally/financially accountable
Key principle:	Contractual justice (professional responsibility and respect for client)

parties in addition to matters of contractual justice. While the covenant model places the emphasis particularly on respect for the patient's autonomy, it must also involve the exercise of due care. Finally, the charter model like the contract model requires respect for the rights and autonomy of the customer in addition to issues of justice.

Historically the *reactive crisis intervention model* of healthcare has tended to set the agenda for nursing ethics and the ethics of healthcare generally, rather than the model of proactive intervention (e.g. in screening, prevention and health education). It is important to be aware that the reactive and proactive stances involve different ethical rules, assumptions and responsibilities. For example, in crisis intervention and consulting roles that are mainly *reactive* to a presenting problem or crisis, the nurse is required to exercise a primary duty of care that is one of protective beneficence, and doing no harm. By contrast, the nurse is expected to be *proactive* in the different situations of screening, health promotion and health maintenance, for well persons, on the one hand, and in providing 'continuity of care' for people who have enduring physical or mental health problems or whose condition is terminal, on the other. Here the nurse is required to show particular regard or respect for the rights and dignity of the patient or client. In these latter roles the nurse seeks to anticipate problems, to identify available options, to actively suggest solutions, and to continue to offer support when curative therapy is no longer effective, and the patient is dying. Apart from the roles being different, namely in moving from a predominantly reactive to a proactive mode, the functions of the nurse in health education and terminal care might be regarded as *supererogatory*, that is, as involving responsibilities to the patient that 'go beyond the call of duty'. These situations of proactive intervention raise ethical issues of a quite different kind from those which arise for nurses in the exercise of their usual clinical roles, including the need for quality assurance, and charters of patients' rights.

Code (Fig. 4.1)

Historically, each of the caring professions in formulating its professional ethics has tended to do so first in terms of a *code of practice*. Codes of practice or conduct tend to be preoccupied with consideration of what duties professionals must exercise when they are required to intervene in a crisis, particularly where the client or patient (sufferer) is unconscious or unconsultable, or incompetent by virtue of youth, or incapacity (e.g. as defined by the Scottish Adults with Incapacity Act 2000, and similar legislation being developed in England). On the one hand, codes tend to justify intervention in a crisis by appeal to the protective duty of care, which the carer has for the vulnerable, incompetent and incapacitated, and to protect them from harm (the principle of beneficence *or* non-maleficence). On the other hand, because they are in charge, carers are assumed to have fiduciary responsibility for the well-being of the persons committed to their care. Consequently, codes also seek to prevent malpractice or abuse of clients, and to protect the carers themselves from unfair claims or demands being made on them by those for whom they provide care (or their representatives).

CODE — crisis intervention

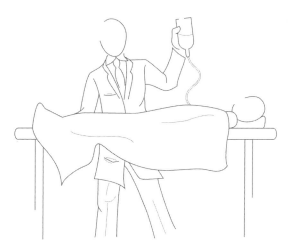

Patient

- Very dependent and may be unconsultable, e.g.
  — unconscious
  — mentally disordered
  — infant or young child
  — incompetent or senile

Health carer

- In position of power
- Total responsibility
- Acts *parens patriae* or *in loco parentis*

Key principle: BENEFICENCE or duty of care

Figure 4.1 Code model.

The law and ethics may often speak of the carer as acting in such situations '*in loco parentis*' (in place of the parent) or '*parens patriae*' (as a parent on behalf of the state). This quasi-parental duty of care carries with it the risk of becoming patronising and of creating and perpetuating dependency in the patient or client. This is because the professional takes it upon themselves to take decisions on behalf of the person dependent on them for help – exemplified by the phrase 'doctor/nurse knows best'. Resulting patronising, professional attitudes and practices have been criticised for tending to 'infantilise' people, to compromise their dignity and disregard their rights.

Codes can serve to entrench the power of the profession over clients, by assuming that the professional is the expert, and the client ignorant, the professional the agent and the client the dependent patient. Codes can be used to specify what is meant by the professional's duty of care to the client. However, they also serve to safeguard the professional's right to clinical autonomy. The statutory requirement that a profession must have a code of ethics in order to be formally registered as a profession has led professions to claim the right to regulate themselves and to have exclusive access to their 'own' confidential client records. Thus, a code can be used both to regulate professional conduct, but also to justify it, because its main focus is on the duties of the professional, rather than on the rights of the client or patient.

However, the duty of care is legally and ethically fundamental, and we cannot dispense with protective beneficence for it remains an important professional value or personal virtue. Because we are all extremely vulnerable at certain times in our lives we will always need others to help and protect us when we are weak or ill, or to decide what is in our best interests when we are unable to do so ourselves.

Contract (Fig. 4.2)

In the *client-initiated consultation*, the client voluntarily approaches the carer with some problem, seeking help. The carer is assumed to have the knowledge, expertise or access to resources to give the necessary help. The carer, in offering a service, is involved in direct negotiation with the client about the nature and scope of the help required and, in the process, establishes either a formal or informal *contract to care*. The client, by voluntarily entrusting himself or herself into the care of the carer, accepts the *responsibility to cooperate* with the carer in the help or treatment given, for example, by giving relevant personal details, allowing physical examination or other kinds of tests and assessments to be made. This is their part in the contract, namely to adhere to or comply with the treatment or advice given. (The term 'concordance' is often used now, to denote a more equal partnership and mutual understanding between patient and healthcare professional in the contract to care. The term 'non-compliance' was previously used (and still is) but 'non-adherence' is now preferred, as a less 'patient-blaming' phrase.)

The carer accepts the duty, or *fiduciary responsibility*, to respect the trust shown by the client by providing a competent service, protecting the patient's dignity and observing the requirements of confidentiality. This contractual relationship, like other commercial and legal contracts, is governed by the demands of natural justice and recognition of mutual rights and duties. Although the relationship between the person with the problem and the person with the power to help is an inherently unequal one, the same is likely to be true of our relationship with any service provider – accountant or lawyer, plumber or motor mechanic – from whom we seek help in a crisis.

However, these situations are different from those where one is completely helpless and/or given help

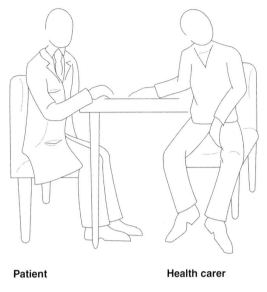

CONTRACT — request for help

Patient

- Independent and able to negotiate terms of care, e.g.
  — lucid and competent
  — mobile and continent
  — voluntary request
  — cooperative

Health carer

- Offers expert help
- Contracts to care
- Acts on fiduciary responsibility

Key principle: JUSTICE — mutual rights/duties

Figure 4.2 Contract model.

without being consulted. The fiduciary responsibility of the carer, as we have explained, is based on the fact that clients entrust themselves into the hands of their carers and agree to bear the cost of that commitment (and do not default on payment – where this is appropriate). Carers have a contractual moral and legal duty or responsibility to perform their service to the best of their ability, with knowledge, skill and consideration for the clients' rights and interests, and not to abuse or exploit their vulnerability. These are obviously requirements of natural justice.

Covenant

In order to clarify what we mean by personal rights (particularly the rights of patients or clients) it is instructive to consider a third type of situation, which we may call a *covenantal relationship*. The need to recognise this different kind of relationship becomes poignantly necessary in situations where the patient is conscious and consultable, but has a long-term or terminal illness. In providing continuity of care in such situations, where there is no hope of cure but only amelioration of symptoms, a different kind of commitment is required on both sides. Here the so-called 'contract to care' may need to be renegotiated and modified to take account of the changed situation.

Where the presuppositions of the original 'contract to care' are based on therapeutic optimism, the client's expectation is that the carer has the necessary knowledge, skills and resources to provide the therapy required. If this situation changes so that the client's condition has become chronic and/or is deteriorating, and if the carer can offer only palliative care or personal support, then the nature of the new situation ought to be acknowledged. What is required is a new kind of agreement that is less formal than a contract, but which expresses an explicit commitment to provide continuity of care, but on terms to be negotiated with the patient and modified if necessary as their condition changes. Because the carer/client relationship changes from a focus on therapy to an emphasis on care, and a shift from *what* is to be done, to *who* does it and *how* and on what terms it is to be done, the emphasis is more on the nature of the interpersonal relationship between client and carer, its open-endedness and the kind of personal commitment involved. For these reasons, the term 'covenant' seems more appropriate than 'contract', to describe this new kind of caring relationship.

Here, because the circumstances applicable to the original 'contract' have changed, the terms of the contract and the client's rights also change. If an ordinary patient has a right to know, the terminally ill should have an enhanced moral right to full information on their condition, so that their right to accept or refuse the form of palliative care being offered is fully respected. They also should have the right to appropriate privacy in negotiations about these matters, The carer, therefore, has a duty to make clear what is being offered. If this is emotional and spiritual support, counselling or just a commitment to 'care to the end', this should be understood on both sides, as involving a change in the terms of the 'contract', and should not be given or imposed against the patient's will (Fig. 4.3).

The new kind of caring relationship which needs to be negotiated in such situations, and which requires a kind of supportive friendship or commitment of mutual fidelity. requires a different name. May (1983) suggested 'covenant', following the biblical meaning – of a commitment of mutual fidelity and unconditional regard for the other. If care is not to be officiously given, or continued without due regard for the patient's views or personal rights, the changed situation must be openly recognised. Further, if the patient is to be prevented from becoming more

COVENANT — terminal care

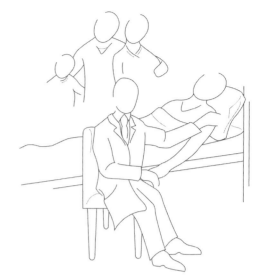

Patient

- Condition chronic or actually terminal,e.g.
  — lucid but very frail
  — mobility limited
  — needs much support
  — cooperative

Health care

- Offers palliation, care (therapy not appropriate)
- Befriending and advocacy role
- Acts on supererogatory duty to promote patient's autonomy and dignity

Key principle: RESPECT— care for person

Figure 4.3 Covenant model.

dependent and either parasitic upon or exploitative of the care given, then despite the vulnerability of the patient, the scope and nature of the continuing care contract needs to be reviewed and renegotiated. Another kind of situation to which covenantal ethics would seem to apply is that of non-directive counselling. Carl Rogers (1961) classically described one of the main ethical requirements for the counselling relationship as being a non-judgemental attitude of respect for the client or one of 'unconditional regard'. This compares with Paul Ramsey's description of the relationship as one of 'covenant-love' (Ramsey 1970).

The principle of respect for persons, which underlies this concept of covenantal ethics, is concerned with protecting the rights and dignity not only of the patient or client, but ultimately those of the carer as well. If the carer's exercise of the supererogatory duties that they take on in these circumstances is not to become a burden to the carer, or to be taken for granted by the patient, then these services cannot be demanded, but have to be freely given by the carer, on the basis of reciprocal trust and friendship.

The different principles of beneficence, justice and respect for persons, which underlie each of these three models respectively, often stand in a relationship of tension to one another, and we must address their competing demands. However, they are not usually mutually exclusive but often make complementary demands on us. Just as there are areas of overlap between the three different kinds of situations, so there are interconnections between beneficence, justice and respect for persons. In crisis intervention, beneficence has to be complemented by considerations of justice and respect for the rights of persons, if its exercise is not to lead to patronising attitudes to patients, and practices that may foster long-term dependency. In the voluntarily negotiated contract to care, the client's vulnerability may still need to be protected, and here beneficence demands that the professional respects the patient's right to properly informed consent and does not exploit their vulnerability. In some situations the needs of a group of patients may be compromised, in the short term, by an individual patient's acute care requirements. Conversely, the rights of individuals may have to be restricted out of consideration for the common good, as in the case where patients may have to be quarantined to protect others, e.g. in the recent severe acute respiratory syndrome (SARS) epidemic. Here the demands of justice and respect for the rights of individuals may appear to be in conflict in the exercise of the general duty to care, and these conflicts need to be addressed and resolved in practice.

Charter

The fourth model we have mentioned is of a client's *charter*. There has been in the past century a major change in the pattern of morbidity in the industrialised countries, with greatly increased life expectancy, due to improved standards of living, better public health and control of the killer infectious diseases. As a result, health professionals have adopted a more proactive approach e.g. to screening for cancer and prevention of lifestyle-related diseases. With this shift from reactive to proactive healthcare, health protection and health promotion, and more proactive marketing of healthcare, it has been necessary to engage the public more directly in negotiation over health policy and priorities in the delivery of healthcare. This has given much greater importance to the views of consumers and taxpayers. The focus in ethics has shifted from the professional's duty of care, to consumers' rights and the need to take account of consumer's preferences. This has led to a demand for quality assurance in the provision of services, and a new emphasis on charters of patient's rights.

Public attitudes to the Welfare State, and the UK NHS, have changed from uncritical acceptance of paternalistic forms of medical authority and a socialised form of healthcare delivery to a demand for more consumer choice: between different medical consultants, treatments offered and the hospital where one receives treatment. Different economic models for the funding of healthcare have also favoured the introduction of various forms of 'internal market' where different providers have to compete for the delivery of the services required by general practitioners or medical consultants for their patients. This in turn has meant that providers have had to guarantee the quality of services they supply.

The demand that health and social services should be operated on this kind of 'business ethic', rather than the more traditional 'service ethic' or 'caring ethic', is driven by several different kinds of moral demand. The primary ethical demands, within this model, are for '*respect* for consumers' rights' and '*justice* to taxpayers' – based on a guarantee from 'providers' to deliver value for money – rather than the model of the state exercising a protective duty of care towards its citizens (Fig. 4.4).

We may ask whether or not the interests of patients are best served this way and, secondly, whether politicians, local or national, are the best advocates for or interpreters of 'consumer's rights' when large contracts are matters of potential patronage! It may be debated whether this should be the case, rather than health professionals making decisions about the best use of scarce medical resources, based on their clinical expertise. Here, health professionals would need to be publicly accountable for the equitable, honest and economical use of public resources.

In the UK there has been pressure from patient support groups, with encouragement from the Government, to make practitioners and managers more accountable, by encouraging health authorities to take account of lay perspectives and to make provision for user participation in developing strategy (Young & Cooke 2001). Most UK health authorities now have a patient involvement group. While this may represent a form of progress, it is debatable how 'representative' individuals who serve on patient involvement groups really are. According to Davies (2001), some appear to be 'professional lay representatives' as they may serve on a number of patient involvement groups, and in the case of the General Medical Council (GMC) and NMC, they have tended to come from a very small 'gene pool' of predominantly white, middle-aged, middle-class, educated professionals (or retired professionals). Selection processes are not always fully transparent, and, prior

CHARTER — health promotion

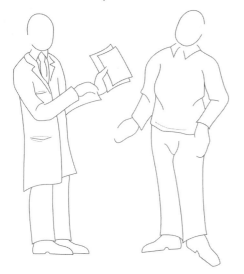

Patient	Health care
• Healthy but at risk because of lifestyle, e.g. — competent and lucid — able to reject advice or accept need for help and freely cooperate	• Proactive professional advice and training • Confidential counsellor and expert 'helper' • Acts on *supererogatory duty to promote patient's health and well-being*

Key principle: RESPECT— empowerment

Figure 4.4 Charter model.

to serving, these patient representatives tend to undergo a process of 'induction' into the nature of their role, which is given by the authority appointing them, e.g. the Scottish Executive Health Department (SEHD), GMC, NMC or Local Health Authority. This induction involves some degree of socialisation into the frames of reference used by the organisation whose functions they are expected to monitor and to which they supposedly provide a lay perspective! (The *Nolan Commission on Standards in Public Life*, recommended that lay people serving on regulatory bodies should be recruited by public advertisement or through the National Audit Office (HMSO 1995, 1996, 1997).

POWER RELATIONS IN INTERPROFESSIONAL TEAMWORK

Power structures and professional status

Few people, with the exception of a small number of self-employed practitioners, work on their own, and even the single-handed practitioner, doctor or nurse, as their workload increases, is likely to require support staff. Most people in their working lives are employed in institutions of some kind and have to learn to work together, and make decisions together, with other people in teams. These teams would almost of necessity be comprised of people with a variety of professional backgrounds and expertise – this diversity, like that of a football or hockey team, being the basis of the strength of the team, but also the source of its potential weakness. Our power can be enhanced by working in teams. We can do more together by cooperation, by pooling our resources and by a sensible division of labour, than we can do unassisted and on our own. However, lack of trust, professional rivalry, non-cooperation, confusion of roles, and inability to share power effectively, can be a disaster – like a football team where a few 'stars' want to 'hog the ball', or the limelight.

To understand the nature of ethics in professional life, we need therefore to take account of the power structures, within our working environments and the complex dynamics of interprofessional relationships as well as the personal relationships we have with our colleagues. To address this complexity the philosopher and social scientist Dorothy Emmet pointed out that the traditional approach to ethics that focuses on the individual and their exercise of decision-making responsibility is inadequate. She suggested that in order to do justice to the complexity of ethical relationships in any functioning moral community (or social institution) we need to distinguish four aspects that she called: *roles*, *rules*, *relations* and *arbiters*. She argues that the way that power is organised and shared, and responsibility and accountability determined, requires that we abandon simplistic models of individual ethical responsibility and decision-making:

> In any formal institution there must be some people who, in virtue of their office, are responsible in the sense of answerable for decisions, policies and their outcomes. This need not mean that they had a major share in making the decision (they may even have their own reservations about it, or not have been able to prevent what happened). They have however, to be prepared to take public responsibility without disclosing their private reservations or giving away confidential matter on how the decision was taken (for some things must be discussed confidentially), and particularly they must be prepared to 'carry the can' if things go wrong. This is a feature of the nature of constitutional responsibility in institutional life. (Emmet 1966, p. 201)

Using her analogy of a play, where actors are assigned different roles (and perhaps more than one role, if the cast is small), it is necessary that each 'player' not only 'knows their lines', but understands and can enter into their role – be it king or beggar, scheming usurper, soldier, courtier, grand lady, or flirtatious maid – for if they are to play their role properly and convincingly they must be able to identify with the role, and follow the rules of behaviour that apply to it.

In a hospital ward the *dramatis personae* (besides the patient) may comprise not only the 'team' of senior and junior doctors, staff nurse (and other nurses), members of allied health professions, but also social worker, chaplain and perhaps patient advocate. Each has a different role to play in the 'drama' and their roles are subject to different rules related to their different responsibilities. Each will be accountable to different 'arbiters' of their performance.

For the smooth and efficient functioning of a hospital, health centre, or any other kind of healthcare provider, that employs a variety of medical, nursing, paramedical, and administrative, technical and service staff, there has to be some clear division of labour, with a clearly understood hierarchy of power and authority, roles and responsibilities. In large hospitals or community health centres, this can be complicated by the involvement of part-time staff based in outside organisations – such as social workers or chaplains, hairdressers and podiatrists, counsellors and even entertainers. In hospitals and other institutions, where teaching of undergraduate and postgraduate medical nursing and allied health professionals takes place, the competing commitments to service and education may create tensions.

Clarifying the roles and responsibilities of each 'player' is necessary before we can proceed to take decisions or to act responsibly as a team. Like a sports team we may need some practice to get it right. We need to know and to understand the different roles and functions of each member of the team, including the implicit or explicit rules applicable to these roles, and to be clear about the lines of accountability of team members to those who are arbiters of their work. Like a stage cast for a play, or a symphony orchestra, there also has to be some direction, some means of conducting and managing the various functions of groups and the contributions of individual 'players'.

In order to do justice to this complexity of ethics in institutional life, we suggest that it is necessary to take account of what we have called *'the four Rs'* – roles, rules, responsibilities and lines of reporting (adapting Emmet's categories). These four dimensions serve to define the ethical aspects of our work in both multidisciplinary teams and in complex institutions – where there is a necessary division of labour and specialisation of roles and functions.

Many of the tensions and sources of conflict in hospital and primary care teams may well be due to lack of clarity about the scope of the responsibilities attaching to the roles performed by their various members, or lack of clarity about what rules apply and who is responsible to whom for what. Research on teamwork in healthcare settings suggests that doctors, nurses, paramedics and administrative staff are generally ill-prepared to work in teams with other professionals – segregated as they are from one another in basic training (Barr 2003a, 2003b, Rushforth 2004, Hanson 2005). Put another way, many professionals are trained as 'soloists' rather than as players in a symphony orchestra, and are ill-equipped or lack experience in sharing power and responsibility. As in the production of a drama, or in training a football team, the right kind of shared learning environment may be critical in team-building, as well as appreciation of the contributions or expertise which each 'player' can bring to the team. Those involved in the education and training of health professionals are increasingly aware of what real team-building requires, and, generally speaking, greater emphasis is being placed on shared learning, communication skills and teamwork in training of doctors, nurses and allied heath professionals (Browne et al 1995, Gallagher 1995, Edward & Preece 1999, Tunstall-Pedoe et al 2003, Rushforth 2004).

Modern hospitals and healthcare institutions, especially in major cities, can be very large and complex institutions. We may lament the fact that relations with patients or clients within such institutions tend to become impersonal and 'institutionalised'. While the attempt to re-invent cottage hospitals and smaller nursing homes may help restore a degree of intimacy to healthcare for some conditions, we have to accept that the trend is towards the concentration of healthcare facilities in ever larger institutions especially to deal with complex problems. It appears to make sense economically and logistically to concentrate resources in one location rather than to disperse these, and to avoid duplication or fragmentation of infrastructure. However, the risk is the creation of what WHO has called 'disease palaces' removed from the needs of people on the ground. The challenge is to make these institutions more accessible to people and to 'humanise' them.

Day clinics where patients can undergo minor surgery or other medical procedures that allow same-day discharge may appear to improve 'productivity' and reduce waiting lists in hospitals, but unless there is good follow-up by the primary care team to provide continuity of care, relatives may find themselves having to cope with the provision of nursing care

Player	Role or function	Rules that apply	Responsible for	Reporting to
Nurse manager or matron				
Other grades of nurses				
Consultant or other doctors				
Paramedics or therapists				
Manager or administrator				
Service staff, cleaners etc.				
Social worker or chaplain				

Figure 4.5 The 4 Rs: roles, rules, responsibilities and reporting.

for patients which they are ill-equipped to provide. Similarly the use of various forms of tele-medicine (such as the NHS24 telephone advice service provided by nurse practitioners) has met with consumer resistance. While these sources of help may give immediate reassurance and advice, to some anxious enquirers, recent surveys in the UK suggest that the majority of people find these impersonal forms of service very frustrating: (a) because they experience many problems with making contact in the first place, and (b) because most want a competent medical opinion rather than that of a nurse, however well trained, and often get referred back to their GP anyway.

However health services are delivered, there is a great need for improved interprofessional communication and teamwork to ensure that well-coordinated services are provided by what is an increasingly mobile, and often part-time professional staff.

It may seem trite to say that one of the primary tasks in leadership of any team is to undertake role clarification, that is, clarify the structures of power, authority and responsibility on the team, and to determine how power is to be shared in practice between members of the team. This means the boundaries of roles and ground rules for their performance need to be carefully and explicitly negotiated, clarifying the scope of each player's responsibility and their line of reporting or accountability to the members of the team. As a means of team-building and to help prevent a lot of misunderstanding, tension and even conflict on a team, it may be useful for members to work

together to complete a grid such as the one illustrated in Figure 4.5.

In the process of working through such a model, the areas of overlapping responsibility, competition or potential conflict can be identified. The team can then determine what ethical ground rules they would need to put in place to resolve disagreements or conflicts. In many cases the confusions which give rise to misunderstanding or conflict within a team may be due to a number of possible factors: novel or unusual developments or unexpected circumstances, or the arrival of a new member of the team who has not been through induction into the 'ward culture' or different tacit or explicit ethical conventions operating within a team.

Consider Case Study 4.1, which illustrates some of the complexities that may arise in a crisis with unexpected developments in the case. While this scenario dates from 1979 we consider that the issues it raises are still relevant. Despite changes in many aspects of hospital management and changing roles and responsibilities, the problems that it highlights, about the need for improved interprofessional communication on ward teams, remain valid.

In the debriefing with the staff involved in this case, which caused great distress to all 'players' in the drama, the following were some of the issues identified as causes of tension and conflict within the 'the team':

- The unexpected reaction of the parents upset the whole team, doctors, nurses and support staff.

case study 4.1

'David' – The boy who broke his neck

David, aged 13 years, was the only child of middle-aged parents. He was attending a local public school as a 'day boy'. Playing a 'banned' game – a special form of 'leap-frog' – another boy landed right on his neck, causing spinal cord transection, ischaemic, progressive and permanent damage.

Day 1: On admission to the paediatric neurosurgical unit, there was already very clear evidence of spinal cord damage, with loss of movement and sensation in lower limbs up as far as the lower abdomen. The patient was a handsome boy, large and obviously physically very fit, and fully conscious and very anxious.

Over the next few hours his condition deteriorated, the level of loss of function rose. A tracheotomy was performed under local anaesthetic, to enable a respirator to be used. David, responding to sedation and constant reassurance from the medical and nursing staff, coped extraordinarily well with this unpleasant procedure.

The consultant, who was pessimistic about the possibility of recovery of the cord from the damage, had a long session with David's parents. David was kept fairly heavily sedated and given 'constant care' nursing.

Day 2: David suffered total loss of all sensation and function of the upper limbs. The parents visited and asked if there was any hope of recovery. They were told as gently as possible by the consultant that he believed there was no hope. He discussed David's possible future as a quadriplegic. The ward sister was also present. The parents saw David and went out for lunch.

They returned after several hours, and asked to speak to the consultant. They requested that no further efforts should be made to prolong David's life and asked that he should not be allowed to suffer. The consultant was surprised and disturbed by their response and suggested a second opinion. The parents did not feel this was necessary, but the consultant insisted. The second opinion confirmed the same diagnosis and prognosis.

The consultant convened a 'case-conference' – involving the ward sister, staff nurse, registrar and the anaesthetist who operated the respirator. The team eventually reached the decision to discontinue antibiotics, to provide suction to the tracheotomy only if the patient was distressed, and to increase sedation.

Day 3: David was found wide awake, alert and very anxious. The night nurse had withheld two doses of sedation, because he was asleep (in spite of formal instruction that 'sedation to be given 4-hourly'). She said it was against her religion to give drugs unnecessarily. David asked to see the ward sister as soon as she appeared on duty. He asked her directly if he was dying. This she denied vehemently and spent some time with him talking to him.

The parents visited later in the day and when he was asleep they came to say goodbye. They never returned. David slept most of the day and sedation was given regularly. He had ice cream and 'sherry and lemonade' to drink when he was awake, as this was his favourite tipple. That night there was a different night nurse on duty, because the consultant had intervened and had the other nurse removed.

Day 4: No sedation needed. David died at approximately 1 p.m.

From: Thompson (1979a) Dilemmas of Dying.

- The lack of confidence of the consultant, upset by the reaction of the parents, and the resulting confusion caused by his apparent abrogation of responsibility to give decisive leadership.
- The poor communication between the nurses, day staff and night nurses, over the agreed care plan, creating a crisis of conscience for the night nurse, lack of support for her, and resulting disarray on the team.
- Lack of clear focus to the case conference for members of the ward team (without including the parents), and whether it was a means of sharing responsibility, or avoiding it.
- It was not clear whether the case conference was designed to reach consensus, or a device for the consultant to seek personal support and reinforcement for his decision.

Thus, many ethical problems, interprofessional and intraprofessional tensions and even interpersonal conflicts, may have their origin, as in this case, in both the traditional structure of power relations, between medical, nursing and other staff, and also in the actual way in which power is exercised or shared within 'the team'. Understanding the ethics of such complex situations may have more to do with analysing the power relations involved, than questions of disagreements of principle.

Power structures and gender roles

Given traditional gender roles and more traditional occupations reserved to men, it is perhaps not surprising that in modern industrialised societies, the services provided by the *caring professions* (e.g. nursing, physiotherapy, occupational therapy, radiotherapy, social work, counselling and primary school teaching) are provided mainly by women. It is also the case in these professions that while men represent only a small proportion of staff, they still tend to predominate in senior positions and in management. Much attention has been given recently to the contribution of gender-role stereotyping to the social construction of the identity and character of nursing as a profession. This is reflected both in studies of the history of nursing (see Bullough & Bullough 1984, Allan & Jolley 1982) and sociological studies from a feminist perspective (Davies 1995).

In Bowden's illuminating analysis of the ethics of caring, she makes the observation of nursing in healthcare:

> The most outstanding feature of this functional organization and its hierarchical ranking is its sex-defined roles. Nursing practices are overwhelmingly carried out by women, and the activities, responsibilities and status associated with them call upon the kind of social capacities and standing that women have typically exercised in their traditional domestic roles. Accordingly the gendered social order is a crucial constitutive factor in the practice of nursing. In keeping with the dominant norms of this order, nursing is encumbered with much of the social apparatus that operated to undermine both the value of women's practices in general and the social possibilities of their practitioners. (Bowden 1997, p. 104)

In the past the assumption generally made was that doctors would lead and nurses follow, that doctors would have the power and authority to take decisions, and nurses were expected to be submissive, dutiful and obedient, like Victorian wives. These stereotypical roles in the division of labour in healthcare greatly influenced the way power was exercised and shared (or not shared) in relationships between doctors and nurses in healthcare teams. This in turn has influenced our understanding of nurses' ethical responsibilities to patients and doctors within those roles.

> [Nurses'] relations with patients are closely tied into relations with other members of the institution. Nursing care thus occupies an 'in between' position in the organisation of the public response to the patient's need, and is infused with the tensions of sustaining interdependent but differently focused relations with different levels of authority. (Bowden 1997, p. 104).

Many of the ethical problems which confront nurses in their daily practice are complicated by these underlying gender-related presuppositions which affect the way both power and authority are traditionally exercised in hospitals as institutions. They also complicate the interpersonal relationships of nurses and medical staff as working colleagues. Growe's research (1991) illustrates that 'most doctors see the nurse "as provider of a conglomerate of insignificant services", e.g. "mother, child, secretary, wife, waitress, maid, machine and psychiatrist"'! While nurses sensitised to the sexual politics traditional in healthcare institutions are increasingly able to assert their professional independence and confront these issues with their medical and other colleagues, many still have to resort to informal ways to overcome the 'put-downs', and lack of respect for their expertise by the medical hierarchy. This is especially the case in old and established institutions, with entrenched rules and practices that can result in the oppression and exploitation of nurses.

Other analysts (notably Reverby 1987) have tried to avoid the idealised picture of women as archetypal 'carers' and pioneers of the 'caring professions', and have emphasised that they have been forced (often by economic necessity) to take up these forms of employment due to their exclusion from others where men have had a monopoly. Women, historically, have had to find niches for themselves in the male-dominated labour market – initially in domestic service, in childcare, as governesses and teachers, then as nurses etc. They have had to take advantage of opportunities for employment which did not necessarily require any special education or training (from which they were largely excluded anyway). The great attraction of nursing was that 'caring' gave respectable moral status to the role, while offering training-on-the-job. Bowden (1997) sums this up as follows:

> The key feature of [nursing] history is its profound entanglement with conventional social constructions of women's character and roles. Modern hospital nursing drew on the social virtues of caring as an act of love *and obligation* to the needs of family and friends, held to be embedded in the natural character of women, rather than a vital function of nurses' work, valued by time, expertise and money.

In the final chapter we will have more to say about the 'ethics of caring'. But before we leave the issue of the gender-determined division of labour in healthcare, we will briefly comment on how this has affected the economics and organisation of nursing itself.

As Bowden points out (Bowden (1997, pp. 129–130), the Victorian way of giving respectability to women's work was not to recognise either their need or right to work, but to offer 'training' that was a 'disciplined process of honing womanly virtue'. Drawing on the work of Reverby, she observes that:

> ... hospital administrators were quick to recognise that opening a 'nursing school' ensured a ready supply of low-cost and disciplined young labourers, who were eager to offer their services in exchange for the professional training offered. Frequently, however, the hospital's nursing school and its nursing service were identical.

Because nursing care always has been the major 'service' being offered (or 'product' being marketed to potential 'consumers' by hospitals), the economics of providing nursing services at the lowest possible cost, has driven the quest for profitability of private hospitals, and cost reduction in the public sector. It can be argued that exploitation of nurses, in terms of relatively low wages, long hours and poor working conditions, has been rationalised, in terms of their commitment to a service ethic based on a duty to care, and that this has not only been a feature of the political economy of hospitals and institutionalised healthcare from the beginning, but continues to be the case to a greater of lesser degree. It is only through collective bargaining and the unionization of nursing labour that nurses have been able to achieve better pay and working conditions. However, they remain captive to a personalist ethic of dutiful care to patients and an ethos of subservience to authority that makes it painful and difficult for nurses to go on strike. This

image of nursing tends to be reinforced by the way in which nurses are represented on the media, but this kind of stereotyping is changing due to criticism from nurses.

Davies (1998) provides a scholarly and accessible discussion of the effects that gender has on our understanding of nursing. She explores the implications of this for the status of nursing and demonstrates that nurses' attempts to define and shape their role are frequently marginalised or ignored. Davies proposes that, in conjunction with discussion of managerial efficiency in healthcare, a debate is also required about the *fundamental* organisation of health and social care. This must include identification of what constitutes 'professionalism' and the value accorded to caring work.

The dilemmas faced by nurses, over taking industrial action, strike at the very foundations of the identity which has been constructed for nurses by the healthcare system, the media and public opinion – as 'self-sacrificing angels of mercy' dedicated above all else to 'tending the sick and alleviating suffering'. It has perhaps gone against the grain of traditional thinking for nurses to accept their role as employees in the workforce of a large service industry, rather than as 'professionals'. However, issues of industrial relations, employee rights, fair pay and working conditions become increasingly important to nurses, as public sector employees, with the industrialisation of healthcare.

 further reading

Beauchamp T, Childress J 2004 Principles of biomedical ethics, 5th rev edn. Oxford University Press, Oxford

Davies C M 1998 Gender and the professional predicament in nursing. Open University Press, Buckingham

Freidson E 1994 Professionalism reborn: theory, prophecy and policy. Polity Press, Cambridge

Hursthouse R 1999 On virtue ethics. Oxford University Press, Oxford

Macintyre A 1993 A short history of ethics. Routledge & Kegan Paul, London

May W 1983 The physician's covenant. Westminster, Philadelphia

Professional responsibility and accountability in nursing

5

Chapter contents

AIMS

This chapter has the following aims:

1. To explore the concepts of responsibility and accountability as they relate to nursing practice
2. To discuss the role of codes of conduct/ethics in decision-making
3. To apply a code of conduct/ethics to specific situations
4. To explore the strengths and limitations of codes of conduct/ethics as a means of ensuring responsibility and accountability for good practice.

LEARNING OUTCOMES

When you have read and worked through this chapter, you should be able to:

- Differentiate between the concepts of responsibility and accountability
- Apply your own country's code of conduct/ethics to situations that you encounter in your own nursing practice
- Reflect on the strengths and limitations of codes of conduct/ethics in relation to nursing practice.

INTRODUCTION

In this chapter the focus is on the ethical aspects of responsibility and accountability of registered nurses. It may be possible to argue that some aspects of nursing (e.g. administrative and technical functions) are morally neutral. However, if we consider the overall impact of nursing practice on the health and well-being of patients and clients it can be argued on the contrary that *no* aspect of nursing, or of healthcare as a whole, is ethically neutral or morally insignificant. If, as we have argued, ethics is about how we promote the well-being or flourishing of individuals, then inefficient administration or incompetent technical care will impact adversely on patients' welfare and is therefore ethically important. We operate from the position that nursing practice is, in its entirety, a moral enterprise.

The concept of nurses' individual accountability for their practice has received increasing publicity in the UK since the United Kingdom Central Council (forerunner of the NMC) published *Exercising Accountability* in 1989 (UKCC 1989). This document may be viewed as partially reactive to an expanded nursing remit and as partially proactive, as a 'public relations or marketing exercise' to promote the status of nursing as a profession. However, as emphasised in Chapter 1, public accountability is considered to be one hallmark that differentiates professions from other occupations. In addition, one factor behind the policy of increased emphasis on accountability in nursing was to counteract the historical view of nursing as subordinate to medicine, and to underline the fact that nurses are independently accountable for their professional work.

In many countries there has been a clear emphasis on nurses being accountable for their practice, rather than dependent on other occupational groups to direct them in their work and to 'carry the can' when adverse events occur, or to claim the credit when all goes well. However, as medical practitioners retain *overall* control over most areas of patient care, structural limitations are imposed on the extent to which nurses can be fully autonomous agents and thus completely accountable for their practice. The tensions that we have previously identified (in Chapter 3) between the *structures* within which care is delivered and nurses' individual *agency* within those structures are of relevance here. It is the case nonetheless that neither continued subordination to medicine, nor the requirement to work within a line-management structure, exempt registered nurses from individual accountability for their actions. However, despite the rhetoric that individual accountability enhances professional

and ethical aspects of care provision, it is arguable that at least some employers have used an emphasis on practitioner accountability to reduce their own.

In this chapter we emphasise the importance of the social context within which healthcare is provided, and would stress that any attempt to define accountability must take into consideration its relationship with other concepts, for example those of autonomy, power and executive authority. Nursing practice does not take place within a social vacuum and the implications of continuities and changes within society will be discussed. We will also be concerned with the different competencies required for nursing practice (e.g. technical and psychosocial), and the fact that these are interrelated and must be addressed holistically in addition to examination of their individual elements. Finally, we would emphasise that the concept of autonomy is multifaceted and, whilst the focus in this chapter is on the *ethical* aspects of accountability, its other dimensions (e.g. legal and professional accountability) must form an integral part of the discussion.

Codes of ethics, or codes of conduct, have been developed by nurses' regulatory and/or professional bodies in different countries, and in the millennial year the International Council of Nurses (ICN) revised its code, which is intended to provide generic guidance to practitioners globally (ICN 2000). The function of such codes is to provide a yardstick against which nurses' practice may be measured, to provide information about the standards required of nurses to other occupational groups and to society in general. In this chapter we explore the use of such codes in assisting nurses to deal with the situations that they may encounter in their practice.

ACCOUNTABILITY: WHAT DOES IT MEAN IN PRACTICE FOR NURSES?

In the UK the Nursing and Midwifery Council (NMC 2002b) found that many queries received from nurses about their practice identified uncertainty about accountability and that many allegations of professional misconduct result from nurses' lack of knowledge about the nature or extent of their own accountability for practice.

Savage & Moore (2004), in their section on defining accountability, note that the term has many shades of meaning; for example, while accountability is frequently used to emphasise openness and transparency in decision-making it is arguably related more to compliance with externally imposed criteria than to the practitioner's own judgement. Other writers like Hunt (1997) argue that accountability must involve the judgement of professional practitioners themselves, independently of the structures within which they work. When Savage & Moore (2004) asked the participants in their study what accountability meant to them, many conflated the term with responsibility and the two terms were viewed as virtually synonymous. There was also a lack of clarity as to the translation of the concept into practice.

Accountability may be defined in a variety of ways, not least by nurses' regulatory bodies in different countries. Some regulatory bodies appear to view the concepts of responsibility and accountability as virtually synonymous and interchangeable (e.g. the Canadian Nurses' Association 2002), whereas others differentiate clearly between the two (e.g. American Nurses' Association 2001).

Eby (2000) suggests a number of different aspects of accountability and the one of particular interest to the focus of this book is that of *ethical* accountability, which is distinguishable from practitioners' professional accountability to a regulatory body and is distinct from their legal accountability. Ethical accountability relates to the *moral* requirement to be answerable to their patients, within a practitioner/patient relationship. Eby examines the basis on which this form of accountability is founded. Accountability's foundation links with deontological approaches in that it focuses on the *duty* of practitioners to be accountable to patients, but it also links with utilitarian approaches in examining the *consequences* of practitioners' actions and with virtue ethics in emphasising the importance of the *character* of the practitioner. Eby also relates accountability to the ethical *principle* of truthfulness and honesty.

Who is accountable and to whom?

To be identified as accountable or responsible, *to* anyone, or *for* their actions, individuals must be independent moral agents despite the fact that they may work within hierarchical organisational structures. These individuals must have the capacity to *give an account* of what they have done and provide a rationale for their actions (or omissions). Accountability is usually owed to specific individuals, groups of people, or may be owed to society as a whole. Individuals who have overall accountability may also delegate responsibility to others, for whose practice they nonetheless remain accountable. One example of this is when a registered nurse (RN) in charge of an area delegates care provision to another person. That person may then be *responsible* for their own actions, or omissions, but it is the RN who is in charge of the delegation who remains *accountable*.

Registered nurses are accountable to their patients/clients, their professional regulator (in the UK, this is the Nursing and Midwifery Council (NMC)), their employer, their colleagues and the law. Nurses are also accountable to themselves in upholding their own ethical standards. This means that, overall, nurses may be viewed as accountable to society. Whilst the different aspects of professional accountability are interrelated, in this chapter the ethical dimension of accountability will be the main focus of discussion.

The accountability of students of nursing

Regulatory bodies have expectations of students, as future practitioners. However, this differs from *professional* accountability, as will be seen in the situation outlined in Case Study 5.3. For example, the NMC (2002a) states that students are not *professionally* accountable to the NMC, but may nonetheless be called to account by their educational institution, the managers of placements within which they acquire practice experience and by the law. Later in this chapter the accountability that registered nurses have in relation to student assessment will be discussed.

Accountable for what?

In Chapter 3 we provided a general definition of accountability. In an earlier section in this chapter we identified those *to whom* nurses may be deemed accountable but it is also necessary to address *for what* they are accountable. Accountability goes beyond activities that relate to technical or cognitive competence although these are clearly important aspects of nursing care. Accountability extends to the attitudes of practitioners and the actions, or omissions, which may arise from these.

All individuals have attitudes, beliefs and values, but nurses' codes of ethics require practitioners to focus on the needs of patients and to ensure that their own value judgements do not impede care provision and delivery. This holistic perspective, which includes the attributes of nurses, links with virtue ethics, mentioned in Chapter 2 and discussed more fully in Chapter 13. Virtue ethics proposes that morally competent or 'virtuous' individuals are those who have internalised values that promote general human flourishing. This requires critical appraisal of their personal attitudes and beliefs. If these qualities or competences are fostered throughout life, and within the preparation for practice of nurses, then the habits and character traits that practitioners acquire, maintain and enhance should facilitate a patient-centred approach to care.

CODES OF ETHICS AND CONDUCT

Introduction

Groups of practitioners, or regulatory bodies, who wish to reassure the public that they are trustworthy may develop codes (or ethical policies), setting out standards against which the public may measure the behaviour and attitudes of individual practitioners. The aim of codes is also to reinforce for practitioners the standards expected of them and to provide a yardstick against which employers and the regulatory bodies may measure individual and group performance. Occupational groups who aim to gain and/or to maintain professional status may use a code as a promotional or 'marketing' tool to gain public trust and respect. Nurses' regulatory bodies in most countries have set out guidelines to which practitioners are expected to adhere. Sometimes these are referred to as 'Codes of Professional Conduct' (e.g. the UK's NMC 2002c) whereas others are called 'Codes of Ethics' (e.g. American Nurses' Association 2001, Australian Nursing Council 2002, Canadian Nurses' Association 2002). In the UK the NMC has recently added a subtitle to their code (NMC 2004), which now reads: *Standards for Conduct, Performance and Ethics.*

For a comprehensive overview of codes of practice/ethics, please see website links at: http://evolve.elsevier.com/Thompson/nursing ethics.

Many nurses' regulatory bodies state that, in addition to their responsibility for clients, registered nurses are expected, both within and outside their actual area of employment, to promote the health of the community generally and to justify the trust and confidence placed in nurses by the public. RNs are therefore individually accountable for their behaviour in both their private lives and in their professional practice, irrespective of the advice, directions or practice of others. In this section we shall explore some of the implications of these standards for practitioners.

The ICN *Code of Ethics* for nurses

Most countries have their own code of nursing ethics but the International Council of Nurses (ICN 2000) published a code that was intended to transcend national barriers and to be of relevance to nurses globally. The ICN code identifies four areas of responsibility for nurses:

- promotion of health
- prevention of illness
- restoration of health
- alleviation of suffering.

In assuming responsibility in these areas, nurses should respect human rights, including rights to life and dignity, without consideration of the care recipient's age, colour, creed, culture, disability, illness, gender, nationality, politics, race or social status. The ICN code specifies four areas where nurses are responsible:

- to people (which includes ecological and environmental responsibility)
- in their practice
- to their profession
- to co-workers.

For website links related to this topic, please see http://evolve.elsevier.com/Thompson/nursing ethics.

The strengths and limitations of codes of ethics in assisting nurses to make decisions and in providing the public with a means by which to evaluate practitioners will be discussed in what follows. Some examples will be provided to illustrate underpinning themes.

Professionalisation

As was suggested earlier, from the perspective of 'public relations' or the 'marketing' of a profession, codes of ethics are important, for they serve as a public proclamation of the trustworthiness of the profession. In this connection it is perhaps useful to think of a profession's standards as follows:

- at the micro level codes stipulate standards to which individual members must adhere in their relationships with patients, colleagues and members of the public
- at the macro level codes set out the values upheld by the whole profession.

In discussing codes of ethics it is important to address both these levels at which codes operate.

In practice, codes of ethics have strengths, but also limitations, and cannot be seen as an infallible guide to dealing with moral issues. What such codes can do, however, is to set out aspirational ideals and the general rights, duties, values and policies that should govern professional practice.

Most codes of conduct (or ethics) require nurses to be accountable for their behaviour not only when at work, but also in their personal lives. The regulatory bodies' rationale for this is usually enhancement, or at least maintenance, of the reputation of nursing as a profession. Nurses are therefore expected by their regulatory bodies to be accountable for behaviours that may not impact directly on their performance during their paid employment. The challenges that this may create are the focus of the situations outlined briefly in Case Studies 5.1 and 5.2. Whilst the UK's NMC (2004) code will be used as a framework for discussion, readers may find it useful to refer to their own country's code, or to that of the ICN (2000).

Application of a code to specific cases

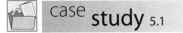 case study 5.1

Over the limit

A woman who was a registered nurse and who was on holiday was stopped whilst driving and found to have a blood alcohol level that was over the legal limit. She received a fine and was banned from driving for a specified period.

Either on your own, or in discussion with others, identify this person's position in relation to her employer and her regulatory body.

Case Study 5.1 – discussion

It might have been the case that this person was on holiday from her employment and, as driving was not a prerequisite for her job, she did not have any accountability to her employer. However, within the UK, all criminal convictions are automatically notified to the nurses' regulatory body (the NMC). (Similarly, the General Medical Council (GMC) receives notification of medical practitioners' convictions.) It is then for the NMC to decide whether a formal investigation is required to ascertain whether a practitioner's behaviour constitutes misconduct.

The NMC code states (NMC 2004, clause 1.5) that nurses must adhere to the laws of the country in which they practise, but this clause is likely to relate to actual nursing practice, for example legal frameworks that govern the administration of medicines. In clause 1.2, however, there is a requirement to protect and support the health of the wider community. As driving whilst over the legal blood alcohol limit may endanger the health and welfare of others, the nurse may be held accountable on this count. Later in clause 1.2 it is stated that nurses are required to act in such a way that justifies the trust and confidence of the public and that they should uphold and enhance the good reputation

of the profession. In clause 7.1 this is expanded upon when the NMC state that behaviour compromising nursing's reputation may call the practitioner's registration into question even if the behaviour is unconnected directly with the nurse's professional practice. It would appear from the above that the RN is accountable to the NMC for behaviour that occurred whilst she was not at work. However, this does not imply her driving offence would compromise her ability to deliver competent care in the course of her job.

The underpinning theme of the situation in Case Study 5.1 is that nurses are expected to behave in certain ways in conducting their lives both within and outside their working environment and that failure to do so may impact on their registration. Removal of a practitioner's name from the register precludes their subsequent employment as a registered nurse. The personal qualities stipulated by the NMC as prerequisites for registered nurses can therefore be seen as integral to the behaviour required in *all* aspects of the individual's life, i.e. they are part of the person's *character* rather than confined to skills identified in their job description.

The ethical implications of the behaviour of the person whose situation was outlined in Case Study 5.1 are that she has potentially endangered the health and well-being of others and that registered nurses have an obligation to avoid this, even whilst on holiday from work. There is also the potential for diminishment of public trust in nursing as a profession if RNs who receive criminal convictions escape professional censure.

Following notification of a practitioner's criminal conviction, the NMC carry out a preliminary investigation. This may result in referral to the NMC's Professional Conduct Committee, whose subsequent judgement depends on a number of factors. The RN's past behaviour and character, both within and outside the work environment, are taken into account and statements requested from those considered well placed to provide such evidence.

It may be seen from the situation in Case Study 5.1 that the clauses in the NMC *Code of Professional Conduct* set the standards for practitioners' performance and ethics, and these are aimed at protection of the public in the widest sense of the word, rather than confined to protection of patients and clients. The discussion of the situation in Case Study 5.1 identifies that registered nurses are not 'free agents', even when apparently without obligations to deliver nursing care to others. Case Study 5.2, however, outlines a situation in which care was required, but occurred outside the RN's workplace.

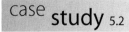

case study 5.2

To give or not to give first aid

A registered nurse was reported to the NMC by a member of the public who had witnessed the collapse of a middle-aged man onto a city centre pavement. The member of the public had recognised the registered nurse from having seen her in a hospital setting and noted that the RN had walked past the collapsed man without stopping.

Either on your own, or in discussion with others, identify what you consider to be the registered nurse's legal, professional and ethical responsibility and areas of accountability in this situation.

Case Study 5.2 – discussion

As in the situation in Case Study 5.1, this situation occurred outside the registered nurse's work setting. She therefore does not owe a *legal* duty of care to the man who had collapsed. The law within the UK is usually based on non-maleficence rather than on a requirement to be beneficent to others. Indeed, in a litigious culture the legal advice might be that providing assistance is ill-advised because if the care provided is inadequate legal action might be taken against the nurse. Legal advice might recommend avoidance of involvement. However, from the NMC's point of view, as outlined in the *Code of Professional Conduct* (NMC 2004, clause 8.5) nurses have a *professional duty* to provide care in an emergency situation, whether they are at work or not.

From the situation as described in Case Study 5.2, the nurse's motivation in passing the man without stopping is unknown and this might arguably make a difference in the judgement made by the NMC of her action. The nurse might, for example, consider that she did not have the skills necessary to provide first aid or resuscitation in such a setting. In deciding not to assist she might then be seen to be acting in the light of the *Code of Professional Conduct* (NMC 2004, clause 6.2), which states that nurses must acknowledge the limits of their competence and implement only activities for which they are qualified. It is not stated whether other passers-by had stopped to provide assistance. A qualified first-aider might be better placed to deal with such emergency situations than healthcare professionals who are used to having resources, including equipment and qualified staff, immediately to hand.

However, the requirement in such a situation is not for 'super-nurse', but for the care that an ordinary registered nurse could reasonably be expected to provide, given the circumstances. This requirement is based on a legal judgement within the UK (*Bolam v. Friern Barnet Hospital Management Committee* 1957) that was subsequently expanded upon in *Bolitho* (House of Lords 1997). The latter judgement stated that 'reasonable' denotes that practice is evidence based, in which an assessment of risk has been carried out and that potential benefits and harms have been balanced prior to action.

According to the NMC's code, the RN had a *duty* to stop and to provide some form of emergency assistance in the situation in Case Study 5.2. The fact that she was 'off duty' did not relieve her of this obligation. Doctors, however, would probably be seen to have a similar professional obligation to provide assistance if called upon to do so. This requirement clearly goes beyond the public's expectation of most occupational groups. Lawyers, accountants, plumbers or teachers, for example, are not obliged to assist those requiring services that they may be in a position to provide, unless in the course of their paid employment. (It is also the case, of course, that assistance to a casualty may have highly significant consequences for the future health and well-being of the individual concerned.)

The expectation that registered nurses have similar obligations to medical practitioners may, at least in part, indicate the NMC's desire for the public to perceive nurses in the same light as members of the medical profession. The NMC's guidance indicates that it considers RNs (and/or wishes the public to perceive RNs) as individuals who are willing to go above and beyond what might be considered the required behaviour of the majority of occupational groups.

The registered nurse in the situation described in Case Study 5.2 is accountable to the NMC, i.e. required to provide an explanation for her actions. The explanation should address not only her *professional* responsibility but also her *ethical* responsibility. Part of the RN's justification for her non-intervention might relate to a decision that she was not competent to deal with the situation. This is an ethical as well as professional decision as it involves the principle of non-maleficence, i.e. a concern that unskilled intervention could cause harm. As in Case Study 5.1, the NMC's judgement of the situation would also involve an assessment of the nurse's known character and behaviour and relevant references might be requested. As was discussed in Chapter 2, virtue ethics places emphasis on character and competence.

It might be seen from supporting references that the nurse possessed the character or virtues that are prerequisites for morally competent practitioners.

The situation in Case Study 5.2 may be viewed ethically from a variety of perspectives. It may be viewed from the point of view of the relevant ethical *principles*, specifically those of beneficence (and non-maleficence). It may be perceived from the viewpoint of ethical *theory*, e.g. utilitarian theory that would assess actions in terms of their consequences, or deontological theory that would identify the duties (obligations or responsibilities) of the individuals concerned. The perspective of the NMC code, like most codes, is *deontological*, i.e. focused on the nurse's duties, though in practice the *consequences* of her actions cannot be ignored. The NMC would have to take into account the effect on the victim and on the profession's reputation if its practitioners fail to provide assistance in emergency situations. In so far as the character of the nurse is taken into account by the NMC in reaching a decision about whether misconduct had occurred and whether action should be taken in relation to the nurse, then aspects of *virtue ethics* become relevant.

Whilst the situation in Case Study 5.2 relates primarily to the nurse's *duty* and *responsibility*, she is also *accountable* to the NMC and may be accountable legally, if the casualty sues on the grounds that the nurse had a duty of care, that she was negligent in relation to that duty and that the casualty suffered significant physical and/or psychological harm as a consequence of that neglect.

Usefulness of a code to practitioners

Given that in the situation outlined in Case Study 5.2 there clearly would be no time to refer to the NMC code for guidance and that this restriction would apply in many situations in practice, the example illustrates the importance of nurses being familiar with the contents of codes in advance. In the situation in Case Study 5.2 the expectation of the NMC is clear although whether the NMC's requirement for nurses to assist in such situations is based solely on ethical considerations or because they wish to promote an image of nurses as accepting a supererogatory duty to act in such situations, is open to debate.

Having examined two situations in which the code applied to a practitioner outside their work environment, its application within practice settings will be discussed next with reference to the situation in Case Study 5.3.

Case Study 5.3 – discussion

The RN's position Whilst it was the student who administered the medication to the incorrect patient, it is the RN who is primarily accountable in this situation. She dispensed the medication for the patient and should have witnessed that it had been given to, and taken by, the correct patient. In this instance delegation was inappropriate, despite the fact that her presence was urgently required elsewhere. The RN should have ensured the safekeeping of the medication (e.g. by locking it within the dispensing trolley or a cupboard) and then administered it when she was able to do so, following the correct procedure.

The situation in Case Study 5.3 indicates the different, but closely interlinked dimensions of accountability present in many of the situations that nurses encounter in practice. The RN may be legally accountable, in that the patient who was given the medication could take legal action if he or she sustained harm (physical or psychological) as a result of the drug error. The RN is also accountable to her employers and potentially subject to investigative and disciplinary proceedings if she is shown to have ignored the requirements of the employer's medication policy. The RN would also be accountable for having delegated responsibility inappropriately (i.e. to a student). The student's higher educational

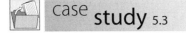

case study 5.3

Emergency cover

In a busy placement that was understaffed due to staff illness, a registered nurse was dispensing medication on her own when a patient in another area of the placement slipped and fell. When this accident was reported to the RN, she asked one of the student nurses to give the medication whilst she, the RN, attended to the patient who had fallen. It was later found that the student nurse had given the medication to the wrong patient.

Either on your own, or in discussion with others:

- identify who is accountable in this situation
- identify to whom that person is accountable
- explore the other issues that are relevant to this situation
- discuss the strengths and limitations of codes of ethics in this situation.

institution (HEI) may also hold the RN accountable for the situation, but the student's position in this situation will be discussed later. The RN may also be professionally accountable, if a complaint is made (e.g. by the patient or patient's relatives, her employer or indeed the student) to the nursing regulatory body (in the UK, the NMC).

The RN's ethical accountability is closely related to these other forms of formal accountability, but might be said to include factors such as abuse of the power imbalance that exists between student nurses and RNs. Whilst the student could (and should) have declined to administer the medication, a refusal might be difficult for students in such a situation. Students usually wish to 'fit in' to placements and are dependent on RNs for satisfactory placement reports. Students may assume that instructions from RNs are correct and may be eager to assist in difficult situations.

Aside from the legal duty of care owed by RNs to patients there is an ethical requirement to ensure that vulnerable individuals are protected from harm and that their welfare is promoted. All patients may be classed as vulnerable by virtue of their care requirements and dependence on nurses for competent provision of care. In the situation in Case Study 5.3 the RN did not fulfil this ethical duty of care.

The RN, as nurse in charge, would also be accountable for the other patient's accident and would have to provide written documentation of this event. Again, it is possible that the patient or relatives might take legal action if the patient suffered damage (physical or psychological) as a result of the fall. The RN is further accountable to her employers, and also to the professional regulatory body, for maintaining a safe environment for patients and for ensuring assistance and supervision for patients if required.

It was stated in Case Study 5.3 that the placement ward was short-staffed. It might then be the case that the managers of the area within which the placement was situated would also be accountable. Adequate staffing levels are required in order to ensure patient safety and it is management who are accountable for this provision. It is important that RNs report inadequate staffing levels to management (i.e. those which might jeopardise patient safety). The information in Case Study 5.3 does not state whether the RN had done this. Whilst such a report on inadequate staffing levels might be verbal, it is desirable that verbal reports are witnessed and subsequently documented. It would be good practice for the RN to make a written record of the request for help and management's response to this (NMC 2003).

The student's position The student nurse also has a degree of accountability, although the NMC (2002a) makes it clear that students are not *professionally* accountable to the regulatory body as that accountability lies with the RNs under whose supervision they work. Students are, however, accountable to their higher education institution (HEI) and to society under the law. The HEI should clarify to students on commencement of their programme, in writing, that they must carry out care only under RN supervision. (This does not mean that RNs must invariably be physically present whilst students provide patient care.) Students must, however, ensure that they are familiar with the policies that relate to the areas in which they undertake placements; in this instance the policy on administration of medication. Students should have received preparation for practice prior to undertaking placements, including advice on the correct procedures. The student's actions in Case Study 5.3, in administering medication without having gone through the checking and dispensing process with the RN, means that she acted beyond her remit. She might thus be liable for discipline by the university and, should the patient suffer harm (physical or psychological) as a result of receiving the incorrect medication, the patient or the patient's relatives might bring legal action against her as well.

Having briefly discussed the students' position in relation to accountability, we shall now examine the accountability of RNs in assessment of students' competence in practice placement settings.

ACCOUNTABILITY FOR ASSESSMENT OF STUDENTS

Students undertaking practice placements within the UK have their performance assessed against a series of competencies or learning outcomes that reflect their stage within the undergraduate programme. During placements students are allocated a registered nurse as a 'mentor'. The designated RN should receive a formalised preparation for this role, although it is usually short and may have been achieved by a distance learning programme or indeed as a component of the consolidation stage of the RN's own pre-registration programme. Mentors should work with their allocated students on a regular and frequent basis during students' placements, should be the main assessor of students' performance and should provide written reports about students to their higher education institution (HEI).

Either on your own, or in discussion with others, please undertake the activity in Case Study 5.4.

case study 5.4

Mentoring

A registered nurse, who was mentoring a second year student, was concerned about the student's performance and attitude during her placement.

Identify the RN's accountability in relation to student assessment. Discuss the options available to the RN and select that which you consider to be the most appropriate. Provide the rationale for your decision.

(The *DECIDE* model of ethical decision-making will be discussed in detail in Chapter 12; you may find it useful to use it as a guide for your discussion.)

Case Study 5.4 – discussion

RNs are accountable for their assessment of students, and they are accountable to:

- the student's higher education institution (HEI)
- the student
- themselves
- their work colleagues
- nurses' regulatory body (in the UK, the NMC)
- ultimately, to society as a whole, in stating whether or not the student is fit to practise as a nurse.

Each of these areas of accountability will be discussed following identification of the options available to the RN. Some of the options available are that the mentor:

- takes no immediate action and subsequently awards a pass to the student on completion of the placement despite reservations about their competence, or fails the student on completion of the placement
- speaks informally with the student about the areas of concern
- provides a written interim assessment that identifies specific instances in which the student's practice was unsatisfactory and clarifies the improvements that need to be made to achieve a satisfactory final assessment
- liaises with the student's HEI to discuss the above
- liaises with colleagues to ensure that, when the mentor is not present, the student will be supervised by another RN
- continues to provide feedback on performance to the student

- passes or fails the student at the end of the placement in the light of the student's response to the interim assessment.

Having identified some of the options that are available to the mentor, it is useful to discuss those to whom the mentor is accountable.

Accountability to the higher education institution (HEI)

Within the UK, undergraduate nursing students divide their time approximately 50:50 between theory and practice and undertake assessments in both. Whilst HEI lecturers are linked to specified practice placement areas, this is usually to provide support for mentors and/or students and as a liaison between the HEI and the practice placement, rather than working with students and thus being able to assess their performance. It is mentors who are best placed, through working with students on a regular basis, to comment on their students' performance. The HEIs are therefore reliant on mentors to assess students' acquisition of practice placement competencies. A prerequisite for registration is verification by the educational institution (HEI) to the professional regulatory body (NMC) that students have attained the required theoretical and practice placement competencies and are of good character. It may be seen then that mentors are accountable to HEIs for assessments of students' competence in practice settings.

Accountability to students

As students have to acquire competencies in nursing practice they are reliant on mentors to verify that these have been achieved. In situations in which students' performance is unsatisfactory mentors should identify areas of concern as soon as possible, so that students are made aware of the required standards and have adequate opportunity to improve.

Duffy (2004) found that mentor/student discussions about progress were sometimes verbal and informal, with subsequent difficulty in verifying their content and timing. Areas of concern should be identified in writing, discussed between the student and mentor and signed and dated by both. This would allow a clear audit of events. In situations in which students fail a practice assessment, mentors are accountable to students, in that they should be able to explain clearly to the individual concerned why their performance does not merit a pass grade. Duffy's (2004) study found that mentors sometimes gave students in early placements 'the benefit of the doubt' and allowed them to progress. Some of these students did not improve over time and were then devastated in their final year when they failed practice placement assessments close to completion of their programme.

Accountability to self

Mentors are accountable to themselves in that they have to be able to live with decisions that they have made as RNs. As students' progression within the undergraduate programme depends to a significant extent on mentors' decisions about students' competence, mentors may experience disquiet if a student fails. On the other hand, mentors also have to live with decisions to give students 'the benefit of the doubt' and/or to pass students whom they consider incompetent, with the potential consequences for the student, future mentors, patients and clients.

Accountability to work colleagues

As all RNs in the UK are required by the NMC to facilitate development of students' competence for practice, mentors' colleagues may provide input into students' assessments although it is the designated mentor who should complete the documentation. Negotiation with colleagues is then important and mentors are accountable to colleagues for decisions that they make. Mentors are also accountable to colleagues in a wider sense. Students progress through a variety of practice placements within their under- graduate programme and if a mentor in one placement deems a student competent to pass then that RN is, in a sense, accountable to that student's future mentors if they fail to perform up to standard. Duffy (2004) found that when doubts were expressed by mentors about students' performance in the final year of their programme, it was sometimes the case that the student's previous mentors had concerns about the student's performance, but that these had not been documented. Mentors assessing third year students may thus have to contend with problems that should have been addressed at an earlier stage.

Accountability to the NMC and society

In stating that a student's performance is satisfactory or unsatisfactory, mentors contribute to the final declaration by HEIs to the NMC that potential practitioners are competent in theory and practice and are of good character. Mentors thus are accountable for students' assessments and could be called to account if they have allowed students to progress whose practice was unsatisfactory. Mentors therefore should be aware

that they are accountable to the NMC, to meet the requirement that practitioners minimise risks to patients and clients. In allowing incompetent students to progress mentors contravene this obligation.

Duffy's (2004) study appeared to indicate little recognition by RNs that they are accountable to the NMC in their assessments of students' performance. RNs are accountable for ensuring that their own actions do not place members of the public, who might be current or future recipients of healthcare, at risk from incompetent practitioners.

Having examined the situation in Case Study 5.4 in the light of the guidance of the UK's regulatory body, it is also of interest that the ICN *Code of Ethics* (ICN 2000) states that registered nurses carry personal respons- ibility and accountability for nursing practice and also that they should use judgement regarding individual competence when delegating responsibility. RNs are also expected to assume the major role in determining and implementing acceptable standards of clinical nursing practice, management and education. If these standards are used to measure the RN's performance as outlined in Case Study 5.3 then it is fairly clear that the RN did not meet the requirements of the ICN (2000) code. The use of codes of conduct/ethics may be useful for professional regulatory bodies and for the public in making decisions as to whether practitioners fall short of standards. As was identified earlier, however, codes are only of use to RNs if they are familiar with their content in advance of practice. Accessing and evaluating a code is not a viable option once immersed in the busy-ness of everyday practice.

Discussion of the situation in Case Study 5.4 has highlighted the wide-ranging accountability of students' mentors. Ultimately, much of this account- ability is ethically grounded, rather than confined to contractual or professional requirements. It is ethical in that mentors have a duty of care to take decisions to ensure the health and well-being of students' future patients and clients. It may be seen that the *conse- quences* of mentors' decisions need to be taken into account, as does their professional *duty* or obligation to their regulatory body and to the public to avoid placing patients or clients at risk from incompetent practitioners. The ethical *principle* of beneficence (and non-maleficence) is therefore important, as is that of justice. The principle of justice is demonstrated in acknowledging that patients have the right to expect competent care provision. Justice (fairness) also requires that students are made aware, from an early stage in a placement, if aspects of their practice are unsatisfactory. Considerations of *virtue ethics* are also of importance, in that the regulatory body requires verification from educational institutions that students are 'of good character' as a prerequisite for registration. As was discussed earlier, the concept of a morally virtuous character includes, but also goes beyond, attainment of competence in technical skills.

NURSES AND INDUSTRIAL ACTION

Earlier in this book we discussed some of the effects of socialisation on individuals within society. We also explored the tensions that may exist between the ability of individuals to act autonomously (*agency*) and the extent to which this ability is influenced by the *structures* within which individuals operate. *Structures* not only comprise the physical environment within which care delivery takes place but also include, for example, management structure, pay and conditions of employment.

Within nursing practice, situations may arise in which nurses consider that these structures impede their ability to deliver safe and competent care to patients. Alternatively, or additionally, nurses may consider that the structures interfere with their ability to meet the economic and social commitments of their own lives outside work. Whilst individual nurses may be able to achieve little to alter the structures within which they operate, collectively their bargaining power may be considerable. Many nurses are members of professional organisations or trade unions whose function is to represent their interests. The laws that govern industrial action and trade union organisation and activity vary from one country to another and it is not the intention to detail these here. As this is a book on nursing ethics it is, however, useful to examine the ethical arguments for and against 'industrial action', which is a term that covers a spectrum of action (or inaction) taken to pursue a claim when other means, such as negotiation, appear to have failed (Box 5.1).

Box 5.1 **Industrial action**

Either on your own, or with others, identify your personal position in relation to industrial action being taken by nurses. Under what circumstances, if any, would you consider industrial action to be justifiable and what form would you consider acceptable? You should provide the reasons for your position.

In providing answers you may find it useful to refer to the ICN's (2000) *Code of Ethics*, or your own country's code of ethics, to inform your discussion.

Box 5.1: Discussion

For the purpose of discussion we shall, as in the earlier cases in this chapter, use the UK's NMC (2004) *Code of Professional Conduct: Standards for Conduct, Performance and Ethics* to address the issue of industrial action.

Clause 1.2 of the NMC (2004) code states that registered nurses must protect and support the health of individual patients and clients and act in a way that justifies the trust and confidence placed by the public in nurses. It also states that nurses should uphold and enhance the good reputation of nursing. Clause 1.3 emphasises practitioner accountability and clause 1.4 reminds nurses that they have a duty to ensure provision of safe and competent care. Clause 1.5 requires nurses to adhere to the laws of the country in which they practise. Clause 8 stipulates that nurses must act to identify and minimise risks to patients and clients by working with other members of the care team and by reporting and documenting circumstances in the environment of care that could impede safe practice. Clause 8.4 states that the 'first consideration in all activities must be the interest and safety of patients and clients'.

It is arguable that the above clauses from the NMC code might justify some form of industrial action in order to avert potential or actual harm to patients in situations in which other means, such as reporting and documenting concerns, have proved unsuccessful. As the major function of the UK's Nursing and Midwifery Council is protection of the public, the code's focus is on the welfare of patients and clients, rather than on the interests of registered nurses. (It is, of course, arguable that the two are indivisible and that attention to staff welfare issues may increase staff motivation and morale and thus impact positively on patient care. Conversely, ignoring staff welfare may have the opposite effect.)

The underpinning theme of the NMC (2004) code is beneficence (and, by implication, non-maleficence), justice and respect for all individuals who require nursing care. Registered nurses who decide to take any form of industrial action must ensure that they adhere to the advice within the code and, if they withdraw from care provision, they must first ensure that patients will not suffer as a result. The emphasis upon individual practitioner accountability entails that nurses who take any form of industrial action will be expected to provide the rationale for their decision.

In deciding whether industrial action is justifiable in a *specific* instance you may, in addition to referring to a code of ethics, use the DECIDE model (see Chapter 12 for details), as it provides a systematic framework within which to approach difficult decisions and review them.

CODES OF CONDUCT/ETHICS: SUMMARY

It may be seen then that codes of practice serve several functions. One is to ensure that practitioners are aware of the standards expected by their regulatory body. Codes also inform the public, employers and other occupational groups of these standards. They are also a means of highlighting the professional aspirations of nursing as an occupation.

It is clear that issues in healthcare practice are so diverse and complex that no code can address all eventualities. Codes do, however, provide one way of ensuring practitioner accountability and maintenance of competencies.

Accountability and documentation

Formal reporting by means of handwritten or printed documentation is one way in which nurses demonstrate accountability for their practice. Documentation of care should provide a comprehensive account of the patient's journey through a care setting, as identified in Box 5.2.

Box 5.2 Documentation of care

Records that document care should include the following information about patients:

- admission/transfer/discharge
- care planned and provided
- patient consent to procedures
- procedures and therapeutic interventions
- medication administration
- accidents/incidents.

Whilst the contents of Box 5.2 focus on documentation of *care*, the importance of documenting *all* areas for which registered nurses are accountable was highlighted earlier, in the section on student assessment. Within the UK, it is also explicated by the Nursing and Midwifery Council (NMC 2005c).

Post-registration education and practice (PREP)

Not only must professional regulatory bodies ensure that new recruits achieve a certain standard before they are allowed to practise, but they must ascertain that their registered practitioners maintain those standards.

Indeed, the use of practice placements within student nurses' programmes makes it imperative that RNs continually update their practice to ensure that students are exposed to competent, if not best, practice.

At both macro and micro levels, nursing must ensure that its standards of practice are supported by a sound theoretical base. The requirement for continuing educational development following initial registration has become formalised within the UK. The NMC stipulates the requirement for evidence-based practice within its post-registration education and practice (PREP) documentation (NMC 2005b) and for lifelong learning (NMC 2002d). The purpose of PREP is to ensure that all registered practitioners remain competent to practise and proof of continuing professional development and practice is now a prerequisite for periodic re-registration.

Nurses and other healthcare professionals

A variety of occupational groups are involved in the care of patients, both directly and indirectly. The relationships that members of these occupational groups have with patients vary according to the problems and needs of individual patients. Within the UK there is emphasis in health and social care provision on interdisciplinary collaboration and also on increased involvement of patients in their care planning and provision. In the UK one example of interdisciplinary cooperation is the formation of managed clinical networks (MCNs). The purpose of MCNs is to unite different occupational groups in communication that provides 'seamless' care for patients, although this may be an aspiration that encounters challenges in practice.

It should also be noted that any attempt to 'manage' a network which is essentially collegial is problematic. The clinical networks and professional associations of like-minded practitioners form a strong link for intellectual and practice development, for example via conferences, workshops, professional journals and publications. Colleagues who work in different organisations may derive their professional stimulation from these clinical networks and, whilst their ties to these networks are weak compared with the more formalised connections that they have with their employing authority, the influence of collegial networks should not be underestimated (Granovetter 1973).

Lapsley & Melia (2001) describe the effectiveness of the clinical network in their study of financial constraints in the ICU. They note that:

> These social networks, however, work at two levels. There are tight, socially cohesive, highly democratic

multi-disciplinary teams working within ICUs. But there is also a weaker social network, based on the clinicians in the ICUs in different hospitals. This is not such a tightly functioning group which meets regularly. At this level the network exhibits the characteristics of weak connections in terms of contracts, but demonstrates the Granovetter thesis, that weak ties can often lead to strong network actions.

This form of professional activity, following Freidson's (2001) 'logic of professionalism', serves patients' interests. The politicians who drive the health service managers to produce results through managed clinical networks have agendas that extend only as far as the next election. The healthcare professionals, on the other hand, have a different kind of commitment. One element of this is their professional ethic – moral principles – which lead them to want to act in their patients' best interests and in the interests of securing a good reputation for the profession. The 'logic of professionalism' serves this kind of end, 'sheltering' it, as Freidson argues, from market and managerial demands (see Chapter 1).

Additionally, whilst policy initiatives address explicitly the need to foster *inter*disciplinary collaboration there appears to be an assumption that *intra*-occupational cooperation is unproblematic. Smooth intradisciplinary provision of care may in practice prove at least as challenging as that within inter-disciplinary teams.

There is a link between good teamwork and an open approach to the moral aspects of healthcare. In a study of ethical issues in intensive care it was argued that the teamwork found in the ICU can serve as a blueprint for the organisation and for the practice of care more generally across the health service (Melia 2004). Teamwork in intensive care works largely because of the nature of the specialism and the condition of the patients:

> The working practices of those committed to teamwork provide a good basis for the same kind of joint approach to understanding and discussion that is necessary for ethical debate. (Melia 2004, p. 120)

A main theme of the NHS modernising agenda in the UK is that healthcare professionals should work together. This entails professional boundary blurring and the development of new and/or expanded roles with consequent ethical implications that need to be explored.

Ethical issues are integral to all aspects of healthcare, but it is worth noting Wanless's (2002) UK government report on the future of the health service, which states that the fewer hours available from the number of professionals in the service (as a result of European Working Time Directives) will entail a less productive service. Wanless (2002) focuses on the fact that a high percentage of health service resources will be spent on provision of care for older adults. The report notes that public expectations of healthcare are growing, in part because of medical and technological advances, but that the number of workers has reduced and that there is greater workforce regulation. There is an increase in the number of older adults in the population, but fewer workers. Wanless also notes that people who inhabit remote communities have needs that may not be met by an increased focus on centralised and specialised healthcare provision. These are all issues that require further ethical examination and debate.

There are several moral paradoxes in the solutions offered to address the workforce shortfall – in terms of their costs and of unintended consequences. One 'solution' has been to expand the roles of nurses to compensate for the reduction in the hours worked by junior medical staff, but this may be the cause of many unfilled nursing posts – for example inadequate pay and conditions. Some registered nurses work for 'nursing banks', or for agencies for better pay. The use of 'nursing banks' and agencies may, however, result in nurses working excessive hours. The end result may then be that the fatigue of junior doctors reappears as fatigue in another part of the healthcare system. When healthcare professionals are expected to work together in new ways, the interests of patients are often cited as the motive. However, it must be remembered that the best use of resources is also an important concern. Both of these are of course moral issues.

There is a conundrum with this idea of boundary blurring, i.e. how may boundaries be blurred and crossed if they no longer exist? In order to blur or cross a boundary you need a clear idea of what it comprises in the first place. The challenge is to produce professionals who can work flexibly, yet retain a sense of their own discipline's identity without tribalism.

In 1951 Everett Hughes noted that:

> Seen in one way, the nurse's job consists of all the things that have to be done in the hospital and which are not done by other kinds of people.

Hughes was discussing status and job content and the study of occupations. We have moved on and nursing is now in one sense on an even footing with medicine in the UK, insofar as education programmes are situated within universities. In reality, however, it is very clear that many distinctions remain between the occupations in terms of power and culture. Additionally, there is a striking similarity with the 1951 position insofar as nursing is to a large extent perceived as the solution to the workforce problems that the modernisation of health services entails.

Public involvement in healthcare provision and regulation

Occupations regarded as professions, or with ambitions to be such, claim possession of specialised knowledge and skills that enable their practitioners to provide a service to society. The fact that the service is of a specialised nature with a theoretical base makes it difficult for the public to judge the performance of professionals. This is one reason why professions have sought to develop ways of assuring the public that they will be protected from the potentially undesirable consequences of professional monopoly. The role of regulatory bodies was outlined earlier in this chapter. Regulatory bodies set and strive to maintain standards of practice (frequently formalised in codes of conduct/ethics), to provide an educational framework for recruits (e.g. NMC 2005a) and to regulate membership of the profession. The arguments for self-regulation are founded on the premise that specialist knowledge is required in order to understand the dynamics of professional practice. One difficulty, however, is that the 'closed shop' nature of self-regulation prevents independent critical viewpoints being brought to bear on the profession's practice.

It might be considered that the fact that no professional is above the law should alleviate public anxiety about the potential for abuse of privileged positions. Law courts provide one means of holding professionals publicly accountable. The extent to which the law is able to carry out this function is, of course, dependent on the transparency of professional practice that enables cases to be brought to court.

Allegations that professional bodies (whose *raison d'être* is ostensibly protection of the public) are more concerned to protect practitioners than their clients or patients, have led in the UK for demands for 'root and branch' reform of medicine's regulatory body, the General Medical Council (GMC). This demand increased following the findings of the Bristol Royal Infirmary Inquiry (HM Government 2001b), the Royal Liverpool Children's Inquiry (HM Government 2001a) and, most recently, the Shipman Inquiry (HM Government 2005a).

Professional regulation has also been reviewed under the modernising agenda in the UK because of the latter's patient-centred focus and standard setting for recognition of competence. The aim has been to set up a modernised professional regulatory system alongside the Quality Assurance arrangements within the NHS. This is not to say that the government is trying to move away from self-regulation, but it stipulates that a rigorous and robust modernisation of the system is required. In relation to the redesign of jobs around the needs of patients, the consultation noted that:

> focusing roles and tasks on what patients actually need in terms of their clinical care raises serious questions about the effectiveness and relevance of the present uni-professional structure of self regulation.

The Health Professions' Council was established in the UK in 2002. An ideological emphasis on working together and learning together requires regulation that encompasses all practitioners within healthcare professions and thus the need for cooperation between the regulatory bodies of all occupational groups.

Public awareness and concern about specific cases in which professionals have abused their powerful position in society have been accompanied by greater public access to information (e.g. via the internet). Recent decades have been marked by a decreased deference towards traditional 'authority' figures and by an increased readiness to question professionals' judgement and practice and to articulate concerns and complaints about treatment.

One way in which attempts have been made to provide increased transparency of decision-making in professional practice has been by a greater focus on public involvement in healthcare planning. This includes increased numbers of lay representatives serving within professional regulatory bodies in the UK and also patient and public participation at national and local levels. The degree to which members of the public who serve in this capacity are actually *representative*, in any quantitative sense, of the population as a whole is debatable. A study by Davies (2001) found that many lay representatives serving on the committees of regulatory bodies were middle-aged, had high socio-economic status and a current or past occupation as a professional.

CONCLUSION

In this chapter we have developed the discussion of accountability and responsibility that was begun in Chapter 3, when it was applied to specific aspects of nurse training and practice. We have explored registered nurses' accountability for their practice and the strengths and limitations of codes of conduct/ethics. We have also discussed the appraisal of nursing students as the registered practitioners of the future.

It can be seen that codes of practice have a number of functions. They provide information for healthcare practitioners and the public, about the standards of practice that are expected of registered nurses. Whilst the issues that arise in healthcare settings are so complex and diverse that no code of ethics can encompass all eventualities, codes nonetheless provide one kind of framework against which nursing practice may be evaluated. The role of nurses within multidisciplinary teams has been discussed in relation to both patient care and professional regulation. The increased involvement of lay members of the public in development of healthcare policy was noted although the degree to which these people are 'representative' of all sections of the community is questionable.

 further reading

Davies C M 2001 Lay involvement in professional regulation: a study of public appointment-holders in the health field. Open University, Milton Keynes

Freidson E 2001 Professionalism: the third logic. Polity Press, London

ICN 2000 Code of Ethics. International Council of Nurses, Geneva

Melia K M 2004 Health care ethics: lessons from intensive care. Sage, London

Savage J, Moore L 2004 Interpreting accountability: an ethnographic study of practice nurses, accountability and multidisciplinary team decision making in the context of clinical governance. Royal College of Nursing, London

Wanless D 2002 Securing our future health: taking a long term view. HM Treasury, London

PART 3

Nursing ethics – issues in clinical practice

Classical areas of controversy in nursing and biomedical ethics

6

Chapter contents

AIMS

This chapter has the following aims:

1. To explore the various meanings of 'care' and their relevance to understanding the ethics of 'nursing care'
2. To consider the moral issues of clinical nursing practice within the wider context of health as a personal and social value and the 'medicalisation' of life
3. To analyse some of the classic 'big issues' in biomedical ethics, to illustrate the general ethical concerns which they raise from a nursing perspective.

LEARNING OUTCOMES

When you have read and worked through this chapter, you should be able to:

■ Explain and illustrate what 'care' means in the context of professional and institutionalised nursing practice

■ Explain and illustrate with concrete examples why nursing ethics must pay attention to the demands of specific cases

■ Distinguish between the justification of particular decisions and giving reasons for a general rule or ethical policy

■ Give an account of the relationship between 'health' and 'disease' as personal and social values and how we construct the 'problems' of nursing ethics

■ Demonstrate ability to discuss the 'pros' and 'cons' of different approaches to at least one of the classic issues of: abortion, euthanasia, truth-telling, compulsory treatment, or resource allocation

■ Indicate what are some of the common ethical features of the classic 'dilemmas' and how they differ from one another.

WHAT ARE THE 'BIG ETHICAL DILEMMAS' FOR NURSES?

In previous chapters we have explored the general nature of ethics, the social context of nursing values and the various kinds of professional relationships and institutional contexts in which we have to exercise moral responsibility and make ethical decisions. In this chapter we begin to examine what are perceived to be some of the classic ethical dilemmas in healthcare, such as the perennial issues of abortion, euthanasia, truth-telling, prohibition of sexual relations with patients, compulsory treatment of people who have mental health problems and the allocation of scarce resources.

While these issues demand proper treatment in any textbook on ethics in healthcare, it can be disputed, however, whether these are the most important ethical issues for nurses to address. Judging from the nursing press, from discussion with student nurses, and looking at typical curricula in nursing ethics, it would appear that these *are* the 'big dilemmas' to be addressed. Why is this the case? There are three kinds of reasons why these issues are perceived to be so important: The *first* is that there is a long history of debate about these issues in the literature of *medico-legal ethics*. Four of these are even mentioned specifically in the earliest known code of ethics in healthcare, namely, the Hippocratic Oath (*c.* 420 BC). They obviously raise critical issues in the doctor–patient relationship, and perhaps the importance these issues have for doctors has determined the importance they are given by nurses. *Secondly*, these particular issues attract media attention because of their 'human interest' value as news stories, and the emphasis given in the press and TV to these issues influences entrants into nursing as well as registered practitioners in their perception of what are 'typical ethical issues'. *Thirdly*, these classical 'dilemmas' do raise important questions of principle and policy that we must get clear if we are working in healthcare, before we address the more specific responsibilities we have as nurses. The Hippocratic Oath gives classic expression to the three fundamental principles discussed in Chapter 2, namely, *beneficence* or the duty to do good, and not to harm patients – the duty of responsible care for patients, including the duty not to take advantage of the vulnerability of the patient, sexually or in any other way; *respect for human life* and, in this context, the specific prohibitions against abortion and euthanasia, and respect for the patient's privacy and secrets; and, *justice or fairness* to patients in not pretending to have expertise one does not have, and in not discriminating against patients because of their status, gender or age (Phillips 1988, pp. 89–90).

While these broad issues of principle are undoubtedly relevant to the nurse–patient relationship, as well as the doctor–patient relationship, most nurses are unlikely to be *directly* responsible for decisions to terminate a pregnancy, to terminate treatment or to assist a patient to die, in the compulsory treatment of mentally ill patients, or in the allocation of medical resources; but nurses do face the same questions and responsibilities about not abusing or exploiting vulnerable patients. However, whilst not directly responsible for clinical decisions in these situations, nurses are frequently the people who are left having to counsel patients or their relatives, and having to deal with the 'fallout' from such decisions, in caring for them afterwards. Nurses may have strong convictions about the ethics of abortion, euthanasia and compulsory psychiatric treatment, and may feel frustrated that they cannot do more to influence the outcome of decisions. They cannot be indifferent to the ethical quandaries involved, because they are not mere bystanders when decisions are taken. They may be consulted as members of the team about particular decisions, and they may be instructed to do something for a patient following a decision with which they disagree.

While nurses cannot take over direct responsibility for making the difficult decisions in cases of termination of pregnancy, or termination of life support, or compulsory psychiatric treatment, they will be expected to contribute their observations to the clinical assessments that are made, and they certainly can and should seek to influence general policy and decision procedures on these matters, to ensure that the ethical concerns of all stakeholders are taken into account, before decisions are taken.

Given their subordinate role in ethical and clinical decision-making in these situations, the real moral dilemmas for nurses arise in practice in relation to their subsequent involvement in providing care for the patients or relatives affected by the decision, e.g. direct nursing care for women having terminations or in recovery. Here the issues relate to the conflict of duties they may experience between what they are instructed to do and what they believe is unethical. The issues to be addressed concern who should have the power to determine clinical and ethical policy and who has ultimate responsibility for decisions about who does what and under what conditions. Some of the issues that need to be addressed are ethical questions about the limits of legitimate and competent authority and the nurse's duty of obedience, in relation to the nurse's legal and moral rights.

Nurses should be alert to the differences between doctors' and nurses' responsibilities here. They need to attend to the specific issues that relate to their own particular roles and responsibilities, and be on their guard against medical preoccupations 'setting the agenda' for nursing ethics. Given the fact that the roles and responsibilities of nurses are different, it is the business of a book like this, on nursing ethics, to attempt to clarify the differences (cf. Melia 1987, *Learning and Working: The Occupational Socialisation of Nurses*).

Before we address some of the classic 'big' ethical dilemmas in healthcare, we must therefore first clarify some of the general ethical presuppositions underlying nursing ethics, and issues to which nurses have contributed insight from the distinctive perspective of nursing care:

- the general nature of the *concept of care*, in the context of *nursing care*
- the *use of 'typical cases'* – a 'casuistic' approach to ethics, based on cases and precedents
- the relationship between *general* rules and *particular* moral decisions.

CARING AND THE DUTY OF CARE IN NURSING ETHICS

First of all, what do we mean by 'care'? The meanings associated with this term go deep into the roots of Western culture. It is related first to the Latin term *carus* = dear, designating something that is valued or expensive because it is scarce. By derivation it came to mean *loved, desired or esteemed* because of the intrinsic value of the object of care. The co-option of the term 'caritas' by Christian thinkers, like St Augustine (354–430 AD), to express the meaning of the Greek term *agape* (for other-regarding love), capitalises on these earlier associations of the word, and enriches it by applying to it the meaning of unconditional love, or self-less concern for the well-being, health and salvation of our neighbour. For Christians this love has its origin in God and is demonstrated in the redemptive forgiving love of Christ. More directly the English word comes to us from the Old English and Teutonic *caru* meaning *sorrow, or to be anxious for, or solicitous for the welfare of someone*. The term 'care' thus combines several meanings, which make it peculiarly apt to express our deepest concern for our fellow human beings and their physical, emotional and spiritual well-being (Barnhart 1988).

Caring for people means that you act for their good – help restore their autonomy, assist them to achieve their full potential, attain their goals in life and reach personal fulfilment. In theological language, the ultimate goal of *caritas* or *agape* is the salvation of the other person, and the word 'salvation' means 'to be made whole'. In that sense, the goal of caring is always to help others to be made whole, to achieve their optimum fulfilment as human beings. For the person who has been injured (and are we not all injured in some way or other?), the need is for healing, to be made whole. For the person who is sick, the need is to be restored to health. Patients need to be 'put back on their feet', to recover their independence where possible, and helped to feel that they are in control of their lives again.

Obviously, we are all vulnerable, and we may even be afflicted by the same problems as the patients we care for. This is not necessarily a bad thing. In fact, the experience of suffering may not only make us more sympathetic (from Greek *sum*, with, and *patheo*, to suffer) but it may also help us to empathise with our patients, that is, to view the world as they see it, from the inside. While sympathy is a spontaneous feeling we either have or do not have for people, empathy, the ability to put ourselves 'in someone else's shoes', is an art that can be learned, an exercise of imagination that can be practised. Furthermore, we need to develop insight into the desires and feelings that attract us into nursing and other caring professions in the first place. While these feelings (and needs) may be powerful motivators, they can also get in the way of doing our professional duty. This is because we may be determined more by our own unconscious agendas, our own need for help, our own fear of illness or death, than by motivation to do a skilled and professional job (Feifel 1967, 1977, Becker 1997).

This is part of what is expressed in the following extract from T.S. Eliot's *Four Quartets*:

The wounded surgeon plies the steel
That questions the distempered part;
Beneath the bleeding hands we feel
The sharp compassion of the healer's art
Resolving the enigma of the fever chart.
Our only health is our disease
If we obey the dying nurse
Whose constant care is not to please
But to remind of our, and Adam's curse
And that, to be restored, our sickness must grow worse.
The whole world is our hospital
Endowed by the ruined millionaire,
Wherein, if we do well, we shall
Die of the absolute paternal care
That will not leave us, but prevents us everywhere.
(Eliot 1944)

Studies of the helping personality show that personal experiences in childhood, or suffering and bereavement in adolescence, may be powerful motivators in the type of person attracted to 'caring' for other people. If we choose nursing to fulfil a personal need, or just an unconscious form of auto-therapy, to deal with our own problems or anxieties, then patients may suffer as we work out on them our own agendas, or 'act out' our own 'scripts' (Eadie 1975, Smithson et al 1983, Green & Green 1992, Branmer 1993).

'Caring' can be damaging to others if we do not understand its true dynamics, that is, the complex psychological forces that come into operation when we are in the powerful position of being 'helpers' to weak and dependent 'patients' or 'clients'. This is why, for example, psychiatrists and psychiatric nurses in training are encouraged to undergo personal psychoanalysis, or to participate in group therapy, as this process obliges the carer to explore his or her deeper feelings and often hidden ulterior motives for wanting to be a carer. While the care and attention of a good nurse can be beneficial, care can also be overprotective, intrusive, overbearing and infantilising (Mackay 1989, Lawler 1991, Laschinger & Goldenberg 1993). Like the corresponding forms of bad parenting, this can be very destructive. It has been well said that our greatest virtues are also the potential sources of our greatest weaknesses and vices. Just as parental strength and authority can be used in a protectively beneficent way, it can and has been used to justify all types of subtle oppression in family life (Campbell 2004).

From a more prosaic point of view, nurses are also employed to get certain work done as efficiently and effectively as possible. As a result, considerable limitations and practical constraints may be placed on the time available for 'caring relationships' and attention to the needs of particular patients. This means that in practice 'care' has to be more impersonal and altruistic. Furthermore, as Campbell points out in *Paid to Care* (1985), the care provided by nurses and other caring professions is not based entirely on disinterested altruism. Nurses enter nursing to care for people, but they also nurse to earn a living. Like any other employees they will have concerns about their own pay, shifts and working conditions, as well as being concerned about the well-being of their patients. As we shall see in the following chapter many of the issues raised about the nurse's 'right to strike' revolve around the ambiguities that arise because the nurse is supposed to be first and foremost a carer bound by the duties of caring, and perhaps only secondarily a paid health service employee. In the third chapter of this book we discussed some of the differences between lay care, and the professionalisation of caring services. 'Care' takes on new meaning and subtly different nuances in the context of paid-for services – whether paid for directly by the patient, or indirectly through state-provided healthcare services.

Thus, when we speak of nursing, we also have to take account of the moral and legal concept of 'a duty of care', namely the duty owed by all those with fiduciary responsibility for other people or their affairs, to protect their interests, health and safety. The moral aspects of a nurse's 'duty of care' are spelled out in the various codes of ethics for nurses, and specified in the rules and procedures nurses are expected to follow in a hospital. The legal duty of care of all those working in the 'caring professions' derives from the nature of the implicit or actual contract between the carer and the person for whom they care – into whose hands they have committed their lives, their children, or their personal affairs and property. To fail in one's duty of care as a professional is not only to be morally blameworthy for a breach of trust, but also may be legally actionable for breach of contract and culpable negligence. Interpreted in this way, as a requirement of both natural justice and contract law, 'care' becomes a matter of implementing the rules and fiduciary obligations implied in contracts-to-care.

In the history of ethics in the caring professions there has always been a tension between the demands of love and the demands of law. Care, in the context of nursing care, combines two different senses of caring:

- sensitive regard for the unique needs of the individual person, as valued in themselves, and recognition of the demands of their particular circumstances
- the general duty of care based on contractual and institutional duties and rules, designed to protect the vulnerability of those who depend on the care and protection of others.

The history of Judaeo-Christian ethics itself illustrates the problems of reconciling the demands of a universal justice and moral rules that are applicable to everyone with the demands of mercy and love, namely, that we address the particular needs of individuals in their unique circumstances. People have been exhorted to: 'follow your conscience', 'love your neighbour', 'do to others as you would have them do to you', and 'consider the effects of your actions on others'. On the other hand, people are charged 'to follow the Ten Commandments', 'to obey the Law of God and of the Church', 'to respect the God-given and inalienable rights applicable to all human beings'. Ramsey addressed these issues in his classic book *Deeds and Rules in Christian Ethics* (Ramsey 1983). These tensions, between the universal demands of moral laws and the specific claims of respect and care for individuals, have their counterparts in the practical counsels of most other cultural and religious traditions too. In tension with the demands of the formulated moral laws of the society, we find emphasis in these different traditions on compassion, respect, tolerance and love which focuses on the needs and rights of the particular person. Their significance is that they attempt to ground ethical obligation in various ways that also give some direction for action.

In the attempt to do justice to the needs of specific people in particular circumstances, the Judaeo-Christian love ethic has emphasised the kinds of obligation that are rooted in caring for others, rather than a more legalistic approach. In fact, St Augustine (354–430 AD) summed up Christian ethics in the challenging phrase 'love, and do as you like' (Clark 1984). An ethics of caring (or *agapeistic* ethics) which strives to determine what is the most loving thing to do in the circumstances serves three different kinds of purposes (see also Chapter 13).

- First, it offers an alternative to an impersonal rule-based ethics of duty, emphasising that the obligation to care for individuals, as we would want to be cared for ourselves, is more important than obedience to formal rules.
- Secondly, it emphasises that caring love demands that in decision-making we pay attention to the specific individual rather than to society in general, to the particular circumstances rather than universal conditions and requirements.
- Thirdly, it underlines the fact that our actions have to be measured by their effects on particular people and situations rather than their conformity to general rules and duties.

Discussion of the possibility of an 'agapeistic ethics' or love-based ethics is not restricted to Christian moral theologians, but has been taken up by secular moral philosophy as well, for whether or not one is a believer, or has faith in a God of love, the challenge of love and mercy to legalism is a perennial theme of ethics. Modern debate about 'situation ethics' has focused on these issues, with philosophers like Fletcher (1967) advocating a love ethic, or ethics of caring, which would do away with rules entirely (although saying that there are no rules is, of course, in itself a rule!). Ramsey (1983) argued that love has its own rules, and that even as it directs us to the uniqueness of each situation, and each existing individual, it is not arbitrary or capricious, but has to be consistent with the given structures and dynamics of being.

More recent discussions of a caring ethic, and its particular relevance to nursing, have been dominated by feminist critique of patriarchal institutions and the masculinist ethics that supposedly supports them. Some of this arose out of the debate sparked by Kohlberg and Gilligan. Kohlberg (1973, 1976) claimed to have established in his research – on the stages of moral development in children – that the highest stage of moral development is a form of altruistic justice orientation or rational ethics based on universal principles. He also made the further highly controversial claim that women rarely reach this highest stage of moral development. Gilligan (1977, 1982 and also 2nd edn 1993), on the basis of her research, published empirical evidence to show that women express their understanding of ethics 'in a different voice'. This feminine ethic is not one that is inferior to Kohlberg's male idealisation of an organising and controlling ethic, but is rather an ethic concerned with conflict resolution, the acceptance of responsibility and caring – something she argues Kohlberg failed to do justice to in his categorisation of developmental stages.

Some nurses (Noddings 1984, Larrabee 1993) and other writers have seized upon Gilligan's work and attempted to claim that caring is a quality native to the make-up of women and is the basis of a different feminist ethic and approach to moral responsibility. Views on ethics have become perhaps unhelpfully polarised between 'the caring perspective' and the 'justice perspective' with some nurses attempting to appropriate the caring perspective as their own, claiming that it is what is different about the approach and values of nurses and nursing care. Bowden (1997, p. 6) sums up the difference between the two approaches:

> The *caring perspective* is distinguished by a concern for care, responsiveness and taking responsibility in interpersonal relationships, and by a context-sensitive mode of deliberation that resists abstract formulations of moral problems. According to the *justice perspective,* emphasis is placed on rights, duties and general obligations, while moral reasoning is marked by schematic understandings of moral problems that allow previously ordered rules and principles to be applied to particular moral cases.

Useful though it may be to reappraise, from a feminist perspective, the presuppositions underlying our public institutions, and healthcare institutions in particular, there is a risk that emphasising the distinctive character of the 'feminine voice' in ethics may simply reinforce male/female stereotypes and strengthen sexist prejudices rather than bring about appreciation of the contribution of both men and women to broadening and deepening our understanding of ethics and the human condition (Davies 1995). The attempts to mobilise 'phenomenological method' to prove that 'empathy', 'embodiedness', 'capacity for tenderness', 'listening skills' are distinctively feminine traits can also be seen as tendentious and unhelpful. The value of moral education and ethics itself is undermined if we follow this course. Instead we need to address the challenge of how we collaborate with one another to develop agreement on the means to educate men and women to transcend their social conditioning and thus enable us to become more competent moral agents and more rounded human beings.

It is thus arguable that the polarisation of the 'caring perspective' and the 'justice perspective' not only risks entrenching male/female stereotypes and prejudices, but also is a distraction from the real task of ethics and moral education. This is admirably summed up by Bowden (1997, pp. 1–2): 'Caring expresses ethically significant ways in which we matter to each other, transforming interpersonal relatedness into something beyond ontological necessity or brute survival', and expresses her concern that attempts to 'penetrate the essence of care' will distract us from the 'radical call to attend to the complex ethical possibilities of interpersonal relationships'. She further observes that while it has been the task of feminist criticism of conventional ethics and systems to draw attention to the way individuals disappear into the anonymous institutions which seek to base their ethics on universal rational rules, there is a risk that we may fall into the trap of 'grand theory-making' in attempting to construct a general 'feminist ethics' – with one 'grand theory' simply supplanting another grand theory (see McAlpine 1996).

To set up caring and justice as antithetical to one another is dangerously misleading, for there can be no real care where the basic requirements of justice are not met, and no real justice where there is no care for the accused (or the victim), no due attention to the specific case, and no scope for mercy, or recognition of excusing conditions or diminished responsibility. St Thomas Aquinas himself suggested that talk about care and individual rights is a luxury, and somewhat meaningless, unless the basic structures of justice are in place. This is equally true in the most intimate of our personal relationships as it is in society in general. Put very simply, we cannot say we care for someone if we treat them unfairly, and infidelity to one another, including sexual infidelity, is basically a violation of justice rather than a failure of love.

THE VITAL IMPORTANCE OF THE SPECIFIC CASE

In applied ethics generally, and in nursing ethics in particular, we look at *typical* cases of moral problems and dilemmas in the hope that we may learn from the way others have thought about or dealt with similar problems. In ordinary life, it is important that we should be able to learn from our own past experience. Similarly in nursing, the accumulated practical wisdom or common sense of the profession, of our colleagues and wider society can give us some general guidance on how to act. However, this general knowledge, like the principles of the common law, does not tell us what precisely we should do in a particular situation. Casuistry – or the ethical approach based on the study of cases and precedents – can be helpful in ethics, as it is in law, but does not decide things for us, any more than does the charge nurse's anecdote of how she/he dealt with a 'similar' case, in the past, or says 'we've always done it this way'. We have to decide for ourselves, but knowing what others have thought or done prevents us from having to start from scratch.

Casuistry is an attempt to help us bridge the gulf between the universal and the particular, between moral absolutes and the relativities of everyday life, general moral rules and specific problems in concrete cases. Historically, casuistry developed as an approach to hard cases with attempts of confessors to deal with the problems presented to them by penitents in the confessional. Casuistry also evolved in the attempt to mediate between the seemingly absolute demands of Christian ethics and the canon law of the medieval Church, and the complex, contingent, and often tragic, circumstances of particular people, trying to live by the counsels of love and perfection.

The term 'casuistry' acquired a derogatory meaning at the time of the Reformation, as thinkers as different as Pascal and Luther criticised the Church for abandoning strict ethical principles, by appealing to precedents and particular cases and to 'prudential ethics' – to justify making all sorts of compromises with the absolute demands of the Gospel. The Protestant Churches in the 16th century claimed to be defending absolute moral principles against moral scepticism on the one hand and compromise on the other. Paradoxically it is the Roman Catholic Church that appears rigid today in its defence of moral truths which it claims are universal and absolute, and the Protestant Churches that seem to have come round to advocating the need for flexibility, and prudence. There has recently been a revival of interest in casuistry, not merely in the domain of religious ethics, but in secular ethics as well. What this debate highlights is the need in applied ethics not for abstract and general discussion of moral theory, but for guidance on how to act in particular circumstances, how to deal with actual moral decision-making.

Jonsen & Toulmin (1988) use the example of the abortion debate in the United States to illustrate the need to rediscover a practical, case-based, approach to ethical decision-making as represented in the tradition of casuistry:

> Behind the contemporary [abortion] debate, with all its topicality and newsworthiness, there lies a deeper intellectual conflict between two very different accounts of ethics and morality: one that seeks eternal, invariable principles, the practical implications of which can be free of exceptions or qualifications, and another, which pays closest attention to the specific details of particular moral cases and circumstances ...
>
> The public rhetoric of the abortion controversy has increasingly come, in recent years, to turn on 'matters of principle'. The more this has happened, the less temperate, less discriminating, and above all less resoluble the debate has been. Too often the resulting argument has boiled down to pure 'head-butting': an embryo's unqualified and unconditional 'right to life' being pitted against a woman's equally unqualified and unconditional 'right to choose'. Those who insist on arguing the abortion issue on the level of high theory and general principle thus guarantee that on the practical level the only possible outcome is deadlock. (Jonsen & Toulmin 1988, pp. 2–4)

Jonsen & Toulmin argue that neglect of practical and applied ethics, of training in ethical decision-making and problem-solving skills, and practice in dealing with real cases has opened the way to what they call 'the tyranny of principles'. Pretending that all moral issues can be settled at the level of theoretical discussion of principles has encouraged debate to become polarised – between antithetical and dogmatically held viewpoints, or dismissed as simply a matter of 'personal taste in morals'. This damaging view of ethics has been reinforced by the adversarial manner in which current moral issues are presented in the mass media. They describe three kinds of outcomes resulting from this trend:

- 'Much more widely, people at large tend to talk as though *ethical principles* or *moral rules* were exhaustive of ethics: that is, as though all that moral understanding requires is a commitment to some code of rules, which can be authoritative.'
- 'The central problem in philosophical ethics (has become) simply to explain what makes certain kinds of rules count as *moral* rules as contrasted with, say, the rules that govern sports or games, the rules for prudent investing, or the rules of social etiquette.'
- '[Principlism] leaves little room for honest conscientiously based differences of moral opinion (on the interpretation of the rules or the facts) ...

Once we accept rules and principles as the heart and soul of ethics, it seems no middle way can be found between absolutism and relativism.' (Jonsen & Toulmin 1988, pp. 6 and 7.)

However, as they point out, 'Taken by themselves, the general rules and maxims that play a part in people's ethical deliberations are only rarely matters of serious dispute ... these things are typically *beyond dispute*.' But what is more interesting, and what people do dispute about, is whether a given case falls under some general rule (e.g. is this a straightforward case of 'lying', 'murder', 'infidelity', etc.?) and whether one or more rules apply in the given case. In the case of two apparently conflicting duties, the debate is not generally about whether the duties are valid duties or not, but rather about the scope and priority of the conflicting duties involved. These are all matters that do vary from context to context and from case to case, even if the general principles are universal in nature (Toulmin 1958).

In this and the following two chapters we shall be discussing a number of cases in the attempt to clarify what some of the key ethical issues are in familiar cases, and to discuss the merits and weaknesses of the decisions taken. In that sense we will be employing a kind of casuistic (or case-based) approach throughout, and, as we explained in the Introduction, we have deliberately left the discussion of general moral theory to the end. However, questions of moral theory arise from time to time, and are dealt with as best we can in the context. We also return to 'casuistry' in another sense in Chapter 9, where we discuss practical methods and approaches to decision-making in ethics, and in particular discuss a number of problem-solving models that may be of value to nurses in dealing with everyday problems.

GENERAL RULES AND PARTICULAR MORAL DECISIONS

Scientific knowledge is general, and concerned with discovering universal laws. Ethics, however, like love, is concerned with particulars. Nurses, because they deal directly and intimately with individual patients, are only too well aware that rules are abstract and general, but decisions have to be made in concrete circumstances with reference to specific cases and particular people. There is a celebrated passage in Dostoevsky's novel *The Brothers Karamazov* where Fr Zossima criticises a young revolutionary, saying of him that 'He loves everyone in general and no-one in particular' (Dostoevsky 1927). There is a similar risk that ethics can get lost in theory and 'head-talk', and lose touch with reality, if it fails to address the fact that ethical decisions always relate to the specifics of particular cases and concrete situations. Moral rules and principles are of their nature general, moral decisions are always particular. Moral rules are intended to apply universally – to human life in general and to all people – but decisions involve applying general rules to specific situations, and can only be responsible decisions if they are a response to the actual needs and demands of a specific situation. We may take *policy* decisions about matters of a general nature, for ourselves, for a professional group, or for an institution, but policy *decisions* as decisions, are not general. They always relate to a specific context, or to a specific professional group at a particular time in a particular country, or to a particular hospital or institution.

Paradoxically, in the study and teaching of ethics, we tend to start by examining general issues and typical cases. This is to illustrate general moral rules and to clarify the universal principles we use to guide us in everyday decision-making. However, discussing typical cases cannot help us decide what to do in a specific case, even if the case material may have once upon a time related to a specific situation (like all the cases discussed in this book). By discussing 'hypotheticals', 'typical cases', general situations, or even specific past case histories (where we do not personally know all the relevant details), we can only reach general conclusions, not a specific conclusion relevant to a specific case.

In this chapter, we will discuss some of the general ethical issues raised by a number of typically recurrent human situations, where healthcare workers and nurses face conflicting moral duties and responsibilities. All of the following situations can give rise to moral quandaries for nurses:

- assisting with antenatal care and childbirth
- dealing with neonatal death and abortion
- advising parents on child and adolescent nurture and development
- helping people cope with physical and mental disability
- care and containment of people who have mental health problems
- counselling related to sexual dysfunction
- assisted reproduction and infertility treatment
- coping with ageing and enduring dependency
- care of the dying and bereaved.

We will argue that the skills and experience we need to make sound ethical decisions, here as elsewhere, cannot be learned by discussion of 'dead' and 'past-tense' cases. To do so encourages the view that ethical decision-making is retrospective, that is, about finding rationalisations after the event for what we, or others, have already done. By contrast, *making ethical decisions is prospective, that is, we must confront problems for which we do not have ready-made answers, and still have to find solutions in the future.* This is what makes decision-making challenging, difficult and sometime scary, even if we base our decisions partly on what we have learnt from past experience. The difficulty lies not in deciding *what* general rules or principles might apply, but rather *how* they should be applied in this particular case. If we think decision-making is about the former, then we are liable to get lost in theorising and 'head-talk', whereas the practical challenge is to make a decision that leads to appropriate action in the actual situation.

So what practical use is the discussion of general ethical problems or typical cases in our moral formation and training in responsible ethical decision-making?

In order to orientate ourselves in life and the world of moral experience, we perhaps need something equivalent to tourist guides and maps to help us find our way. The information we can gain from a tour guide is indirect. It is the second-hand knowledge of someone who has been to the place before and has learned to find their way around. A map can also help us orientate ourselves by giving us general bearings and directions, but it is no substitute for traversing the terrain and discovering its attractive and dangerous features for ourselves. Although a map is always a map of a particular place, the information it contains is general, abstracted from reality and represented in a different medium – say on paper – by means of formal conventions, techniques of projection, scales and colour codes, etc.

Approaching the subject of ethics by discussing general ethical problems and issues has the same kind of value to us that studying geography from textbooks has, namely, that it gives us general knowledge of what kinds of things we are likely to encounter in that territory. Using typical cases, or other people's case histories, is more like relying on an experienced guide to show us around, but ultimately you only learn to find your own way about by venturing out on your own. Other people's experience can be no substitute for your own. With the best manual in the world, you cannot learn how to swim without getting into the water yourself!

These remarks need to be borne in mind, as you read this chapter and the following three. You can learn some general knowledge of ethics from textbooks, but you cannot learn skills or wisdom in ethical decision-making from a textbook. You may learn what is involved in making ethical decisions, and what is required to give a sound practical or theoretical justification for some course of action, but you can only learn how to become skilled in these areas by practising the skills, exercising practical responsibility, and developing competence in applied ethics in real life, and in relation to real-life moral problems.

THE 'BIG ISSUES' IN A WIDER NURSING CONTEXT

In examining some of these classic dilemmas it is important to stress again, as we said in Chapter 2, that ethics is concerned not only with 'dilemmas', but also with how we learn to deal in a skilled and professional manner with those recurrent moral problems to which the bulk of our routine moral decisions relate. Further, it is important to stress that nursing ethics is not confined to dilemmas or problems of clinical nursing, but must include discussion of a much wider range of ethical issues. For example:

- how 'health' and 'disease' are matters of personal and professional value judgement
- how to manage conflict and promote cooperation in interprofessional relationships
- how to develop corporate ethical policy in hospitals and other healthcare institutions
- how to address general ethical issues in the political economy of healthcare.

To illustrate how the real ethical issues may differ from the apparently important ones, we might cite the example of the Edinburgh Medical Group study of professional attitudes and values in the care of the dying and the bereaved (Thompson 1979a, Chs 2 and 8). The Group set out to examine some of the classic moral problems in terminal care, such as 'to treat or not to treat', 'to tell or not to tell', and euthanasia and the right to die. What came to light in the course of the study was the fact that in practice these issues were less important (especially for nurses) than a host of other issues around care of the dying – e.g. interprofessional communication and conflict, 'buck passing', and institutional constraints on good practice – issues that tend to be neglected in most discussions of ethics. While society, forms of healthcare provision, and nurses' and medics' preparation for practice have changed considerably, the general point remains relevant, namely that we cannot accept at face value what conventional wisdom, or the media, suggests are the most important ethical questions. Observation and research in nursing has brought to light the fact that the issues perceived as important by practitioners and patients may be quite different from those perceived as important by the public (Broekmans et al 2003, DoH 2001a).

In particular, we have argued (in Chapter 2) that there are at least four different levels at which we need to address specific features of situations in nursing ethics: namely, what we have called the micro, macho, meso and macro levels, or collectively, the 'Russian dolls' model of ethics, for each level is nested within a more encompassing level (see Boxes 2.1 and 2.2). In Box 6.1 we attempt to disaggregate some of the ethical issues that we have to address at the different levels of nursing practice, management, policy-setting and inter-agency cooperation.

It is for these kinds of reasons that it is important not to restrict the scope of nursing ethics to examination of the *micro-ethical* issues involved in clinical nursing. We must examine the following range of questions around interprofessional relations and teamwork: questions of professional dominance and professional autonomy, individual roles and responsibilities, the accountability of teams, questions of leadership and who ultimately 'carries the can'.

Box 6.1 Micro, macho, meso and macro issues in the ethics of healthcare

Micro issues (clinical nursing ethics)

- Ethics of one-to-one nurse–patient relationship
- Ethics of clinical nursing in home or hospital
- Ethics of nursing people who have enduring or terminal conditions
- Ethics of health screening/well-person clinics

Macho issues (professional nursing ethics)

- Professional codes and professional dominance
- Nurse–doctor–nurse roles and responsibilities
- Teamwork – leadership and accountability
- Primary care/hospital team membership

Meso issues (ethics of managing nursing services)

- Nurse manager/nursing and general staff relations
- Employment policies, work allocation, grievances
- Corporate ethical standards and quality assurance
- Human resource management and resource allocation

Macro issues (political ethics of health policy)

- Health service policy, management and scarcity
- Nursing research and health promotion strategies
- Political ethics of health authority/region cooperation
- 'Politics' and 'economics' of the National Health Service

These are what we refer to as the *macho* issues. The third level at which important ethical issues arise, the *meso level*, is the level of internal management of healthcare institutions and the relationships of the various parties or 'internal stakeholders' that have a vested interest in the outcome of any management decisions. The fourth level, or *macro level*, relates to that of the political economy or political ethics of healthcare and applied social policy. We can become involved in ethical disagreements at each of these levels because we differ in our personal philosophies of health and the value we invest in our health as a society; or in relation to: our professional values, the ethical culture and policies of institutions and hospitals; the performance standards, policies and methods of quality assurance adopted; and in relation to local and national health policy (Campbell 1985, White 1985).

Pedagogically, to focus first on the moral quandaries in clinical situations is probably sound, both because of their immediate appeal, and also because they focus directly on the nurse–patient relationship. These quandaries also serve to illustrate the tensions experienced by nurses in accepting responsibility for the well-being of patients, between their personal feelings and moral beliefs on the one hand and their professional responsibilities on the other. These issues are important and cannot be avoided, but it should perhaps be emphasised that as a professional carer, paid to provide care, the nurse also has wider social responsibilities in this public role as a kind of public servant, hospital official or health service employee.

The moral problems and dilemmas which arise, in the exercise of the public office of 'nurse', are no less important and, in senior posts, often involve much heavier responsibility. Special ethical issues arise in the exercise of the wider responsibilities of nurses to groups of patients, relationships with colleagues, and in accountability to employers and the general public. These areas of responsibility are often regarded as more 'political' but are really continuous with the direct and intimate problems of patient care. Perhaps by regarding them as 'political' we implicitly recognise that they raise questions at the macro level about our commitment to wider ideals and beliefs about society – our ideological commitments. By contrast, the more familiar clinical dilemmas relate to the micro level, that is, to specific problems or dilemmas raised for us by conflict within our personal systems of beliefs. Problems of cooperation, and conflicts, with other professions (doctors, social workers, chaplains and allied health professions), may not be merely problems of the pecking order of the various professions in the ranks of professional dominance,

or who 'calls the shots'. There may also be specific difficulties which arise because of the different theoretical perspectives from which each profession defines '*the problem*', different '*diagnoses*' and different kinds of interventions or '*treatment*' of the problem, as well as different expected '*outcomes*' (Downie 1971).

In dealing with a difficult case or complex situation it may be useful to use the grid shown in Box 6.2 with the parties involved, to clarify the conflicts of values and expectations involved.

OUR DIFFERENT VALUE JUDGEMENTS ABOUT HEALTH

We cannot avoid making value judgements about our health or debating matters of ethical policy in relation to healthcare since the whole question of our health and well-being – as individuals, in family life, in our work and in society – is not a matter of indifference to us. Anthropologists have pointed out that there is a wide variety between different societies in what they regard as 'health' or what they define as 'disease', but however we define these terms, we all desire good health and seek to avoid pain and injury, disease and death. The illness or disability of a parent or one family member can affect the well-being of all the others. Work-related accidents or absenteeism caused by illness affects the productivity of organisations and industry, often more seriously than strikes. The cost of caring for the sick, the injured, people with mental health problems, those who are severely handicapped, have dementia or are dying, is a burden on any society – a burden not only on those in families who bear the brunt of most of the anxiety and direct care, but also on the state in providing primary care and hospital services, and on the professional staff who are paid to care.

Following the UK Community Care Act 1990, government policy encouraged care in the community as an alternative to hospital-based care, and the estimated number of informal carers in the UK was estimated by Department of Health in 2000 as 5.7 million (DoH 2000a). While critics of the government considered that this was done simply to cut public expenditure, there was a groundswell of public support for 'normalisation' for those in long-stay institutional care that was used to justify this policy. The debate was in part about values, about the meaning of 'health' and 'quality of life' and what constitutes 'normal' living for those with disabilities.

'Health' and 'disease' are terms with several meanings – scientific and medical meanings, and more popular meanings that relate to ideal states of personal

| Box 6.2 Proforma for distinguishing professional perspectives and value bases |||||
Key player or STAKEHOLDER	Professional VIEW or VALUE BASE	Definition of 'THE PROBLEM'	Proposed action or INTERVENTION	Hoped-for result or OUTCOME
1.				
2.				
3.				
4.				
Areas of difference				
Areas of common ground				
Elements in possible joint action plan				

and social well-being or states of personal and social disorder we wish to avoid. Even in physiology and pathology, 'health' and 'disease' are normative terms, that is, they describe the state of an organism as approaching ideal or optimum functioning or varying degrees of malfunctioning or dysfunction – within a continuum where health is at one pole and disease at the other. At a more personal level, we do not have to be 'health freaks' in order to want to be healthy, because most of the things we do are more enjoyable when we are fit and healthy than if we are unfit, ill or injured. Good health is something we value. It is an ideal and a goal we strive to realise for ourselves (and perhaps for others). So, too, disease is an evil we try to avoid or prevent, or failing both, to cure. The classic WHO definition of health expresses in ideal and aspirational terms this sense of health as a personal and social value, and disease as a dis-value, by stressing that 'health is complete physical, mental and social well-being and not just the absence of disease, or infirmity' (WHO 1947). In attempting to define health we raise fundamental ethical, political and even religious questions about values and lifestyles, even before we get into specific questions about the personal and moral responsibilities of nurses and other health professionals in paid service to others (Seedhouse 1986). Our expectations about our health and treatment of disease and disability give rise to wider policy debate about the nature of health services and the best systems for effective and efficient delivery of healthcare (Robertson et al 1992).

In making decisions about our personal health, we have to make both practical and moral choices about our behaviour and lifestyle – if we are to live healthy lives and avoid accidents, injury, disease or premature death. Alternatively, while we may tend to regard attempted suicide as a sign of mental disorder in an individual, the decision to end one's life prematurely, either by direct suicide or by taking risks that may result in death, is also a moral choice. We do not exist in splendid isolation and our lives touch and interlock with those of others in many different ways: in family life, in our friendships and love affairs, in our work and recreation. Just as an attempted or actual suicide can cause intense pain and grief to many other people, so too in a less dramatic way illness, injury or personal distress can and does affect other people.

Society is and has to be interested in the health and well-being of its members. First, because we are part of one another; second, because the whole human family may suffer if we are unable to make or are prevented from making our own contribution to society; and third, because of the additional burden and cost of care and treatment that may result. Consequently, government public health measures (including health education, immunisation, screening, the imposition of quarantines and travel restrictions, compulsory notification of diseases, and general controls on sanitary supply of food and water, sewerage/waste disposal and environmental controls on housing, provision of public amenities and health services) are all undertaken by the state in order to prevent disease and to promote the health of society. These measures are intended to promote better health for people, and to reduce the cost of ill-health to individuals and the state.

From the outset there is a potential conflict here between our personal liberty to do what we want in pursuing the lifestyle of our choice, and the well-intentioned but often officious and interfering attempts of family, friends, school and health professionals, mass media and political agencies to change or redirect our health behaviour. These tensions relate to basic ethical questions about the relations of personal rights and social responsibility, of personal well-being and the wider good of society, and these also have general relevance to nursing ethics. As front-line health educators with a professional responsibility to prevent disease as well as to care for and treat those who are ill, nurses have to face contradictions between their own health behaviour (e.g. with regard to smoking, drug or alcohol abuse, diet, fitness, responsible sex) and what they are advising their patients or clients to do. The issues are not only about the public's expectations relating to the nurse or health professional as a role model, but also about their credibility as health educators or agents of social control.

For example, health education can be presented in such a way as to encourage us to know more about healthy living, to make informed choices and to take responsibility for our own health and choice of lifestyle. Alternatively, health propaganda may seek to redirect our behaviour, either by persuasion, or by subtle means or not so subtle legal coercion. Aggressive promotion of healthy lifestyles by state agencies is implicitly justified by endorsement of a kind of healthist ideology, whereas traditional preventive medicine simply sought to prevent disease. This is not necessarily to be condemned, but rather we should be clear about what kind of values are being promoted and should be willing to examine and challenge these.

On the one hand, millions of pounds are spent annually by the tobacco, alcohol and junk food industries on advertising and sponsorship to promote the sale of products that are damaging to health. On the other hand, we increasingly see the alliance of health propaganda with commercial interests in the marketing of health (sports equipment and clothing, public spectaculars and mass participation in spectator sports). The public fashion for jogging, health foods, diet and fitness is not just a product of individual people's desire to be fit and healthy. It is the result of a deliberate marketing of health – using peer pressure, personal interest, and raised awareness of health as an issue in people's lives – but also of an orchestrated attempt of political and commercially controlled media advertising to 'market' health as an ideology and to change people's health behaviour and lifestyles accordingly (Tones 2001).

When the World Health Organization (WHO) adopted *Health For All by the Year 2000* as a policy objective in 1978, this was dismissed by many cynics as wildly optimistic, impractical and unattainable. However, by setting such a goal, the WHO has encouraged UN member states to formulate specific attainable objectives and action plans to achieve this target. As a result, member states have adopted and begun to implement programmes of health promotion, disease prevention and reorientation of resources to primary care that may well improve the health status of millions of people around the world and change the face of healthcare well into the 21st century (WHO 1981, 1999b). This has come about, and is coming about, through attention to the ethical and political implications of good health being pursued as something of personal and social value. If we start by recognising that 'health' and 'disease' are normative terms, then we will be obliged to see that discussion of moral problems and responsibilities around direct patient care fall within the broader commitments we make as individuals, professionals and members of society to achieve good health. These may include individual and pressure-group activity either to promote good health for all and to encourage people to help themselves to health, or to raise public awareness and mobilise public support for fiscal, legal and other controls on the advertising and marketing of products which will damage our health. In this context the development of the internet has served both as a platform for advertising health and health products, but also as a means for groups to rally support for health causes, e.g. free or cheaper drugs for treatment of HIV/AIDS.

As nurses become more active as front-line agents of health education and health promotion, the ethics of this kind of activity requires more careful attention and debate. Some argue that state-initiated health promotion carries with it the risk that health professionals will be co-opted to become 'health police', invading the privacy of households and intruding into the lives of ordinary people. Major national health promotion campaigns or programmes can also be seen as experiments in health and social engineering. Perhaps they should be subject to ethical review and controls like any other forms of medical or nursing research, as required by the Declaration of Helsinki (WMA 1996), or review by Research Ethics Committees. To prevent health promotion becoming authoritarian, officious and inclined to blame the victim, ethical guidelines are required. The WHO itself has sponsored workshops and issued discussion papers on the subject (WHO 1981, Robertson et al 1992).

THE 'MEDICALISATION OF LIFE' AND THE 'BIG DILEMMAS'

It is not these broader ethical issues related to public and community health that we think of first when medical or nursing ethics is discussed. Although the issues around prevention and positive health promotion are increasingly important in nursing, it is the ethical issues related to the treatment of injury, disease and death that have greater prominence in public debate and professional training. The popularity of hospital-based TV 'soap operas', including police dramas with a focus on forensic medicine, reflects perhaps a morbid preoccupation of a healthy population with the ever present threat in life of suffering and death, but for whatever reason, the dramatic 'ethical dilemmas' of medical fiction grip us more than the ethics of healthy living. Further, medical students and trainee nurses perceive the dramas of clinical medicine to be important, because they are the issues which first challenge them when they enter the extraordinary world of hospitals and the crises they observe in acute medical and surgical wards, and in accident and emergency medicine.

The reasons for the focus on clinical medical ethics are complex and various; for example, most health professionals are trained within the crisis-oriented treatment services rather than in prevention. The so-called 'health' services are in practice more concerned with the treatment of disease; and, indeed, despite the encouragement of the WHO to shift emphasis in healthcare to primary care (with an enhanced role for nurses), and despite recent government policy favouring a shift of resources to primary care and general practice, nevertheless the evidence is that the bulk of the money and resources is still going into clinical research and therapeutic services. So, it is not surprising that power and prestige tend to be concentrated there (Baggott 2004, Ch. 10).

McKeown, in his classic study (1979), argued that diagnostic and treatment services have contributed less to improving the health of society than have improvements in housing, food supplies, income, clean water, hygienic sewerage disposal and general public health measures. However, the image of high-technology medicine and intensive care nursing remains more attractive to those attracted to working in healthcare, and the focus on individual patients and their problems has more human appeal. Similarly, although the majority of nurses will be employed in long-term care of elderly people, those with enduring health problems, or mental illness, it is midwifery, neonatal and paediatric nursing, acute medical, surgical and terminal-care nursing that enjoy higher prestige and glamour. These factors influence our perception of what issues are ethically most important.

All the big ethical issues of common concern to health professionals relate to the way power (or control) is exercised over people, or power shared with people – whether people seek their help voluntarily or are committed into their care by relatives or other authorities. Questions of respect for patient autonomy have become increasingly important as we have moved away from a position where the authority of the doctor or nurse was beyond question, and pressure has built from various special interest groups to defend patients' rights. While the division of responsibility and/or authority may differ in the ward or in the primary care team, and while many of the frustrations of nurses may focus on the fact that they often have responsibility without executive authority, it would be a mistake to overlook the very real and proper responsibilities carried by nurses, as distinct from doctors.

The ethical issues of greatest concern to nurses tend to be those that relate directly to their spheres of personal responsibility in either direct patient care or management roles, rather than the more general and intractable issues where they feel they can personally do very little or which are beyond their control. Issues around communication with patients (truth-telling and confidentiality) and conflicts with doctors, other carers and relatives over patient care tend to predominate. Nurses may well have an intellectual interest in, and need to be informed about, a wide range of current moral issues in healthcare, and some nurses may have particular reasons to conscientiously object to assisting with abortions or be worried by requests from patients for euthanasia, but in practice they can also distance themselves from some of these issues as not being their responsibility but the doctor's.

In many cases nurses may feel relatively powerless insofar as others in more powerful positions (e.g. doctors or the competent legal authorities) take decisions that affect the admission or discharge of patients or the form of treatment they are to receive. In this sense nurses are not in control and inherit responsibilities which flow on from decisions taken by others, and which they may feel powerless to change or influence. Most of the classic big dilemmas are problems in law or medical ethics before they become problems for nurses. However, this is not to say that these problems and dilemmas do not present in a different way in nursing, or that nurses do not have unique and distinctive responsibilities, or that nursing ethics does not have a unique contribution to make to the debate about these issues. In fact, if nurses were to focus their concern and frustration on their perceived powerlessness relative to doctors, and were to see nursing ethics only as a kind of commentary on or vicarious participation in medical ethics, then it would be hardly worth pursuing.

In reality, nurses do have considerable power over patients, and even influence over doctors. The way they organise staff time and ward or community resources can directly influence both the quantity and quality of care given to patients. They can influence the patient both directly and indirectly by the way they change or manipulate the patient's environment. They can influence the decisions of doctors, paramedics and other carers, by their reported observations about patients and the appropriateness or inappropriateness of treatment, levels of pain control, compulsory detention in hospital or discharge. The nature and quality of their observations regarding the patient's physical, emotional and psychological state may be critical in the patient's management. They can also influence nurse and hospital management about necessary organisational and institutional change, or campaign for more resources, and in general have a responsibility to maintain the quality and standards of patient care.

While individual nurses may have reason to object to carrying out doctor's orders, whether in administering drugs with potentially fatal side-effects, assisting with abortions, offering euthanasia or administering ECT (electroconvulsive therapy), the real focus of concern in nursing ethics should be rather on those areas where nurses have specific responsibilities that are different from those of other health professionals or social workers. These areas relate to such matters as the organisation of the patient's day, observation and communication skills, skilled attention to the patient's physical, psychological and spiritual needs, making the environment more patient-friendly, and counteracting institutionalisation and dependency. These nursing issues are often overlooked while more attention is given to the big dilemmas of medical ethics.

One explanation of how abortion, euthanasia, truth-telling, compulsory psychiatric treatment and the allocation of scarce resources have become big issues in medicine and nursing in modern life is to see this as a consequence of the historical process which Illich (1977) called 'the medicalisation of life'. According to his analysis, the concentration of human popu-

lations in cities, the loss of extended family support and the increasing isolation of the nuclear family have led to the deskilling of ordinary people in the ability to deal with suffering, illness, injury and death in the community. As a result, we have all become more dependent on doctors and other health professionals to cope with the problems of living. Doctors, he argues, have effectively become the priests of modern society, presiding over and controlling all the crucial rites of passage from birth to death, with nurses as their acolytes. The whole of life and all its stages, from the cradle to the grave – health and disease, reproduction, birth, maturation, death and bereavement, and mental disorder – has been medicalised.

This 'medicalisation of life' has meant that health professionals have inherited increasing power and control over matters of life and death, which in more traditional society have been the domain of lay-carers, priests and religious healers. Faith in religion and in divine judgement or providential care has to a large degree been replaced by faith in secular science and the 'miracles' of modern medicine. Illich argued that health professionals tend to preside over the rites of passage at all key life events, and have thus acquired awesome, even god-like, responsibility for making life-and-death decisions. Public preoccupation with the classical ethical dilemmas of healthcare can be seen partly as a critical response to this medical control of people's lives and an attempt to reiterate their own rights in these areas. Furthermore, some of the ethical problems can be seen to be 'iatrogenic', that is caused by this medicalisation and institutionalisation of people and their life problems. Other problems have been created for professionals, in this vast, growing, and now multinational 'health industry', because commercialisation of healthcare and the division of labour have also complicated interprofessional relations by making them compete for clients. At the macro level, major political and fiscal problems have been created for governments by public expectations of total care of people by the healthcare services.

Illich's critique of this process of medicalisation sparked a powerful reaction worldwide, and this has resulted in a much greater emphasis on patients' rights, the need for patient advocacy, and representation of lay people on many management and policy-making bodies in local and national healthcare. Nurses have often used his arguments to reinforce their criticisms of the arrogance and assumed moral superiority of doctors 'playing God' and to support attempts to humanise the environment of care.

However, the implications of Illich's analysis go much further and relate to the role of nurses too in the process of medicalisation of healthcare – whether in the traditional role of 'doctors' handmaidens' or as modern self-consciously independent health professionals with distinctive roles and responsibilities of their own. In both cases nurses are part of the process and the system that has resulted in this medicalisation of life, with its corresponding removal from ordinary people of the power of decision-making and responsibility for their own lives. While it is arguable that the power of priests and religious healers was limited by acknowledgement of a transcendent divine power and authority to which they felt ultimately accountable, secular healthcare is subject to no such limitations. It has remained for patient advocacy groups to campaign for patients' rights, and to influence governments' policies to recognise and promote 'consumer choice', not least on the basis that they pay, directly or indirectly, for the services they receive, and have a right to hold health professionals accountable.

Some of the big dilemmas arise as a direct consequence of the responsibilities health professionals have acquired in this process of the medicalisation of life. For example, medical science had created expectations that a 'magic bullet', or technical 'fix' can be found to every human problem. The high risk and high cost of many of these life-saving interventions, and attempts to deal with human distress and unhappiness, have created their own crop of unprecedented ethical quandaries. This is obvious in the case of the side-effects of treatment and the questions that arise about the extent to which patients should be informed of all the possible consequences of treatment, and of the difficulties of obtaining fully informed consent from anxious, traumatised and perhaps ill-educated patients. There are also questions about the use, in situations of extremity, of untried remedies that have not been subject to proper randomised controlled trials.

The quest for miracle cures has driven science to extraordinary lengths to find new (and commercially profitable) ways of treating diseases such as cancer or multiple sclerosis. Bioengineering has resulted in the production of the most amazing range of aids to assist people with various disabilities, or loss of limbs, eyesight etc. As means are discovered that might enable painful conditions to be treated or prevented, the question arises whether scientists have a duty to try these out, regardless.

The development of biochemistry, genetics and methods for genetic screening have raised hopes that by means of genetic engineering and gene 'therapy', genetic disorders will be eliminated, infertility treated, in vitro fertilisation and embryo transplant made safe and routine, organ 'donation' and replacement reliable, and chemotherapy for all kinds of human distress and mental disorder found.

Some of the issues are not new, as routine screening for sexually transmitted infections in the past has shown (in relation to questions of contact tracing etc.), but this has additional poignancy if the patient is discovered to have HIV/AIDS. Genetic screening may identify an individual (or their offspring) as liable to inheritance of genetic defects or fatal disease, such as Huntington's chorea. This not only presents the healthcare worker with the dilemma of whether or not to tell the person involved, but also presents the subject with a terrible choice if they wish to have children.

While assisted reproduction techniques such as in vitro fertilisation (IVF) of previously harvested ova, or intracytoplasmic sperm injection, in severe cases of male infertility, may result after several attempts in a successful live birth, there is also a high failure rate for these expensive procedures. They not only involve serious additional risks to women in the 'harvesting' of sufficient numbers of their ova for experimental purposes, but also raise serious questions about the long-term genetic and health consequences, and costs relative to benefits, of interventions to assist individuals with genetic defects to have children. There are also the questions that arise about the propriety of the long-term storage of fertilised ova, to whom they belong, and who pays for the costs of storage – perhaps even beyond the lifespan of the donors.

Other consequences of the medicalisation of life, to which Illich himself drew attention, were the increasing number of medically induced kinds of pathology or *iatrogenic disease*. Examples where medical treatment has itself created health problems are multiplying. These include: unnecessary surgery; indiscriminate use of antibiotics (creating pathogens that are immune to all available drugs), including the risks of hospital-acquired infections such as MRSA; vast numbers of patients addicted to prescribed drugs, (particularly stimulants, antidepressants and major tranquillisers); the risks of ovarian hyperstimulation in the 'harvesting' of ova in the treatment of infertility; the risks of multiple births and cerebral palsy in low-weight babies associated with IVF; and the risk of unscrupulous pharmaceutical research on vulnerable patients in the attempt to be the first to market new 'wonder' drugs.

Obviously, we need to look at the specific issues raised by each of the big dilemmas, but it may be useful to bear in mind this more general historical perspective and be prepared to consider its broader implications too.

INDIVIDUAL 'HEALTH CAREERS' AND PROFESSIONAL CONTROL

Because ethical decisions usually relate to concrete cases, it is tempting to address the fundamental questions of ethics from a consideration of particular cases. Such an approach gives rise to difficulties when we try to generalise to other cases what can be learned from one specific case. However, there is another difficulty involved in looking at illustrative cases. This relates to the question of *what defines a 'case'* – how much background information, contextual detail, family and social history is relevant? What we may call a case from a medical or nursing perspective can be easily caricatured by phrases like 'the case of the burst appendix in bed number 6' or 'the hysterectomy patient in side ward 3'. What the caricatures illustrate is not only that 'being a case' from the patient's point of view means something rather different from the concerns of health professionals, but also that the aspects of reality that are considered important to illustrate a medical or ethical point of view constitute an abstraction from life for the person involved, a person with a past and an ongoing history.

A 'case' may appear to be relatively self-contained too from the medical or nursing perspective – an example of a particular problem or pathology. From the patient's point of view the crisis which gives rise to the need for medical treatment or nursing care is just one episode in the ongoing drama of their life. It is too easy to forget the whole human and social context in which the health crisis or illness episode occurs, and to perhaps forget the real person in the process, and the fact that the health crisis may be of life-shattering importance to them, affecting their whole future life and prospects. To achieve a balanced ethical judgement about a specific situation it may be just as important to *understand the background* of the person involved, as it may be important from a nursing perspective not only to know the patient's medical, but also her *personal and social history*.

The concept of a 'health career' – a concept derived from developmental psychology – may be useful here, for each 'case' or 'incident' has to be seen in the context of the person's health career. As we grow from infancy through childhood to maturity and decline into old age and die, our life passes through a series of ups and downs which comprises our particular life or health career. From a medical or nursing perspective, episodes of illness or health crises need to be located in this dynamic context of 'before' and 'after', if their full significance is to be grasped. Listening to the patient's story, however, is not just useful and perhaps

comforting to the patient, but it is also essential if we are to acknowledge and respect the dignity of the individual in genuinely 'patient-centred' nursing. The concept of a health career has proved very important in health education, particularly in understanding patterns of both health-promoting and dysfunctional health behaviour (first used by Baric 1974, and Dorn & Nortoft 1982).

For example, the acquisition of a smoking habit, or a disposition to heavy drinking or drug addiction involves a 'career' of initiation or introduction to the practice, repeated reinforcement of the habit through practice and then developed dependency, attempts to cut down or quit, relapse, maintenance, reinforcement and so on (Prochaska & DiClementi 1992). Such a dynamic view of human life crises can be just as illuminating for ethical decision-making as it is in arriving at clinical judgements, whereas the 'typical case' tends to be frozen in time, abstracted from the developmental and historical context.

If we represent the whole of our life career by a parabolic curve, starting with conception, rising to the peak of our physical and mental development and curving down to meet the horizontal axis again at death, then along that line, our progress is not necessarily smooth; it has its 'ups' when we are healthy and things are going well for us, and its 'downs' when we are sick, suffer injury or external factors limit and arrest our development (Fig. 6.1A). As we get better, or get over a crisis in our lives, so we regain some of the lost ground and our development continues. As we get past middle age or suffer severe illness or disabling injury, so our capacity for recovery becomes more limited and our general condition may decline, until we finally succumb to the disintegrating effect of disease, injury and the wear-and-tear of old age, and die. Some people may live a long time with a very steady rhythm, other people's lives may be marked by numerous crises, others may be cut short tragically by sudden, accidental or violent death. It is possible to examine the medicalisation of life across the whole span of an individual's health career, but it is also illuminating to apply it to the specific analysis of smaller sections of people's lives or individual episodes of illness, injury or mental disorder.

If we map the course of an episode in a person's life career, from a state of relative health and independence through some health crisis where the person becomes relatively or completely dependent on help from others, and then recovers and returns gradually to something like their former state of health and independence, this process can be illustrated on a simple graph by an inverted parabolic curve. On such a graph the horizontal axis would represent the

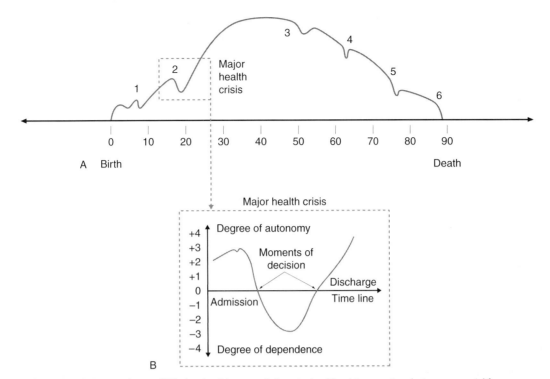

Figure 6.1 A: A person's overall lifetime health career. B: A major health crisis occurring during a person's life career.

continuous time-line. On the vertical axis we could represent various degrees of autonomy above the line and various degrees of dependency below. Such an episode relative to one's life career could be illustrated as in Figure 6.1B.

What is ethically significant about health and illness for the person involved is that normal physical and mental health means growth towards greater autonomy. Illness and injury usually involve loss of autonomy and greater dependence on other people. 'Making a good recovery' usually means recovering more control over our lives, and 'being able to stand on our own feet again'.

When a healthy person who is, say, lucid, mobile, continent and independent, experiences some health crisis (through injury, disease or environmental insult) she may rapidly decline into a state of relative or deep dependency on others, from which she has to be assisted to recover. The process of assisting people to get back on to their feet we call 'rehabilitation'. *The deeper the downward curve, the more total will be the carer's responsibility for the person entrusted into his care*, but as she is assisted to recovery, or recovers spontaneously, then the carer has to assist her back to recovery and independence, not keep her in a state of perpetual dependence. There are at least two points of 'crisis' in

this process ('moments of decision', from Greek *krino*, to judge or decide): first, when the individual hands over responsibility, or is handed over, to the carer; and second, when responsibility is handed back to the patient or client. The crossing of the horizontal axis by the downward and upward movement of the line illustrates these points in the episode, making these crisis points on the boundary line between autonomy and dependency on the parabolic curve.

What is important about this model for illustrating a person's health career is that it emphasises that there is a dynamic process, or movement, or *shift in responsibility from the patient to the carer, and back again*. This is clearest in cases where individuals have emergency admissions for major injury, or for severe mental health problems, but even in the minor illnesses or ups and downs of life there are considerable fluctuations in our need for help and support, and our capacity to stand on our own feet. Problems arise for patients and clients when professionals are either reluctant or too eager to take on responsibility for them when they are in a crisis or need help. Alternatively, professionals may be slow to give up the control which they acquire over people's lives, or too readily abandon them before they are able to take control of their own lives again.

The effects of institutionalisation in reducing the capacity of people to cope with responsibility for themselves and their health, and in reinforcing the dependency-creating attitudes and behaviour of carers, have been well studied from a psychological but not always from an ethical point of view. Goffman's classic study of 'total institutions' in his book *Asylums* (first published in 1961, and reissued in 1993) explored the effects not only on inmates of their institutionalisation, but also how carers become institutionalised themselves. While much has been written about institutionalisation from a sociological and psychological point of view, the ethics of institutionalisation requires more attention. This applies both to the inmates and to staff, to the way care is routinised and also how carers acquire unwanted moral responsibilities as a result of taking on people in need. Where the health crisis requires emergency treatment, the pressures on the carers to take urgent life-and-death decisions may be considerable. They may well find it emotionally costly and physically exhausting. Without respite or adequate support they may risk 'burn-out'. Alternatively they may soldier on, but resent being left carrying the can, and then may feel exaggerated guilt if things go wrong.

Ethical codes in the caring professions have focused mainly on the responsibility the carer accepts for the client; few have stressed the importance of the commitment the carer must make to return control to the client as soon as she is again capable of being independent. We are not aware of any existing medical code of ethics which stresses that the doctor has a primary moral duty to assist (where possible) the rehabilitation of the patient. It is significant, however, that the original draft code of ethics of the Royal College of Nursing (1979), the International Council of Nurses (2000), and the Nursing and Midwifery Council Code of Professional Conduct (NMC 2004) have all emphasised the responsibility of the nurse to work to restore autonomy to the individual who has lost it as a result of illness, injury or mental health problems. These statements emphasise a value fundamental to nursing ethics which appears to arise out of reflection on the distinctive nature of nursing care.

SOME CLASSICAL ISSUES IN BIOMEDICAL ETHICS

Abortion and the 'right to life'

From the dawn of time women have sought assistance to terminate unwanted pregnancies, whether or not this has been permitted by law or morality. If help has been refused or unavailable, women have attempted by an extraordinary variety of means to effect an abortion themselves or have resorted to infanticide. Some societies have tolerated abortion, but it has generally been prohibited and those seeking to procure or assist with abortions often have been severely punished. In a sense it is only with liberal legislation, which has decriminalised abortion, that the issue has become, strictly speaking, a matter of clinical and moral responsibility for nurses. Of course, nurses have had to grapple with the problem before the Abortion Act in Britain, for example, and nurses also will have had views on the morality or immorality of abortion before 1967, but it is only since that time that nurses, as nurses in Britain, and particularly in the National Health Service, have had to face the issues as a direct challenge to nursing ethics. For the nurse, or midwife specifically, it might be argued that there is an immediate, and apparent contradiction between the responsibility to protect, nurture and save the life of the child, and the responsibility for the wider care of the woman for whom an unwanted pregnancy is a personal disaster.

The issue of *abortion* (or more strictly *deliberate termination of pregnancy*) is usually debated from the pro-life point of view in terms of the sanctity of life or the rights of the unborn child. From the point of view of those that favour further liberalisation of the law and moral attitudes on termination of pregnancy, the issue is about women's rights and in particular their right to control their own fertility, including securing a termination. Relatives and wider society tend to enter the debate in an attempt either to protect the rights of the unborn child or to defend the rights of the woman. Here the issues tend to be discussed in terms of the tensions between popular morality (represented by different pressure groups) on the one hand and the law and social policy, on the other. The passionately held and opposing moral beliefs of those representing say the Catholic Church, or other faith communities, and those representing women's rights are not necessarily in disagreement about fundamental values, but rather about which values, as a matter of policy, are to be given priority. It is not generally the case that one group believes termination of pregnancy is an absolute wrong and the other that it is absolutely right, for both groups would probably regard it as neither a good nor an ideal solution in general, but where the differences arise is about what discretion may be allowed in dealing with specific cases, which may be devastating for the individual woman.

It is important to distinguish two very different levels of moral argument in relation to termination of pregnancy:

- debate about the right or best (or least harmful) thing to do in a specific case, given the circumstances
- debate about how termination of pregnancy should be dealt with in society in general, as a matter of law and social policy, given the widely differing cultural and religious attitudes to these matters.

Of course, religious and other specific interest groups have a right in a democratic society to campaign to have their views more widely accepted, and to influence social policy and the law. However, it cannot simply be assumed that the morality of a particular faith community can be legitimately imposed on the whole community, even in societies where they represent the majority. Considerations of justice and equity, as well as respect for the rights and freedom of conscience of individuals, make it necessary that there is scope for dissent; otherwise the society is on course to become an authoritarian society, whether the position entrenched in law and social policy is an extreme libertarian one or strictly anti-abortion.

The health professionals may get left out of 'the abortion debate', except where they are called in as expert witnesses, but in reality they are often left playing 'piggy in the middle'. The duty to care for both mother and child leaves them in an impossible situation, for example where they have to choose between the life of the one or the other. The conflicting demands of such a situation cannot be resolved for carers either by consulting the law (which may be a convenient 'cop-out') or their personal consciences, about which individual (mother or baby) is owed a greater duty of care. Other considerations of personal rights and justice have to be taken into account, and the tension between these conflicting values in real life is what makes these problems so painful and faces us with apparently unsolvable dilemmas (see Johnstone 1994).

The sanctity of life argument that so easily leads on to claims that 'abortion is murder', raises both fundamental issues and insuperable problems in ethics. If all life is sacred, where do you draw the line? With the newborn, the fetus, the conceptus, the ovum or individual sperm ... or where? Is it only human life that is sacred or is animal and vegetable life sacred as well? If we say human life, when does life become human in the continuum between individual cell and adult person? Attempts made to legislate that human life begins at conception do not solve the problem, nor did the position adopted by St Thomas Aquinas in the 13th century, that the fetus acquires legal and moral rights at 'quickening' (when ensoulment was supposed to take place); nor does the modern legal limit of 28 weeks' gestation. Why not at birth, or at puberty, or at age 21 years? What all these attempts to find a secure biological foundation for the definition of a 'person' fail to recognise is that they beg the question: 'What is a person?' This is *essentially a moral question* and a matter of value judgement, namely, a judgement about what in particular is to be valued about human persons as such. The debate about what we mean by 'a human person' is not a scientific, but an ethical question, and the various ways different societies and religions define personhood directly influence how we give concrete meaning to the legal concept of a person as 'a bearer of rights and duties' and how we define the scope and limits of membership of the 'moral community' (see Kerridge et al 1998).

What is distinctive about the Judaeo-Christian and Muslim faiths is the high value placed in these traditions on the value of fetal life, and on the 'right to life' as a God-given natural right. In European philosophy, since the Protestant Reformation and the Enlightenment, the emphasis has been placed on the exercise of individual moral responsibility and rational choice as essential prerequisites for any claims to moral rights. As a result, liberal humanists have tended to regard our entitlements to rights and our obligations as increasing with our growth in maturity and responsibility, with the exercise of personal moral autonomy. So, within this tradition, neither rights nor duties would be attributed to prenatal life. In complete contrast with both these European traditions, traditional Hinduism and animistic religions, around the world, regard all life as sacred – respect for the rights of animals and even plant life means that the moral community is expanded to include all living things. Taken together with the doctrines of re-incarnation and of Karma, all living things are bound together in one chain of being, one moral community of reciprocal rights and responsibilities, and our progress up or down the hierarchy of more or less complex forms of life is dependent on one's Karma – on how well or badly one fulfils the responsibilities of one's fate or station in life.

Dogmatic definitions simply foreclose rational debate and exploration of these complex questions to which fundamentally different answers have been given in different societies and cultures. In Hinduism, where all living things are regarded as sacred – and strict vegans would not kill any animal or eat animal products – the moral community is so broad as to include all living things as having rights. At the other extreme, the Nazis sought to restrict the moral community to pure Aryans, and other 'lesser' races were denied fundamental moral rights or even the protection of the law – with terrible consequences.

In Western culture we tend to have regarded only human beings as having moral rights or qualifying as members of the moral community and have extended protection to animals on the grounds that cruelty to or abuse of animals is inhuman, not that animals as such have rights. The animal liberation movements have sought to challenge this view. Furthermore, within our own culture we have been very confused about whether all human beings – including women and children, slaves, and people with mental health problems or learning disabilities – should enjoy the same rights. The present legal debate about in vitro fertilisation is bedevilled by confusion in many countries about the legal status of the unborn, and where we draw the line in experiments with embryos, or the storage of embryos. English law, for example, acknowledges on the one hand the right of the unborn child to inherit property or to recover damages for injury suffered in utero, but on the other hand abrogates the unborn child's right to life by permitting termination of pregnancy, under specific conditions.

This analysis is not meant to decide the abortion or deliberate termination of pregnancy issue one way or the other, but rather to raise a fundamental series of questions in ethics. What do we mean by a 'person'? What do we mean by respect for personal dignity and rights? What is the scope of the 'moral community'? What criteria do we apply to determine membership of the moral community? What rights and responsibilities does membership entail?

Ironically, those who campaign for women's rights, and the 'right' to termination of pregnancy on demand, rest their claims upon similar presuppositions about the nature of the rights of members of the moral community to those raised in the defence of the moral and legal status of prenatal life. The dispute is not so much about the nature of rights as to whom they apply, and the boundaries of the moral community. Whether the unborn child and the mother's rights are equal and apply in the same way and on the same level are questions about the scope and limits of our definitions of personhood and the terms on which we qualify for full membership of the moral community. These are all issues which relate back fundamentally to the principle of respect for persons and how we define the rights and responsibilities of members of the moral community (Rumbold 1993). Consider some of the conflicting rights of the parties involved in Case Study 6.1.

Issues round euthanasia and compulsory psychiatric treatment relate to extremes in the balance of

case study 6.1

The question of termination of pregnancy to a mother with AIDS

Vicky is a student who is 18 and has a boyfriend, Jack, who has been using drugs. She is very fond of him and they have been living together for some months. Vicky misses a period and goes to her local health centre for a pregnancy test. She is shocked to discover that she is pregnant, but after a few days makes up her mind that she wants to keep the baby at all costs. She does not initially tell either her boyfriend or parents. When she goes to the maternity hospital for an antenatal examination, routine blood tests reveal that Vicky is HIV-positive. Her boyfriend is worried and insists that she should have an abortion. Vicky is upset, mainly because she says her parents 'will go berserk' if they know she is pregnant. However, she still wants to keep the child regardless. Her boyfriend's argument for her having an abortion is that there is a risk the baby will be born with AIDS and then die, and he 'wants to protect her from that'.

If you were the community midwife caring for Vicki, how would you support Vicki and try to assist her in reaching a responsible decision about her baby?

power between carer and client and the tensions which such situations generate – between the requirements of the duty to care, to protect the vulnerable and incompetent, on the one hand; and respect for the autonomy and personal rights of the patient or client, on the other.

Euthanasia and the 'right to die'

Euthanasia is a term used rather loosely. It comes from two Greek words: *eu* meaning good and *thanatos* meaning death. The term 'euthanasia' is sometimes used to cover both the situation where a carer on his own initiative assists the patient to a good death – whether that involves withholding treatment (passive euthanasia) – and the intentional killing of the patient by administering a drug or treatment hastens death (active euthanasia). In either situation a carer would probably justify the action as an extension of their duty to care – to prevent unnecessary suffering, for example. However, the term 'euthanasia' is also used where a patient requests assistance to put an end to their suffering (assisted suicide), or has requested in advance (perhaps in a sworn statement or 'living will') that they do not wish their life to be artificially prolonged if their condition is terminal. This kind of 'voluntary euthanasia' involves the patient insisting on respect for their personal wishes and claiming the 'right' to die, or at least demanding to be consulted about the scope and limits of what we euphemistically call 'terminal care'.

Infanticide, murder, intentional killing or assisted suicide, with or without the instructions of the victim, is prohibited in almost every jurisdiction around the world. Therefore the legal definition of euthanasia as 'the intentional termination of a patient's life, by act or omission, in the course of medical care' makes the practice problematic morally and legally, regardless of what may be the overwhelming desire of the carer to see someone who is suffering a painful death put out of his misery. Where the carer feels compelled to act to put an end to the hopeless suffering of a patient, there is also an inevitable clash between the ethical duty of protective care the carer owes to the patient – to do good (beneficence) and to avoid doing harm (non-maleficence) – and respect for the patient's autonomy and right to choose.

Alternatively, nurses may feel pressurised by patients who demand respect for their 'right' to die, while nurses may feel that nursing care is about sustaining life, not about assisting patients to kill themselves or to hasten their death. The fundamental question is whether we do in fact have a 'right to die'. It is difficult to see how this right could be justified or enforced. Nurses (and doctors) generally feel that no patient has any entitlement to impose on them the duty to assist them to terminate their life. This raises a crucial philosophical question about the difference between liberties and rights.

The UK Voluntary Euthanasia Society has long campaigned for the legalisation of voluntary euthanasia, but there seemed to be insuperable legal obstacles as long as attempted suicide was illegal. When the Suicide Act of 1961 was passed, suicide ceased to be a criminal act in England (it had never been so regarded in Scotland). Supporters of the Voluntary Euthanasia Society claimed a moral victory and argued that the Suicide Act created a legal 'right to die'. This argument was based on a misunderstanding

---

Box 6.3 Rights and duties

What do we mean by 'rights'?
Generally speaking, moral and legal rights are justified claims that entitle us to demand that other people act, or desist from acting, in certain ways; that is, our 'rights' impose either positive or negative duties on others.

- *Negative rights:* the right to demand that a person desist from doing something to you is generally stronger than the positive right to have something given to you or done for you.
- *Positive rights:* your right to some personal or social benefit will depend on the generosity of others as well as the available resources or benefits.

Rights may also be particular or universal, depending on their moral and legal foundations:

- *Particular rights:* these arise where we make promises, bets, vows or enter into contracts with particular people, where only the contracting parties have rights and duties to one another.
- *Universal rights:* these rights which we claim are applicable to all human beings regardless of race, sex, creed or age (e.g. the UNO Declaration of Universal Human Rights) and are based in claims that we all share a common species being – e.g. rationality, sociability or freedom – which makes the possession of these rights essential if we are to lead a recognisably human life.

'Rights' and 'duties' relate to one another
My rights impose duties on you, and your rights impose duties on me, so my rights are relative to your rights and your rights limit mine. Thus no rights can be absolute, while they may nevertheless be inalienable to me as a human being.

- *Moral rights:* these only have such force as the accepted rules and consensus of the moral community give them, may depend on available resources, and are often not enforceable.
- *Legal rights:* these may be enforceable through civil or criminal courts, both in the case of particular contractual rights and fundamental human rights, such as the right to privacy or freedom from assault, with the sanctions of fines or imprisonment applying in some cases.

Rights and responsibilities
On what basis do we praise or blame people for their actions? Or hold them responsible for their actions?

- If they knew what they were doing (i.e. are not ignorant or insane).
- If they acted voluntarily (i.e. are not acting under compulsion).
- If they had other options (i.e. are not powerless to act otherwise).

Persons can only be said to have rights and duties in the strict sense if they are responsible for their actions and thus capable of being responsible to other people. Other 'rights' are rights by analogy (e.g. rights of animals) or they are 'rights' by proxy (e.g. the rights of children).

of the permissive nature of this particular piece of legislation, as an 'enabling' Act. What the legislation did was to decriminalise suicide and attempted suicide. The Act is permissive in that people are *allowed the liberty* to take their own lives without suffering the penalties of the criminal law. But did the Act create a positive legal right to die? (Box 6.3)

Generally speaking, *moral and legal rights are justified claims that entitle us to demand that other people act or desist from acting in certain ways – that is, our 'rights' impose either positive or negative duties on others*. Although we argue passionately about our moral rights, they may be unenforceable, because they only have the strength which existing social consensus and convention give them, and impose only moral rather than enforceable legal obligations on others. We can in some cases seek the assistance of the courts to uphold our legal rights, for example where there is a breach in our contract of employment or invasion of our privacy, but the enforceability of our moral rights involves persuading enough people to support us and act in our interest (Box 6.3).

In the strong sense of 'right', the UK Suicide Act 1961 does not create a right to die, nor one which is legally enforceable, in the sense of imposing on anyone else a legal duty to assist anyone to die, nor could the law impose a duty not to intervene to prevent someone taking their own life. In fact the Homicide Act of 1957 specifically precludes the former by making assisted suicide a form of criminal homicide, and some mental health legislation imposes on professionals who are directly responsible for patients a legal duty to act to prevent patients from committing suicide. The provisions of both English and Scottish mental health legislation make it possible for both health professionals and lay people to take action to have persons detained in hospital compulsorily if they are considered a serious suicide risk.

In the weaker sense of 'right', where the individual is allowed the liberty in law to attempt suicide, it may be argued that in cases of patients dying in extreme pain or undignified circumstances, nurses or other healthcare staff, may *feel an obligation* to assist the patient to an easy or good death. However, feeling obligated would not be sufficient grounds to make such an action legal (or ethical), as most societies would argue. The action would have to be taken at great personal risk and as a lonely, individual and ambiguous act of compassion. Although there has been growing public support and sympathy for such acts in individual cases (e.g. of spouses assisting one another to 'an easy death') and the courts have tended to take a lenient line on charges brought against doctors and nurses who have practised active euthanasia. The conviction in the United States on a charge of murder of Dr Kevorkian, who openly practised euthanasia, and the overturning by the Federal Court of Australia of the Rights of the Terminally Ill Act 1995 introduced in the Northern Territories, may indicate a swing to a more conservative legal position on euthanasia. The attempt in the Australian Northern Territories to legalise euthanasia on demand may have failed, as much as anything, because it attempted to create a legal *right* to die, rather than simply introduce a permissive act allowing people the *liberty* to seek assistance to terminate their lives, under specified conditions (Kerridge et al 1998).

In general, neither law nor public morality concedes that anyone has a right to demand the assistance of another person to terminate their life. In practice, some nurses (or doctors) may feel moved to stop treatment or life support, or may actively intervene to terminate the life of someone in extreme suffering by the administration of drugs or by other means. However, such action would be illegal, whatever the circumstances, and in most cases would not be morally sanctioned either, because carers are expected to sustain life not to end it, and most societies have in fact moral principles forbidding suicide except in the most extreme circumstances (Beauchamp & Veatch 1996). (Permissive legislation, said to 'legalise abortion' in Britain and many other countries, has not, with the possible exception of Hungary and Western Australia, created a legal 'right' to termination on demand – at least not in the sense of an enforceable right, nor as a duty which can be imposed on individual doctors and nurses.)

The provisions of the law and the constraints of public morality may or may not suffice to help the nurse in a particular case to decide whether to refuse the desperate request from a patient for deliverance from a living death. The 'legalisation' of euthanasia in the Netherlands is a case in point. Like the Abortion Act in Britain, it is permissive legislation, intended to formally decriminalise acts of euthanasia under certain defined conditions. No law permitting voluntary euthanasia can impose on doctors and nurses the duty to perform euthanasia against their will or conscience, and neither can legislation remove the painful tension, for the doctor or nurse, between their duty to care and respect for the dignity of the suffering patient in a particular situation. Neither could such legislation adequately prevent the misuse of euthanasia by unscrupulous individuals who might benefit from another's death. Arthur Clough's ironic wisdom remains relevant: 'Thou shalt not kill, but needst not strive officiously to keep alive' (Clough 1951).

There have been several attempts to legalise euthanasia in Britain but the arguments which have invariably prevailed are: (a) that it is impossible to build in adequate safeguards to prevent the misuse of euthanasia by unscrupulous doctors or relatives, or both in collusion with one another, to take advantage of someone in a situation of extremity; (b) that introducing permissive legislation to permit 'voluntary euthanasia' will inevitably lead 'down the slippery slope' to 'non-voluntary euthanasia' or intentional killing of the terminally ill.

Evidence over a period of 15 years from the Netherlands, based on official statistics, two large-scale surveys and critical analyses of both specific cases and interviews with practitioners, suggests that these fears may indeed be well grounded. In the first survey in 1991 there were 2300 officially notified 'euthanasia deaths', 4000 cases of 'physician assisted suicide' and 1000 cases where euthanasia was performed without evidence of a specific request from the patient. All in all there were 10 500 cases where withdrawal of treatment or increased use of drugs had 'shortened life'. Given the specific conditions prescribed in the Netherlands, if euthanasia was to be performed legally, there was less than 25% compliance with one or other of the following requirements (Keown 1995):

- the patient must have made an explicit and voluntary request for euthanasia
- the patient must be suffering unbearably and euthanasia should in such cases be a last resort
- the physician must have consulted with another medical practitioner regarding the case, and
- the doctor must submit an official report that he/she had complied with the law.

Another line of approach to the question, illustrated by the 1999 Council of Europe Working Party on Euthanasia, identified the following rights of the terminally ill (Council of Europe 1999):

- the right to adequate and competent palliative care
- the right to self-determination of the dying, rooted in their human dignity
- the right to be protected from involuntary euthanasia, or intentional killing by any person.

In order to ensure these rights are protected, the Council of Europe Working Party identified areas of need where action is necessary by member states if the rights and autonomy of the dying are to be properly respected and protected from neglect or abuse (Box 6.4).

The detailed and specific recommendations to member states of the Council of Europe are classified in the report under the headings of the basic rights

---

Box 6.4 Measures required to protect the rights of the terminally Ill (Council of Europe 1999)

- To ensure adequate access of all people to expert palliative care and good pain management.

- To ensure skilled treatment of physical suffering, and care for the psychological, social and spiritual needs of dying patients.

- To avoid artificial prolongation of the dying process either by using disproportionate medical measures, or by continuing treatment without a patient's consent.

- To ensure adequate funds and training facilities for the continuing education and psychological support for health professionals working in palliative care medicine.

- To provide means for the care and support of relatives and friends of terminally ill or dying patients, both for their own sake, but specially to alleviate the suffering of the dying patient.

- To help alleviate the fear of patients of losing control of themselves, and becoming a burden to or totally dependent upon relatives or institutional care.

- To provide a suitably quiet and private space, within institutional environments, where a dying person can take leave of his/her relatives or friends.

- To ensure adequate allocation of funds and resources for the care and support of the terminally ill or dying.

- To educate people, including healthcare staff, to overcome the social stigma of weakness, terminal illness, death and bereavement, and the associated discrimination against the dying.

---

listed above. These include requirements that member states should ensure legal protection for the following rights of the terminally ill:

- the right of access to appropriate and skilled palliative and terminal care
- the right to truthful, comprehensive yet compassionately delivered health information
- reaffirmation of the right (enshrined in Article 2 of the European Convention for the Protection of Human Rights and Fundamental Freedoms), namely 'everyone's right to life shall be protected by law and no one shall be deprived of his life intentionally'.

In addition, the Council of Europe recognises that there are very practical things that need to be done to ensure the improvement of the general standards of terminal care, namely adequate funding for terminal care facilities, both institutional and mobile home-care services, for training and supportive services. In addition, it emphasises the importance of formal recognition of palliative care as a proper area of specialisation in medicine and nursing, of skilled training of healthcare staff and evidence-based research in the area. With increased life expectancy, death has become increasingly unfamiliar to the majority of people, and public opinion requires to be educated about the needs of those dying, whether from degenerative diseases or old age.

One of the most commonly expressed fears of the terminally ill is the fear of losing control – of their bodily functions, of their lives and personal affairs, and of the process of dying itself. Death itself therefore might be defined in terms of progressive loss of control. Being alive means having some degree of control over one's life and decisions: bodily functions are maintained in a balance, albeit precarious, of homeostasis, and one has some control over one's finances, property and relationships. Part of the pain of death is that it is something that happens to us, it is beyond our control, bodily systems disintegrate or 'self-destruct', our bodies corrupt and dissolve, we lose control over our futures and fortunes. There is even a paradox in suicide, as Sartre (1969) pointed out, in the fact that by attempting to remain in control, to assert our autonomy by taking our own lives, we put an end to our autonomy. We all wish to retain control over our lives for as long as possible. Glaser & Strauss's early research (1965) showed that the healthcare team do not like to feel that they are losing control of the process and have difficulty giving in to the inevitable. From this perspective, voluntary euthanasia may appear to help both the patient and the health professional to maintain the illusion of being in control in the face of death and it may amount to a form of collusion to avoid facing the fact that death itself ultimately means loss of control. This is not to make light of the painful issues faced by carers and their patients in situations of terminal illness. Some of these anxieties would appear to be present in Case Study 6.2.

Commenting on this case, Karen Lebacqz remarks that the most remarkable and disturbing thing about this case was the absence of controversy or protest about the judge's decision and the fact that this may indicate that popular opinion in the United States is moving towards acceptance of the concept of 'a time to die', without examining critically the position of the patient and the contribution to the suffering of the patient of his circumstances of inadequate social support. However, the recent case of Terri Shiavo in Florida might indicate otherwise, for public opinion (including that of President Bush), driven by media

case study 6.2

A time to die?

The difficulty is to know when it is 'time'. Consider the following case:

Kenneth Bergstedt was 31. A quadriplegic with injuries to vertebrae C1 and C2, he had been on a respirator for 20 years. He spent his days lying on a hospital bed, watching television, and writing poetry on a computer by blowing into a special device. He was cared for by his father, who was 65 and in failing health himself. Through the agency of his father, Kenneth Bergstedt applied to the courts to have his respirator turned off so that he could die. An affidavit filed with the court said '[he] has no happy or encouraging expectations to look for from life, receives no enjoyment from life, lives with constant fears and apprehensions, and is tired of suffering'.

A psychiatrist interviewed Kenneth and found him 'alert and intelligent'. The psychiatrist further found that Kenneth's 'quality of life' was 'very poor' and that his future 'offered no relief'. Kenneth's judgement was considered good and not unduly influenced 'by impulse or emotion.'

Faced with this evidence, the judge ruled that Kenneth Bergstedt's life support could be turned off and he could be allowed to die. Further, this action would not constitute suicide and thus no laws would be broken. The judge then ordered the case sent to a higher court, so that a legal precedent might be set to assist other disabled people who sought to end their lives. One reporter suggested Kenneth Bergstedt's wish to die, and his father's desire to help him do so, 'probably are the greatest gifts of love either man could give the other'.

Example used by Karen Lebacqz (Berkeley) (Quoted with permission from Biomedical Ethics Vol. 4, 1999, No. 1, p. 16.)

hype, was against termination of life support for Terri. However, some surveys in the US indicated that, in contrast to the media hype, the majority of people were in favour of terminating life support in Shiavo's case, and it is perhaps not surprising that the US Supreme Court finally ruled in favour of the husband who had petitioned that his wife be allowed to die.

Karen Lebacqz quotes Carol Gill, a disability psychologist, who says: 'In the vast majority of cases, when a severely disabled person persists in wanting to die, there is an identifiable problem in the support system.' Lebacqz continues:

Social structures are crucial to the meaning and purpose that people find in their lives. Kenneth was taken care of almost exclusively by his father. Two consequences of this care-giving arrangement are significant. First, Robert Bergstedt had recently lost his spouse and was ruminating on his own death. The father's grief and preoccupation with death undoubtedly influenced the son to seek his own death. Second, and more important, all his future possibilities came from his father. Robert Bergstedt painted a bleak picture of what would happen to Kenneth if Robert were hospitalised or died. Kenneth believed that if his father died, he would die from lack of care, or be placed in a nursing home. He was never told that people with his severe level of quadriplegia and need of respirator support can live active and productive lives. His entire view of the world – and of its possibilities for someone with his disability – was filtered to him through his father's eyes. At no time did anyone from a disability rights movement have access to Kenneth, whose friends and outside contacts were controlled by his father. The social structures that might have made a difference to Kenneth's understanding of the meaning of his life were not provided.

However, another kind of irony emerges in the ethics of terminal care in hospice care. The more staff seek to respect the autonomy of dying patients, to discuss the implications of their imminent death with them, to support them through the anticipatory grief and distress, to consult them and respect their wishes regarding how, when and where they are to die, then good terminal care, which was supposed to be an alternative to voluntary euthanasia, actually approximates to it. If good terminal care is not 'assisting patients to a good death', what is it? The pain and the dilemmas do not go away, although each case may be sensitively handled in a quite different way. In the case of a major disaster or where, for example, a person is crushed and trapped in a burning motor vehicle the doctor or nurse may feel there is no alternative but to end the victim's misery, but where a patient has been so well maintained by 'good' terminal care that their death has become unduly protracted, where they have outlived their death sentence, it may be much more difficult not to press on regardless with treatment. What should be done and how it should be done, and by whom, can all be agonising questions. The situation may demand that something is done, and even non-action is a form of action. No universal prescriptions are possible in such situations, nor would they be appropriate (Doyle 1984).

Dilemmas of truth-telling and confidentiality

Francis Bacon once remarked that 'knowledge itself is power' (Bacon (1561–1626) 1996). The doctor's or nurse's knowledge of health matters gives them *power to help* people in distress, but also gives them *power over them*. People give or withhold information about themselves in communication with health professionals depending on whether they trust the people involved, and believe they will use the information for their benefit, for the better diagnosis and management of their problems. While people are generally willing to disclose sensitive and private information about themselves to doctors and nurses, they also realise that they make themselves vulnerable by doing so, and are aware that possession of this information gives health professionals further power over them. Legal safeguards for confidentiality of patient records and information are required to protect the vulnerability of patients, and to ensure that possession of secret information about people is not abused by those caring for them, or inappropriately disclosed.

On the other hand, the amount of information about a patient's medical condition, diagnosis, treatment and prognosis that is or should be disclosed to the patient is also a matter of sensible and responsible judgement. The control of information and its selective disclosure is part of the power exercised by doctors and nurses over patients, and can be used as a tool to secure their adherence to treatment. It is also a grave responsibility for nurses and doctors to decide when, how much, and by whom, information should be disclosed to patients. Refusal to disclose relevant information may deprive people of the power to make important decisions affecting their lives. If 'knowledge is power' then to be kept in a state of ignorance is to be kept in a state of impotence, infantilised and controlled.

While in the past medical staff might have been reluctant to tell a patient their prognosis, it has become the usual practice now in the UK to give patients information about their condition, unless they have specifically asked not to be given further information, or if the responsible doctor considers that disclosing information would cause the patient psychological harm. However, 'telling the patient the truth' is not simply a matter of 'stating the facts', for callous imparting of a fatal diagnosis would not only be insensitive and irresponsible, but could constitute a form of abuse of a vulnerable patient and as such an inappropriate expression of professional power. The real question may be whether healthcare staff are adequately trained and skilled to communicate with patients sensitively.

Dilemmas of truth-telling and confidentiality arise because of apparent or actual conflicts between the patient's right to know and the carer's duty to care. The classic situation of whether and when to tell a dying patient that their condition is terminal illustrates the tension between two opposing moral concerns:

- respect for the patient's autonomy and right to know their condition, on the one hand, and
- the feeling of the carer that she should protect the patient from news which might shock and distress them, perhaps causing them to give up in despair.

It may seem simplistic to say that what such situations require is honesty, but if we interpret honesty as demanding that we *honour*, that is, show sensitive regard for the particular patient's needs and their capacity to assimilate the information at the time, then maybe we can 'learn to titrate the truth to the pain and needs of the individual'. Responsible and compassionate truth-telling requires maturity, experience and counselling skills on the part of the nurse or doctor.

The situation may be further complicated in practice by the intervention of relatives demanding to know or forbidding communication with the dying. Here, in the absence of permission from the patient (if they have the capacity to give consent), disclosing information about their condition amounts to breach of their rights to confidentiality. The various parties involved, including staff, may not be willing to acknowledge failure or to relinquish control. They may simply wish to protect themselves from the emotional burden of the dying patient's grief. Communication with the dying requires great sensitivity, and depends on the patient's trust and confidence in the nursing staff. The issues involved are not susceptible to universal prescriptions and the predicament of nurses may be that, in practice, they are caught in the middle and prevented by 'doctor's orders' from doing what they believe to be the best in the circumstances. What makes these issues perennial dilemmas is that they bring opposing rights and duties into painful conflict. Whether priority should be given to the patient's right to know or to the professional's duty to protect the vulnerability of the dying patient cannot be decided by mere appeal to principle but has to be worked out in the complexity of each unique situation, in the way that seems most caring and responsible at the time (Thompson 1984).

Respect for a patient's secrets, their right to privacy, is again complicated by the often overriding duty to care and to do what is in the best interests of the patient. This may involve the carer in passing on confidential information to another professional in the hope that it will assist in the better care of the patient. Ideally carers have a duty to seek the consent of persons who have confided in them before sharing their secrets, but if it is not possible to get their consent, then the dilemma arises: which is to take

precedence – the patient's right to privacy or the professional's duty to provide the best possible care for the patient? Dilemmas of confidentiality generally do not arise out of careless disclosures of patients' secrets, but rather when the responsibilities of nurses to their patients, for example, come into conflict with the requirements of team management of patient care or in sharing information with relatives. The issues are further complicated by the problems of shift work and lack of continuity in care, where carers need to have crucial information if they are to provide appropriate care.

Being in possession of sensitive confidential information about clients or patients is often both a burden and privilege of carers, but it also gives them a special relationship with those in their care and subtle power over them. It can be a burden where it is difficult to set limits to the process of self-disclosure in a patient with a compulsive need to 'tell all'. Here the nurse may have to negotiate clear boundaries with the patient about what information is relevant and what is not, what information is strictly secret and what can be passed on to the rest of the care team. Doctors and nurses sometimes may be inclined to guard jealously 'their' confidential information about patients, and are reluctant to share it with other members of the team, because it means compromising the special relationship they have with 'their' patients/clients. Situations also change within the carer/client relationship, for example, as the client enters a crisis and becomes increasingly dependent, so the carer acquires greater power and control over the life of the client. Part of this control consists in management of the flow of information to the client, from the client and about the client. Giving or withholding information can also be a powerful way of encouraging cooperation or compliance and maintaining control in the caring relationship. Because knowledge is power and to be kept in ignorance is to be kept in a state of dependence, the manner in which the information and confidences are shared is a sensitive indicator of whether professional attitudes are creating dependency or are used to assist clients towards autonomy, to enable them to retain some control of their lives (Thompson 1979b).

Compulsory psychiatric treatment – for whose benefit?

The dilemmas of confidentiality and truth-telling, as well as general conflicts between protective beneficence and respect for a person's rights, arise in the most acute form where the patient or client has become incompetent. This is particularly the case where the patient is psychotic and rendered practically and legally incompetent by virtue of a severe mental health problem.

Treatment of people who are suffering from what political correctness demands we call 'a severe mental health problem' has varied dramatically in Britain and Europe from the Middle Ages to the present day. Some of these changes are reflected in the range of terms we have historically applied to those whose mental states have resulted in bizarre and often dysfunctional behaviour. In the Middle Ages the mentally ill were treated as 'holy innocents' or 'possessed of devils', depending on whether their condition seemed socially benign or evil. In the Enlightenment people were deemed to have 'lost their reason' and were subjected to floggings and other indignities to help them 'regain their senses' (e.g. 'mad' King George III). Other terms, such as 'lunatics', 'nutter', 'crazy', 'cuckoo', 'mad', 'insane', 'imbeciles', 'mentally ill', reflect the history of changing attitudes to people suffering from different kinds of mental disorder. Significantly all these terms originally had neutral meanings, but have tended to acquire derogatory meanings and stigmatising effect over time. These examples illustrate clearly Wittgenstein's observation that 'language shift' usually signals a shift in both social values and explanatory paradigms. For example, the use of the term 'lunatic' implies that insanity is caused by the moon; 'nutter' from the Latin word 'to nod, stagger' suggests a diagnostic sign of some forms of disorder; 'crazy' originally meant 'broken or shattered'; 'cuckoo' that one's reason has been usurped by some other power; 'insane' simply meant 'not whole', 'imbecile' meant 'weak'. What all these terms illustrate is our deep ambivalence about disordered or deranged mental states – both fear of the strange and unknown, and awe in the presence of something extraordinary or paranormal.

Treatment of individuals who have severe mental health problems has also varied around the world from the compassionate tolerance of some societies to persecution and even execution in others. Even in modern times there have been wide divergences between psychiatrists themselves in the classification and definition of types of mental diseases. Most striking in the recent past have been differences in the definition of schizophrenia by American and European psychiatrists. One of the great achievements of psychiatric epidemiology, sponsored by the WHO, in the past twenty years has been research evidence of broadly similar distribution of the classic psychotic disorders around the world, and the achievement of a remarkable degree of consensus in the universal classification of psychiatric disorders (WHO 1992, Scull 1992).

Definition, as Aristotle noted two and a half thousand years ago, is not only an essential tool of scientific method, but it is also a means by which we gain control over the world, over other people and our subject matter. Precise names help to define people and things as individuals and as being of distinct kinds. The word 'definition' comes from the Latin word *finiens* for a fence or boundary. By naming and defining things, we draw boundaries around them so as to order our knowledge, and thus control reality better, both conceptually and practically. Thus knowledge gives power. Stokeley Carmichael, the American Black Power leader, said of white racism: 'Definition is the primary instrument of the white man's will-to-power over blacks' (Stokely Carmichael, in his address to the World Council of Churches Consultation on Racism, held in Notting Hill, London, in 1969). By the same token, we establish boundaries to intimacy with people by determining what names, titles or forms of address they are permitted to use in speaking to us. Clinical labels, as observed in Chapter 3, have both value to the healthcare worker in defining the problem and to the patient in legitimising their access to treatment and being off work etc. However, these same labels, e.g. 'schizophrenic', 'HIV positive', etc., can all be seriously stigmatising and affect people's status and rights in society. The power of definition carries with it serious ethical responsibility for all professionals, namely, to exercise it for the benefit of those in their care (Scull 1992, Boudreau & Lambert 1993).

The legal power of definition may be illustrated in the fact that given a psychiatric diagnosis of severe mental health disorder or mental incapacity, society may require that the affected individual is taken into hospital against his will, and even subjected to compulsory treatment. Deciding whether an individual should be compulsorily detained in hospital may be relatively easy in cases of severe dementia or florid mental ill-health, but the vast majority of psychiatric problems are not so clear-cut. The general legal requirement in most jurisdictions, that individuals must be 'a danger to themselves or others', leaves the mental health officer in an extremely difficult situation, for 'dangerousness' is notoriously difficult to assess in practice. To avoid public criticism, or legal action for negligence, caring staff may tend to err on the side of caution and thus compromise the rights of individuals when the degree of danger would be virtually impossible to prove. Furthermore, individuals admitted in a severely disturbed state may recover without treatment, or may have periods of reasonable normality and periods where they are clearly incompetent. Whether the system is sensitive enough to respond to these fluctuating changes in the moral status of detained patients and to respect their right to information or to be consulted about their treatment, may be doubted. The disabling effect of mental health problems, in affecting a patient's competence to exercise responsibility to control and/or direct their life, makes it peculiarly difficult to decide at what stage in the rehabilitation process it is appropriate for the carer to relinquish control. Conservatively protective and defensive practice on the part of carers may seem to be common sense, but it may keep patients in a state of chronic dependency.

There are several peculiar features of the medical treatment of mental illness which create moral difficulties or dilemmas for nurses. These problems arise because of ambiguities in the diagnosis, treatment and rehabilitation of people with mental illness (including senile dementia and severe mental handicap). These ambiguities are to be found in all of the following:

- the moral/legal status of the patient
- the scope of definitions and diagnosis of 'mental illness'
- the variety of activities which count as 'treatment' in psychiatry and rehabilitation
- the definition of which patients are the carer's responsibility.

The status of the 'patient'

The ambiguous moral/legal status of someone suffering from a mental disorder is reflected in the fact that health professionals have unique legal powers to detain and treat patients who are regarded as 'incompetent' because mentally ill. The central moral paradox of psychiatry is that people may have to be deprived of their liberty and treated against their will in the hope that this will make it possible to restore their autonomy and enable them to take control of their lives again. To legitimate the use of these extraordinary legal powers by professionals, most legal systems require proof that a person is either a danger to others or a risk to himself. Assessment of these risks is necessary to justify detention of a patient for treatment, and this action is justified morally both on the basis of a duty of protective beneficence towards the patient (in protecting their health and safety, and ultimately their rights as well), but it is also a requirement of justice to wider society (in maintaining lawful order, preventing others from harm and defending the common good). Ensuring adequate safeguards for patients' rights becomes a difficult ethical issue in these circumstances.

Mental health legislation varies considerably around the world, from the most libertarian (as has been the case in Italian experiments with community psychiatry) to the most authoritarian and repressive in the old Soviet Union and some traditional societies. These differences are reflected both in the stringency or laxity of requirements for proof of 'mental disorder' or 'dangerousness', and also in the controls placed on compulsory detention and treatment of patients against their will. Concerns about the abuse of psychiatry not only in the USSR during the Cold War period, but also in the USA during the Vietnam War, to control political dissidents by having them certified insane, led the UN World Psychiatric Association to introduce the Declaration of Hawaii on the ethics of psychiatric practice and protection of the rights of psychiatric patients in 1977 (see Boyd et al 1997).

To protect the rights of the patient, various legal safeguards and rights of appeal tend to be built into mental health legislation and there is generally some kind of recourse to the courts or mental health tribunals for independent review of patients and their care. But serious questions may be asked about whose good the system serves, whether (with a few exceptions) people who have mental health problems are really a danger to others, and whether legal action is justified to restrain attempted suicide by 'mentally ill' patients, if attempted suicide is not a crime for 'normal' people.

As an example of how difficult it is to protect the rights of people with mental health problems, we might take a case from Scotland. The Mental Health Scotland Act 1964 made provision for an independent Mental Welfare Commission to review all cases where patients were detained in hospital on long-term compulsory orders, on a regular basis. Patients or their representatives could also appeal directly to the Commission where they felt a patient's rights were not receiving appropriate treatment or were being inappropriately detained in hospital. This provision was widely hailed as a welcome means to protect patients' rights. However, research undertaken in 1983, as part of a review of the Act, showed that these provisions failed to provide adequate protections for patients' rights. This was mainly because emergency detention orders, (for up to a week), were being applied without these safeguards. The system was being abused, either by discharging patients prematurely, or by simply applying successive 'emergency orders' to circumvent the need for court appearances and mandatory visits and reporting on cases by the Mental Welfare Commission. The practice of defensive medicine here undermined the operation of the measures meant to protect psychiatric patients' rights.

These abuses took place against a background of the supposedly liberal move to greater community care for people with mental health problems. Ironically this was made possible by the success of new pharmacological treatments for schizophrenia and bipolar affective disorders, which allowed patients on long-acting depot drugs to return home. The condition of such patients was described by some nurses to the Edinburgh Medical Group Research Project Review Team, as 'a cheap solution – keeping patients in a 'chemical straitjacket', rather than keeping them in hospital for more labour-intensive and expensive treatment. Again, the ethical pros and cons of such measures need to be debated more openly by nurses, as they often find themselves as both the gatekeepers and supervisors of patients in the community.

What came to be called an 'open-door' policy in mental hospitals (or 'revolving door policy' as it became in fact) also suited the prevailing mood of economic rationalism in government, which favoured quicker bed turnover and 'community care' as this was thought to be a cheaper way of delivering mental health services. A decade of experiment with the deinstitutionalisation of people with mental illness has resulted in serious problems in many countries adopting this approach, because resources to support community-based services have been nowhere near adequate and psychiatric patients have tended to be simply recycled back into institutions, through prisons and the criminal justice system. Criticism of 'community care' as a solution to the problem of mental health treatment services and the protection of the rights of patients, in Italy, Britain and Australia, has led to renewed demands for adequate mental hospital services and 'the right to asylum'. Typical would be the critical Australian Burdekin Report on the inadequacy of the mental health services provided in Western Australia, a society with a very high per capita income and one which prides itself on its general standard of healthcare, but where community mental health services were considered unacceptably low (Burdekin et al 1993). In the USA and Canada there have been considerable variations between different states in views regarding compulsory community treatment, or community commitment. These are critically reviewed by Boudreau & Lambert (1993).

The definition of mental illness

The notorious imprecision of definitions of 'mental illness', and even serious disagreement between psychiatrists as to whether mental illness exists – as distinct from physiological disorders, or emotional distress and problems of living – led to considerable debate in the 1970s about whether we should refer to 'mental illness' at all. Laing & Esterson (1970), in *Sanity, Madness and the Family*, argued that 'mental illness' is a response to dysfunctional parenting, and Thomas Szasz (1974), in *The Myth of Mental Illness*, argued that mental illness is a social construct to categorise a range of maladaptive behaviours causing people to deal ineffectively with problems of living. These approaches contrasted sharply with the current attempts to explain mental illness in terms of disturbances in the biochemistry of the brain or malfunctioning brain metabolism. There may be more agreement today about the causes of different types of mental disorder, and about the methods of classifying types of psychiatric disorder, and this may make the furious debates about the definition of mental illness in the 1960s and 1970s seem somewhat passé. Nevertheless there remains a considerable degree of medical and scientific uncertainty about the predisposing conditions and aetiology of mental illness.

This uncertainty makes it at least questionable whether individuals who are diagnosed as suffering from some kind of 'mental' ill-health should be singled out for special legal sanctions, deprivation of liberty and the denial of their fundamental rights. Examples of the rights of individuals who have mental health problems that may be compromised are (Szasz 1987):

- the right to be adequately informed and to give voluntary consent to treatment
- the right to privacy and confidentiality (which may be compromised in group therapy and team management)
- the right to refuse treatment and/or to discharge themselves from hospital (where even voluntary patients may fear imposition of a compulsory order if they do not comply)
- the right to vote in general elections, to emigrate or in some cases even to go on holiday abroad.

Western Australia, which well into the 1990s had some of the most conservative mental health legislation, might serve to illustrate how concern for patients' rights over the past 30 years has resulted in greater caution being exercised over the involuntary admission of people to a mental hospital and the provision of safeguards to protect the rights of psychiatric patients. For example, the West Australian Mental Health Act 1996 sets much more stringent conditions which must be fulfilled before a patient can be deprived of their liberty and treated without their consent. In *A Clinician's Guide to the Mental Health Act 1996* (Health Department of Western Australia 1997), the criteria justifying compulsory admission are set out as shown in Box 6.5.

Box 6.5 **Conditions for compulsory psychiatric treatment (HDWA)**

- The individual must have a mental illness, as described by the Act, requiring treatment.

- The treatment can be provided through detention in an authorised hospital, or through a Community Treatment Order, if this is necessary in order to:
  protect the health and safety of that person or any other person
  protect the person from self-inflicted harm, which includes financial harm, and lasting or irreparable harm to any important personal relationship caused by damage to the reputation of any of the parties
  prevent the person doing serious damage to property.

- The person has refused, or is unable to give consent to treatment.

- The treatment cannot be adequately provided in a way that would involve less restriction.

What is significant about this is that the Act does not attempt to define different forms of mental illness or syndromes in clinical terms, but rather *in terms of observable behaviour* and the extent to which the person's behaviour would be seen to be bizarre, even within his or her unique cultural milieu (Health Department of Western Australia 1997).

The 'benefits' of a psychiatric diagnosis (asylum, access to care and treatment, relief from the burden of family or work responsibility) have to be counterbalanced against the 'costs' of the disabling and stigmatising effect of being labelled 'mentally ill' or as a 'psychiatric patient', and denied some fundamental human rights – even if no longer called a 'lunatic' or imprisoned.

The limits of 'treatment'

In psychiatry, there is a further irony related to interpretation of 'consent to treatment' for 'voluntary patients', for the extent to which their participation is voluntary can be debated, and the consent they are required to give amounts to almost 'writing a 'blank cheque'. What counts as 'treatment' in psychiatry possibly covers a wider range and is perhaps more inclusive than in any other area of medicine – ranging from protective asylum to being 'straitjacketed' in a locked and padded cell, from one-to-one psychotherapy to group therapy of various kinds. Also included is an enormous range of other 'therapies'

ranging from chemotherapy, ECT and psychosurgery to behaviour therapy, physiotherapy and occupational therapy (including art, music, dance, and sheltered employment). It is by no means clear to the average patient (or nurse for that matter) what the patient is consenting to or what will be included in the scope and limits of 'treatment' in the case of any specific patient. There is a risk that health professionals will arrogate to themselves the right to simply decide what therapies are in the best interests of the patient without consulting the patient or relatives. For the compulsorily detained patient, cooperation and compliance can be elicited by the mere hint of the extension of compulsory powers, or implied threat of their reimposition. Nurses are intimately involved in the whole complex of relationships which operate and sustain these systems of social control in psychiatric and psycho-geriatric institutions. Since the first publication of Goffmann's book *Asylums* in 1961, and his research on 'total institutions', we have become more aware of the effects of 'institutionalisation' on both patients and staff in psychiatric hospitals. While much can be done to 'humanise' the environment of institutions, the fact remains that in the sphere of mental health in particular, nurses perform a dual role, as carers and as agents of social control. Popular films such as *One flew over the cuckoo's nest*, while they may exaggerate the punitive and repressive nature of mental institutions, nevertheless bring out the unavoidable conflict there is for nurses between a caring ethic and their role in policing the behaviour of people compulsorily detained in hospital. It can be argued too that incarceration of patients in institutions creates conditions that predispose to abuse or at least mistreatment, as discussed by Wardhaugh & Wilding (1993).

Community psychiatry, which involves not only the supervision of psychiatric patients in the community but also the investigation of the 'social supports' or family background of the patient, raises serious new ethical questions for the nurse in dealing with the family. Who is the patient? How many family members are included within the scope of the responsibility of the community psychiatric nurse? Has the nurse the right to intervene in the family life of the patient, to draw other family members into the therapeutic net? Again, the situation is without parallel in nursing (except perhaps in contact tracing in HIV or sexually transmitted disease). Do health professionals have a right to seek out undisclosed pathology, or undeclared 'patients' who have not recognised that they have a problem? Because the legal powers taken in psychiatry are extraordinary, they raise all sorts of difficult ethical questions about the scope and limits of professional responsibility and the rights and status of patients/family (Reed & Lomas 1984).

A further complication in psychiatry is that people with mental health problems are consistently portrayed in a negative light in the media, and in films and TV the danger represented by people with psychiatric disorders is frequently exaggerated and even caricatured. While serious efforts have been made to balance this distorted view of mental ill-health in sensitive docu-dramas and documentaries, there remains a high level of prejudice in the minds of the public towards people with mental health problems, leading to their isolation and often discrimination when they seek employment.

Management and allocation of resources

All the previous 'classical dilemmas' we have discussed tend to occur within one-to-one relationships in patient care, where the primary tension is between the professional's duty to care for and protect the patient, and the demand that the carer respects the dignity and rights of the patient/client as a person. There is a whole class of other ethical problems and dilemmas which arise for nurses when they move from one-on-one clinical nursing responsibility into ward or hospital management, or into teaching and research roles. In these situations they are responsible for groups of patients and staff, for the allocation of staff time, administration of drugs and equipment and general allocation of resources as well as for the well-being of a whole institution. While we will discuss other examples of these kinds of one-to-many ethical responsibilities in later chapters, the ethical issues which are raised most frequently in discussion are on the borderline between problems of direct patient care and management.

The critical decisions which doctors face when there are scarce resources have been the subject of much attention, from television dramas and discussions in the popular media to more serious academic debate. Such crises are often illustrated by situations where there are two or more patients urgently requiring kidney dialysis and only one available machine, or where there is a patient needing a heart transplant and there is a shortage of donor organs. While the crises over limited resources facing nurses may not be so dramatic, they are often left having to give support to the patient waiting for dialysis, or a transplant, and their families. Resource allocation issues that are common in nursing are such as a registered nurse having to decide between keeping to the agreed ward routine for staff or mobilising more staff to deal with an emergency affecting one particular patient.

In more prosperous countries where hospitals are reasonably well funded, the ethical crises for nurse managers over allocation of scarce resources may not be of major proportions; but in poorer, developing countries these problems and dilemmas may be acute where there may not be enough routinely prescribed drugs to go around, where disposable hypodermic syringes and scalpels are unknown and those used must be regularly sterilised, and even bandages may have to be boiled and reused, and where there may be a shortage of beds. Determining who gets the treatment or resources may not be so simple as the application of 'triage' methods in an urban road traffic accident. The sheer volume of need may be so overwhelming that the ethical question might be whether a nurse should perhaps give up her job in the field and return to the USA or Europe to campaign for resources for 'her patients'. A moving example of this was a British nurse working in Uganda who appealed at the 1990 World AIDS Conference 'not for facilities to test for HIV, not for drugs to treat AIDS, but for calamine lotion and means to palliate the suffering of AIDS victims, where the cost of treating 100 of the 1 000 000 AIDS victims with AZT would consume the entire national health budget'. Recent public attention, directed by popular musicians at mass pop concerts to the predicament of many African countries, has resulted in pressure on G8 countries and their commitment to make AIDS drugs freely available to all by 2010. Raising the awareness of pop musicians to the needs of people in Africa, and elsewhere, has been due in large measure to the campaigning work of health professionals, particularly groups such as Médecins Sans Frontières.

In our more prosperous societies, the resource allocation 'dilemmas' may have more to do with the possible diversion of resources from 'hi-tech' expensive treatment for a few patients to larger groups of patients with enduring conditions, mental health problems or the growing number of frail elderly people. In dealing with these problems, technical clinical considerations may be relevant to determining what may be done, and might in some cases help to decide the issues, but the fundamental moral questions to be addressed are ones of justice and equity.

Generally, the ethical problems in allocation of resources have less to do with the traditionally opposing moral demands of the professional duty of care versus the rights of the patient. Here the problems concern the tensions between equality of opportunity, for all groups in society, to gain fair access to the best available healthcare and the right to anticipate equal treatment and outcomes. Applying a simple utilitarian calculus to determine 'the greatest happiness for the greatest number' will inevitably mean that minorities are disadvantaged, whether it is those marginalised in society by intellectual disability or mental ill-health, or ethnic minorities. This is not only a problem in Britain, where studies have shown the relative disadvantage suffered by immigrant populations, but in Australia where white Australians enjoy one of the highest standards of healthcare in the world, but Aboriginal people (1994 WHO World Health Report) have to make do with Fourth World standards of health and healthcare services.

Another issue that has become urgent in most developed economies is the impact on health services and health budgets of the demands of immigrants, whether they are legal or illegal economic migrants, or asylum seekers escaping from repressive regimes. Linked to this is the problem of the unprecedented number of refugees created by war and revolution in the past half century, not to mention the millions of people affected by the Asian tsunami, and the question of whose responsibility it is to care for these people. The ethical challenges facing health professionals and health services, related to the needs of all such displaced persons, range from the question of what the front-line medical or nursing staff do when such people present for treatment, to what hospital and health service administrators do about the impact on their limited resources of extra demands of this kind, to what we do to pressure our governments, the United Nations and WHO to address these global problems. These issues of social justice arise at many levels.

The ethics of resource allocation concerns the right of everyone to equal access to appropriate care and treatment, particularly in a system of healthcare to which all contribute by taxation directly or indirectly. The claims of certain individuals, because of their special needs, have to be balanced against the common good. The priorities determined by professionals on their own criteria for giving certain clients preference over others because 'in need of greater care' may also have to be challenged or questioned in the name of justice, if others suffer neglect as a result (Boyd 1979, Ch. 3, Campbell 1995).

The dilemmas of responsibility and accountability in nurse management roles are not restricted to dilemmas in the allocation of limited resources or reconciling conflicting needs of different patients. There are some prosaic and routine problems about the management and deployment of staff, the management of time and resources in the routine care of large groups of patients, and the rational ethical

choices which have to be made between the balance of time spent on patient care and/or patient education, teaching or research and evaluation.

Current concern with quality assurance, research, evidence-based practice, and individual assessment and corporate performance review is at its best the application of research criteria and principles of rational justice to the responsible management of resources. While nurses may feel passionately about the care of individual patients and feel that 'research-driven' or 'evidence-based' practice is impersonal and ignores the needs of the individual, they have to realise that resolving, even in particular cases, the difficult tension between the competing demands of care and justice requires evidence not hunches. Managing the tensions between the demands of beneficence, justice and respect for the rights of individuals is at the very centre of routine administrative responsibility.

Even the economic thinking which gave rise to the 'internal market' where hospitals and healthcare staff became part of the purchaser–provider 'contract culture' was driven by ethical concerns to ensure the most fair and cost-efficient use of public resources and protection of the common good. But, given the culture in which nurses begin their careers in a clinical context, these issues all raise important new ethical problems for management of staff and resources. Some of these issues will be further addressed in Chapter 8, but suffice it to say at this point that a very individualistic, personalist, even 'privatised' morality based on one-to-one relations in clinical settings does not translate very well into dealing with these broader issues relating to the well-being of groups of patients or to management and service of the public health and common good of wider society. The former 'privatised' perspective tends to see all moral issues in personalist terms within the tensions between the duty to care and respect for patients' rights. The wider issues of distributive justice and equity in healthcare, of effectiveness and efficiency in the responsible administration of public resources, require not only a different perspective on things, but different kinds of skills in management, team-building and teamwork, committee procedure and 'political' action.

We have stressed earlier that to be a professional is to exercise a public office and carries 'political' responsibilities. This is all the more true of management and administration. These roles are inherently political – political in the sense that they involve balancing interests and powers of various kinds. These may be within the institution or involve negotiating with higher authority outside the institution about policy, staffing, wages, and resources. It may involve using collective action through professional or union organisations to seek better working conditions for nurses or to maintain or achieve better standards of patient care. Such 'political' action may generate new kinds of moral conflicts, e.g. issues of the rights of patients versus the rights of nurses; of the duties of nurses and the duties of patients; of justice in the sense of non-discrimination against individuals, and equality of opportunity and outcome for groups; of the duty to care for vulnerable patients, and the duty to care for staff. These all involve the same fundamental moral principles and require skills in balancing or resolving the tensions and conflicts between them. The demands of justice and the common good may limit the liberty of doctors and nurses in the exercise of unlimited clinical autonomy (e.g. not just which drugs they may prescribe, but on larger matters of where patients may be referred for treatment). Similarly the rights and autonomy of patients may have to be compromised in the interests of public health, not only in circumstances of emergency or life-threatening epidemics, such as cholera or AIDS, but also where scarce medical resources do not permit priority to be given to things like cosmetic surgery, assisted reproduction or transplant surgery (White 1985).

The moral problems in the remainder of this book will be examined within a structure where we move, in ever widening circles of responsibility, from consideration of the personal moral issues in direct nurse–patient relationships, to consideration of problems in managing groups of patients and finally the wider responsibilities of nurses in institutional settings, in relation to society, and the national and international political order.

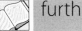
further reading

Beauchamp T, Veatch R 1996 Ethical issues in death and dying. Prentice Hall, New York

Branmer L M 1993 The helping relationship, processes and skills. Allyn & Bacon, Boston

Campbell A V 1995 Health as liberation. Pilgrim Press, Cleveland, OH

Davies C 1995 Gender and the professional predicament in nursing. Open University Press, Buckingham

Goffman E 1993 Asylums: essays on the social situation of mental patients and other inmates, 2nd edn. Penguin, Harmondsworth

Green J, Green M 1992 Dealing with death: practices and procedures. Chapman & Hall, London

Johnstone M J 1994 Bioethics: a nursing perspective. Saunders/Baillière Tindall, Sydney

Keown J 1995 Euthanasia examined: ethical, clinical and legal aspects. Cambridge University Press, Cambridge

Kerridge I, Lowe M, McPhee J 1998 Ethics and law for the health professions. Social Science Press, Katoomba, NSW

Larrabee M J (ed) 1993 An ethic of care: feminist and interdisciplinary perspectives. Routledge, London

Scull A 1992 Museums of madness. St Martin's Press, New York

Tones K 2001 Health promotion: effectiveness, efficiency and equity, 3rd edn. Nelson Thornes, Cheltenham

Direct responsibility in nurse–patient relationships 7

AIMS

This chapter has the following aims:

1. To explore the reciprocal nature of rights and duties within any moral community, in relations of nurses and patients, and in determining the nature of patients' rights

2. To clarify the difference between liberties and rights, positive and negative rights, institutional, legal and moral rights, and particular and universal rights

3. To explore the value and limitations of 'rights talk' as a basis for deciding in difficult cases: disclosure of information, resuscitation, sedation and involuntary treatment of patients in crisis situations.

LEARNING OUTCOMES

When you have read and worked through this chapter, you should be able to:

- Give a coherent account of the particular rights arising from our contractual commitments and acceptance of the rules which apply in the community where we work

- Explain the nature of and the basis for 'universal human rights', demonstrating ability to discuss specific examples and their justification

- Illustrate the nature of patient's rights by discussing examples of particular cases from your own experience of nursing where issues of patients' rights arise

- Demonstrate ability to tease out the conflicting rights and duties of patients, staff and other stakeholders in analysing work-related case studies

- Demonstrate ability to discuss the general policy issues involved in the protection of patient's records and personal confidences

- Demonstrate ability to recognise how changes in the level of dependency of the patient and the power relations of nurse and patient impact on human rights.

INTRODUCTION – THE RIGHTS AND DUTIES OF PATIENTS AND NURSES

In the previous chapter, before discussing some of the classic ethical dilemmas in healthcare, we examined the difference between the ethics of caring for a specific individual in a particular case and the question of developing general ethical policies to deal with types or classes of problems. Part of the chapter was devoted to discussing a number of preliminary questions relating to the moral environment within which we make ethical decisions in healthcare. These were: the different ways we construe 'health' and 'disease'; the different levels at which we encounter ethical problems (viz. personal, team, institution, health service); the issues raised by the 'medicalisation of life'; and the need to consider the whole 'health career' of an individual (and not just isolated episodes or health crises) when making decisions about them in the real world. Having considered these prior general and methodological questions, we can now proceed to look at how ethics bears directly on specific cases in the one-to-one relationship of the nurse with the patient, in hospital or community. We will begin with some remarks on the concepts of 'rights' and 'duties' and consider how these apply in a variety of different situations in nursing.

Given the power nurses have over people when they are at their most dependent and vulnerable, and the privileged and intimate access nurses have to people, both to their bodies and to their private lives, the 'duty of care' and other general 'duties' of nurses have rightly been emphasised in nurse education since the beginning. Talk of patients' rights in the context of such relationships is a relatively new phenomenon. Several factors have contributed to this recent emphasis on patients' rights.

The human rights movement, which had its roots in the European Enlightenment and gained momentum in the 19th century, was undoubtedly given considerable impetus by publication of the Universal Declaration of Human Rights (UNO 1948). The popular demand for rights of more equitable access to health and social services, after World War II, led to the establishment of welfare states in a variety of countries around the world. However, it was the increase in litigation over cases of alleged medical malpractice, particularly in the United States, and campaigns by consumer rights and patient advocacy groups that did most to raise awareness of 'patients' rights' in the latter part of the 20th century. A typical response to this was the American Hospital Association's attempt to codify a bill of rights for patients (American

Hospital Association 1992), and other local statements of patients' rights and 'Patients' Charters'.

Clamorous demands for rights by or on behalf of one group often lead to counter demands from those from whom responsibility and recognition of their rights is being demanded. Pope John XXIII (1963) stressed that we should always pay attention when people start clamouring for their rights, because this usually signals deeply felt injustice for which people are demanding redress. Not surprisingly, demands by patient advocacy groups for patients' rights have been met by counter demands from nurses for recognition of the 'rights of nurses' as well. Expected to be 'always dutiful', nurses have found themselves becoming more militant in campaigning for their own rights, e.g. as their wages and working conditions have often failed to keep up with the general standard of living and improvements in the economic and social conditions of other workers. The unionisation of nurses and their willingness to take industrial action is due to this growing awareness of their rights.

Legally and morally, nurses clearly share the individual and industrial rights of other workers, but they also have specific rights and duties in the context of healthcare where they work, in relation to doctors, nurse managers and patients. Rumbold (1993) devotes a whole chapter of his book to the discussion of the rights of nurses, and clearly this area of ethical debate is becoming of increasing importance to nurses. However, we must pause and ask whether 'rights talk' gets us very far, and whether it is an adequate basis from which to examine nursing ethics (Johnstone 1994, Ch. 13).

In Chapter 4 we distinguished between several kinds of different situations in which nurses deal with patients, namely, *crisis intervention, voluntary requests for help, nursing individuals who have enduring conditions, and dealing with terminal illness and/or with proactive screening and health promotion*. In each of these situations the degree of independence or powerlessness of the patient affects the ethics of the situation, and the weight given to the duties of the nurse relative to the rights of the patient and vice versa. Just as in family life the balance of duties and rights between parents and children changes as children grow from infancy to adulthood, so in nursing the balance of rights and duties will change with the degree of dependency or autonomy of the patient. For example, the patient's right to know will be differently interpreted if the patient is unconscious, insane, very distressed or anxious, compared with when they are conscious and in full possession of their faculties. In the accident and emergency department, the nurse's first duty to a vulnerable patient is to respond immediately to the patient's right to adequate care and treatment. Because 'rights-talk' has to be interpreted differently in relation to changing situational demands, it is necessary before we proceed to discuss ethical decision-making in specific cases that we clarify what we mean by 'rights' and 'duties', how are they related and distinguished, and how they apply in nursing contexts.

The meaning of 'rights' and 'duties'

In the previous chapter, in discussing abortion and euthanasia, we briefly distinguished between liberties and rights and introduced a number of preliminary distinctions between positive and negative, particular and universal, moral and legal rights (see Box 6.3). In that context we said: *Moral and legal rights are justified claims that entitle us to demand that other people either act, or desist from acting, in certain ways – that is, our 'rights' impose either positive or negative duties on others.* Rights and duties are thus connected, but what is the nature of this connection?

The literal meaning of the word 'right' – from the German *recht* for rule – has to do with what a rule entitles us to expect, or allows us to do. The word 'duty' – from the French *due* for what is owed – relates to what obligations we owe to others or responsibilities we have under the rule in question.

If rights are 'justified entitlements', the first question to ask is how are our rights to be justified? This immediately raises some difficult theoretical questions about the nature of human rights and their philosophical rationale or foundation. We discuss 'rights theory' in Chapter 13, but here we simply need to clarify the use of the terms 'rights' and 'duties' in everyday usage.

Most simply put, particular rights and duties exist where we are subject to rules or agreements with other people. This applies in every kind of moral community to which we belong and in which we act as responsible members. For example, the rules of a sports club impose certain *duties* on members (e.g. to pay subscriptions, to support the club's aims, to participate in club competitions, to dress and behave appropriately, etc.), but they also give members certain *rights or entitlements* (e.g. to gain access to club amenities, to be included in club competitions, to represent oneself as a member of the club, to bring guests, under specified conditions, etc.). Similarly, if I wish to drive a motorcar in Britain, I am required by the Highway Code to drive on the left. It is my *moral and legal duty* to do so, to prevent accidents which might be caused by uncertainty on the part of other drivers, who would otherwise be unable to predict my behaviour. On the other hand, I have a *legal right*, or justified entitlement, to expect that you will drive on the opposite side of the road, and will not collide with me because you decide to drive towards me on 'my' side of the road!

The rights and duties of members of a sports club do not apply to non-members. The rights and duties that we enjoy as motorists in Britain do not apply in other countries where the rules of the road may be different. These rights and duties are first of all *particular rights and duties* in the sense that they are peculiar to those who are participating members of a particular society. The rights and duties involved do not apply to everyone, but only to those who agree to abide by the rules of that particular community.

These specific agreements give rise to specific obligations and justified entitlements for those involved in the agreement, and not to outside parties. *Particular rights* – as opposed to universal rights – arise as a result of a number of different kinds of agreement between individuals or groups of people. Some philosophers have suggested that *promises and promising* are the foundation of all rights and duties. If Jack promises to take Jill out to dinner, and does not turn up as arranged, Jill has a right to be annoyed because Jack has a moral obligation to keep his promises – on pain of never being trusted again. Here, only Jack and Jill have rights or obligations to one another, related to the promise. They are particular to them, and no other party is involved. However, if Jack fails to keep his promise because of some overriding duty (say to go to his mother's bedside if she has had a stroke), or if he had a motor accident on the way to meet Jill, then we might say that he could be excused from his obligation to meet Jill. Similarly, a promise made by a nurse to a patient will create an expectation in that patient that the nurse will recognise an obligation to keep his or her promise, and failing to do so will undermine the patient's trust in that nurse, and possibly in nurses generally 'who do not keep their promises'.

Other types of agreements where we acquire particular rights and obligations are *vows*, *bets* and *contracts*. The obligation to pay up if you lose a bet could be enforced through the courts, provided there were witnesses to the bet having taken place. Solemn vows, such as those sealing a contract of marriage, create both moral and legal obligations, breaches of which give rise to much conflict and litigation in the divorce court, and often at high legal cost. Contracts of employment and business contracts with suppliers of goods and services again give rise to moral and legal duties and entitlements, where the breach of a contract can lead to civil court action – to either enforce the right, or to seek compensation for the breach.

Claims that we enjoy certain *universal and inalienable rights*, as human beings, cannot be justified by appeal to social agreements or conventions, or they would not be universal or inalienable. These *fundamental human rights* or *universal human rights* form a different class of 'rights' or 'entitlements', which have to be justified in a different way. The ancient Greeks, and particularly Stoic philosophers and lawyers, argued that we all share a common human nature, and common needs, as rational beings or members of the species *Homo sapiens*. They, as well as modern rights theorists, argue that universal human rights exist on the basis that certain conditions must obtain if we are to achieve our full human potential as members of our species, and that all human societies must recognise this. Universal human rights purport to express necessary conditions without which we cannot flourish or develop as human beings, nor lead anything like recognisably human lives. It would be claimed that violation of these universal rights results in oppression, discrimination and subjection to forms of life that are degrading and inhuman or sub-human. It is not difficult to think of forms of treatment of patients that are degrading and inhuman, such as the treatment by Dr Mengele of prisoners in the Nazi concentration camps, or conditions where the sheer lack of resources and amenities means that patients cannot get the most basic forms of healthcare. In the former case, the Nazi doctor and Third Reich were responsible for the violation of human rights. In the latter case we may contribute ourselves to the deprivation of basic human rights in the developing world by our failure to deal with poverty, debt and unfair trade terms.

The claim, expressed in the Preamble to the United States Constitution, that all human beings are created equal and independent, and from that inherent equality possess the inalienable rights to 'the preservation of life, and liberty and the pursuit of happiness', is rooted in this tradition. The ancient belief and moral claim that because we all share certain characteristics and needs in common as rational human beings we are therefore entitled to fundamental 'human' rights – like freedom of speech, conscience and association – rests on certain general metaphysical assumptions about the unique nature or essence of human beings, as well as specific beliefs about what particular characteristics and needs are definitive of our species and distinguish it from other animals.

While there is an interesting range of theories, and much debate, about what is *the* most essential defining characteristic of the human species, there would not be much disagreement about the fact that we are really different, for example, from crocodiles and giraffes (that are visibly different from us) but that we are also distinguishable from the higher apes (or hominids) whom we resemble in so many amusing ways. How we understand human rights and duties will depend on how we define a 'human person'. The terms 'person' and 'personality' serve to define what we mean by humans, both as members of our species and also as individuals. The term 'person' comes from *persona*, the Latin word for a mask, and signifies the role or identity we assume in life. Immanuel Kant (1724–1804), in his *Groundwork of the Metaphysic of Morals* (Kant (Paton, tr) 1969, reprinted 1991) argued that the term 'person' is foundational for ethics, and that without it ethics cannot get off the ground. Why is this? There are two kinds of reasons:

- The 'mask', or 'masks', we assume in the drama of life define both our role or identity and also public expectations of the normal rights and obligations that go with the various roles we play.
- The way we define a 'person', or specify the defining characteristics of 'personhood', sets the boundaries for the 'moral community' and determines who qualifies for membership.

In its most general and abstract sense, the term 'person' has been interpreted in law from the earliest times as simply 'a bearer of rights and duties'. Individuals that are 'bearers of rights and duties' may not only be individual people, but, as in Roman law, the term can also apply to corporations, individual partnerships, clubs, businesses or public associations. In this sense, the term 'person' is a formal and empty concept until we fill it with some meaning. It is like a 'blank cheque' until we 'cash' it, by filling in some value in the blank space, by defining what we mean by a person in this context.

How we define personhood will determine what we regard as 'universal human rights'. The emphasis we place on certain essential attributes in our definition of human nature, or the way we specify the defining characteristics of our species, will profoundly affect how we interpret and apply concepts of universal human rights. Thus different human rights will be given priority depending on which characteristics we value most and regard as definitive of human nature. Different traditions have emphasised different characteristics as definitive of human nature. Greek philosophy emphasised that 'man is a rational animal' (Aristotle); the Bible, that 'we are made in the image of God, who is love'; Marx, that 'man is *homo faber* – man is man the worker or maker of things'; existentialist philosophers, that 'to be human is to be condemned to be free' (Sartre). When 'cashed out', each of these definitions has different practical implications, as each embodies different social and moral values, leading to different rights being given priority.

If we invest 'rationality' or 'critical intelligence' with ultimate importance and value in human life, as we have done in modern Western society, then this has considerable impact on our view of what education is about, the priority given to science and technology in society, and to the value given to IQ scores and academic grades in defining who and what we are. This affects us both positively and negatively. Intellectual ability and academic achievement have enormous positive value, and intellectual disability and mental illness a corresponding negative dis-value. This is reflected in the priority given in the allocation of funding for education, science and technology and the relative paucity of funding for mental health and mental disability. It also leads to the relative marginalisation of, and discrimination against, people with mental disorder or learning difficulties. Similarly, if we overemphasise a capacity for sociability, or productive work, or autonomy, then we will devalue people who have difficulty relating to others, or who are unemployed, or those who do not have the education, resources or opportunities to exercise any meaningful kind of autonomy. The variety of claimed universal human rights based on these definitions are illustrated in Box 7.1.

While these definitions of human nature and the corresponding human rights derived from them appear to differ considerably from one another, they are not mutually inconsistent or incompatible with one another – unless interpreted as exhaustive defini-tions in themselves. Thus the UNO Universal Declaration of Human Rights (UNO 1948) represented to some extent a combination of several complementary views of what is fundamentally important to us in defining what it is to be human.

In distinguishing 'liberties' and 'rights' we pointed out that if we concede that other people have certain 'rights', then recognition of their rights imposes certain 'duties' or 'obligations' on us, but the same is not true of our freedom or liberty to do something. For example, smokers frequently claim that they have a right to smoke. If this were the case then other people would have a duty or obligation to enable them to indulge their habit. Here it is incorrect to speak of having a 'right to smoke', for no-one is obliged, if they do not want to, to provide us with cigarettes or smoking breaks or rooms in which to smoke. If, however, we are over the legal age we do have the liberty to purchase and smoke cigarettes (and damage our health) without being interfered with or prevented by others (unless our habit is irritating or harming them). The unjustified claim of smokers that they have a right (as distinct from the mere liberty) to smoke has delayed the restriction of smoking in restaurants and public places, but recently in the USA, in Ireland and in some locations in the UK, new legislation is being introduced to prohibit smoking in public places (in the interests of public health and the common good).

While there is a reciprocal and complementary relationship between rights and obligations, there is no positive reciprocal relation between liberties and duties. A liberty is something we are permitted to

---

Box 7.1 Universal human rights derived from universal human attributes

If to be human is to be a *rational animal* then certain conditions or rights must be satisfied before we can become fully rational beings, e.g.:

- the right to know, to information
- the right to freedom of conscience
- the right to freedom of speech
- the right of access to education and training.

If to be human is to be a *social being*, characterised by the capacity to love, for social intercourse and social cooperation, then other requirements have priority:

- the right to be nurtured in a human community
- the right to freedom of association
- the right to freedom of movement
- the right to marry and found a family.

If to be human is to be a *worker*, defined by the capacity for creative work, and to be able to transform the world and humanise it, key rights would be:

- the right to work, to contribute to society
- the right to profit from one's labour
- the right to own land and property
- the right to emigrate to seek employment.

If to be human is to enjoy *freedom* or *autonomy*, then in order to be able to realise one's freedom and express it in one's life and work then one would require the following rights:

- the right to freedom from oppression or discrimination
- the right to freedom of opportunity for self-development
- the right to freedom of cultural self-expression
- the right to participate in political activity.

do without being subject to sanctions or physically prevented from doing it – provided it does not interfere with the liberties of others. For example, as we saw in Chapter 6, if termination of pregnancy is permitted, or has been decriminalised, then a woman has the *liberty* to terminate a pregnancy and to request others to assist her to do so, without being prosecuted or physically prevented from exercising this liberty. However, such 'permissive' legislation does not create a 'right' or entitlement of a woman to demand that termination services are provided as a public duty. Only in Hungary and in Western Australia has the state recognised an obligation to provide such services.

Here it is important to stress the difference between positive and negative rights. In general our negative rights are stronger than our positive rights, and most negative rights are, or can be, secured by law.

A negative right is an entitlement to demand that someone *does not do* something to you, or desists from doing something to you. In a sense, negative rights do not cost other people anything, for they do not have to do anything to observe your negative rights. The rights involved, for example demanding not to be tortured, not to be assaulted, not to be raped, not to be abused, and not to have one's privacy invaded, are all *negative rights* and are all rights protected by law.

We all regard the negative rights listed above as fundamental human rights, and express outrage when these rights are violated. Yet, hospital patients are constantly at risk of having these rights compromised or abused, because of their 'captive' state as inmates of institutions of various kinds, particularly the frail elderly, patients with advanced dementia or with severe mental health problems. The doctors and nurses who performed experiments on prisoners in Nazi concentration camps were rightly condemned by the Nuremberg War Crimes Tribunal. There have been highly-publicised cases of assaults on patients in psychiatric and mental handicap hospitals (and no less serious assaults on staff by patients). Examples of the rape or sexual abuse of patients by staff, their physical and emotional abuse, invasion of their privacy, have all been reported in the press in the past decade. Not surprisingly, the courts take a very serious view of crimes of this kind because nurses and other healthcare staff are expected, in addition to respecting the rights of patients, to exercise a protective duty of care or fiduciary responsibility towards patients committed into their care.

However, there are other important negative rights of patients where doctors and nurses may sometimes feel that in the interests of a patient these rights may have to be compromised. Such rights are the right to refuse treatment (or the right not to be treated without one's consent), and the right to not have private information shared with a doctor or nurse, or divulged to anyone else without one's permission. These negative rights of patients are also subject to legal safeguards, in so far as treatment without consent is treated in law as a form of criminal assault – regardless of the good intentions of the nurse; and breach of a patient's confidences may be subject to claims for damages in a civil court. Nevertheless there are borderline and difficult situations where doctors and nurses may have to decide to treat a patient against their will, or pass on confidential information, where the patient's competence is in doubt or there is grave risk to the life of the patient, or sharing the information with a colleague is essential for their proper care and treatment.

A positive right is an entitlement to demand that someone *do something for you* or *give you something you need*. Such rights are weaker than negative rights, because they depend on the ability, generosity or willingness of others to do what you ask, and also depend on available resources. While some positive rights may become entrenched in law, such as the right to free healthcare, at the point of delivery, for UK citizens on the National Health Service, and the right to education and welfare, other positive rights are unenforceable, such as 'the right to employment'.

Even within the UK and other wealthier nations these are not unlimited rights, and, some would argue, even these rights are being progressively circumscribed. General entitlements to free dental and optical treatment were removed some years ago (although some exemptions apply), and many more exotic medical treatments may not be available on the NHS because of the cost and the scarcity of medical resources to deal with more essential matters of life and death. Debate about whether cosmetic surgery or in vitro fertilisation (IVF) for infertile couples are essential treatments and should be available on the NHS will depend not only on available resources, but on the seriousness of the condition and how much it is seen to affect the person's ability to lead a normal life in society. What is possible in Europe may be quite unimaginable in Africa, so how much leverage we have in claiming our positive rights, even those listed in the Declaration of Universal Human Rights, will depend on where one is living and the resources available. This in turn is a reason why people are often motivated to migrate to countries where better opportunities for education, employment or healthcare are available.

Finally, although some people claim there are some rights that are absolute, this seems to us to be a difficult position to defend, and that for two reasons. First, because my rights impose both direct and indirect duties on you, and my rights impact upon your rights and limit your rights. Secondly, because human generosity and resources are limited, and entitlement to claim our positive rights will always be relative to what is available. My negative right not to be assaulted restricts your freedom to assault me and imposes on you a duty to respect my right (even if you want to assault me), because I can seek redress if you do. My right to education is not unlimited, but limited by what free education the state can afford to provide. While most countries attempt to guarantee primary education for all, and some secondary, virtually no country guarantees access to tertiary education, but may provide bursaries, scholarships or loans to deserving candidates. Thus, it follows that all rights are relative because my rights limit your rights and yours mine. We work within a world of compromise.

Institutional, legal and moral rights

Broadly speaking, we may distinguish between institutional and legal rights, on the one hand, and moral rights, on the other. Consider Case Study 7.1, summarised from a 1987 Public Enquiry Report of the child abuse controversy in Cleveland. Although the events occurred nearly 20 years ago, similar situations recur in other places, and this case still serves well to illustrate the variety of conflicting 'rights' that are claimed by the various stakeholders. This should perhaps make us cautious in thinking that appeal to rights can resolve the difficult issues that have to be addressed in cases where there is alleged or proven abuse of children.

In this case, several parties claimed that their rights, or those of others, had been violated or infringed. However, if we look carefully at each use of the terms 'right' or 'rights', we will see that they do not all mean the same thing. In the first instance, the term clearly has a legal meaning, referring to the legal authority of the social services to issue care orders and to have children taken into care. This also applies to the authority of the paediatricians to examine the children. Here the *legitimacy of their authority* was being questioned.

With reference to the parents' 'rights', the term is being used in a double sense – both a legal and a moral sense. The legal sense relates to whether their proper entitlement to a second medical opinion, or appeal to the High Court, has been taken into account. However, public interest in this case and the Official Enquiry that followed, was stimulated by the insinuation in the media that the general moral rights of parents were

case study 7.1

Whose rights are being abused?

In Cleveland Health Authority, between January and July 1987, 110 children were taken into care by the social services, on the advice of two paediatricians, because of suspicions that these children were subjected to sexual abuse at home. Legal representatives of the parents contested the right of the social services to take these children into care. In seeking leave to appeal to the High Court, it was claimed the rights of the parents had been infringed. Furthermore, it was claimed in evidence that the children had been subjected to several painful and humiliating examinations of their genitalia and other private parts, that repeated examinations involved violation of the children's rights (to privacy and respect for their persons), and that the doctors had not shown due care for these vulnerable patients. The local police surgeon complained that the right of the police to be consulted by the paediatricians, before care orders were signed, had not been respected. Also at issue were the rights of the paediatricians, their duty of care as responsible medical officers to protect the safety of the children, and their right to examine the children to establish the facts, and, if necessary to recommend they be taken into care. They claimed the right to give evidence in court and to be given a fair hearing in the Public Enquiry.

being threatened – such as their right of access to their own children. The rights of the children that it was claimed were not respected were fundamental moral rights, based on the principle of respect for persons – in particular their rights to privacy, dignity and proper care and treatment. What is of particular interest here is that the doctors and social workers claimed that they were exercising a proper duty to care in having the children medically examined and placed under care orders, to protect their rights, that is, to protect them from further sexual exploitation or abuse. What we have here is two different parties seeking to protect the children and basing their arguments on appeal to different rights.

Finally, the right appealed to by the police surgeon is what may be called an *institutional right*, that is, an accepted protocol or courtesy exercised in the relationships of doctors, social workers and police. The rights of the paediatricians – to give evidence in court and to be given a fair hearing – would ordinarily be protected by institutional provisions, for their legal representation by their employing authority. Failing that, they would be defended by the Medical Defence Union. However, their 'right' to a fair hearing could be said to be a right to which we are all entitled as a matter of natural justice, a fundamental moral right, but it is a right which may also be guaranteed in law, as a legal right as well.

Each of these different kinds of 'rights' and 'duties' has a different kind of justification. Like our positive and negative rights, positive and negative duties may be legally enforceable or may depend simply on the agent recognising the moral duty to act or to desist from acting in a particular way. Because of this important practical connection between rights and duties and the fact that we often have reciprocal rights and duties to others, it is important to understand that different kinds of rights and duties will be subject to different kinds of justification (Waldron 1984, Wellman 1995).

Institutional rights are created by and can be abolished by decisions of people with competent authority. For example, the rule that only members of the Marylebone Cricket Club (MCC) have the right to use the club facilities or to introduce visitors to the members' bar is decided by the elected and life members of the governing body of the MCC. While some women cricketers argued on legal grounds that their exclusion from membership of the MCC constituted sex discrimination, this did not succeed because the Sex Discrimination Act 1975 did not apply to private clubs. However, women did succeed in gaining access by an appeal to broad moral rights and by mobilising the media to support their cause.

Legal rights must be enacted by competent legal authorities, such as Parliament, regional or local authorities; or must be based on bills of rights such as the United Nations Universal Declaration of Human Rights (1947) or the European Convention on Human Rights (Council of Europe 1950). Alternatively, they must be based on common law or natural law, that is, the body of principle and precedent embodied in the legal tradition of the country.

The first kind of legal rights, *statutory rights*, are explicitly enacted in law, and in most cases are legally enforceable – in the sense that individuals can claim their rights or seek redress for the violation of their rights through the courts. The second kind, general *human rights*, based on bills of rights, may be enforceable through appeal to an international agency such as the International Court of Human Rights, provided the country of the person making the appeal respects its jurisdiction. However, these 'human rights' may be expressed in general terms and it would be the task of constitutional or international lawyers to

interpret the constitution, or bill of rights, to see if the particular claim of the individual was justified in terms of the universal principles embodied in these statements of human rights. Claims based on common law, or principles of natural law, may also have to be interpreted in this way, as both embody general statements of a moral rather than a legal kind. Their application in specific cases may have to be a matter of appeal to precedent, or some specific legislation may have to be introduced to make the principles applicable to the type of case in question.

In fact, if we consider the way that the term 'rights' is used in political life, in the general rhetoric of politicians and in the activity of pressure groups, it is significant that both groups are seeking as a rule to clarify or extend the scope of the law, or to mobilise public opinion to change the law. Thus debate about the 'woman's right to choose' (to terminate a pregnancy on demand), or the 'right to employment', or the 'right to a living wage', or the 'right to free healthcare', or the 'rights of the unborn child', or the 'right to die', are all concerned with the actual or possible reform of the law in the light of what people believe are their moral rights, or ones they claim on behalf of other people.

On what basis, then, do we justify *moral rights*? Generally, people appeal to their 'rights' when outraged by some injustice, or are protecting their human dignity when faced by degrading social conditions. In fact, appeal to moral rights presupposes the existence of fundamental moral principles, or at least a consensus about fundamental moral principles. Thus appeal to 'the right to adequate care and treatment', or 'the right to protection' (for children, frail elderly people or people with mental health problems or physical disabilities) is based on the assumption that society, and the law, will recognise the fundamental *principle of beneficence* (or the duty to care). The appeal to 'the right to equality before the law', to 'the right to freedom from discrimination on the basis of sex, class, religion or political affiliation', and the claimed 'right to equality of opportunity', or 'equal rights of access to healthcare', is based in each case on appeal to the fundamental *principle of justice*. Similarly, appeal to individual rights, such as the 'right to know', the 'right to privacy' and the 'right to refuse treatment' is based in these cases on appeal to the fundamental *principle of respect for persons*.

We can argue that human rights, particularly universal moral rights, rest on belief in some general concept of human dignity, of what it means to be human, and what minimum conditions would have to be satisfied for us to live fully human lives that enable us to develop our human potential. Alternatively, we can argue that universal moral principles are decided by society on the basis of a kind of social contract or consensus. Here, moral rights would be derivable as practical implications of these social contracts for the lives of ordinary people as moral agents.

Whether human rights can be regarded as 'inalienable', and in what sense, will depend on whether you believe that fundamental moral principles are God-given, grounded in the nature of things or determined by social convention. Whether human rights can ever be regarded as 'absolute' is debatable. However, it is more plausible to argue that the fundamental moral principles from which rights are derived, rather than the moral rights themselves, can be treated as absolute or unconditional moral demands.

Thus in the interests of justice and public health, our rights may have to be subject to limitation to protect the common good, e.g. the freedom of movement or association of people may have to be limited in times of epidemic, natural disaster, or war. People may also have to be subjected to compulsory immunisation in similar circumstances. In another case, we may not give treatment to a patient, which is seemingly required by our duty of care, when a patient has refused treatment while being of sound mind.

RIGHTS AND DUTIES OF NURSES IN DEALING WITH PATIENTS

If we consider practical examples of recurrent moral dilemmas in nurse–patient relationships we shall see that many of these raise fundamental questions about the rights of patients and the scope and limits of the responsibilities of nurses. Quandaries such as to tell or not to tell, to treat or not to treat, to limit the patient's freedom in his best interests, and which patient's interests or needs take precedence all raise questions of this kind.

Patients' rights form a subclass of general human rights, but how do we derive the rights of people as patients from their general human rights? How do patients' rights relate to the fundamental moral principles of beneficence, justice and respect for persons? It is to these questions that we must now turn.

One approach would be to attempt to derive patients' rights from their general human rights (e.g. from the UN Declaration of Universal Human Rights). The UNO Declaration now includes certain health rights, but more specific rights of people as patients would have to be derived from these general rights. However, another approach might be to start with the contract-to-care between the carer and client, nurse and patient, to examine the implicit assumptions involved in such 'contracts' and to analyse their moral and legal implications.

In what follows we shall adopt the latter approach, looking at the way contractual obligations arise in consulting relationships, and then considering the rights and duties that flow from these formal and informal contracts between people in need and their professional carers.

In general, when people with health problems seek help, they go first to a doctor. If the doctor agrees to take someone on as a patient, then that general agreement is first formalised by the patient registering with the doctor's practice. This arrangement constitutes one kind of 'contract'. The subject of the initial consultation relates to the boundaries of another kind of contract, namely the doctor's negotiation of the right to interview the patient and to record the patient's details and the medical (and perhaps family) history, and the right to undertake a physical examination of the patient and perhaps to do a series of tests. The patient's agreement to this process involves recognition of the duty to cooperate.

All this is essential, but preliminary to the more formal 'contract-to-care'. The 'contract-to-care' only comes into operation once the doctor has offered a diagnosis and suggested a possible course of treatment, and the patient has accepted the doctor's medical opinion. The (informed) consent to treatment by the patient is an essential part of the contract. The patient 'entrusts' himself/herself 'into the doctor's hands'. The doctor then assumes responsibility for the care and treatment of the patient and decides what form this should take. The doctor may prescribe treatment directly, refer the 'patient' to hospital or to a specialist, or the doctor may refer the patient to a nurse for continuing care. Although it is increasingly common for patients to consult directly with nurses, particularly in well-person clinics and community settings, nevertheless the 'contract-to-care' is usually made initially with the doctor, and the nurse usually has derived, rather than direct, duties following from the 'contract' with the 'patient'.

Despite these considerations, it may be useful to think through the process by which a person negotiates the help they require from a specific carer, and what assumptions underlie the agreements made. In general, the specific rights of people as 'patients' flow from the kind of relationship into which they enter with healthcare staff. When a patient is lucid, ambulant, continent and able to approach the health services independently for help, there is a kind of contract set up in which the patient agrees to cooperate in investigations, treatment and rehabilita-tion, in return for appropriate therapy and supportive care. The situation is rather different if the patient is brought in unconscious, or is unconsultable because of the specific nature of his disease or injury, or by reason of severe mental illness. Here the health professionals have to assume total responsibility for the patient and must fall back on their own and their professional moral code for guidance. A third situation is where the carer is involved with the patient as a friend – either through previous association, special circumstances of shared confidences, or because the person is dying and needs care and support rather than further therapy. Here the relationship may take on a more intimate form and the moral commitment in the contractual relationship may need to be renegotiated as something more personal and informal.

In Chapter 4 we described four possible models for carer–client relationships, namely, *code*, *contract*, *covenant* and *charter*. The relationships between the rights and duties of client and carer vary in each type of situation. The *first type* of situation – which has traditionally been taken to define the relationship between carer and patient – is one of crisis inter-vention, where the person is incompetent and the professional carer is expected to exercise a quasi-parental and protective duty to care towards the vulnerable patient, governed by the *code of practice* of the profession. The *second type* of situation, where a person independently approaches the health services for help with a health problem, is one in which an implicit or explicit *contract-to-care* is established by negotiation. In such a contract there will be rights and duties on the part of the patient and corresponding duties and rights on the part of the carer. In the *third type* of situation, which we have suggested is *governed by a covenant* of friendship, special consideration may be given to the rights of the patient as a person, and the patient may feel able to make unusual demands on the carer in the knowledge that he/she is prepared to act over and beyond the call of duty. Likewise, in the *fourth type*, where services are ostensibly based on 'customer-focus', *priority is given to the rights of the 'customer' or 'client'* – their right to choose, their right to guaranteed quality control in services, and their right to value for money.

When a person approaches a doctor or nurse for help, the practitioner has the right to refuse to help that particular person. They might legitimately refuse for several kinds of reasons. For example:

- if they are related to the client or the client is in a dependent relation to them
- if they have such a heavy caseload already that

they could not provide adequate care and support to the particular person
- if they do not believe they have the necessary competence
- if the person is being abusive and unpleasant, and they do not wish to have that person as a client.

If carers refuse clients on such grounds, they would be exercising their ordinary moral rights, but they would also have a professional duty to at least refer them on to someone else who might be willing and able to help them with their problem.

Refusal in the first case would be justified on the grounds that carers have the right not to be exploited or to have heavier demands imposed on them than they could reasonably be expected to cope with. Furthermore, carers have a duty, in justice to their clients, not to take on more clients than they could possibly provide with adequate care. So, too, in the case of difficult clients, refusal to take them on may be in the clients' best interests as well as the carers. In these examples the rights in question would appear to be derivable mainly from considerations of justice, although respect for persons comes into it as well.

Once the carer agrees to take on the person seeking help, the carer acquires fiduciary responsibility for the client, that is, a responsibility to look after a client's interests and to protect his rights. This responsibility of the carer follows from the trust the client shows in the carer, but the client also has responsibilities towards the carer. This is shown as soon as the carer proceeds to interview the client or patient.

In a medical consultation, a doctor would not only ask the patient a well-rehearsed checklist of questions about the patient's health and any adverse symptoms. He would also take down a medical history and, if necessary, would probably proceed to physical examination as well. Making a psychiatric assessment and taking a social history may also be indicated. A nurse, in making an assessment of a patient in order to develop a proper care plan, would quite likely follow a similar series of steps. The general assumptions underlying the exercise of these rights by the carers are that they are *entitled* to these privileges of intimacy because they are exercising a beneficent *duty to care*, in the best interests of the patient. Patients have a corresponding *obligation* to answer truthfully the questions asked by a doctor or nurse about them and their problems, and a duty to cooperate in treatment, if they are to be *entitled to* medical assistance or nursing care.

Doctors and nurses not only have a fundamental fiduciary duty to protect the interests of and to care for people who have entrusted themselves into their care, but they also have an obligation to give patients relevant information in return for their cooperation (concerning the diagnosis of their problem and the proposed methods of care and treatment), to enable them to make an informed choice whether they wish to continue with treatment. Here the health professionals have a fundamental duty to ensure that the consent to treatment given by the patient is both 'fully informed and voluntary'.

This means that the information must be given in a simple and intelligible form, preferably both verbally and in writing, and written material should be tested for readability for people of average reading age, not that of professionals. The patient's consent must not be obtained under pressure, when the patient is confused, or when subject to extreme stress of anxiety, as he is unlikely to be able to assimilate the necessary information, even if he is capable of understanding it. Health professionals have a duty to give clients all the information they require to make an informed decision about their treatment options, or the drugs or procedures involved in their treatment, including the degree of risk and possible complications involved.

On both counts it may be difficult to determine in practice whether the consent obtained is truly voluntary or fully informed. On the one hand, it can be argued that to be under the duress of pain or anxiety, or trussed up in a hospital bed, may place considerable limitations on your liberty to dissent from what the doctor or nurse proposes by way of treatment for you. On the other hand, who decides how much information is enough? And how fully must *all* the possible risks of treatment or side-effects of treatment be discussed with a patient? And when would failure to meet these criteria amount to culpable negligence?

For some time, within the sphere of jurisdiction of English law, the Bolam principle has been applied to determine whether or not a health professional is negligent in the discharge of his or her duty to a patient. The principle was enunciated to the jury by McNair J in the English case of *Bolam v. Friern Hospital Management Committee* (1957), viz:

> A doctor is not guilty of negligence if he [sic] has acted in accordance with a practice accepted as proper by a responsible body of medical men skilled in that particular art. (Kerridge et al 1998, pp. 109–113)

What this means is that in the past it has generally been assumed that the courts would follow the guidance of responsible members of the medical or nursing profession in deciding whether a particular doctor or nurse acted responsibly or not. This principle was further reinforced by the judgement of Lord Scarman in the Sidaway case (*Sidaway v. Board of Governors of Bethlehem Royal Hospital* and others [1985] AC871) in which he stated that:

> a doctor is not negligent if he acts in accordance with a practice accepted at the time as proper by a responsible body of medical opinion, even though other doctors may accept a different practice. In short, the law imposes the duty of care: but the standard of care is a matter of medical judgement.

As Kerridge et al (1998, pp. 110–111) pointed out, the Bolam principle has been challenged repeatedly in the Australian courts where the 'courts have tended to opt for standards of care that are defined by the courts, rather than the profession itself'. However, what has had a considerable influence in confirming this trend and changing legal policy on the rights of patients to fully informed consent, as determined for them by the courts rather than by the professional group involved, is the 1992 case of *Rogers v. Whitaker*, 175 CLR 479. The issue was that Mrs Whitaker, who was nearly blind in her right eye, had developed an extremely rare condition of her remaining good eye. She was referred to Dr Rodgers for advice on possible surgery. She was told that he could operate to remove scar tissue from her right eye, probably improve her sight in that eye, improve its appearance and help prevent the development of glaucoma. Following successful surgery, Mrs Whitaker developed an inflammation in the treated right eye which infected her left eye as well, resulting in the total loss of sight in her good eye and virtually total loss of vision. Because Mrs Whitaker had specifically requested reliable advice about the risks of the operation and had not been told that there was a risk of cross-infection between the two eyes, she sued for damages for not having been properly informed, and won. In his defence the doctor argued that the known risk of this complication was 1:14 000 cases and he had not considered it significant. He appealed to the Bolam principle in his defence. However, commenting on their verdict, the learned judges remarked:

> Further, and more importantly, particularly in the non-disclosure of risk and the provision of advice and information, the Bolam principle has been discarded, and, instead, the courts have adopted the principle that, while evidence of acceptable medical practice is a useful guide for the courts, it is for the courts to adjudicate on what is the appropriate standard of care after giving weight to the paramount consideration that a person is entitled to make his own decisions about his life.

Further clarification was provided in the case of *Bolitho v. City and Hackney Health Authority* 1993 (House of Lords 1997), to the effect that what is meant by 'reasonable' is the capacity of those responsible to demonstrate that specific risk assessments were made, based on evidence-based practice, and the benefits to the patient against the potential harm were weighed up.

Kerridge et al observe that while the judges in this case reaffirmed that doctors have a duty to disclose and warn patients of material risks to their health and well-being, they rejected use of the expression 'informed consent', arguing that it was misleading, and suggested the use instead of the phrase 'duty of disclosure'. Kerridge et al point out that given the broad terms in which the principle was expressed by the court it was clearly intended to cover other professions besides medicine, and hence is of relevance to nurses as well. They proceed to describe the fundamental elements enabling informed and valid consent as consisting in (a) competence and (b) voluntariness. Whereas elements that enable a person to be informed are (a) disclosure of relevant information and (b) understanding and acceptance of the information by the patient. In communicating information to patients about their care and treatment, nurses would do well to note these criteria, and apply them (Kerridge et al 1998, p. 145) (Box 7.2).

Box 7.2 Kerridge's criteria for information transfer

Requirements for information transfer in clinical practice
- Diagnosis (including degree of uncertainty about this)
- Prognosis (including degree of uncertainty about this)
- Options for investigations/treatments
- Burdens and benefits of investigations/treatments
- Whether the intervention is conventional/experimental
- Who will perform the intervention
- Consequences of choosing or not choosing treatment
- Significant expected short-term and long-term outcomes
- Time and cost involved

Information given may have to be modified by considering:
- the seriousness of the patient's condition
- the nature of the intervention
- the degree of possible harm
- the likelihood or risk of harm
- the patient's needs, attitude, understanding

Source: Kerridge et al (1998), p 145.

THE RIGHTS OF PEOPLE AS PATIENTS

One of the earliest attempts to formulate a Bill of Rights for Patients was put forward by the American Hospital Association (1992). The Patient's Bill of Rights of the US Advisory Commission on Consumer Protection and Quality in the Health Care Industry set out the following rights (US Com 1998):

- **Information Disclosure.** You have the right to accurate and easily understood information about your health plan, healthcare professionals, and healthcare facilities. If you speak another language, have a physical or mental disability, or just don't understand something, assistance will be provided so you can make informed healthcare decisions.

- **Choice of Providers and Plans.** You have the right to a choice of healthcare providers that is sufficient to provide you with access to appropriate high-quality healthcare.

- **Access to Emergency Services.** If you have severe pain, an injury, or sudden illness that convinces you that your health is in serious jeopardy, you have the right to receive screening and stabilization emergency services whenever and wherever needed, without prior authorization or financial penalty.

- **Participation in Treatment Decisions.** You have the right to know your treatment options and to participate in decisions about your care. Parents, guardians, family members, or other individuals that you designate can represent you if you cannot make your own decisions.

- **Respect and Nondiscrimination.** You have a right to considerate, respectful and nondiscriminatory care from your doctors, health plan representatives, and other healthcare providers.

- **Confidentiality of Health Information.** You have the right to talk in confidence with healthcare providers and to have your healthcare information protected. You also have the right to review and copy your own medical record and request that your physician change your record if it is not accurate, relevant, or complete.

- **Complaints and Appeals.** You have the right to a fair, fast, and objective review of any complaint you have against your health plan, doctors, hospitals or other healthcare personnel. This includes complaints about waiting times, operating hours, the conduct of healthcare personnel, and the adequacy of healthcare facilities.

In the UK the Citizens Advice Bureau, has a website (www.adviceguide.org.uk), setting out NHS patients' rights, with linking sources of information for Scotland and Wales.

Earlier attempts were made by the authors to derive a simpler list from consideration of general contractual and moral rights. For example, the Edinburgh Medical Group Working Party on the Care of the Dying and the Bereaved (Thompson 1979a) suggested three fundamental rights of people as patients:

- the right to know
- the right to privacy
- the right to treatment.

The right to know

Patients, it has been argued, do not disinterestedly give doctors or nurses access to private information about themselves, nor allow intimate physical, psychological or social investigations without the expectation that the carers will give them some indication of their diagnosis, tell them what they propose to do by way of treatment, and to give them sufficient information to enable them to make an informed decision.

The normal expectation of clients is that the carer will discuss their problem with them and give an opinion as to its nature; that the carer will discuss the proposed course of treatment or management of the problem; and that they will discuss the possible options and outcomes. Thus it can be argued that the right to know is implicit in the contract with the carer who is being consulted by the patient, and is predicated on the trust shown in the carer. Similarly, the requirement in law and medical ethics, as we have seen above, that a patient should give informed and voluntary consent to treatment (unless the patient is incompetent) presupposes his right to know. However, in this case the right to know tends to be based on wider considerations of the rights of the individual as a person (in the legal sense), that is, as someone who can be held responsible for his actions since he is capable of making informed and voluntary choices for himself.

When a patient is recruited to be a 'volunteer' in a clinical or drug trial, especially if that patient is unlikely to benefit directly from the experiment, or there is a significant element of risk involved, the requirements for obtaining properly informed and voluntary consent are more stringent than in the case where the direct treatment of the patient is involved. This is not only because of the specific ethical requirements for medical research involving human subjects (see the Declaration of Helsinki, WMA 1996), but also because the nature of the contract is different.

When a patient is dying or when news of a bad prognosis has to be communicated to a patient, a health professional may feel that he has a duty to protect the patient from knowledge which may be too painful to bear or which she is not yet ready to receive.

In such cases there is a tension between the patient's right to know and the professional's duty to care. How this tension is resolved in practice may be decided on an individual basis. It may be further complicated by relatives who demand that the patient should not be told. In such cases, whose rights are to be given priority? However, even if a professional decides that providing the patient with the diagnosis is contraindicated because it may cause physical and/or psychological damage to the patient, this does not justify a professional deciding to breach the duty of confidentiality by telling the patient's relatives the diagnosis.

However, the question of the patient's right to know has been given new poignancy and practical urgency for health professionals, as we have discussed above, because of the court finding, in the case of *Rogers v. Whitaker*, that Dr Rogers was negligent in failing to give full disclosure to his patient of the risks entailed in her operation. Writing in the *Journal of Medical Ethics*, Australian judge, Michael Kirby, commenting on the significance of the *Rogers v. Whitaker* case, argues that times have changed and greater weight should be given in English and American law to the rights of patients rather than retain the 1958 Bolam principle and defend the entrenched privilege of doctors:

> We must see the moves towards ... the provision of greater information to patients in the context of the wider social developments that affect society and the law. All professions, including the judges, are now more accountable. ... The difference between the standards expected in England and in the other countries is not large. But it is significant. And at the heart of the difference is an attitude to the fundamental rights of the particular patient. Those rights should take primacy both in legal formulae and in medical practice. (Kirby 1995)

What is at stake here is not only the question of the relative importance of the rights of doctors versus the rights of patients, but the question of how far we can go with the concept of rights in determining moral choices in particular situations. The strength of the justice perspective, reflected in law and in the moral theory of rights and duties, is that it purports to be objective. However, in a case, like that of the unfortunate Mrs Whitaker, the question of sensitivity to the needs of a particularly vulnerable but intelligent woman might have resulted in a more honest disclosure of information and less reliance on medical judgement and formal procedural rules.

While it has become increasingly necessary for nurses to be aware of the requirements of the law affecting healthcare practice, what this case demonstrates is that the exercise of professional judgement requires practical wisdom, discrimination and sensitivity to the values applicable in a given situation, and cannot be made a matter of law and regulation. Hence the study of law can never be a substitute for understanding of ethics and skills in its practical application. In fact, it is ethical considerations that are more fundamental than legal ones, for we always have to test the integrity and fairness of any law by consideration of whether it can be squared with the demands of the fundamental ethical principles of beneficence, justice and respect for persons. It is a strength of the tradition of English law that it rests on the common law, which embodies consideration of case and precedent in the light of the principles of natural justice. Similarly, Scots and Roman-Dutch law is based on the principles of natural law, which served as the foundations for classical ethics.

The right to privacy

The right to privacy covers both the right to respect for the dignity of the person (physical privacy) and respect for their secrets (confidentiality). The right to privacy does not mean the right to have a private ward, or the right to private medicine, although in some circumstances it may include that. For example, an elderly single woman who has never shared a room with another person may be emotionally distressed at having to be nursed in a public ward, and might prefer to pay extra health insurance to ensure that she can get the privacy so important to her. While most people entering hospital may expect some general loss of privacy, it often comes as a shock to people to realise how little privacy they have. Patient advocacy groups and Health Councils have claimed that hospital staff often show scant consideration for people's sensitivities or need for privacy, particularly the needs of those who are dying. While individual nurses may differ in their sensitivity to a patient's needs, the routines and physical environment in overcrowded or mixed wards may not provide sufficient safeguards for patient privacy, or scope for them to hold confidential conversations with family members or medical and nursing staff. There can in practice be a tension here between the scope for individual agency and structural constraints. Even if staff do recognise, and wish to meet patients' desires for privacy, the structures – physical and managerial – within which care is provided may prevent this.

Generally people are prepared to share their secrets, expose their bodies and reveal their vulnerabilities when they need help and when they feel they can trust the person from whom they are seeking help. In such a situation, sensitive carers will respect the patient's confidences and privacy. Carers should also recognise that the information is to be used only for the benefit of the patient, and that they thus acquire duties of advocacy, to protect the rights and interests of the persons in their care, in the light of what they have learned about them.

The right to privacy, to have confidences kept, is not an unlimited right (NMC 2004, clause 5.3) When the interests of justice require that evidence is brought before a court to establish the guilt or innocence of an accused, it is generally assumed that the principle of justice and the common good takes precedence over the individual's right to privacy. In Britain, only lawyers enjoy professional privilege, that is, the right to refuse to disclose information in court (e.g. information which may compromise defence of their client). Contrary to popular belief, priests and journalists, doctors and nurses do not enjoy this privilege, and if they refuse to divulge secrets of patients or penitents because they may feel obliged to protect their clients' confidences, they may have to suffer the penalties of the law for being 'in contempt of court'. In practice the court may not insist on the disclosure of information or sources if the confidant is adamant, but as the law stands, it is entitled to impose fines or send a person to prison for refusing to give evidence.

Similarly, when the public interest is threatened, for example by a serious epidemic, the nurse may be expected to divulge information to the responsible authorities if a patient's condition is likely to put the lives of other people at risk. In the context of the AIDS epidemic, if a nurse learns that a patient is having a sexual relationship with a person who is HIV-positive but is not prepared to disclose this to her doctor, what is the nurse to do? The patient's personal right to privacy has to be balanced against protection of the right to life of others and the question is: which right is to be given priority? Many other cases could be considered to illustrate the same moral quandaries in less dramatic circumstances, e.g. the epileptic who discloses to the nurse that he is a long-distance lorry driver, or the unemployed and 'disabled' patient who reveals to the district nurse that he is falsely claiming benefits when he is actually making a good living on the side. The disclosure of information by a nurse, to another health professional involved in a patient's care, may be expressly forbidden by the patient. In such circumstances, especially where the patient's safety or welfare is at stake, the nurse may have to decide, on the principle of beneficence, that her duty to care takes precedence over the patient's right to prohibit disclosure of vital facts (NMC 2004, clause 5.3).

A different kind of problem can arise for the nurse when clients use the sharing of secrets or self-disclosure as a device to establish a kind of intimacy with the nurse, and to create a kind of obligation on the part of the nurse towards them, which they can then manipulate. Being at the receiving end of people's secrets can create burdensome problems for carers, for example when the intimacies shared are irrelevant to the management of the patient's health problems. Similarly, health visitors can be faced with a conflict of duties when they discover on domiciliary visits that patients/clients are concealing the true nature of their problems, or that they, or someone living with them, are breaking the law or have some contagious disease. Setting in advance boundaries to confidentiality, or limits to information-sharing with patients, may be helpful, and may be in the best interests of both patient and nurse.

The guidance given by the British Association of Social Workers (BASW) to their members, more than 30 years ago, namely that social workers should seek to establish with clients explicit 'confidentiality contracts', remains fundamentally good advice for all professionals in consulting professions. In the most recent version (BASW 2003), this is has become: 'Consult service users about their preferences in respect of the use of information relating to them.' This may not be easy in hospital practice, although it may be particularly important on domiciliary visits. The extent to which it is possible to negotiate explicit confidentiality contracts will vary with the context and setting. In a public hospital ward confidentiality means one thing, in the privacy of a consulting room or a patient's home, another. Here, as with many other moral rules, the context may be very important in determining the scope and applicability of the rule.

While patients may share secrets in an attempt to gain some influence over their carers, it is also true that knowledge of their secrets gives professionals great power over people. This power can be used for the patient's benefit, but it can also be abused. Direct breach of a patient's confidences is not only a serious breach of trust, but is a serious legal offence. Abuse of a patient's trust by using information given in confidence for the purposes of blackmail may be an uncommon occurrence, but it does happen from time to time and is also a serious criminal offence that can lead to heavy penalties against professionals. However, a more subtle abuse occurs when practitioners use knowledge gained from the patient in confidence as leverage to get patient compliance. This is more difficult to prove, and in some cases the carer may feel that their action is justified. Doctors and nurses are given great power to help or hurt people by the secrets people share with them, and with this power goes a great responsibility on the part of all those in the consulting professions (Windt et al 1989, pp. 160ff., Kerridge et al 1998, pp. 128–140, Keatings & Smith 2000, pp. 142–134).

The right to care and treatment

The right to adequate care and treatment can again be argued as a fundamental human right, as it is in the UN Declaration of Human Rights, Article 25, where it is implied that without basic health protection people cannot survive, let alone lead a full human life or exercise any of their other human rights. In Britain, the National Health Service Act of 1947 also created the legal right for citizens to claim medical treatment, which should be free at the point of delivery (although financed by general taxation).

However, the right to adequate care and treatment can be argued on different grounds, namely as a particular right that is a direct consequence and implication of the contract-to-care negotiated with the doctor or health professional. Every person who has been taken on by a doctor or nurse as a patient has a right to expect proper care and treatment. The doctor or nurse is employed to provide a service, or offers a service on a fee-for-service basis, and patients are entitled to treatment in fulfilment of the deal made with the doctor or nurse to whom they have entrusted themselves. Malpractice and negligence is not confined to incompetent, dishonest or faulty practice. It also applies to the failure to provide due care, in fulfilment of the contract-to-care.

In reality, the right to treatment is based, for all practical purposes, on the contract, formal or informal, between the particular doctor or nurse and a specific patient. This right is not absolute, however. Patients cannot demand whatever drugs or treatment they fancy – even if they are in a position to pay for these. It is for the doctor or nurse to decide whether the treatment requested is appropriate. Besides, it may not be possible to give particular patients the special treatments which they request without detriment to the interests of other patients. Furthermore, while the patient has a fundamental moral right to adequate care and treatment, that 'treatment' may in certain circumstances be neither drug therapy nor surgery, nor any other active intervention. In the case of the dying patient, 'treatment' may simply mean tender loving care and settling for comfort rather than therapy. The fact that the term 'treatment' covers both palliative care and therapy can be a source of confusion in discussions about stopping treatment. While it may be appropriate to stop therapy, it would never be right to stop palliative care, such as the alleviation of pain or treatment of distressing symptoms. There are three points which should be emphasised about patients' rights, as with human rights in generally:

- having rights does not mean that one is bound to exercise them
- having rights does not mean that they are absolute and their exercise is unlimited
- patient's negative rights are in general stronger than their positive ones.

Thus having the right to know does not mean that one has to exercise it. One may not wish to know that one is dying, for example; or, even if one suspects that one is dying, one may not wish to discuss it; or one may not wish to discuss it with a particular doctor or nurse. One has a right to be asked, but one is not obliged to accept unwanted information or even 'counselling'. The right to privacy is not an unlimited right, because the demands of caring for others in similar need, with limited staff and resources, may require that patients sacrifice some of their privacy, and consent to be nursed in public wards. While doctors and nurses are encouraged to regard confidentiality as an important moral duty, it is generally recognised by hospital staff (and often by patients themselves) that team management necessitates the operation of a kind of 'extended confidentiality', which includes other members of the caring team. While the right to treatment is a fundamental right of patients, it does not include the right to demand particular therapies. However, the negative right to refuse treatment is a much stronger right – in law it is virtually an absolute right – unless the patient is mentally disordered. The treatment of patients against their will, as we have already said, has long been treated as criminal assault and is actionable in law.

TELLING THE TRUTH TO PATIENTS OR RELATIVES

Consider the situation faced by a staff nurse in a paediatric hospital, in Case Study 7.2.

The staff nurse in this case recognised that knowing the truth that Mary was dying imposed certain responsibilities on her, to protect Mary's vulnerability (a feeling she shared with Mary's parents), but she also recognised that Mary had a right to know the truth. The dilemma she faced was the conflict of loyalties to Mary and to her parents, because of the trust and understanding that had grown up between her and Mary on the one hand, and between her and Mary's parents on the other. The problem was made more difficult by her uncertainty that it was right to tell

case study 7.2

When is a child no longer a child?

Mary, aged 13 years, was admitted with acute myeloid leukaemia. Over the next two and a half years she was in and out of hospital at increasingly frequent intervals. The permanent ward staff established a good relationship with Mary and her family during this period. Initially her parents did not accept the diagnosis, but with much support and reassurance eventually accepted the situation fairly well.

Two and a half years after her first admission, Mary was admitted for terminal care. Throughout the course of her illness her parents had been adamant that Mary should not be told what was wrong with her. This was still the situation when Mary was admitted for the last time. We tried to point out to her parents that Mary was no longer a child and that if she enquired, it might help her to know the truth, but they still refused to let her be told.

Three days before she died, Mary asked outright if she was going to die. She said she felt she was getting worse rather than better, and she asked directly what it was like to die. In spite of her parents' views, I felt that I had to be truthful with Mary as she was no longer a child, but 15 years old. We talked about death and I explained to her that everyone had to die sooner or later. I was with her when she died, as were her parents, and she died peacefully and calmly. I felt I had done the right thing in telling her, but felt that I had betrayed the trust of her parents, which had been built up over nearly three years.

Mary because she was technically still a minor, and her sense of guilt at going against the wishes of Mary's parents. On the other hand, she was also aware of having been specially chosen by Mary as the one to ask this momentous question. Was it not possible that the distraught parents, faced with loss of their daughter, were using the staff nurse in a vain attempt to reassert their rights over their daughter? In such a situation, which does the nurse put first: the rights of the parents or the rights of the patient?

It is questionable whether doctors or nurses, or relatives, ever have a right to keep information from a dying patient. Whose death is it anyway? If the dying patient does not have a fundamental right to know that they are dying, who has? However, in this case the patient was a child, 12 years old when myeloid leukaemia was first diagnosed, and only 15 when she died. Both the nurse and the parents assumed that they had a duty to protect Mary from the knowledge of her impending death because she was a child. But did they have the right to deny her this knowledge? Because Mary was so young, at first the staff nurse felt that the parents were right to protect her from the painful truth, but as Mary grew older and asked more searching questions the staff nurse's attitude changed. However, did Mary have any more right to know at age 15 than at age 12? Are parents or relatives of dying patients entitled to withhold the truth from them however young or old they are (Melia 2004, Ch. 5)?

In general, the right to know is derived from the principle of respect for persons. If people are to be treated as persons with rights – for example the right to make informed choices, the right to autonomy, that is, to be in control of their own lives – then they cannot be denied the knowledge or information which will enable them to make important life choices. We say glibly that 'ignorance is bliss', but many studies show that dying patients are often frightened because they do not know what is going on, are aware of the conspiracy of silence around them, and are too afraid to ask. More than thirty years ago, research by Parkes (1966) and Hinton (1979) showed that, contrary to common belief, dying patients are often reassured by knowing their prognosis, as the anxiety based on doubt and uncertainty is ended, and there is evidence that the condition of patients may improve, and they may enjoy remission of their symptoms, once they 'know the score' (Parkes & Markus 1998).

The policy of openness adopted by hospices for the dying is based not only on the belief that the patient has a right to know (particularly if the patient asks), but that good terminal care presupposes the knowing cooperation of the patient. The conspiracy of silence around the dying patient deceives no one – except perhaps the conspirators themselves. Several studies involving terminally ill patients have shown that in units where the policy was not to tell, more than 75% of patients nevertheless did know that they were dying (Parkes 1972/1996). As a consequence of this kind of research, it has become much less common, in the UK at least, to withhold information from patients. Not surprisingly, patients pick up this information anyway from various sources: by comparing their symptoms and treatment with other patients, by what they learn from conversation with other patients and hospital staff (including cleaners and porters), by observation of their own deteriorating condition and what they infer from the non-verbal communication of nurses and medical staff (hushed voices, telling looks, silent passing of the bed, over-solicitous care). Hinton's research showed that patients do not 'give up', 'turn their faces to the wall', 'go to pieces', when

told their condition is terminal, provided they are given adequate emotional support, and time to come to terms with dying (Hinton 1979).

However, it is not such pragmatic considerations which are of fundamental importance in this argument, but rather the fact that knowledge is power. Deliberately keeping another person in a state of ignorance is to deprive them of power, which results in a state of dependency and powerlessness. The attitude of Mary's parents had the effect of infantilising her, depriving her of the opportunity to discuss with them her grief and anxiety at facing death. Their protective paternalism mirrors the attitudes often adopted by doctors and nurses – in being more concerned to protect patients than to respect their rights as persons to know and choose for themselves.

Consider another case, taken from an obstetric ward, where a mother has to be told that her baby, born by caesarean section, was stillborn (Case Study 7.3).

case study 7.3

Death in the obstetric ward

A nurse midwife is caring for a mother who has had a stillborn baby, by caesarean section, just recovering consciousness and asking to see her baby. How, when and where does the nurse tell the mother that her baby is dead? Should she call for the doctor and get around the difficulty that way? Should she tell the absent father first? Should she avoid telling the mother till the father is present and can comfort his wife? Should she arrange for the couple to see the baby? How does she cope with her own grief, her own feelings of failure, her need to appear strong in order to comfort the parents and to continue providing care for the mother?

Here, the mother not only has a right to know, but is bound to know sooner or later. The grief cannot be avoided. However, the nurse cannot simply 'tell facts as they are' without considering the consequences for the mother (and father). Truthfulness carries with it the burdensome responsibility of deciding how much truth a person can take at a given time, and how full disclosure should be in the circumstances. The questions for the nurse are: whether she can cope with being the one who tells, who shares the mother's grief and the mother's likely sense of her own failure, and who is available to provide ongoing support afterwards. The inhibition which the nurse feels about sharing the truth in this situation, particularly if there is no convenient way out of facing the challenge, probably has more to do with her fear of accepting the responsibility for telling the truth, than any uncertainty about the mother's rights. Sharing the truth can be a costly business. Once the midwife accepts the responsibility to tell the mother she implicitly commits herself to share her grief (and that of her partner as well). If the nurse knows anything about loss and bereavement she will also know that telling parents that a longed-for baby has died will not only cause them immediate grief but will initiate a process which may take many months to work through. She will also know that she has a duty to continue with support for as long as possible, while they deal with their bereavement. Truth-sharing means accepting responsibility to share the pain and grief, anger and despair, shock and depression which knowing the truth may cause. If there is not well-established understanding, trust and caring, if there is no possibility that the nurse can provide continuing support to the individual concerned, then 'telling the truth' may be cruel and irresponsible (Doyle 1984, 1994).

Sharing painful truth requires great sensitivity and skill in judging how, when and where it is appropriate to tell. Once the midwife accepts the responsibility to tell the mother, she also has to face the difficult practical decisions, requiring tact and judgement, whether the mother will be most helped by being allowed to cuddle her dead baby, or needs to be protected from an experience which may be too painful for her to bear, or for which she is not yet ready. Being *honest* with other people is a measure of how much we *honour* them – how much we trust and respect them as persons. Honesty, or truthfulness, is being sensitive to 'where other people are at', in their own present experience and ability to cope. In making an assessment of a patient the nurse will not only have to rely on her own common sense, but also on the opinions of her colleagues and perhaps the relatives. But the nurse can never shelve her responsibility by relying on, or being tied by, the opinions of others. Sooner or later all nurses have to face situations where they have to accept responsibility for sharing the painful truth with patients, and this means becoming as skilled at 'titration' of the truth to the needs of the patient, as in administering appropriate doses of painkilling drugs.

A different but related problem about sharing information arises when the patient knows the truth yet refuses to let the medical or nursing staff tell his wife or family. Here in no direct sense do the relatives have a right to know since it is not their death that is at issue; but as people who are intimately involved and likely to be affected by the patient's death, the nurse may feel that they ought to be told. As we do not exist in isolation from other people, least of all from our families in most cases, family members also have a right to know (though in an extended sense of 'right') – based on both considerations of compassion and the reciprocal responsibilities which obtain in families and close communities.

Faced with such a situation, a nurse may be helped by discussing the matter with the persons prohibiting the disclosure of information, to make them aware of how the interests of others are involved, to help them see what comfort may be gained by sharing the truth and the grief together. For example, Mary's parents might have been persuaded to tell Mary themselves (with or without the support of the medical and nursing staff); the husband might be persuaded and assisted to tell his wife about the stillborn baby himself, with the midwife providing support; the dying patient might need to be encouraged and assisted to share his anxieties about dying with his wife and family and to set his affairs in order. However, if they still refuse, the nurse may be able to gain moral support from discussion with other members of staff. But in the end, the nurse may have to make her own painful decision whether or not to tell. Here she has to balance several conflicting interests and duties: her responsibility to her patient against her wider responsibilities to the family and other concerned parties. If this course is taken by nurses, they have to recognise that they have breached their duty of confidentiality and may be called to account by their regulatory body, e.g. the Nursing and Midwifery Council (NMC 2004, clause 5.3). There is also the possibility of disciplinary action being taken by the nurse's employer if a complaint is made either by the patient or by medical staff. In such cases there is also the possibility of legal action taken by the patient in relation to the breach of confidentiality.

In the cases considered, it can readily be seen that dilemmas about truth-telling relate to the rights of patients (e.g. the right to know and the right to privacy) and to the tensions between these rights and the duties of nurses (e.g. the duty to protect the vulnerable patient from knowledge too painful to bear, or the duty, in fairness to others, to share information that may affect them). Here we see that considerations other than respect for persons and their individual rights come into play. The principles of beneficence and justice are also involved, and it is precisely this actual or apparent conflict of principles which makes these present as moral dilemmas, and which makes decisions in these areas difficult, painful and uncertain.

DECIDING BETWEEN THERAPEUTIC CARE AND PALLIATIVE CARE

As already indicated, the right to treatment is a fundamental right of people as patients, regardless of their age and whether or not they can speak for themselves. Problems arise in interpreting this right, because of the varying degrees of competence of patients to make decisions for themselves. Not only do different patients differ in the degree of competence that can be attributed to them, but depending on the severity of their illness, injury or mental disorder, their degree of competence may vary from one stage of their illness to another.

The least problematic situation is where an independent adult, in full possession of his senses, enters into a contract for treatment with a doctor, or the caring team, when he becomes their patient. In principle, infants, people who have learning difficulties, and frail elderly patients have the same rights and are entitled to the same standards of medical and nursing care as anyone else. When, by reason of physical or mental illness, a patient is in a very dependent and vulnerable condition, decisions have to be taken about their care and treatment by others. A lucid, independent and ambulant patient can actively claim the right to treatment or refuse treatment. Confused or unconscious, bed-bound or unconsultable patients are in a different situation, depending entirely on others to protect their rights and dignity, to ensure that they get adequate medical treatment and proper nursing care. An infant born with serious physical or mental problems also needs to have their interests safeguarded by others. Just as special tribunals are set up to oversee the care and management of compulsory psychiatric patients, so the courts have a special responsibility to protect the rights of individuals who are not competent to defend themselves, owing to physical or mental infirmity, old age or infancy.

These safeguards are put in place not because healthcare workers cannot be trusted to care for their patients in a responsible fashion but because they need protection, as much as their vulnerable patients do, from criticism and litigation or dismissal. A patient who is not consultable needs an independent advocate to represent their interests, where there may be doubt and uncertainty about the right course of treatment, or there is conflict between doctors and nurses about whether the patient's rights have been protected.

Part of the difficulty centres around the ambiguity of the word 'treatment', when we speak of the 'right to treatment'. 'Treatment' can be taken to embrace every kind of medical intervention and every form of nursing care. So it is important for nurses to be clear, in negotiations with patients, about what 'treatment' is being referred to in a particular context, as there are important ethical differences, for example, between the justification for therapeutic measures or palliative care, for compulsory hospitalisation and/or asylum. In certain contexts the purpose of an operation may be to cure, by repairing injury, removing diseased tissue or preventing the spread of infection. In another context surgery may be purely palliative, to relieve pain or to delay the spread of malignant disease. Alternatively, the operation may be strictly unnecessary for medical reasons, but indicated for psychological or social reasons, as, for example, cosmetic surgery, sterilisation or 'gender realignment'. In each case, the 'right to treatment' will have different ethical significance.

Because 'treatment' often is taken to include both 'cure' and 'care', it may in practice be difficult to separate the one from the other. When a patient has a potentially fatal disease, which might be curable or at least treatable, it may be extremely difficult for the ward team to decide when further therapeutic measures are no longer justifiable and it is time to provide palliative care. For the caring team to be clear about when a patient has reached the pre-death stage is vitally important for good terminal care. But if a change of management from a therapeutic regime to palliative care is indicated, the patient has a right to be consulted about this step. The contract with the patient to provide therapy may not cover 'palliative care', and may need to be renegotiated. A conspiracy of silence about the true condition of the patient may also lead to conflict between members of the care team (i.e. conflict may be intra- as well as inter-occupational, between nursing staff and doctors) about which type of 'treatment' is appropriate. This may be particularly difficult if the patient or relatives are desperately demanding that everything possible should be done, or that all treatment should be stopped (Doyle 1994).

We now consider three different kinds of problems/dilemmas relating to the 'right to treatment: (a) resuscitation of a baby with a severe heart defect (Case Study 7.4); (b) struggles between nurses and doctors over sedation (Case Study 7.5); and (c) treatment without consent (Case Study 7.6).

Resuscitation of a baby with a severe heart defect

There are broadly speaking two schools of thought in this case – the one that emphasises the rights of the baby and the one that emphasises the responsibility of the medical team. In principle, the baby has the same

case study 7.4

Birth of a Down's syndrome baby with a congenital heart defect

When I was a student midwife, a baby with Down's syndrome and a severe heart defect was born to a 38-year-old mother and a 42-year-old father. Both parents were unable to accept the baby. The father expressed the wish that the baby should not be resuscitated if a crisis occurred. Soon afterwards the child suffered cardiac arrest, and a junior member of the medical team initiated resuscitation. The baby died, however, several weeks later.

right to life and right to treatment that any adult has, and the law should safeguard these rights as it does those of other vulnerable individuals. An outside party (e.g. a social worker) should have the right to appeal to the courts to ensure that the child's rights are protected. Although all citizens have a moral duty to protect the rights of others – thus protecting their own rights – certain professionals, such as social workers and hospital chaplains, have special responsibility to act as advocates for those whose rights may be compromised or neglected. The parents do not have a moral right to refuse the treatment that their child requires for survival, but neither can they be forced to care for the child. If, as a society, we recognise that the child has a right to treatment, then we must also recognise that society has an obligation to provide adequate care and support for the child (and possibly for the parents as well) (Melia 2004, Ch. 3).

In practice, the situation is often more complicated. The social provision for the care of severely handicapped children in most societies is inadequate, and support for affected families insufficient to prevent hardship and distress. Compassion for the parents, who, understandably, may feel unable to cope, and compassion for the medical and nursing staff, who are faced with immediate decisions about care and treatment for the child, may point to letting nature take its course and allowing the child to die. In reality, the hospital team and the parents have to try to resolve the situation in the most responsible way. In this case the risks of medical intervention are that the child would still be left severely handicapped for life, and would require constant nursing care and medical attention. The parents would almost inevitably have to carry the main burden of caring for the child because of the lack of practical alternatives.

Issues of social justice are involved as well, because the painful reality is that the child's right to treatment and the medical team's duty to care have to be reconciled in most cases where there is inadequate social provision for the care and support of such children and their families in the community. This places unjust pressure on the family to accept responsibilities greater than they may be able to cope with themselves, and pressure on the medical and nursing team who may not feel free to do what is in the child's best interests. This illustrates how issues of rights cannot be separated from considerations of justice relating to the equitable distribution of resources in society generally.

Clinical decisions in such cases are not un-ambiguous. Past experience may show that there is little hope for such children, or that particular interventions can be successful in ensuring survival and reasonable quality of life. However, medical evidence will not be enough to resolve the moral dilemmas, for technological or medical progress might make possible improvement to the child's quality of life. How objective are assessments of 'quality of life' anyway? These judgements cannot be made solely on medical grounds. Medically it is not possible to decide whether a life of severe physical or mental disability is better or worse than no life at all. We might set up criteria and tests for people with disabilities, to determine their competence and capacity for independent living, but these tests may palpably fail to take account of the patient's own view of things – even where obtaining this is possible. A survey of adults with learning disabilities in Scotland found, contrary to prevailing opinion among medical policy-makers and managers of large institutions for people who have learning disabilities, that over 75% of those in long-stay care wished to and would be capable of living in the community with minimal support (Baker & Urquhart 1987). There are considerable risks in depending on one group of professionals to define what 'quality of life' means for other people. Where the political will to provide adequate community care is lacking, there is the additional risk that medical opinion will be used to rationalise the detention of people who have learning disabilities in special asylums for life.

The infant with Down's syndrome certainly had a right to treatment, but it does not follow that everything possible has to be tried, including the most expensive, untried or dangerous treatments. Treatment, in this case, may mean direct interventions that aim to cure, or it may mean simply the provision of good nursing care and control of symptoms. Deciding which is appropriate in such a case is bound to be difficult and morally ambiguous. It may be tempting to simply 'treat' the parents' distress or the ward team's anxiety by removing the object that is the cause, but that would not represent the kind of moral initiative the situation demands – the courage to act in spite of the practical uncertainty and moral ambiguity and to live with the consequences.

The distinction drawn by moral theologians between 'ordinary' and 'extraordinary' means is often invoked to deal with such situations. The healthcare team are obliged to give a child in such a case the 'ordinary' means of assistance but not obliged to employ 'extraordinary' means in an attempt to save the child's life. However, it is doubtful that this distinction solves the moral dilemma in such cases. There is a need, though, for decisions to be based on common sense, and due regard for the circumstances and needs of the patient, and of all other stakeholders. 'Leaving nature to take its course' seldom means doing nothing more for the affected infant; it would normally mean continuing to give fluids (and possibly food or drugs to suppress hunger) and keeping the infant comfortable and pain free. It could also mean not intervening actively, e.g. by not giving antibiotics, performing an operation with a poor record of success, or resuscitating an infant who suffers cardiac arrest (Glover 1977).

In the case we are considering, the houseman acted decisively to resuscitate the child, but she died anyway. His action was a perfectly understandable one. It was one possible response to a distressing situation, one possible attempt to resolve the painful dilemma. It was an action which had its own possible medical and moral justification. The child did after all survive for several weeks, and this may have been of some help to the parents in coming to terms with their bereavement. However, it might have been no less morally courageous, and possibly more difficult in the face of the pressure to 'do something!', to have left the child to die. Such situations are called dilemmas precisely because there is no way one can know with certainty, or unambiguously, what is the right thing to do in the circumstances (Stinson & Stinson 1981).

Not taking any action to resuscitate a patient who has suffered cardiac arrest, or choked, is sometimes referred to as 'passive euthanasia', in contrast to 'active euthanasia' when someone takes direct action to end the life of a patient. Some philosophers argue that there is an important moral distinction between active killing and letting someone die, in terms of the different intentions of the agent, and that while active euthanasia is not morally acceptable, in some circumstances passive euthanasia may be. Others argue that if the doctor or nurse knows that the patient

will die as a result of discontinuing life support, this amounts to the same thing as killing the patient. The consequences are identical, the patient dies: the intentions 'to kill' or 'to deprive of life support' are virtually indistinguishable. There are complex and important arguments on both sides, but medical and nursing staff faced with decisions to stop treatment or not to intervene, tend to maintain that there is a valid common-sense distinction between actively killing a patient (with or without a patient's consent), and taking no action to save the patient's life when he is dying.

These so-called common-sense distinctions between 'active' and 'passive' euthanasia, and 'ordinary' and 'extraordinary' means, are put under strain when we consider what has been made possible by the development of modern drugs, new anaesthetics and life-support machines. To some extent, the boundaries between 'ordinary' and 'extraordinary' means are changing all the time with the development of more sophisticated techniques and knowledge (as, for example, the definition of 'viability' has had to be changed from 28 weeks for neonates as it has proved possible to keep younger babies alive). These changes do not make decisions in these cases any easier. However, the presence or absence of sophisticated resuscitative equipment can make all the difference to how a case is viewed. Is actively switching off a life-support system to a brain-dead patient being kept 'alive' for transplant purposes, active or passive euthanasia? Or neither? With more precise medical and legal criteria for defining death this particular dilemma may be removed, but, with live and conscious patients who are dying, the problems remain (Harris 1981).

Struggles over sedation

Case Study 7.5 illustrates some of the struggles that may arise over sedation.

In the conflict between the nurses and the doctors over the level of pain control to be given to Margaret, we encounter a common problem in doctor–nurse relationships in terminal care. The problem relates to the different functions of the nurse and the doctor, and their perceived roles in relation to the severely ill patient – the nurse being more concerned with the comfort and well-being of the patient, the doctor with sorting out the medical problems. However, conflicts also tend to arise in the pre-terminal stage when it is as yet unclear whether a patient is dying or their life could be saved. While there is hope, curative measures are appropriate, even to the point of denying pain relief if this may jeopardise the possibility of a cure. Once the situation is recognised to be hopeless in

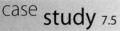

case study 7.5

Pain control in a severely ill patient

In my second year of nursing, during my second spell of night duty as a registered nurse, Margaret was admitted to our ward. She was 23 years old and recently married. She was suffering from oesophageal varices, and the consultant surgeon had used a new technique of portacaval shunt in an attempt to treat her condition.

Margaret's condition deteriorated after the operation and she was in considerable pain. The surgeon insisted she be kept completely drug-free to rest her liver, and the resident doctor consequently refused to sign her up for any painkilling drugs, and instructed me to give a placebo only (whether intravenous or intramuscular). Margaret was in considerable pain and had more and more distressing nights. She was a most charming person and the nurses were very fond of her. This made it very difficult for us, feeling we could not help.

In the mornings the ward sister would come on duty, often very early, and would demand to know whether Margaret had been sedated. When I told her that I had not been allowed to give her any sedation she would become very angry with me and would (to my relief) instruct me to give her sedation. Each day the same battle would go on between the consultant, resident doctor, ward sister and myself – with the nurses concerned to make Margaret as comfortable as possible, and the consultant concerned that his operation should be a success.

The battle continued until very close to her death, when the consultant surgeon finally conceded that she should be given adequate sedation.

---

therapeutic terms, then appropriate palliative care should be given. Deciding when it is appropriate to switch from therapeutic to palliative measures may be difficult and fraught with uncertainty for the doctor, faced with possible charges of negligence if he misses something.

While hospital and medical practice may have changed in some cases, with more ready recognition of the need for palliative care, this historical case still raises the same substantive issues about who decides on the levels of pain-control that are appropriate and under what conditions. The British Medical Association has recently reported that following investigation into the case of Dr Shipman, who was responsible for the premature death of over 200 of his patients, doctors have become reluctant to prescribe major

opiate drugs for fear of being accused of hastening the death of their patients, for whatever reason.

The anxiety of the medical staff not to be found wanting has tended to drive them to do all that is possible, while the anxiety of the nursing staff at having to cope with the distress of the patient (and relatives) may drive them to demand that they should provide palliative care instead. The doctor's experience that patients (especially young patients) may sometimes be 'snatched from the jaws of death' has to be balanced by the insight of experienced nurses that patients have 'turned the corner never to return'. Decisions about the type of management that is appropriate may have to be taken under pressure from rebellious nurses, or by doctors asserting their medical authority. However, decisions do have to be taken by someone, and usually that is a doctor, because of their ultimate legal responsibility.

A common dilemma in such circumstances relates to the use of powerful pain-controlling drugs such as diamorphine, which nevertheless can have dangerous side-effects – such as the suppression of respiration – which may hasten a patient's death or make them more susceptible to infections which may kill them. Some nurses object to giving diamorphine to dying patients even if they are in great pain, because they regard this as a form of euthanasia. Even more nurses are afraid of being the one who administers the last injection and thus appearing to be responsible for the death of the patient. Clearly, a nurse has a moral right to refuse to do something that violates their conscience, but they may not have a legal right to refuse to carry out a doctor's orders.

The *principle of double effect* has sometimes been invoked to help provide common-sense guidance for action in such circumstances. When nurses are confronted with situations demanding action which they can foresee will have two effects, one good (such as relieving a patient's pain) and the other bad (putting the patient at risk of earlier death), they

---

> **Box 7.3 Criteria for applying the principle of double effect**
>
> - The action must itself be a good action, or at least morally neutral.
> - The performance of the action must bring about at least as much good as evil.
> - The evil effect must not be a means to achieving the good effect.
> - The agent must have a justifying and sufficient reason for acting rather than refraining from acting.

would be justified in performing the action subject to the conditions listed in Box 7.3 (O'Keeffe 1984).

Treatment without consent

It may be doubted whether these conditions entirely solve the dilemma, but they may help some people to cope with the painful responsibility involved. Better knowledge of pain control, and experience gained in terminal care units, has shown that proper use of diamorphine and other drugs not only greatly improves the quality of life of dying patients, but can actually give them the determination to live longer. Consider Case Study 7.6, dealing with treatment without consent.

case study 7.6

A child whose parents refuse treatment

A child victim of a road traffic accident, with severe injuries and loss of blood, was brought in by ambulance to the accident and emergency department. The child's parents were Jehovah's Witnesses, and insisted that the child should not be given blood transfusions. The parents were asked to wait while X-rays were taken and other tests made. While these were being done it became apparent that the child would not survive without immediate blood transfusions. The child was given the necessary transfusion. The parents were not informed. The child survived.

This case, of Jehovah's Witness parents refusing blood transfusions for their child, raises in an acute form the questions of whether parents have the right to decide for their children in such vital matters as those affecting their right to life and whether parents' authority can override the ordinary human rights of the child. Leaving aside the merits of the theological and scientific arguments adduced by Jehovah's Witnesses to justify their position, the case is discussed here in order to illustrate some of the issues of parental 'rights' versus the 'rights' of the child.

(Another type of case, to illustrate the problems for professional staff, would be where serious physical or sexual abuse of a child is suspected. Decisions in these cases have been made much more difficult recently by the UK courts overturning the convictions of parents, convicted of infanticide, who successfully appealed the judgements made in a number of highly publicised trials of 'shaken baby syndrome' or 'cot death'. It was considered that the convictions had been rendered unsafe because the testimony of a key medical witness had been discredited. Without going into the merits of the arguments in these particular cases, it must be recognised that they have raised in an acute form the dilemmas facing medical or nursing staff when they suspect non-accidental injury to be the cause of a child's death.)

So far as the law is concerned, a child does have the same right to life as an adult, and in most societies the courts can overrule the authority of parents – where the life or even the mental health of the child is believed to be at risk. In this sense the courts exercise a protective duty of care towards minors and people who are incompetent by virtue of mental illness or mental disability. Those concerned about the well-being of a child can appeal to the court to intervene. However, they would have a duty to prepare an appropriate case for making such an appeal, and the parents would have the right to be heard in their defence.

In the case of the Jehovah's Witness parents, the medical and nursing staff acted as a law unto themselves, whether for the best of intentions or not. In seeking to protect the rights of the child, they could be said to have failed to show due regard for the moral and legal rights of the parents. They colluded in deceiving the parents so as to ensure that the child was given the necessary life-saving blood transfusions. They might have applied to a judge and had the child made a ward of court, and this might have been a more proper procedure, not least to protect themselves from litigation. (Although proxy consent to treatment by parents is often accepted on behalf of a child, the law is not clear on whether proxy consent, as exercised here by hospital staff, is legally adequate, let alone morally acceptable, if staff intervene without a court order (McCormick 1976, Ramsey 1976, 1977).)

However, even if the ward team had obtained the proper legal authority, the action of the doctor and nurses in this case leaves much to be desired. They made assumptions about Jehovah's Witnesses which might in this case have been unfounded, and they failed to address the issue of what the parents might do if they discovered what had been done, without their knowledge or consent. A more sensible course would have been to attempt to persuade and negotiate with the parents about the available options, and, failing all attempts to persuade them, only then would recourse to the courts have been justified.

Where parents and professionals do not share the same beliefs or value system, the interpretation of rights and responsibilities can become a matter of great difficulty. Common examples in work with people of different ethnic and cultural background may arise in relation to dietary or dress taboos or particular sensitivity about issues of privacy or related to sexual health or reproduction. The value of institutions such as the courts is that they remove the problem from the domain of private professional responsibility, and enable discussion to take place in a public arena, where the parties involved in the disagreement both have the right to legal representation and the responsibility to present arguments and evidence to enable the court to make a reasonable decision in the public interest. However, in a life-and-death crisis, the urgency to act may lead the team (as possibly was the case here) to act on their own judgement, but this would be unwise unless they had sought approval from higher medical authority.

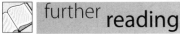

further reading

Exploring the nature of 'rights' and 'duties'

Dworkin R 1977 Taking rights seriously. Harvard University Press, Cambridge, MA

Macintyre A 1988 Whose justice? Whose rationality? Notre Dame University Press, Notre Dame, IN

The rights and duties of nurses

Johnstone M-J 1994 Bioethics: a nursing perspective. WB Saunders/Baillière Tindall, London

Staunton P, Whyburn B 1997 Nursing and the law, 4th edn. Harcourt Brace, New York & Sydney

Patients' rights (and duties)

Beauchamp T L, Childress J F 2004 Principles of biomedical ethics, 5th rev edn. Oxford University Press, Oxford

Charlesworth M 1993 Bioethics in a liberal society. Cambridge University Press, Cambridge

Scope of 'treatment', 'control' and 'care'

Keatings M, Smith O B 2000 Ethical and legal issues in Canadian nursing. W B Saunders (an Elsevier imprint), Toronto

Kerridge I, Lowe M, McPhee J 1998 Ethics and law for the health professions. Social Science Press, Australia

Conflicting demands in nursing groups of patients

8

Chapter contents

AIMS

This chapter has the following aims:

1. To explore the positive meaning of 'moral autonomy' and to distinguish this from the 'absence of external constraint' or mere personal freedom 'to do your own thing'

2. To explore the meaning of the 'common good' and the role this concept plays in our thinking about social justice and the responsibilities of the state for health and welfare

3. To apply these concepts to the analysis of a range of moral choices we face in deciding on the scope and limits of our responsibility for patients, and to intervene in their lives, viz. preventing suicide, behaviour modification, health screening and prevention and 'counselling'

4. To explore the ethics of those situations where nurses have to exercise authority to refuse admission or 'persuade' patients to cooperate, or make difficult decisions about the allocation of scarce resources, in the interests of others.

LEARNING OUTCOMES

When you have read and worked through this chapter, you should be able to:

■ Distinguish theoretically and in practice between the right to freedom of action and one's responsibility as an autonomous moral agent to demonstrate commitment to a clear set of values

■ Demonstrate understanding of the nature of our commitments within any moral community, to promote the health and well-being of others and to protect their interests for the common good

■ Demonstrate insight into the nature of issues of social justice in healthcare, by ability to give examples at ward or community, state and international level, and explain the issues

■ Demonstrate ability to analyse and to critically evaluate the competing 'rights' of various 'stakeholders' in given situations, with a view to reaching fair appraisals of their relative priority in making decisions

■ Demonstrate sensitivity and understanding of the conflicts between the responsible exercise of power and authority and patients' rights.

The previous chapter discussed two classes of moral difficulties in direct nurse–patient encounters; these centred on moral problems related to truth-telling and confidentiality, on the one hand, and the problematic area of deciding between therapeutic and palliative treatment, on the other. While cases of these types could be discussed without particular reference to the rights of other patients and relatives, the moral difficulties examined in this chapter cannot be discussed without taking into account the rights of other people, public health or the good of society. The moral problems we propose to examine relate to setting limits to the 'management' of patients, i.e. the control and direction of their lives, and, balancing the rights of individual patients with those of other patients or third parties.

It may be useful in this connection to remind ourselves of the four different, but related, senses of responsibility that we discussed in Chapter 4 (Box 8.1).

Box 8.1 **Responsibility and accountability**	
Responsibility *for* one's own actions:	(personal responsibility)
Responsibility *for* the care of someone:	(fiduciary responsibility)
Responsibility *to* higher authority:	(professional accountability)
Responsibility *to* wider society:	(public accountability/ civic duty)

When nurses are compelled to weigh their responsibility for individual patients against their responsibilities for groups of patients, conflicts may arise between these different types of responsibility, which nurses exercise both as individuals and as professionals. The authority vested in nurses, to serve the best interests of their patients, may contrast with the actual or relative lack of power they have – depending on their position in the nursing hierarchy or their relationships with other professional staff. What nurses are entitled to do by law, and what they are or are not allowed to do by their union or professional associations, may also have a bearing on the matter. Some of these complex issues of responsibility and authority are examined in this chapter.

PERSONAL AUTONOMY VERSUS THE COMMON GOOD

Championing of individual autonomy and 'the individual's right to choose' has become a hallmark of much contemporary ethical debate. This is evident in changing models of family life where there has been a championing of children's rights and reaction against traditional models of parental authority and over-protective care. It is evident in scepticism towards forms of religious ethics based on appeal to divine authority rather than reason (e.g. to justify policies on contraception, abortion or euthanasia); and in feminist critiques of male-dominated 'patriarchal' society and its moral norms. In both the public and private sectors of the economy and service provision, there has been a shift of emphasis from the authority and duties of the service provider to the rights of the 'customer' and issues of 'client choice'. The adoption in healthcare of models of management and client relations taken from business and professional life has also given impetus to a change in our discourse from talk about 'patients' to talk about 'consumers', 'customers' and 'clients', and a renewed emphasis in ethics on the issue of 'client autonomy' and the 'client's right to choose' (Murley 1995). Here, as elsewhere, we should take note of what Wittgenstein (1958) called the phenomenon of 'language shift', for shifts in terminology often signal changes of paradigms and theoretical perspectives, and embody important value changes as well.

Traditional models of care in the health and human services (including medicine, nursing, ministry, school teaching and social work) tend to have given priority to the principle of beneficence – to the professional's duty of responsible care for the person being cared for. The very term 'patient' suggests that the person is the *passive* recipient of *active* care or treatment given by another person (the agent). From the Latin *patior*, meaning 'to suffer', the term 'patient' also suggests that the person being cared for is in a dependent state due to their pain or suffering. Within this model there is little scope for talk of the 'patient's right to choose', for the 'patient' is regarded as relatively helpless and the doctor or nurse is presumed to know what is good for them.

A focus on the autonomy of the moral agent developed relatively late in the history of philosophy, during the so-called Enlightenment of the 18th century, and the emphasis on patient's rights developed even more recently, in the latter part of the 20th century. The classical philosophers, from Plato and Aristotle to the medieval scholastics, treat autonomy not as given or innate, but as a capacity that has to be developed and which grows with wisdom, experience and maturity. In radical contrast to many modern thinkers who regard personal freedom or 'the right to autonomy' as something given with human nature itself, one could say that for traditional Graeco-Roman and Judaeo-Christian thought, autonomy is something we have to earn by proving ourselves to be responsible and capable moral beings.

Virtue ethics, as we shall see, emphasises that by cultivating the intellectual and moral virtues, knowledge and sound habits or competence in practice, we gain greater control over ourselves, and thus acquire both greater freedom and a capacity to act more responsibly. We are not born free, but become progressively freer as we develop the capacities required to control and direct our own lives. A baby is almost totally dependent and subject to the determining forces of its heredity and environment. Even to learn to walk a child has to be assisted onto its feet by other people before the child becomes capable of walking on its own, and able to determine which direction to take on life's journey. For the classical philosophers (Aristotle in particular) to say that 'man is a rational being' does not mean that we are born with fully developed rational capacities, but on the contrary 'rationality' (and 'autonomy') are capacities that require to be developed through habit and practice. In other words, they do not have a determinate meaning, but are *developmental concepts* which would apply to people to different degrees at different times, depending on their knowledge, experience and maturity (cf. Hill 1991, Mele 1995).

The term 'autonomy' came into prominence in modern philosophy with Kant (1724–1804), who stressed that in order to be held a fully rational, responsible moral agent, one must have freedom to act, to be an autonomous person. 'Autonomy' (from *autos* = 'self' and *nomos* = 'law') means to be a self-legislating moral agent, to be a 'law unto oneself' in the sense that one must demonstrate personal commitment to the moral law, and not just mechanically obey imposed or external authority. A 'heteronomous' law is one imposed on me by someone else. It may be my parents, the Church, or the state, or any other moral authority. Autonomy is the state of moral maturity where one is able to personally acknowledge the validity of the moral law, chooses oneself to live by it and commits oneself to uphold it – not because one is told to do so, but because one chooses to do so of one's own free will. 'Autonomy', for Kant, stands in opposition to 'heteronomy' as a mature attitude to the demands of morality, where the latter means unthinking and uncritical obedience. Autonomy is an achievement of fully adult and developed understanding of one's responsibilities as a moral agent. In this sense, we cannot treat a person as a fully responsible moral agent unless he fulfils the requirements for being an autonomous agent. One must both act freely and without compulsion, and also with insight into and personal commitment to the requirements of the moral law (Paton 1969).

The current tendency in North American bioethics to treat 'autonomy' as an inherent *right* of human beings, or even as a fundamental ethical *principle*, as do Beauchamp & Childress (1994, Ch. 3), when they include 'respect for personal autonomy' along with non-maleficence, beneficence and justice as fundamental ethical principles, presents us with some philosophical difficulties. This classification seems to involve a category mistake – for autonomy is surely not a principle but a *precondition* for one to be able to affirm principles as your own, or the liberty to claim one's rights or the freedom to act as a fully responsible person. Alternatively, it is *the capacity to apply moral principles* with insight and discrimination, not a moral principle as such. Respect for the rights of others would seem to include *respect for their need to act freely* and to make their own moral choices, making autonomy the ground for the principle, rather than a principle itself. If we follow Kant in saying that we should always treat persons as 'ends in themselves' and never simply as 'means to an end', this means that 'respect for persons and their rights' really means 'treating other persons *as if* they were fully autonomous moral agents', even if they are not.

Our Western concept of the 'self' has come under critical scrutiny over the past century, from Eastern philosophies such as Buddhism, which regards the self at best as a provisional construct, and in the end as 'unreal'. It has also been subject to 'deconstruction' in recent postmodernism, where the presumed ontological foundations of selfhood, i.e. its foundations in reality, have been subject to radical criticism. While some may be puzzled why this is of such concern to philosophers, in particular feminist philosophers, the debate raises fundamental questions about our nature as moral agents. Is our nature something determined, fixed or given, which we cannot change, or is our nature something we can shape by our choices and projects? (See Berlin 1969 and also Taylor 1992, who provides a most helpful survey of trends in the discussion of selfhood and autonomy.)

Jean-Paul Sartre (1956, 1973), the French atheist philosopher and existentialist, maintained that if the Creator does not exist, to give us a predetermined nature and purpose for living, then we are totally responsible for ourselves, and 'must make ourselves by our decisions'. (Jean-Paul Sartre gives popular expression to this idea in his play *No Exit*, and in his essay *Existentialism and Humanism*, but his detailed analysis of the phenomenology of the self and selfhood is to be found in his *Being and Nothingness*.) Feminist writers, including Sartre's companion Simone de Beauvoir, have argued that *essentialist* philosophers and theologians who have argued that human nature is given and predetermined all too easily use essentialist arguments to justify sex-role stereotyping and male dominance as 'natural'. In criticising patriarchal structures in society (and perhaps particularly in the world of medicine and healthcare), feminist philosophers like de Beauvoir (1988) and others have been concerned not only to address questions of sex discrimination against women but also to encourage women to see that by the exercise of their own autonomy they can mould and change their identity, both as individuals and as an oppressed group in society (de Beauvoir 1988, Bowden 1997).

In defence of the traditional view of human nature or species being, as something given, it can be argued that I cannot choose to become something other than what I am (e.g. a shark or a baboon). While we might say the behaviour of some lawyers, or money lenders, justifies us in calling them 'sharks' or 'loan-sharks', and otherwise civilised individuals can behave like baboons under the influence of alcohol, we can never actually change our species being however much we may seek to transcend its limitations or may abuse ourselves. This does not mean, however, that we cannot to take control of and direct our lives, shaping our destiny as best we can. In fact as we acquire and internalise the intellectual and moral virtues, so we acquire greater responsibility and capability as moral agents to do so. Existentialism and postmodernism tend to caricature the traditional 'essentialist' view, because Aristotle, for example, does not presuppose a static and unchanging human essence, but speaks of our nature in terms of potentiality and its develop-mental possibilities (which may be unending). Of course, we can get stuck with fixed stereotypes, and these have done great damage in the past. The real challenge is whether or not we actually develop our full potentialities, including our autonomy, through participation with others in a moral community, for we certainly cannot do it on our own.

'Personal autonomy' always stands in tension with the 'common good', for we do not spring ready-made out of nothing, either biologically or psychologically. We are the products of the sexual activity and love (or lack of love) of our parents, and of generations before them. We are moulded and nurtured by our families, communities, schools, religious and political institu-tions. Our maturation as individuals, with an identity of our own, is a product of the interaction of our growing capacities for self-determination with these forces of social determinism. In seeking to express ourselves and to realise our autonomy, we do not do this in isolation, but in action and reaction within our given and the chosen moral communities in which we live and work. For this reason my good can never be intelligibly discussed apart from yours or the common good of society, who are responsible for me and to whom I am responsible. The cult of 'personal autonomy' fails to do justice to this other side of the equation.

When we speak of healthcare, we are concerned with services provided by society, at least in principle, for all its members. While most healthcare systems do in fact discriminate positively in favour of the rich and powerful, and negatively against the weak, poor, elderly and mentally incapacitated (and perhaps against ethnic minorities in some societies), neverthe-less the public resources which are spent on healthcare (and other public services) are meant to contribute to the common good. As it was said in the 18th century, 'the common wealth of the Commonwealth is for the common weal' (where 'weal' meant welfare, suffering or need).

Our modern state-funded or state-subsidised healthcare systems, and in particular modern welfare states, are designed to achieve a greater degree of equity for all, both in access to health services, and also in the distribution of health resources. The source of inspiration for these models can perhaps be traced back to the development of the concepts of 'common-wealth' and 'commonweal' in the Enlightenment, but they also present us with the practical political and ethical challenge of how we develop systems of healthcare delivery that will serve the urgent needs of individuals with critical health needs and also ensure some measure of distributive justice for all in society.

We have pointed out before that there is always a tension in any society between the competing demands of the principles of beneficence, justice and respect for persons, for while the protective duty of care and respect for persons tends to focus on individuals, justice concerns how we share power and social benefits fairly and equitably in society, for the common good. In many respects popular 'medical ethics' and 'nursing ethics' tend to have given undue attention to the 'dilemmas' which arise between the competing duties of beneficence and respect for persons: on the one hand, to promote the well-being of individuals and protect them from harm; and on the other to respect the rights of individuals. This 'bed-face' clinical mentality finds it uncomfortable to address the further demands of social justice – when it becomes a matter of choosing between more or less 'deserving' patients, managing limited staff and resources, undertaking randomised control trials, or dealing with the demands of public health, public screening and health education of the masses.

In discussing the 'common good' it is important to draw attention to two related but different notions of distributive justice, apart from the more commonly understood retributive sense of the word 'justice'. To the extent that 'justice' is understood in its connection with the civil or criminal courts, or the criminal justice system, we tend to think of justice in primarily negative and punitive terms, as exacting retribution, compensation or punishment from those who have infringed our civil or personal rights. However, the courts have traditionally been seen as institutions of last resort in which people seek to achieve fairness in terms of distributive justice (e.g. over breach of contract), when ordinary common-sense interpersonal negotiations fail. Nevertheless our main concern here is with distributive justice in the sense of power-sharing in society, with fair and equitable distribution of benefits and burdens, resources and responsibilities. The two types of distributive justice that need to be distinguished here are:

- fairness in the sense of *equality of opportunity* for individuals
- fairness in terms of equity, *or equality of outcome*, for groups of people (Woozley 1981).

In cultures which emphasise 'the right to personal autonomy' (usually prosperous conservative societies), there is a tendency to focus on the right to equality of opportunity for individuals, and to ignore the question whether or not the circumstances in which individuals find themselves make it actually possible to claim their rights. The fact is that one requires a certain level of education, financial self-sufficiency and social leverage to be able to claim and exercise the 'right to equality of opportunity'. Poverty, lack of parents, social and racial discrimination may so disempower you that you are actually prevented from exercising these rights. Shifting the emphasis from 'justice' to 'equity' involves a shift of emphasis to the means to achieve 'equality of outcome for groups'. The impetus to set up 'welfare states', e.g. the UK National Health Service, systems of universal and compulsory health insurance, and state provision of healthcare in socialist states, are all driven by concern about social inequalities in health and access to healthcare. Each represents an attempt to ensure greater equity in the sharing of healthcare services and resources across the whole of society, so as to achieve equal outcomes or benefits for all groups in society.

Similarly, 'affirmative action' or 'positive discrimination' have been adopted as strategies which attempt to compensate for the inherited circumstances of social disadvantage in which people find themselves and over which they have no control. These strategies have been applied in education and training, and employment policies and legislation in particular. For example, where a large proportion of hospital nurses are black, but few have gained promotion to positions of seniority within the nursing hierarchy, adopting a policy of 'affirmative action' would mean giving preference to a black nurse over a white nurse, with equivalent qualifications and experience, in making appointments until the balance is more equitable. Alternatively, positive discrimination might involve giving preference to a woman rather than a man in making senior appointments to nurse management, in an institution where men predominate, even if the man might appear better qualified.

In the heady 1960s these strategies enjoyed popular political support in many countries, but in the 1990s there was a backlash against these measures (particularly in the USA) because it was argued that they are not in fact fair (to the individual involved). The argument is that affirmative action discriminates against the best candidate in favour of achieving some ideal ethnic or gender balance in organisations, and it is questioned whether there is such a balance and whether this achieves the desired benefits intended. While there is considerable evidence that policies of reverse discrimination have achieved the social goal of greater equity (in access to education, health and social services) in many countries, the arguments based on 'merit first' and 'equality of opportunity for the individual' enjoyed some degree of popularity in the 1990s, possibly connected with economic recession and unemployment affecting the middle classes and economically privileged.

David Thomson, in his incisive paper 'Welfare states and the problem of the common' (1992) and his more controversial book *Selfish Generations? The Ageing of New Zealand's Welfare State* (1991), pointed out that the generation which had grown up with the rights and benefits of the welfare state have become more concerned about protecting their own entitlements than extending the benefits of the welfare state to the younger generation. While the post-war older generation were willing to make sacrifices to ensure that the younger generation had access to education, healthcare and welfare (particularly protection against unemployment), he argues that the beneficiaries of this generosity have not been prepared to show the same altruism to the new generation, that the welfare states have become welfare states for the elderly, at the expense of the young. While his general thesis is hotly contested, he amassed sufficient historical evidence to give us pause for thought (cf. Mishra 1990).

However, in Britain since the return of a Labour government in 1997, there has been renewed emphasis on the rights of minorities, of women and dependency groups, and a renewed attempt to address inequalities in health (Baggott 2004, Chs 1 and 8). Health practitioners, in facing up to their ethical responsibilities in dealing with groups of patients rather than simply with individuals, and the responsibilities of management and administration, public health and research, need to grapple with the tensions between autonomy and the common good, between respect for the rights of individuals and the demands of social justice and equity.

Lars Reuter (1999) argues, in a paper to the Council of Europe symposium on protection of the human rights and dignity of the terminally ill, that the public attention given to the ethical debates about the ethics of abortion and euthanasia is related to the current preoccupation with 'the right to personal autonomy'. He further points to some of the inherent contradictions in the kind of arguments advanced, from a postmodernist point of view, in favour of 'the woman's right to choose' or the 'patient's right to die'. His argument is that if the self is a construct, in Sartre's sense, then it is difficult to argue from the necessary relativity of different chosen forms and expressions of selfhood, to any kind of universal right to abortion or voluntary euthanasia. If we adopt the traditional view that all human beings, as members of the wider moral community, share a common species being, then our claims to universal human rights can make sense on the basis that they also serve the common good. In other words 'rights' cannot be decided on the basis of subjective choices, but need to be acknowledged by others, and our rights are circumscribed by the rights of others as well as the duties we owe to them and to ourselves.

Thus, the woman claiming to exercise her 'right to choose' to terminate a pregnancy is denying any actual or potential right to autonomy to the child or to the father of the child. This begins to sound like Humpty Dumpty speaking to Alice: 'When I use a word [like 'autonomy'] it means just what I choose it to mean, neither more nor less'(Carroll 1954). Similarly, to insist that one has an unconditional 'right' to be helped to terminate one's life ignores the question whether one is entitled to impose duties on others that they would find morally unacceptable. So, we may ask whether it really helps to talk about 'rights' in these contexts, for what are one's corresponding obligations to the moral community?

Setting limits to the control and direction of patients

The 'management' of patients is a complex art, ranging from subtle persuasion to the use of force to subdue violent patients. What gives the nurse the authority to control other people in this way?

In psychiatric wards, in accident and emergency departments and in working with people with intellectual impairment, nurses often encounter violent patients who have to be restrained by physical means, or by the use of drugs or by calling the police and invoking the law. In such cases it may appear that the nursing staff are justified in using 'reasonable force' to control patients simply in order to defend themselves, other patients and staff. However, they may also be said to be acting to protect the patient from injury, self-mutilation or suicide, or, less dramatically, 'acting in the patient's own best interests' (COHSE 1977, UNISON 1997).

The fact is that a nurse is not only responsible for individual patients and their needs, nor can a nurse be simply concerned with the rights of one individual. The nurse also has to protect the interests of other patients, and, as a public officer who is accountable to society at large, has to consider the public good. The rights of individual patients may have to be restricted where the rights and safety of other people are put at risk. In addition, the nurse has a responsibility to protect the interests of a patient who is incapable of understanding what their own best interests are; for example, if a patient is mentally ill, under the influence of drugs, intoxicated or has severe learning difficulties. The nurse has to decide what is in the best interests of the patient and of good patient care. Depending on whether the patient is competent and the circumstances in which the patient comes into care, or is referred to the nurse for appropriate care, nurses may have to interpret their responsibilities differently. (See Chapter 4 for a discussion of models of care based on code, contract, covenant and charter.) In general, nurses exercise fiduciary responsibility for patients entrusted into their care, and they must be guided in their decisions by training and experience, professional code and personal conscience, acting always in such a way as to 'safeguard and promote the wellbeing and interests of patients/clients' (NMC 2004).

Concern with the 'best interests of the patient' means that nurses have to exercise both clinical and moral responsibilities towards their patients. These responsibilities are determined not only by consideration of the patients' rights and respect for their freedom, but also by consideration of the wider health needs of the individual and the community. 'Management' of patients (including those who cooperate fully in treatment) can involve various degrees of control, ranging from physical restraint or legal measures, to behavioural modification through health education or just directive managerial communication. Skill in nursing means, in part at least, learning to control people appropriately and with respect to their needs.

Preventing suicide, and the 'right' to die

Consider the problem encountered by a psychiatric nurse faced with the possible discharge of a patient thought by the doctor to be a suicide risk (Case Study 8.1). Her concern was whether she had a moral or legal duty to prevent the patient from committing suicide.

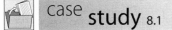

case study 8.1

'Half in love with easeful death?'

On our ward we had a 70-year-old woman who was described as an alcoholic and who had taken several overdoses over a period of two years. The staff feared that if she were to be discharged she would return home to her alcoholic husband and sooner or later would be found dead. However, when she was sober she appeared completely rational and demanded to be allowed home. Her compulsory detention in hospital on the grounds that she might commit suicide seemed to me a flagrant violation of her right to freedom when there did not appear to be adequate evidence that she was mentally ill.

In the above case the moral quandary for the nurse arises because of uncertainty in the given situation about the elderly woman's mental state. Was the woman capable of making rational decisions about her life? The action of the hospital in protecting her might appear overly protective and restrictive of her liberty, but it could be said to be a natural extension of her right to treatment and the contract of the staff to care for and protect her (as well as to offer her such therapy as might be appropriate). Here the nurse has to exercise fiduciary responsibility on behalf of the patient and, paradoxically, that might involve restricting her movements, 'in her own best interests'. This action might even be construed as a demand of protective beneficence, or as required to defend the patient's rights – where the patient appears unable to take responsible decisions for herself. Of course, this argument presupposes that suicide is never in the best interests of the patient. The moving play *Whose Life Is It Anyway?*, about a young quadriplegic who is being kept alive against his will, by artificial means, challenges this assumption – at least as far as the young man is exercising his right to refuse further treatment and wants to be left to die (Clark 1978).

Unlike the questions previously discussed in Chapter 6 relating to voluntary euthanasia and assisted suicide, this case is less concerned with the question of the rights and autonomy of patients than with the scope of the nurse's responsibility to prevent patients from committing suicide, and whether or not the nurse, in this case, should use the legal powers available under the law to detain the elderly woman in hospital against her will, and for her own protection. However, while there are important differences here relating to social attitudes to suicide, which we might wish to discuss, there are some aspects of our discussion of Case Study 6.2 that are relevant. First, there is evidence that the majority of people who commit suicide are clinically depressed or are suffering from some form of mental illness. So, there is a factual foundation to the common-sense view that people do not commit suicide unless 'the balance of their mind is disturbed' – as the coroner's court expresses it. Second, there is important research evidence from both the field of gerontology and the study of people with severe disabilities that people who request assistance to commit suicide or euthanasia generally feel isolated and lack adequate family or social support systems. They tend to be very pessimistic about the future and anxious that they will be a burden to their families (Shaw 1994, Sommers & Shields 1987, Lebacqz 1999, Thompson 1993). Because of this evidence and prevailing social attitudes to suicide, there is still an expectation that nurses and other professional carers, in particular, will take action to prevent people committing suicide.

A less generous construction which could be placed on the action of the hospital in this case is that the nurses were acting less to protect the old lady than to protect themselves – against charges of negligence or the guilt which might result if the patient succeeded in killing herself. The fact is that no matter what precautions are taken, some patients do succeed in committing suicide and that does cause great distress to the staff responsible for their care. Nevertheless, defensive action and conservative measures, though somewhat repressive at times, are morally justifiable. Nurses are entitled to protect themselves, and their professional reputations, from allegations of culpable neglect of patients in their care. The courage to take the risk of discharging a potentially suicidal patient may show admirable regard for their autonomy but can always be attacked as irresponsibility. Achieving a balance between both caring for and protecting patients and respecting their freedom, between defensive medicine and attempted rehabilitation, is always difficult. It is a matter of risk often complicated by the threat of legal action.

Throughout history most societies have condemned suicide, unless in extreme circumstances – e.g. to avoid capture by one's enemies, or to avoid being sold into slavery. Many societies have applied extremely severe penalties to those who attempt suicide, and in Europe those who committed 'self-murder' could not be buried in 'Christian' cemeteries or in 'hallowed ground' but were buried at the cross-roads. Although we tend to be more compassionate today towards suicides, and seek to explain or excuse their actions as due to psychiatric causes, nevertheless we still react with involuntary horror at the news that an acquaintance has ended their own life. G.K. Chesterton's comment in Chapter 5 of his book *Orthodoxy*, that 'the suicide refuses to take the oath of loyalty to life', or the belief that the suicide acts in a way that 'contradicts our natural instinct for self-preservation', might partly explain the reason for popular disapproval of suicide (Chesterton 1927). In Roman times, for a man to commit suicide was regarded as a crime against the state, depriving the state of a potential soldier. In a somewhat similar vein, Lenin argued that suicide was a crime because it deprived the state of a worker! While we might not want to endorse such simplistic views, we may recognise that there is more than a grain of truth in these ideas, for we do not exist in isolation; but are involved in and are part of the extended human family. We only have rights as members of a moral community, but responsibilities to one another as well.

There have been attempts to justify acts of suicide, or to even regard them as heroic acts of defiance in the face of overwhelming fate. The Roman Stoics maintained that a person was justified in taking his own life, not only as a soldier in war might do to prevent his being tortured for information, or taken prisoner and sold into slavery, but rather if circumstances were such as to totally overwhelm the person's ability to make rational choices. Stoics were encouraged to cultivate their freedom and power of self-determination by developing an attitude of *apatheia*, i.e. of emotional detachment and indifference to pain, suffering and desire, in order to achieve self-mastery and a life that could be lived in conformity with nature, ruled by purely rational principles. Our modern ideal of personal freedom and moral autonomy might be said to have its roots in this Stoic philosophy. Regarding suicide, the cultivation of an attitude of indifference or *apatheia* to both life and death was supposed to enable the Stoic philosopher to choose with complete freedom between them, as Seneca suggested, 'like a man calmly leaving a smoke-filled room'. Or, as Tillich (1952, Ch. 1, pp. 9–17) emphasises, 'suicide as an escape from life, dictated by

fear, contradicts the Stoic courage to be'. More recently the Lutheran theologian, Bonhoeffer (1955), said:

> Suicide is a specifically human action, and it is not surprising if it has on this account repeatedly been applauded and justified by noble human minds. If this action is performed in freedom it is raised high above any petty moralizing accusation of cowardice and weakness. Suicide is the ultimate and extreme self-justification of man as man, and it is therefore, from a purely human standpoint, in a certain sense even, the self-accomplished expiation for a life that has failed. … Suicide is a man's attempt to give a final human meaning to a life which has become humanly meaningless. The involuntary sense of horror which seizes us when we are faced with the fact of a suicide is not to be attributed to the iniquity of such a deed but to the terrible loneliness and freedom in which this deed is performed, as a deed in which the positive attitude to life is reflected only in the destruction of life.
> (Bonhoeffer 1955, p. 123; cf. Aldridge 1998)

Paradoxically, however, the atheist philosopher Jean-Paul Sartre, who argued that existence is freedom, argues that a person must be deluded to think that to take one's life is a supreme act of freedom in which one can triumph over fate, for it is the ultimate absurdity to use one's freedom to end one's freedom (Sartre 1973).

Thus, our attitudes to suicide are ambivalent, and this is reflected in the fact that there is generally no legal obligation on people as citizens to prevent someone attempting suicide, although they may feel that they are duty-bound to do so if they can, for a variety of moral reasons. However, the law takes a different view of the responsibilities of doctors, nurses and other health professionals who have charge of patients. As long as a person is in a nurse's care, the law requires the nurse to protect the patient from harm including self-inflicted harm. In fact, a nurse can be charged with negligence if one of her patients succeeds in killing himself. The nurse has this legal duty towards patients in her care in spite of the fact that suicide is no longer illegal in Britain. Because the law assumes those who attempt suicide are mentally unbalanced, they are no longer prosecuted for attempting to take their lives but nevertheless health professionals are expected to intervene if they threaten suicide. The fact that the law allows people the licence, or liberty, to attempt suicide without prosecution does not mean that the law or morality recognises that persons have a right to kill themselves. We ordinarily understand by a 'right' (as discussed in Chapter 7) the entitlement to demand that other people either assist us in particular ways or desist from acting towards us in particular ways. In this sense of 'right', the so-called 'right to suicide' is not a right. There is no way we can appeal to the law or to morality to compel others to assist us to end our lives. Whether we can extend the use of the term 'right' to cover personal entitlement to act in a particular way, for example to attempt suicide, will depend on our understanding of the reciprocal obligations we owe one another, as members of the moral community.

Behaviour modification

Another type of control which raises ethical problems is the use of rewards and punishments to reinforce behaviour modification in long-term psychiatric patients. For example, money or cigarettes may be given as rewards to encourage better self-care among institutionalised patients – for washing, shaving, dressing, bed-making, care of living area. Alternatively, sanctions may be applied – by the removal of privileges such as access to television, opportunities for exercise or recreation. Is it ethically justifiable to extend the definition of 'treatment' to include the retraining and rehabilitation of patients by these means?

Healthcare staff, trained to standards of cleanliness, order and tidiness, may find the slovenliness of some patients intolerable. (In the same way that community nurses may find offensive the behaviour of elderly people with Diogenes syndrome, who accumulate rubbish and live in a mess.) It is easy to rationalise the use of retraining measures for such patients on the grounds that it is necessary, for reasons of hygiene, to avoid fire hazards, and to protect other patients' interests. 'Retraining' patients to care for themselves and their environment may also ease the burden on the nursing staff and make the institutional management of such individuals easier and more pleasant for everyone. The use of aversion therapy in the treatment of some phobias and to help people – e.g. to give up smoking, stop abusing drugs, or alcohol – can be justified reasonably easily in practice because the patient generally wants to overcome the phobia or dependence on addictive substances and, as a rule, can be consulted about treatment and can give informed and voluntary consent. Each of these kinds of reason may carry some weight in justifying the use of behaviour modification techniques, but unless balanced by respect for the patient's right to non-cooperation, they can lead to abuse (Matthies et al 1997).

When the patient is competent to give consent, these cases are reasonably straightforward. However, the situation is much more complicated when the patient has a severe learning disability, severe mental health problem or dementia, or is suffering the consequences of long-term institutionalisation. Here there may be serious doubts whether consent can be either informed or voluntary in any true sense. It becomes a matter of interpreting what the 'duty to care' means in these circumstances for the healthcare staff. They have to fall back on other kinds of justification: arguments that such measures are ultimately in the best interests of the patient (in the attempt to restore some degree of autonomy to the patient), or that the retraining is necessary to protect the rights (health and safety) of others, or that the staff cannot be expected to work in intolerable conditions (Ross 1981, Hamberger et al 1997, UNISON 1997). The legal position of healthcare staff in giving treatment to patients who are unable to give or refuse consent has been clarified by the Adults with Incapacity Act 2004 in Scotland, and in the new draft Mental Capacity Bill for England and Wales; the key principles of the bill are stated as:

- *An assumption of capacity:* every adult has the right to make his/her own decisions and must be assumed to have capacity to do so unless it is proved otherwise.
- *Capacity is decision specific:* an assessment of someone's capacity must be based on the actual decision to be taken at the time it needs to be taken – no blanket label of incapacity.
- *Participation in decision-making:* everyone should be encouraged and enabled to make their own decisions, or to participate as fully as possible in decision-making, by being given the help and support they need to make and express a choice.
- Individuals must retain the *right to make what might be seen as eccentric or unwise decisions*.
- *All decisions must be in the person's best interests:* decisions made on behalf of people without capacity should be made in their best interests, giving weight to the decision being what they themselves would have wanted.
- Decisions made on behalf of someone else should be those which are *least restrictive of their basic rights and freedoms*.

The argument that something is in the best interests of the patient is acceptable if, and only if, it is informed by a proper respect for the dignity of individual patients, by a concern to rehabilitate them, improve their quality of life or environment, or at least to improve the general standards of patient care. Respect for the dignity of persons will obviously set limits to the degree of coercion or forms which are employed, and even the use of cigarettes as inducements may be ruled out on the grounds that they may damage the health of patients. There is always a risk that the assumption of fiduciary responsibility may lead to overprotective treatment or even abuse of patients if it is not limited by respect for persons. Older people who have mild dementia are often assumed, by neighbours and anxious caring professionals, to be at risk from house fires – a common argument for their being put into 'sheltered accommodation'. Studies in Edinburgh of the extent of fire hazards with elderly people have shown that the risk is much less than it has been imagined to be and that the use of alternative forms of heating can sometimes circumvent the need for institutionalisation of older people. Research by the Department of Geriatric Medicine at the University of Edinburgh does not support the common view that demented people living at home constitute a serious fire risk to themselves and others. On the contrary, available evidence from the Chief Fire Officer for Lothian and Borders points to most domestic fires being associated with alcohol abuse; and, over a period of 10 years up to 1982, not a single fire in the Region occurred in houses or flats occupied by patients known to the psychiatric services as demented.

It is far too easy for health professionals to rationalise their prejudices against people who adopt different lifestyles or standards of cleanliness, and to impose a regimen on patients for their own convenience rather than the real benefit of patients. If this risk is recognised, then the use of behaviour modification techniques for the rehabilitation of those whose standards of self-care have deteriorated through illness or institutionalisation, may sometimes be justified on the kinds of grounds already discussed. The rights of nursing staff members to decent working conditions are important, but these are not so important as to justify coercion of patients to conform to staff demands, when perhaps collective action by nurses may be required to ensure better staffing levels, modernisation of equipment and the provision of adequate resources.

Health education

Health education itself, in so far as it seeks to change people's attitudes and behaviour, raises ethical questions as well. Are nurses entitled to tell people that they should stop smoking, should not drink so much or that they should go on a diet? Or, more controversially, are nurses morally justified in advising people to practise contraception or to seek sterilisation? If so, how directive should this advice be? Should people just be given the facts and left to decide for themselves? Should nurses actively try to change people's attitudes and lifestyles? Should they

be campaigning for legislation to control advertising of alcohol and tobacco? Should they support campaigns, e.g. for compulsory use of seat-belts, laws against driving under the influence of drugs or alcohol, or compulsory fluoridation of water? Should they be involved directly in community development in areas of high unemployment and social deprivation (Downie et al 1996, Tones 2001)?

One of the main difficulties presented to doctors and nurses by their becoming involved in health education, screening and immunisation is that *proactive* preventive health initiatives involve a change of mind-set for the average health professional. Trained to *react to crises* of various kinds and to deal with the presenting symptoms, they are generally loath to seek out undisclosed pathology. To shift from a *reactive mode* of interaction with patients to a *proactive mode* involves not only a change in attitude and practice, but some subtle changes in ethical orientation as well. Crisis intervention and treatment of the symptoms identified by the patient fits comfortably with a service ethic based on responsible care or protective beneficence. Actively seeking out undeclared morbidity, in screening for breast or cervical cancer in women and prostate cancer in men, for example, requires a different kind of ethical justification. Recruitment of people for screening, or suggesting to patients that they should undergo screening, may cause people a great deal of anxiety. If the tests involve biopsies these can be more painful and inconvenient than is generally indicated, and people can experience considerable fear and anxiety until the results are known. Given the doubts which have been raised about the effectiveness of some forms of screening, (e.g. for prostate cancer or breast screening), it can be seriously questioned whether it is ethically justifiable to put people through all this and the inconvenience involved, unless there are serious grounds for suspicion.

The costs of some methods of screening, relative to their actual benefits for patients, can be seriously questioned on both ethical and medical grounds. The ethical justification for such public health measures is generally a utilitarian one, namely that they contribute to improved health for the majority of the population, even if they cause distress or health complications for some individuals (e.g. untypical reactions to vaccines, or anaesthetics used for biopsies, or painful screening procedures). Here the principles of protective beneficence and justice may be invoked to justify interventions which it is claimed will contribute to the common good, but individual interest and individual rights may be compromised. Trained to care for individuals, nurses may hesitate to get involved.

Health education, if it is to be relevant, must be related to the patterns of morbidity and mortality in society. In the past, the infectious diseases and those associated with poverty were responsible for high infant and maternal mortality and the deaths of young people. These diseases have been largely controlled by general improvements in the standard of living (better housing and diet), public health measures (better sewerage disposal, cleaner water supplies), and by medical measures (immunisation and the development of effective drugs). Today in the developed countries, the pattern of morbidity and mortality is quite different. Infant and maternal mortality rates have been dramatically reduced and most dying is done by older people. There has been a vast increase in the proportion of the population over the age of 50 years, and most illness in this group is lifestyle related. Apart from accidental and violent deaths (a small proportion), the vast majority of deaths and morbidity in the population are associated with smoking, alcohol abuse, inappropriate diet and lack of exercise, and here the contribution of alcohol and drug abuse to accidents, domestic violence and suicide is considerable. While poverty and social deprivation can be aggravating factors contributing to poor health status, the epidemic of chronic and disabling diseases of middle and later life is clearly lifestyle related. If the major causes of premature death are to be eliminated, then people's attitudes, values and lifestyles have to be changed (WHO 1999b, Tones 2001).

The key ethical questions about health education concern the *question of means and methods*: How are people's attitudes, values and lifestyles to be changed? What methods, inducements or sanctions is it ethically permissible to use to achieve the long-term goal of reduced morbidity and mortality in the general population? Is it legitimate to exploit our knowledge of psychology and of people's vulnerability to play on their anxieties, to use subliminal advertising, to actively promote alternative lifestyles along with commercial marketing of 'health products'?

More subtle, but just as important, is the question of the style of 'education' to be used. Is it to be authoritarian and guilt-inducing; take-it-or-leave-it 'scientific' information-giving; focused on developing individual knowledge and life skills for more competent living; or about community development and mobilising the resources in local communities to help themselves (WHO (Ottawa Charter) 1986, Downie et al 1996, WHO 1998)?

Obviously, the major ethical justification for health education is the same as that which was invoked in the 19th century to justify compulsory immunisation, notification of infectious diseases, and compulsory public health measures. This was to appeal to both the principles of beneficence (to protect the health and safety of people) and justice or the common good (to ensure people have equal opportunities of access to healthcare and good health). Such action was felt to be justified even if it meant restricting the rights of some individuals and dissenting minorities. (Compulsory seat-belt legislation and fluoridation raise similar questions.)

The problem facing most governments is that legal and fiscal measures cannot be forced on a community entirely without their consent, even in a totalitarian state. Public opinion has to be informed and persuaded, a consensus created, and that is a task of health education. If health educators are not to give offence they have to respect the rights and autonomy of individuals, and their right to decide on their own values and lifestyle. People cannot be forced to take responsibility for their health. They may be given inducements to do so, or subjected to various forms of sanctions if they do not do so, but not otherwise.

If health education is to be effective, it may be necessary to use a wide variety of health education measures. It will not be sufficient just to give people the facts and leave them to make up their own minds. Other forces come into play, influencing people's health choices, such as peer-group pressure and mass media advertising of products damaging to people's health (such as tobacco, alcohol and junk foods). It will not be sufficient to promote the value of positive health and healthy lifestyles through the education of individuals, when some people's social conditions mean that health has low priority in their scale of survival values, and where housing, food, clothing and employment are more urgently needed. It will not be sufficient to try to influence health behaviour through taxation and legal measures when there are huge vested interests, in terms of company profits, retrenchment of staff and government revenues in relation to the tobacco, alcohol and food industries. Advertising may need to be controlled, funds may have to be allocated for community development and the combating of social deprivation and poverty. State subsidies and tax incentives may need to be given to companies to diversify and phase out the production of things damaging health (Thompson 1987a, Robertson et al 1992, Tones 2001).

If we accept the World Health Organization definition of health, as 'complete physical, mental and social well-being, and not merely the absence of disease or infirmity', then all health professionals have a fundamental responsibility for the prevention of disease, as well as its treatment (for 'prevention is better than cure'). The UK National Health Service, for example, was not intended to be simply a national *disease* service but to improve the nation's health (Seedhouse 2001). So-called 'health professionals' have both a moral and professional duty to be health educators. Nurses, in particular, whether on the ward or in the community, should be committed, as nurses, not only to the treatment of disease but also to active health promotion. Nurses and other health professionals therefore have a special responsibility to act as role models. Doctors or nurses who are heavy smokers or abuse alcohol cannot expect their advice to be taken seriously. Their credibility as health professionals is called into question. The tobacco industry regard them as the best possible advertisers of their products – 'one doctor or nurse who is a smoker is worth a hundred advertisements elsewhere'!

This does not mean that all nurses have to be positive role models, but their example in taking responsibility for their own health is important because it is closely observed by their patients. The high cigarette consumption among nurses as a profession, although now on the decline, may have many explanations, including the alternating periods of stress and boredom which characterise their work. However, the example of doctors in giving up smoking has not only had a dramatic effect (among other factors) in reducing the incidence of heart disease and lung cancer in their ranks, but seems to have impressed their patients, who have given up smoking in large numbers (Pender 1996).

Health professionals, as a body of people with public responsibility for maintaining the health services, cannot simply rest content with passive implementation of health policies decided by other people. As those who see the casualties on the wards and in the community every day, they have a responsibility to try to use their political influence actively to shape health policies. Through their professional associations and unions, nurses have the power to influence public opinion and so to achieve by political, legislative and fiscal means what cannot be achieved simply by counselling individuals – important and effective though that may be for individual patients. However, respect for the rights of individuals must be maintained, when pressure is being exerted on individuals and nations to change their lifestyle. The ultimate justification for health education is that the rights of patients demand it – especially the right to know and the right to treatment – for good health empowers people to claim and exercise their other rights.

Communication and 'counselling'

Communication with patients is not only important as a means of discovering or conveying information, and as a means of expressing sympathy, encouragement and personal interest, it is also the single most important way of securing their cooperation in treatment. In other words, communication plays a vital role in the management and control of patients (Bradley & Edinberg 1990, Porritt 1990, Balzer-Riley & Smith 1996).

It has become fashionable to talk about the importance of communication in medicine and nursing, and to explain the failures in relationships with patients as being due to 'poor communication'. This explanation is misleading if it implies that health professionals are poor communicators. Experienced doctors and nurses are highly skilled at certain forms of directive managerial communication – using language and the selective disclosure of information as a means of securing the cooperation of patients, and as a means of controlling them. However, qualified practitioners may be much less skilled than their junior colleagues at listening to patients, communicating with patients as persons, understanding their personal needs, responding to their different levels of comprehension of information.

Early research in health education showed up major problems in the attempts of health professionals to communicate with ordinary people (Fletcher 1971, Bennett 1976, Baric 1982). Several reasons emerged: their use of specialist jargon, their different educational level and level of literacy as compared with average patients, and their quite different life expectations. Simple tests for readability and comprehensibility can now be applied to written material, such as patient information sheets and consent forms, and this becomes a moral imperative when one takes into account the high levels of functional illiteracy in the average population, despite increasing use of the internet. It is therefore both a professional and moral duty of nurses to ensure that patients can in fact read the information they are given, particularly when informed consent is required for treatment or participation in a clinical controlled trial.

In the attempt to meet some of these difficulties, recent government policy in the UK has stressed the importance of lay involvement in developing healthcare policy, representation on health committees, and consultation with 'consumers', by using focus groups and surveys to get their feedback on the quality of services and the need for improvements.

Research on communication with patients in hospital, regarding their treatment or the likely effects of surgery, showed wide discrepancies between the levels of actual comprehension and recall by patients and that attributed to them by nurses, and doctors in particular (Ley 1976, Faulkner 1984). The form of training to which health professionals are subjected, the demands of institutional life, and the need to 'manage' large numbers of patients may make nurses and doctors less sensitive, with the passage of time, to the way manipulative communication can offend patients and create mistrust.

First and foremost, all health professionals need to enlarge their repertoire of communication skills. In some circumstances 'controlling' and 'managerial' communication may be required and appropriate, particularly in a crisis, but the other more sensitive communication skills, associated with 'counselling' and 'helping' patients to sort out their own problems and being assisted to take their own decisions, require quite different training and the development of quite different skills. On the whole, the traditional forms of education and training for health professions, as well as clinical experience, do not equip health professionals with these skills – if anything, the available evidence suggests that, in the process of their training in patient care, there is 'serial desensitisation' of nurses and doctors to the need for these skills (Porritt 1990, Horne & Cowan 1992).

While psychiatric nurses tend to have specialised training in techniques of psychotherapy, group work and counselling skills, and an increasing number of other nurses are introduced in basic training to the methods of 'client-centred' and 'non-directive' counselling, the wide application of these methods is relatively recent. However, competence in these forms of communication is increasingly being required of nurses working in areas such as terminal care, midwifery, genitourinary medicine, family planning, screening for cancer or genetic disorders, and in dealing with people with HIV/AIDS. (In relation to counselling people with HIV/AIDS, there are particular legal issues that need to be addressed by counsellors (McCall-Smith 1991).) The ethics of the counselling relationship could be the subject of a special chapter on its own, because it involves a very different orientation from that most commonly practised in nursing. Much communication between nurses and patients is necessarily directive, and often involves giving specific advice or warnings, and it is generally legitimised in terms of the nurse's duty of protective care. Professional counselling is the antithesis of 'advice-giving' or the 'counselling' or 'formal cautioning' which is part of the disciplinary process, and counselling in this sense requires more specialised training.

Within the classic schools of psychological counselling, associated particularly with the names of Carl Rogers and Gerald Egan (Rogers 1961, Egan 1986), 'counselling' is a term that has come to be applied to the process whereby a helper facilitates clients to communicate more effectively about their concerns, so as to enable them to first clarify the nature of their problem/s, to spell out what options they have, and to assist them to find their own solutions to their problems. 'Client-centred counselling' requires the nurse to restrain herself from giving advice, or trying to 'help' a patient by solving their problems for them, and to learn skills in the following: attentive listening, focusing and clarifying, challenging and presenting of options, and teaching problem-solving skills, to help patients to address their own life problems, and to empower them to exercise more control over their own decision-making.

As an intimate exchange of often very sensitive private information, the first ethical requirement for the counselling relationship is one of clearly negotiated and agreed boundaries of confidentiality. Secondly, the counsellor is bound to exercise a protective duty of care towards clients, both in terms of protecting their vulnerability and privacy, but also for a counsellor to recognise the limits of her own competence and to be prepared to refer the client to a psychiatrist or other appropriate specialist, if necessary. Thirdly, the counsellor has a fundamental duty to respect the individuality and opinions of the client, even if the client disagrees with what the counsellor is saying. This non-judgemental attitude (what Carl Rogers calls 'unconditional positive regard') is essential if clients are to feel free to explore their feelings and conflicts without fear of disapproval or subsequent discrimination. The fourth requirement of empathy (the ability to put yourself in the other's shoes) is often cited as another ethical as well as functional requirement of counselling. This is not equivalent to sympathy, which can often be condescending, but an attempt to put oneself professionally in the client's position and to understand it on their terms and within their frame of reference (even if this may need to be changed as part of the therapeutic process).

Several counselling organisations have developed codes of ethics and practice for counsellors, and the latest nursing codes include terms that relate to the counselling role of the nurse (NMC 2004). In particular, we would recommend the British Association for Counselling and Psychotherapy's Ethical Framework for Good Practice in Counselling and Psychotherapy (BACP 2002), which has wide general relevance to nurse–patient communication as well.

In general, communication between nurses and patients can raise two kinds of ethical problems: first, when communication fails to express respect for the patient as a person; and, second, when the patient's right to know is ignored. The first kind of problem arises, for example, when hospital staff members 'talk over the heads' of patients or, more seriously, fail to respect their confidences. The power relationship between a patient and a health professional is an unequal one, and communication can be used to talk down to or to control patients rather than to relate to them as persons. Sick or injured patients are often anxious and distressed because they do not understand what is happening to them or why it is happening. They are vulnerable and dependent. Not only do they need the reassurance which nurses or doctors can give them, but they need information to be able to exercise any degree of control over their lives. Medical and nursing staff consequently have a responsibility to share with the patient their knowledge and specific information about that patient, and to share it in the most helpful and caring way.

BALANCING THE RIGHTS OF PATIENTS WITH THE INTERESTS OF THIRD PARTIES

In general, and for very good reasons, the focus of training in nursing and medicine is on direct patient care, on the one-to-one relationship between carer and patient in the clinical situation. Less attention is given to the wider responsibilities in management, research and health promotion. Clinical practice is grounded on the more individual, or 'personalist', values of beneficence, and respect for persons. The values on which the other functions of healthcare are based are the more universal values derivable from principles of justice. In practice, nurses – like doctors and paramedical staff – usually have obligations to several patients at the same time. Because each nurse 'has only one pair of hands' and 'cannot be in two places at once', they have to make decisions about which patients should be given priority while doing the best for all their patients. These more universal considerations of justice and the common good may suggest different responses to a charge nurse as a manager than those the charge nurse would take into account when dealing with individual patients. The same could be said of doctors: the demands of teaching, administration, research and public health all introduce more universal obligations to be balanced against their duties to individual patients.

Health professionals often feel most comfortable in making ethical decisions of a personal kind relating to individual patients and their health needs. Their expertise and clinical experience relate best to the treatment of individual patients and decisions about their management. A personalist ethic, based on 'caring', appears most appropriate to such situations.

The doctor may well feel that his expertise (unless he is an epidemiologist or trained administrator) is not applicable to decisions about the general allocation of manpower and resources. Nurses, on the other hand, while sharing the same personalist ethic, may have more experience in managing large groups of patients and feel less uneasy about making decisions based on the general good. The conflict between these different kinds of values, personalist and universal, comes out most clearly where the rights of individual patients have to be balanced against the interests of third parties. The situations that may serve to illustrate some of the problems and dilemmas are:

- decisions to refuse admission to a patient, either because of risk to other patients, or lack of a bed
- persuading patients to 'volunteer' as research subjects in clinical trials and/or non-therapeutic research
- the use of patients as teaching material for the education of nurses
- decisions about allocation of resources within the hospital or in the community.

It is to the discussion of these issues that we now turn, before looking at some of the wider 'political' responsibilities of nurses, both as individuals and as a profession.

Refusing to admit a patient

A classic dilemma facing a charge nurse may be whether they can accept responsibility for another patient when there is an acute shortage of nurses or resources, or where a patient is very disturbed and disruptive, or where there are too few staff to ensure management of a ward. The conflict here is between the charge nurse's straightforward duty to care for a patient who has been brought to the ward and the nurse's duty to provide adequate care for the other patients on the ward (and perhaps to consider the other nursing and auxiliary staff, and what it may be reasonable or unreasonable to expect of them in such a situation). An alternative way of viewing the problem is to see it as a conflict between the right to treatment of an individual patient being admitted and the rights of those in the ward already receiving treatment. Either way there is a dilemma to be faced.

In Case Study 8.2, the issues faced by the charge nurse concerned the relative weight to be given to the rights of the various patients in her care and the conflict between her responsibility to a whole ward of acutely ill patients and her duty to help a particular woman who clearly needed urgent psychiatric attention. At one level, the charge nurse's decision might appear sensible and possibly the only thing to do in the circumstances. She did not perceive it as a moral dilemma in the strict sense, but rather as a moral problem which she solved by giving priority to the demands of justice to her staff and the ten patients on the ward. The young doctor clearly saw the problem differently and gave greater weight to the needs of the suicidal woman, perhaps because he felt responsible for taking the legal decision to have her admitted on an Emergency Order and perhaps because he felt he could do something about her problem. The tense and difficult situation gave it the proportions of a 'crisis' for the overstretched staff, and this atmosphere of crisis was aggravated by the differences between the charge nurse and the doctor. In such circumstances it becomes difficult to make sensible and responsible moral choices, and the moral issues may in fact be secondary to other agendas between the nursing and medical staff or between them and the hospital administration.

However, it is important to tease out what moral issues are involved and to develop models for sensible decision-making in such circumstances (see Chapter 11). Some of the most critical decisions faced by healthcare staff occur in situations where there are numerous people in need of urgent attention and limited staff and resources to deal with the emergency. Part of the problem may relate to factors of a non-moral nature, such as the youth and inexperience of the doctor, or the sense of helplessness of the charge nurse faced with staff shortages and an unsympathetic health authority, and the arrival of another patient, being 'the last straw' (Case Study 8.2).

The moral questions raised by this case are of various kinds. There are the questions which relate to the rights of the various patients involved, the apparent conflict between the rights of one acutely disturbed patient, and the rights of others. Clearly here no one patient's rights are paramount. As indicated in Chapter 7, our rights are not absolute or unlimited. Provision of treatment or a bed for one patient, for example, may mean that another patient is deprived or that there are fewer resources to go around for others. Sensible decisions have to be made in the best interests of all. In some cases this demand of distributive justice may mean that a patient cannot be given treatment at a particular time because all available resources are committed. Alternatively, in some situations of extreme emergency, where the life of a patient is at risk, less-ill patients may have to

case study 8.2

'I've only got one pair of hands'

Recently, when I was doing night duty as charge nurse in the acute admissions ward of the local psychiatric hospital, I was faced with a very painful decision. We were short of staff. This was due to the freeze on vacant posts – seemingly part of the policy of 'cuts' imposed by the local health authority, but also aggravated by an epidemic of 'flu which had affected several nurses and medical staff. We had been operating for several days below what I would regard as safe staffing levels. The duty doctor was a young trainee psychiatrist with little experience of the application of the Mental Health Act, but we managed because we had most of the patients well under control and had not had a new admission for several days.

On the night in question, one of the patients on the ward, Mrs M, was upset by an accidental injury caused to her by another patient and became very disturbed and violent towards other patients and staff. I called for help from the duty doctor, as I had only one staff nurse and an auxiliary to deal with the demands of 10 disturbed patients. We had difficulty subduing Mrs M and

persuading her to take some medication – a powerful tranquilliser – and were trying to calm down the other patients, who had become very agitated, when we were informed that the police were at Reception with a woman who was hysterical, had attempted to slash her wrists and was being abusive and violent towards the police. They were demanding that she be admitted under the relevant section of the Mental Health Act which gives police the authority to detain people who, in their opinion, are mentally disordered.

The young doctor was undecided whether we could cope with the new admission, but felt we ought to accept the woman because she was in a bad way and needed immediate medical treatment. In the circumstances I felt I had to refuse, as I knew we could not cope and that the care of the other patients might be put at risk. The doctor was angry, although he later admitted that he thought I was right to refuse. The suicidal woman was given the necessary first aid and some medication and taken to the police cells for the night, until other arrangements could be made for her care.

suffer a degree of neglect for the sake of saving the life of another. In the one case the demands of justice for the common good prevail, in the other case the right of a particular person to treatment.

Both cases could be said to arise from competing demands of justice for individuals or a fair outcome for the group. In theory we may derive most personal rights from the principle of respect for persons, but we may not be able to resolve conflicts of rights between different parties without other considerations based on justice and beneficence.

There are also questions raised by this case about the moral and legal entitlement of nurses and doctors to administer compulsory treatment in an emergency without fulfilling the procedural requirements of the relevant Mental Health Act. Forced administration of tranquillisers in order to subdue a violent patient may be necessary even if the patient has not given consent to treatment. (Some of these questions were covered in Chapter 6, when discussing the ambiguous status of the mentally disordered patient. Other questions raised by this type of case relate to the nurse's right to conscientiously object to assisting in treatments ordered by the doctor – a subject discussed in Chapter 5.)

Another area of concern, on which the Health Service trade union UNISON and the Royal College of Psychiatrists have pronounced, is the matter of the legal responsibility of staff in dealing with violent patients, both with respect to their own safety and in protecting themselves from subsequent litigation if charges of negligence or physical abuse are brought against staff (NIMHE 2004, UNISON 2004). The issues here relate, on the one hand, to the rights of nurses or doctors, their own entitlement to justice – to fair conditions of service and protection from mischievous prosecution when coping with difficult and dangerous patients. On the other hand, they have a duty of public accountability in situations where use of the very legal powers for compulsory detention which are necessary to control disturbed and vulnerable patients give rise to fears that 'captive' patients may be abused or maltreated by staff. The provision of legal safeguards for the rights of mentally ill patients (in particular their rights of access to a Mental Health Tribunal or Mental Welfare Commission in Britain) is necessary because of the extra-ordinary legal powers exercised by health professionals in the case of patients who have severe mental health problems. These powers relate both to their authority to deprive patients of their liberty and to administer compulsory treatment, and to the protection of patients who are vulnerable and 'incompetent' by virtue of severe mental illness.

Finally, there is a whole series of ethical questions to be raised about the marginalisation of mental health and the inadequate resources provided, compared with the acute medical and surgical services – despite the large proportion of patients requiring treatment for mental health problems. In spite of official recommendations to the contrary, the low priority accorded to mental health services generally raises questions about the rationality of health service planning and of justice in healthcare. The kind of crisis which makes a charge nurse refuse to admit a patient demands more of the nurse than merely a gesture of non-cooperation. The wider 'political' responsibilities of nurses are painfully illustrated in such situations, and organised protests to the hospital or health authority, industrial action or 'leaks' to the press may be more effective and successful in drawing attention to the inadequacy of the service for these particularly vulnerable patients – patients who are unable to defend their own rights to have proper care and treatment.

Persuading patients to 'volunteer' as research subjects

Nursing practice, like medical science, can only advance through properly controlled scientific research. The 'controls' required in scientific research are both methodological and ethical. Research that is not conducted according to rigorous scientific methods is valueless, and research that is not conducted with proper respect for the rights of patients may be unethical and result in inhumane treatment of research subjects. The World Medical Association's Declaration of Helsinki (WMA 1996), on the ethical and scientific requirements for sound research involving human subjects, is of general value in discussing issues related to research in which a nurse may be involved, whether as responsible investigator or in an auxiliary role.

In order to be *scientific*, nursing research must be based on sound scientific knowledge and proper scientific methods. This means that the research must satisfy several conditions, namely:

- Initial investigations (e.g. by data collection or literature survey) must establish what has already been done in the field, to avoid unnecessary repetition and waste of public resources.
- New research instruments must be properly pre-tested to establish their reliability and validity, or alternatively, well-tried methods should be used.
- The project must be based on sound research design, approved by one's professional peers and independent assessors, and undertaken by properly qualified research staff.

- The findings of the research must be disseminated, to inform future practice, e.g. by publication in a peer-reviewed journal.

These requirements are not only scientific but ethical. The researcher has an obligation in justice not to engage in research that is valueless, and a waste of time and resources. This is not only because most research is funded from public money and involves the use of public resources, but also to protect research subjects from unnecessary investigations of no benefit to them or to anyone else. Here nurses have particular responsibilities to patients in their care, whether they are conducting the research themselves or assisting in someone else's project.

In order to be *ethical*, nursing research must be based on prior critical consideration of the ethical basis and implications of the research, namely, whether the proposed research satisfies the demands of beneficence/non-maleficence, justice and respect for persons:

- The duty of protective beneficence demands careful prior assessment of the potential risks to patients from their participation in the project, and clarification of what benefits the research may bring directly to research participants and/or to the wider community. No research is ethically acceptable when the risks outweigh the benefits. If clinical research involves potential risk to research participants, then prior laboratory tests and animal experiments are demanded to satisfy any researcher's duty to care for their research participants, and to protect their rights.
- The principle of justice demands that no research should involve abuse of or discrimination against particular patients, or groups of patients (whether on grounds of race, gender, social class, captive status, or the medically 'interesting' nature of the complaint being investigated); and further, that it should potentially benefit the whole population.
- The principle of respect for persons means that for research to be ethical, it must ensure that the patient's rights to know, to privacy and to treatment are respected:
  - Patients should not be involved without a fully informed understanding of the nature of the research, and their free and voluntary participation. (Where patients are not competent to give consent, special safeguards must be established to protect their rights; e.g. proxy consent or tribunals to monitor research in the interest of patients.)
  - The physical privacy and confidentiality of the research participants must be protected by appropriate procedures and protocols; e.g. within the UK this entails scrutiny and approval by an approved and competent multidisciplinary Research Ethics Committee.
  - The patient's right to proper care and treatment should not be compromised nor their health put at risk by participation in research (e.g. involving placebo or in randomised controlled trials).

Clinical research may be therapeutic or non-therapeutic. Therapeutic research is directly related to the patient's complaint and the patient stands to benefit directly from the treatments or procedures used. Non-therapeutic research is where patients participate in general investigations, e.g. research aimed at improving patient care, techniques of management, nurse–patient communication, or general knowledge of the physiology or pathology of particular complaints, where the investigations are of a general nature and have neither any specific therapeutic purpose nor are of any direct benefit to the research participant. In practice, the distinction may not be so clear-cut, for patients may stand to benefit in the long run from even the most academic studies of sociology or psychology, as they may from laboratory studies of the composition of the blood or the biochemistry of the brain. Furthermore, in randomised controlled trials using placebos, some patients may receive potentially therapeutic drugs or treatment and others no effective treatment at all, and yet no progress can be made without such trials. The claimed effectiveness of drugs cannot be proved by mere accumulation of evidence without testing the 'evidence' in rigorously controlled experiments, to exclude other possible explanations of why the health of some patients appears to improve with their use (Buchanan & Brock 1989).

However, in broad principle the distinction between therapeutic and non-therapeutic research is a useful one even if only to emphasise that the ethical safeguards in the latter type have to be more stringent. In general, the greater risks taken in clinical research are justified on two grounds, first that there may be direct benefit for the patient and, secondly, that the research may contribute to the benefit of humanity even if it does not directly benefit the patient. The right of the patients to treatment includes the implicit assumption that they will cooperate in the trial of various procedures, yet have the right to withdraw if they believe they are suffering harm, or that the responsible researcher will withdraw them from the study if they are at risk of harm.

It has been argued that the right of a patient to benefit from research carries with it a corresponding duty to assist in research that may be of benefit to other patients too. On the other hand, the patient's right to care and treatment cannot rest solely on this premise. Our entitlement to treatment cannot depend on our capacity to barter for it by payment in time served as a research participant. Our entitlement to adequate care and treatment must rest on some more fundamental right – related to our right to life and membership of a moral community that cares not only for the strong, but also for the weak and vulnerable too. The 'duty' to assist medical research by participation in clinical trials, if it is a moral duty, is so in an extended sense of the word 'duty', and may or may not be recognised as such by the patient. It is not a duty that can be forced on anybody (McCormick 1976, Hellman 1995). Patients have a right to be properly informed and to give their consent without coercion or moral blackmail. Patients also have a right to be informed of the risks and possible benefits, and to withdraw from any trial or research project without prejudice to their treatment. Both requirements arise because a patient's participation cannot be said to be ethical unless it is voluntary, i.e. free and appropriately informed.

The nurse or doctor in charge of patients in research trials has a special responsibility to protect the interests of the individual patients, to act as their advocate advising them about the conditions of participation and their right to withdraw from experiments. Because patients in hospital are to some degree captive, it is important to ensure that they feel quite happy about participation in a trial, particularly if it is not one from which they stand to benefit directly, or where there is a significant degree of risk or inconvenience involved. Research Ethics Committees are increasingly requiring of investigators that independent assessment is made of the quality of consent given by patients, and the degree of discomfort or inconvenience caused, by a competent professional not involved in the research project. However, medical and/or nursing staff involved in the research may also have to persuade patients to cooperate, and here the personal values of clinical practice and the more universal ones justifying research may come into conflict. These may be particularly acute in justifying clinical research involving children, prisoners, or those who have severe mental health problems or learning disabilities. In such cases, legal and institutional safeguards (such as proxy consent) are particularly important, to protect the wider interests of those not competent to give informed and voluntary consent – whether they stand to benefit or will merely be contributing to the welfare of others (Kerridge et al 1998, Ch. 21).

The issue of whether it is ethical to use children as subjects of clinical research has been hotly debated over the years. On the one hand, it has been argued that children cannot be said to give consent that is either informed or voluntary in any proper sense. Children's lack of knowledge and understanding of the implications of medical procedures, and even of the legal significance of consent, may be said to invalidate any attempt to justify their use as research participants on moral grounds. Children's dependency on adults for protection and advice makes them peculiarly vulnerable to moral pressures, and it is doubtful whether their consent could really be voluntary. This approach was classically adopted and argued by Ramsey (1976, 1977). On the other hand, it has been counter-argued that this issue cannot be settled by simply appealing to the rights of the individual child – for advances in the treatment of paediatric disorders often cannot be made without research or clinical trials involving children. Against Ramsey, McCormick (1976) argued that the right to benefit from new discoveries in the clinical sciences carries with it the corresponding indirect moral duty to contribute to the advance of clinical research, and this correspondence between rights and duties applies to children as much as to anyone else. This argument was advanced in the Belmont Report (DHEW 1978). However, in both sources it is emphasised that the researcher has a fundamental duty to protect the rights of children and incompetent adults, to avoid their being put at risk and to prevent their exploitation. Furthermore, the researcher has an obligation to avoid subjecting any human subjects to hazardous procedures, where other procedures involving competent adults or animals as subjects would do just as well, or where the risk outweighs the possible benefits.

Those people who are contemplating research involving children (or individuals who have severe mental health problems or learning disabilities) sometimes fall back on the proxy consent of the parents or a relative. This can be an attempt to safeguard the interests of vulnerable individuals, but the question can be raised too whether the insistence on proxy consent is not more to protect the doctor or institution from legal action than to protect the child. Ramsey (1976, 1977) maintained that it is never permissible to use children as research subjects in non-therapeutic research, and that proxy consent does not make it ethical either. McCormick (1974) argued, on the other hand, that since the ultimate justification for clinical research is that it contributes to the common good, and justice requires that we are prepared to accept risks ourselves if we wish to benefit from medical discoveries (either in the short term or the long term), then we ought to be able to understand the principle of this exchange if we have the capacity. Even if we did not have the capacity, it can be argued by analogy that we would give our consent if we could understand, and should therefore not be deprived of the right to contribute to the common good merely because we are not competent to give fully informed and voluntary consent. In fact, it can be doubted whether even the consent of normal adult patients can ever be fully informed or completely voluntary, and with children it is just a difference of degree.

Clearly this classic moral debate about the ethics of research on children now has to be revisited and reviewed in the light of the legal requirements in the UK of the Children Act 1989 as amended 2004, and the related policy guidance *Every Child Matters* (DFES 2004). The guidance that applies to court orders relating to looked after children apply *mutatis mutandis* to healthcare practitioners with responsibility for the care and treatment of children, including children who are directly or indirectly involved as research subjects or the subjects of research.

Under Section 1(3) of the Children Act 1989 the court must have regard in particular to:

1. the ascertainable wishes and feelings of the child concerned (considered in the light of his age and understanding)
2. his physical, emotional and educational needs
3. the likely effect of any change in his circumstances
4. his age, sex, background and any characteristics of his which the court considers relevant
5. any harm which he has suffered or is at risk of suffering
6. how capable each of his parents, and any other person in relation to whom the court considers the question to be relevant, is of meeting his needs
7. the range of powers available to the court under this Act in the proceedings in question.

There are also more general considerations relating to the consent of children and those unable to give or refuse consent, spelled out in the Council of Europe Convention for the Protection of Human Rights and Dignity of the Human Being with regard to the Application of Biology and Medicine: Convention on Human Rights and Biomedicine (1997):

> CHAPTER II: CONSENT – Article 5 – General rule
> An intervention in the health field may only be carried out after the person concerned has given free and informed consent to it.
> This person shall beforehand be given appropriate information as to the purpose and nature of the intervention as well as on its consequences and risks.

> The person concerned may freely withdraw consent at any time.

> Article 6 – Protection of persons not able to consent
> 1. Subject to Articles 17 and 20 below, an intervention may only be carried out on a person who does not have the capacity to consent, for his or her direct benefit.
> 2. Where, according to law, a minor does not have the capacity to consent to an intervention, the intervention may only be carried out with the authorisation of his or her representative or an authority or a person or body provided for by law.
>   (a) The opinion of the minor shall be taken into consideration as an increasingly determining factor in proportion to his or her age and degree of maturity.
> 3. Where, according to law, an adult does not have the capacity to consent to an intervention because of a mental disability, a disease or for similar reasons, the intervention may only be carried out with the authorisation of his or her representative or an authority or a person or body provided for by law.
>   (b) The individual concerned shall as far as possible take part in the authorisation procedure.
> 4. The representative, the authority, the person or the body mentioned in paragraphs 2 and 3 above shall be given, under the same conditions, the information referred to in Article 5.
> 5. The authorisation referred to in paragraphs 2 and 3 above may be withdrawn at any time in the best interests of the person concerned.

This line of argument was used in the past in the United States to justify experiments using institutionalised psychiatric patients, patients with learning disabilities and prisoners (Hornblum 1997). It would seem a dangerous line of argument to pursue, not significantly different from arguments used to justify the infamous Nazi medical 'experiments' with captive patients. There are, of course, particular problems about whether the consent given by captive patients can ever be voluntary in an ethically satisfactory way, and this is where the argument from analogy becomes suspect and tendentious. Research involving children and people of borderline competence is a highly controversial area in the ethics of clinical research, and while, more often than not, doctors have to take the key decisions, nevertheless nurses may have to cope with the enquiries of both children and their parents, and will therefore be required to have a clear view on where they stand on these issues – especially if it is the nurse who is required to seek the 'consent' of the child, psychiatric patient, or person with learning disabilities (Kerridge et al 1998, Goodare & Smith 1995).

In reality, the health professional has to exercise discretion about how much to tell and to judge whether consent is being given under duress. Respect for persons and the duty to care stand in a relationship of tension to one another here. A degree of protective beneficence is necessary to interpret the needs of vulnerable individuals, to judge their competence, to decide what is in their best interests. But this kind of quasi-parental attitude can become condescending and insensitive to the needs of individuals if it is not based on sensitive regard for their condition and respect for their rights as persons.

The establishment of Research Ethics Committees in Britain, and elsewhere (Institutional Review Boards in the United States) has been hailed as a major step forward in the attempt to monitor research involving human subjects. This came about in the first instance as the result of public concern in the late 1960s over the possible abuse of patients as 'human guinea pigs' and, more seriously, the abuse of captive subjects such as prisoners and the mentally ill in research, not only for clinical purposes, but also by pharmaceutical companies for merely commercial ends (Pappworth 1967, DHEW 1978, McNeill 1993).

Researchers working with human subjects (and even with animals) are now required to submit research protocols for scrutiny by these committees, to ensure that they fulfil the requirements of sound scientific and ethical research. In some cases these committees may insist on direct monitoring of the ongoing research, or may require periodic reports, to ensure that the general guidelines are being adhered to by all concerned. Nurses are increasingly taking a significant part in the work of these multidisciplinary committees. In their role as nurses they have important professional and moral responsibilities, not just to ensure the proper vetting of nursing research but to provide a considered nursing viewpoint on the implications of the research proposed on patient care and well-being, as well as the implications for staffing and resources. Nurses, arguably, also have a responsibility to ensure that Research Ethics Committees actually work and do their business in a conscientious way. Surveys of some such committees suggest that there is a lot of room for improvement, e.g. poor and unrepresentative attendance (Lock 1990, McNeill et al 1990, 1994, National Health and Medical Research Council 1995, 1999).

The new emphasis by the UK government on total quality management and governance in healthcare requires an integrated approach and the application of ethical principles across all levels in the NHS. This includes corporate governance, staff governance, clinical governance and research governance. Here the Royal College of Nursing has set up a Research and Development Coordinating Centre based in Manchester University, which gives detailed advice on research governance policy (for website links related to this topic, please see http://evolve.elsevier.com/Thompson/nursing ethics).

Use of patients as teaching material

Should patients be used as teaching material for the training of doctors and nurses? Should patients with rare or exotic disorders or unusual complications be expected to put up with the additional inconvenience, embarrassment and even discomfort of being examined by students? In a major teaching centre, where the population does not have the opportunity of being treated in non-teaching hospitals, should patients be given the choice of consent or refusal to act as demonstration material for clinical tutorials without suffering prejudice in treatment? And what about the right to privacy of psychiatric patients, and the dying, as subjects of research?

Clinical training without the opportunity to work on real patients would be like learning to swim on dry land. Here the justification for compromising the right to privacy of individual patients is that the patient stands to benefit by having highly trained staff to care for their needs. Alternatively, it can be argued that the common good of all patients is served by having properly trained staff. However, this does not give medical or nursing instructors an unlimited right to do as they like with patients.

The requirements for the provision of sound clinical training for nurses (like the demands of medical research, healthcare planning and public health measures) are such that they tend to give greater importance to considerations of the common good than to the specific needs or interests of individual patients. The nurse on the ward and the junior medical resident with a particular interest in and clinical responsibility for the individual patient may feel protective towards 'their' patients and critical of the insensitivity of those passing through on a 'teaching round' or conducting surveys. The tension between universal and personal values in healthcare is well illustrated here. Neither view is exclusively right. Each needs to be tempered by the other. Institutionalised healthcare imposes some limitations on personal rights, including the right to privacy, but teaching and research institutions and hospitals generally need to be humanised as well (Johnstone 1991).

Justice demands that patients with unusual and 'exotic' disorders should not be unduly exposed to students, with or without their consent. Even unconscious patients deserve to have their privacy respected and dignity protected. Lack of respect tends to breed insensitivity, callousness and lack of consideration in trainees. Some patients, or patient populations, may be at risk of being over-investigated, over-scrutinised because they are 'interesting teaching material'. Some reasonable and just limits have to be set to the demands made on such patients. The 'duty' of patients to participate in clinical teaching cannot be an unlimited demand, and has to be secondary to their own treatment and concern for their general well-being. Apart from the need to preserve the trust and goodwill of patients by not exploiting them or trying their patience beyond endurance, professionals also have a duty to protect the dignity and privacy of those in their care. This is particularly important if the complaint makes them vulnerable (as in cases of mental illness) or liable to embarrassment (as in cases of pregnancy, disfiguring injury and handicap, or sexually transmitted disease) (Goodare & Smith 1995).

It may be questioned whether it can be morally justified to place additional stress on anxious and distressed patients (e.g. disturbed psychiatric patients) by exposure to a group of nursing or medical students, even with the patient's 'consent'. The tutor may have to decide against using particular patients, however interesting, because of their vulnerability. On the other hand, it needs to be stressed that the expectations of people with regard to their privacy vary according to their situation. People tend to expect the greatest degree of privacy and strictest confidentiality to be observed when they are visited in their own homes or see health professionals in a private consultation. However, when people enter public institutions they recognise the implicit restrictions on their rights, for in order to benefit from institutional care, they may be obliged to surrender some degree of their privacy. In an institutional setting, the health professionals may be more anxious about privacy and confidentiality than patients are (where, for example, much intimate information about patients may be common knowledge on the ward). Nevertheless, professionals cannot ignore the need of individuals for privacy, and they have a primary moral duty to protect the rights of the patients entrusted to their care.

Because nurses are in the front line in dealing with patients, whether it be in hospital, community or a clinic, they have a particular moral responsibility to protect their patients, or to advocate on their behalf, when they believe the treatment of patients may be compromised, or they may be put to serious inconvenience, if not risk, by participation in teaching or a research study, whether being conducted by a doctor, outside researcher or another nurse. For example, it may be awkward but necessary for a duty nurse to challenge the research methods of a nursing colleague if she is upsetting patients by her approach.

Allocation of resources

Although the ethical problems related to the allocation of human and material resources in healthcare are discussed more fully in the next chapter, there are some issues which arise here in the context of having to balance the rights of individuals against the interests of third parties. Let us consider a few examples. Should older patients be discharged from hospital to make way for more acute cases if there is any doubt that they will be able to cope on their own, even with domiciliary services and support? Should nursing staff be allocated according to need or according to the number of patients? Should more effort be put into nursing those who have the potential for 'cure', rather than individuals who have enduring conditions? What role should nurses have in decisions to ration drugs and medical equipment where these are in short supply (Gross 1985, Johnstone 1994, Ch. 7, Cummings 1994)?

In real life, decisions have to be taken and these may be both painful and subsequently found to be mistaken or based on inadequate knowledge. All decisions where the rights of one patient have to be balanced against those of other patients or third parties may involve agonising choices. In formal terms it may be a choice between the demands of personal care for the individual patient and justice for a larger group of patients or society. In practical terms, it may be a matter of responding to external pressures and the internal guilt and anxiety generated by an unresolvable tension between conflicting duties. The extreme case may be a medical emergency such as an air crash or train disaster in which many people are injured or dying and there are limited medical supplies and perhaps only one qualified doctor or nurse available. As in wartime, the responsible health professional may have to adopt a policy of *triage* – dividing the victims into three groups: those who must be left to die because they are beyond help, those who can wait for treatment later, and those who must be attended to first because they need treatment urgently and stand to benefit from it most. A question we need to address here is: How do we reconcile the conflicting demands of the principles of beneficence, justice and respect for persons in such situations?

Faced with several patients with renal failure and needing urgent dialysis, but only one dialysis machine available, who is to be given priority? Generally, the decision will be the doctor's, but if there are no obvious clinical criteria which would decide the issue in favour of one patient rather than another, other criteria might have to be considered, and nurses might get drawn into discussion of the available options.

Would the decision be made most fairly by drawing lots or by adhering to a first-come, first-served basis? Would attempts to assess the usefulness, value, importance of individuals be reasonable or invidious? Attempts to involve patients in group decisions about the allocation of a dialysis machine would seem to be very unfair. In such circumstances, a decision by team consensus or by outside assessors might be justified if there were objective grounds on which the choice might be made. However, the judgements would tend in practice to be based either on the assessment of probabilities on the basis of the personal experience of staff, or on the past experience and subjective judgement of professionals. In the case of a real moral dilemma, where there are no practical strategies to avoid the problem of choice, the responsible health professionals would have to be prepared to take a decision and to live with the guilt and anxiety which that responsibility entails. (It has been remarked that doctors are paid well 'to pad their shoulders' in carrying the burden of decision-making responsibility. Perhaps the difficulty experienced by nurses is that, faced with having clinical responsibility for decisions in similar situations, they do not have the necessary padding!)

In making decisions affecting the lives and well-being of individuals in their care, health professionals act as guardians and advocates of the rights of all their patients. They have to make decisions based on their knowledge, expertise and available resources for the common good. They will have to exercise courageous initiative and be willing to take risks as they try to effect the best compromise between the demands of justice, beneficence and respect for the rights of individual patients.

While fit today, we may be ill or in desperate need of treatment tomorrow. Thus all of us are potential patients (including doctors and nurses), so we should have an interest in protecting patients' rights. The right to know, the right to privacy and the right to treatment are all better understood by health professionals who have experienced the impotence and vulnerability of patienthood. Health professionals who take their duties seriously will also be more willing to act as advocates defending the rights and dignity of patients. They will also be aware that as public officers they have a responsibility to uphold the common good and to promote the health of the whole community. These competing duties may indeed give rise to painful and difficult choices.

further reading

Autonomy

Clement G 1996 Care, autonomy and justice: feminism and the ethic of care. Westview Press, Boulder, CO

Lindley R 1986 Autonomy. Macmillan, Basingstoke

Thomson D 1991 Selfish generations? Ageing of New Zealand's welfare state. Bridget Williams Bks, Wellington

Behaviour modification

Braun J V, Lipson S 1993 Toward a restraint-free environment. Health Professionals' Press, Baltimore, MD

Erwin E 1978 Behavior therapy: scientific, philosophical and moral foundations. CUP, Cambridge

Häring B 1975 Ethics of manipulation: issues in medicine, behaviour control and genetics. Seabury Press, New York

Matthies B K, Kreutzer J S, West D 1997 The behaviour management handbook. Therapy Skill Builders, San Antonio, TX

Suicide

Aldridge D 1998 Suicide: the tragedy of hopelessness. Jessica Kingsley Publishers, London

Durkheim E 1952 Suicide: a study in sociology. Routledge and Kegan Paul, London

Health education and health promotion

Gold R S, Greenberg J S 1992 The health education ethics book. WmC Brown, Dubuque, IA

Lipson J G, Steiger N J 1996 Self-care nursing in a multi-cultural context. Sage Publications, Thousand Oaks, CA

Pender N 1996 Health promotion in nursing practice. Prentice Hall International, London

Sidell M 1997 Debates and dilemmas in promoting health: a reader. Macmillan (Open University), Basingstoke

Tones K, Telford S, Keeley-Robinson Y 1994 Health education: efficiency, effectiveness and equity. Chapman & Hall, London

Violence and nurses

Hamberger L K, Burge S K, Graham A V, Costa A J 1997 Violence issues for health care educators and providers. Haworth Maltreatment and Trauma Press, New York

UNISON 1997 Violence at work: a guide to risk prevention for Unison Branches and Safety Representatives. UNISON, London

Communication

Balzer-Riley J, Smith S 1996 Communication in nursing. Mosby, St Louis, MO

Horne E M, Cowan T 1992 Effective communication: some nursing perspectives. Wolfe Publishing, London

Kagan K, Evans J 1995 Professional and inter-personal skills for nurses. Chapman & Hall, London

Nursing research

Burnard P, Morrison P 1994 Nursing research in action: developing basic skills. Macmillan, Basingstoke

Burns N, Grove S K 1999 Understanding nursing research. WB Saunders, Philadelphia

Hellman S 1995 The patient and the public good. Nature Medicine 1(5):400–402

Johnstone M-J 1991 Ethical issues in nursing research: a broad overview. RMIT, Bundoora, Victoria

McNeill P M 1993 The ethics and politics of human experimentation. Cambridge University Press, Cambridge

Nursing dependent elderly people

Benson S, Carr P 1994 The care assistant's guide to working with elderly mentally infirm people. Hawker, London

Couglan P B 1993 Facing Alzheimer's: family care givers speak. Ballantine, New York

McClymont A Thomas S E, Denham M J 1991 Health visiting and elderly people. Churchill Livingstone, Edinburgh

Tice C J, Perkins K 1996 Mental health issues and ageing: building on the strengths of older persons. Brookes/Cole, Pacific Grove, CA

Informed consent

Buchanan A E, Brock D W 1989 Deciding for others: the ethics of surrogate decision-making. Cambridge University Press, Cambridge

Kerridge I, Lowe M & McPhee J 1998 Ethics and law for the health professions. Social Science Press, Katoomba, NSW

PART 4

Ethics in nursing management, research and teaching

Ethics in healthcare management: research, evaluation and performance management

Chapter contents

AIMS

The main aims of this chapter are:

1. To explore the main responsibilities of management in healthcare settings and the need for evidence on which to base planning, direction of operations and evaluation of services

2. To explore the nature of evaluation and its different forms, and how this relates to more formal research whether in service-based action research, or more academic projects

3. To explore the role of evidence-based practice in continuous improvement of the quality of overall management, staff performance and the cost effectiveness of services

4. To explore the strengths and weaknesses of a number of different models and styles of management and their ethical rationale.

LEARNING OUTCOMES

When you have read and studied this chapter you should be able to:

■ Give a coherent account of the different kinds of evaluation that may be required in healthcare practice or management, and the values that underlie each kind

■ Discuss some of the different kinds of research that may be used in healthcare and its function at different levels of operation, from studies of treatment and direct patient care, to studies of service efficiency, standards of staff performance, and overall corporate management and governance

■ Demonstrate understanding of the importance of evidence-based practice and its relationship with service planning, performance management and continuous quality improvement of the whole service

■ Explain the ethical rationale for different kinds of management, discuss the strengths and weaknesses of the different models discussed, and give examples of the different kinds from your own experience and/or observations.

ETHICAL RESPONSIBILITIES IN MANAGEMENT

Research and evaluation as core responsibilities of sound management

We have been concerned to emphasise throughout this book that we do not believe the scope of nursing ethics should be confined simply to study of the ethical issues that arise for nurses in direct clinical relationships with patients, but should also include the exercise of their various roles in leadership and management. For nurses and other health professionals, as they gain in experience and seniority, take on new roles and wider responsibilities beyond the care of individual patients, they also acquire different kinds of ethical responsibility.

As we move on to discuss ethics in management of nursing and other healthcare services, we should perhaps dismiss at the outset the view that management and administration are purely technical and impersonal matters without real interest from an ethical point of view. Nothing could be further from the truth, for ethics embraces the whole of life and all dimensions and levels of our work. Recent developments in quality management have shown how crucial ethics is to good human resource management as well as to corporate strategic management (James 1996).

Furthermore, we will argue in this chapter that *evaluation and research are not subsidiary functions, but core responsibilities of management.* The moral authority of managers does not rest primarily on their right to direct and control operations, but their entitlement to manage, and their authority to do, so rests on their responsibility to promote the flourishing of the organisation as a whole. This includes commitment to continuous improvement of the organisation, to improving the competence and productivity of its staff and the standards of service provided for its customers or clients. This can only be done by systematic evaluation and honest research on all aspects, functions and operations in the organisation. Quite apart from the current emphasis on research and evaluation in total quality management, we would want to stress that there is a general ethical duty on health practitioners to evaluate their own performance and the quality of service they provide to patients, in order to improve their knowledge and skills. While not all practitioners wish to, or are able to, undertake actual research, they all should use an evidence base and research data to inform their practice. These duties flow from the fiduciary nature of their professional responsibilities for patients, and while implicitly required of front-line practitioners, they are explicit requirements for the public accountability of managers of healthcare services (Downie & Macnaughton 2000).

Ethically sound and competent management needs to be supported by appropriate research on organisational systems and processes, and staff performance appraisal grounded in evidence-based practice, if it is to deliver quality services/products for its patients or customers. Good 'people-management' skills will also be necessary to deal with the needs of staff and to ensure a worthwhile environment in which they can work and perform to the best of their ability.

In discussing the role of ethics in evaluation and research, we need first to distinguish between the ethical responsibilities of nursing and other healthcare managers *to do sound evaluation and research* related to their organisation's core functions; and secondly the question of applying scientific and ethical standards *in the conduct of research and evaluation,* generally, and in appraisal of services and staff performance in particular.

Ethical principles in applied research

While both the Nursing and Midwifery Council (NMC 2004) and the Royal College of Nursing (RCN) have developed guidelines for nurses, the focus of these has been primarily on ethical standards of individual conduct, and in 2004 the RCN published its *Research Ethics – RCN Guidance for Nurses.* However, neither the NMC nor the RCN has yet addressed the broader question of ethics in organisational governance and professional audit. Guidance from the World Medical Association in its *Declaration of Helsinki* (WMA 2000) sets out useful general guidance for the conduct of medical research involving human subjects, but the WMA has yet to address the issues of strategic ethical management (WMA 2005). Nevertheless the general principles elaborated by the WMA and RCN which apply to clinical research can be extended by analogy to issues in corporate management. The key principles of the *Declaration of Helsinki,* first adopted by WMA in 1964 and amended several times, remain the basis of more specific forms of guidance on the ethics of research in nursing and allied health professions. These principles relate on the one hand to the ethical requirements for sound scientific research, and on the other hand to ethical requirements for the actual conduct of the research (Box 9.1).

(It should be noted that the UK Department of Health, and, in Scotland, SEHD (Chief Scientist Office) have published guidelines via their websites that provide extensive detail about research governance. They also provide links to related websites, e.g. Central Office for Research Ethics Committees,

Box 9.1 Basic principles for all medical research (reproduced from WMA 2000)

1. It is the duty of the physician in medical research to protect the life, health, privacy, and dignity of the human subject.

2. Medical research involving human subjects must conform to generally accepted scientific principles, be based on a thorough knowledge of the scientific literature, other relevant sources of information, and on adequate laboratory and, where appropriate, animal experimentation.

3. Appropriate caution must be exercised in the conduct of research which may affect the environment, and the welfare of animals used for research must be respected.

4. The design and performance of each experimental procedure involving human subjects should be clearly formulated in an experimental protocol. This protocol should be submitted for consideration, comment, guidance, and where appropriate, approval to a specially appointed ethical review committee, which must be independent of the investigator, the sponsor or any other kind of undue influence. This independent committee should be in conformity with the laws and regulations of the country in which the research experiment is performed. The committee has the right to monitor ongoing trials. The researcher has the obligation to provide monitoring information to the committee, especially any serious adverse events. The researcher should also submit to the committee, for review, information regarding funding, sponsors, institutional affiliations, other potential conflicts of interest and incentives for subjects.

5. The research protocol should always contain a statement of the ethical considerations involved and should indicate that there is compliance with the principles enunciated in this Declaration.

6. Medical research involving human subjects should be conducted only by scientifically qualified persons and under the supervision of a clinically competent medical person. The responsibility for the human subject must always rest with a medically qualified person and never rest on the subject of the research, even though the subject has given consent.

7. Every medical research project involving human subjects should be preceded by careful assessment of predictable risks and burdens in comparison with foreseeable benefits to the subject or to others. This does not preclude the participation of healthy volunteers in medical research. The design of all studies should be publicly available.

8. Physicians should abstain from engaging in research projects involving human subjects unless they are confident that the risks involved have been adequately assessed and can be satisfactorily managed. Physicians should cease any investigation if the risks are found to outweigh the potential benefits or if there is conclusive proof of positive and beneficial results.

9. Medical research involving human subjects should only be conducted if the importance of the objective outweighs the inherent risks and burdens to the subject. This is especially important when the human subjects are healthy volunteers.

10. Medical research is only justified if there is a reasonable likelihood that the populations in which the research is carried out stand to benefit from the results of the research.

11. The subjects must be volunteers and informed participants in the research project.

12. The right of research subjects to safeguard their integrity must always be respected. Every precaution should be taken to respect the privacy of the subject, the confidentiality of the patient's information and to minimize the impact of the study on the subject's physical and mental integrity and on the personality of the subject.

13. In any research on human beings, each potential subject must be adequately informed of the aims, methods, sources of funding, any possible conflicts of interest, institutional affiliations of the researcher, the anticipated benefits and potential risks of the study and the discomfort it may entail. The subject should be informed of the right to abstain from participation in the study or to withdraw consent to participate at any time without reprisal. After ensuring that the subject has understood the information, the physician should then obtain the subject's freely-given informed consent, preferably in writing. If the consent cannot be obtained in writing, the non-written consent must be formally documented and witnessed.

14. When obtaining informed consent for the research project the physician should be particularly cautious if the subject is in a dependent relationship with the physician or may consent under duress. In that case the informed consent should be obtained by a well-informed physician who is not engaged in the investigation and who is completely independent of this relationship.

15. For a research subject who is legally incompetent, physically or mentally incapable of giving consent or is a legally incompetent minor, the investigator must obtain informed consent from the legally authorized representative in accordance with applicable law. These groups should not be included in research unless the research is necessary to promote the health of the population represented and this research cannot instead be performed on legally competent persons.

continued

Box 9.1 Basic principles for all medical research (reproduced from WMA 2000)—*cont'd*

16. When a subject deemed legally incompetent, such as a minor child, is unable to give assent to decisions about participation in research, the investigator must obtain that assent in addition to the consent of the legally authorized representative.

17. Research on individuals from whom it is not possible to obtain consent, including proxy or advance consent, should be done only if the physical/mental condition that prevents obtaining informed consent is a necessary characteristic of the research population. The specific reasons for involving research subjects with a condition that renders them unable to give informed consent should be stated in the experimental protocol for consideration and approval of the review

committee. The protocol should state that consent to remain in the research should be obtained as soon as possible from the individual or a legally authorized surrogate.

18. Both authors and publishers have ethical obligations. In publication of the results of research, the investigators are obliged to preserve the accuracy of the results. Negative as well as positive results should be published or otherwise publicly available. Sources of funding, institutional affiliations and any possible conflicts of interest should be declared in the publication. Reports of experimentation not in accordance with the principles laid down in this Declaration should not be accepted for publication.

Multicentre and Local Ethics Committees within the UK. The Research and Development Offices of Health Divisions, e.g. Lothian University Hospitals Division, also have websites that provide guidance/instructions for those who wish to conduct research.)

The Royal College of Nursing points out in the preamble to its publication *Research Ethics* (RCN 2004, p. 4) that nursing has changed considerably since the RCN first set out its guidance on nursing research in 1977:

> Many more nurses are now participating in research for degree programmes; nurses based in higher education are expected to be active in research; and there are more nursing roles with a research and development element, such as nurse consultant. Many nursing activities involve the collection and interpretation of information from and about patients and staff, from small-scale practice development projects to large, multi-centre clinical trials. People are also much more aware of their right to information and consultation about care, treatment and any associated research. There is, as well, a trend towards greater accountability in health care, and research is a vital part of developing the nursing evidence base.
>
> This guidance considers the ethical issues of carrying out research with human subjects, and the areas which you as a nurse researcher, manager, student, member of a research ethics committee or any other relevant role must consider when setting up or advising on research studies. It is a guide to basic principles, and with its extensive list of internet resources, a gateway to further information.

The document continues to point out most usefully the multiple meanings of 'research' and 'evaluation' in nursing and healthcare:

> What do we mean by 'research'? The many ways of collecting and analysing information are described in

varying terms – research, evaluation, clinical audit, quality assurance or student projects – and will vary in depth and scale. The ethical issues are usually the same. While the specifics of approval for studies by research ethics committees will differ for each organisation and according to the type of investigation, this document provides general guidance for all these forms of investigation.

Nurses and other health practitioners may be involved in research in a number of ways:

> Nurses act in a range of roles in research – including carer, student, manager, investigator, research supervisor, sponsor, ethics or governance committee member. Whatever your role, you have clear responsibilities to patients and their families, and to colleagues, to make sure that research you are involved in, or know about, is of the highest standard. As the United Kingdom Nursing and Midwifery Council states, nurses must 'act to identify and minimise the risk to patients and clients'.

The RCN *Research Ethics* document emphasises that nurses are no different from other researchers in that they are subject to the same common law requirements, the duty to seek ethical approval from a competent Research Ethics Committee, and to accept full responsibility for the conduct of their research in accordance with sound research methodology and fundamental ethical principles.

The RCN document then sets out the main ethical issues in nursing research, and these are identified as *respect for every individual* and *respect for the autonomy of research subjects* (including their right to withdraw from a research project without prejudice to their treatment or standard of nursing care). Next the problems of research involving groups of vulnerable people are discussed, in particular the problems of clinical or nursing research involving children and vulnerable adults – who are not able to fully understand what is being proposed and whose competence to give free and voluntary consent is in doubt. The RCN then gives guidance on how to deal in practical terms with the issues of informed consent, patient confidentiality and confidentiality of health records, and finally, stresses the responsibilities of researchers to make realistic estimates of the risks and potential benefits of the research being proposed, as well as the impact on research subjects, once the research study has commenced.

The publication concludes with very helpful advice to nurses on the preparation and submission of research applications to Local Research Ethics Committees (LREC). There is a reminder that in the United Kingdom the UK Central Office for Research Ethics Committees (COREC) coordinates policy and procedures for National Health Service (NHS) ethics committees, and offers useful guidance on approval procedures. Nurses and others involved in healthcare research are obliged to await approval from the appropriate Research Ethics Committee before commencing their research.

WHAT IS MEANT BY EVALUATION IN HEALTHCARE?

We emphasised earlier that research and evaluation are fundamental ethical responsibilities of sound management that is concerned with the well-being of the organisation, its staff and its clients. It is also a requirement of public accountability for the effective and cost-efficient use and administration of human and material resources, and for maintenance and improvements in the quality of services to clients. Hence, the term 'evaluation' has a variety of meanings and applies at various levels in organisational management and professional life:

- evaluation of day-to-day clinical practice, and nursing processes
- evaluation of the effectiveness of individual and team performance
- evaluation of effectiveness in interprofessional and interdisciplinary cooperation
- evaluation of risk assessments and risk management
- evaluation of the competence of healthcare management
- evaluation of outcomes of the service as a whole
- evaluation of measures for quality control and continuous improvement.

To mean anything, evaluation at each of these levels needs to be grounded on facts, and data collected from

evidence-based practice. However, the very term 'evaluation' contains and implies the application of values in the processes of assessment that we use. The implicit or explicit values, or value frame which defines the standpoint from which evaluation is made, also serve to define the aims and objectives of the specific form of evaluation undertaken. From an ethical point of view the crucial first step in evaluation is to be clear about what values are driving the process and how it is to be applied to people and human organisations.

Important components in evaluation

1. *Sound evaluation presupposes prior clarification of values* – this refers to: (i) analysing the personal and professional values of practitioners that inform the intervention to be evaluated; (ii) resolving conflicts between the values of different stakeholders; and (iii) the formulation of a clear statement of common values and the goals that will inform the intervention proposed and its evaluation.
2. *Evaluation requires the setting of achievable objectives* – for healthcare services these may refer to existing National Strategic Objectives or internally defined strategic and operational objectives agreed by the organisation. These need to be realistic in terms of available time, resources and skills.
3. *Evaluation depends upon having reliable intelligence* – this is usually thought to be the domain of researchers or administrators, but practitioners have a key role to play in gathering data accurately and consistently and for offering feedback about how data systems are used. Practitioners will also have a view on how the data are to be interpreted in the light of the processes/interventions they use. How reliable is the information collected?
4. *Evaluation provides a basis for option appraisal and strategic planning* – the data gathered should be used to inform how services are planned and developed at a strategic and operational level. Practitioners need to see this strategy in action in order to maintain motivation to continue data-collection, which can often seem an arduous task. It is the responsibility of operational managers to ensure service developments are reported back to practitioners. this is referred to as the 'feedback loop'.
5. *Evaluation implies ongoing monitoring processes* – evaluation or audit is a continuous process of updating systems, ensuring data are valid and used to inform service planning and delivery.

Usually managers have responsibility to set up systems and practitioners will be invited to feed their data into monitoring processes for quality improvement purposes.

6. *Evaluation is a learning strategy* – where assessment of outcomes is made with reference to pre-set values and goals. Finally, in a learning organisation all stakeholders need to be engaged in the process of reviewing the effectiveness and fairness of the systems employed. Evaluation will involve assessment of: the quality of services actually provided; the adequacy of the data collected for the purpose of identifying achievements and failures or gaps in services; the usefulness and fairness of methods of performance appraisal; and an congruence between all these and an organisation's values and goals (Rossi et al 1999, Nutley et al 2004, CJSWDC 2005) (Box 9.2).

Box 9.2 Stages of evaluation and questions to address (CJSWDC 2005)

Stages of evaluation
1. Clarify objectives
2. Design the evaluation
3. Decide on the data collection methods
4. Plan how the data collected will be processed
5. Think about how the data will be analysed
6. Consider the best methods for reporting and feedback.

Some useful questions
- Who is the evaluation for?
- What is already known about this service or intervention?
- What do we want to know from this evaluation?
- What theory underpins this service or intervention?
- What are the objectives of the action plan and performance indicators?
- What validated measuring tools can be used for assessment?
- How will reporting and feedback on the evaluation be given?
- What decisions will be based on the outcome of an evaluation?
- What are the time /resource constraints?
- What ethical or legal questions arise out of the evaluation?

Types of evaluation

1. *Outcome evaluation:* Outcome evaluation is about results. Have the service plans or interventions met their predetermined objectives? For healthcare interventions, this may mean evaluating the achievements and failures of attempted service improvements, or the extent that evidence-based practice is shown by the quality of data collected.

2. *Process evaluation:* This focuses on the way a piece of work was carried out and how this may have affected the outcomes. For example, does the intervention show programme integrity? Has the programme been applied to meet the real needs of the patients or clients in question? Has there been intelligence-led targeting of resources? Process evaluation seeks to embody 'What works' principles to achieve best practice.

3. *Cost effectiveness evaluation:* Essentially this form of evaluation ascertains 'value for money'. Are the outcomes of the programme worth the inputs? Could similar results have been achieved for less cost? This is distinct from 'cost–benefit analysis', which relates all outcomes in monetary terms. Improvements in health or well-being cannot be simply quantified in monetary terms. While subjective assessments may be an outcome measure for a cost effectiveness evaluation, they should not feature in a cost–benefit analysis.

4. *Realistic evaluation:* This is a model developed by Pawson & Tilley (1997) and asks the evaluator to theorise the whole process of why a programme might work, i.e. looking at inputs, outputs, the context in which the work takes place. Why does a programme work for one person and not another?
   - External evaluation: to provide information to outside agencies and organisations about the aims, objectives, efficiency and effectiveness of an accountable service.
   - Internal: to provide information to practitioners to enable them to review, reflect and modify programme design to improve efficiency and effectiveness for service users.
   Types of data yielded by research:
   - *Prospective:* The integration of the routine collection of data into the operation of programmes. This will normally include 'before' and 'after' measures.
   - *Retrospective:* The collection of data after the event. This can often clarify unstated objectives of a piece of work, e.g. looking at cases or annual evaluation reports over a 3-year period and identifying interventions which were successful and why.

DIFFERENT TYPES OF RESEARCH DESIGN AND THEIR ETHICAL RATIONALES

Research may be conducted for a variety of reasons or purposes, adopting different methods, and with different kinds of ethical rationale.

Variety in the reasons for research: e.g.

- clinical research may be conducted to test the effectiveness of various treatments
- research on staff working practices may be concerned with finding the most effective way of doing things
- research investigations (e.g. comparing business and public sector models) may be concerned with the cost efficiency of different methods of administration of human and material resources, and audit of corporate and individual performance may be required to meet the government's agendas on governance.

Variety in different research methods: e.g. clinical research may be restricted to investigation of the impact of a particular treatment, or a straight comparative study of the effects of different treatments or interventions, or one that involves the use of placebos or control groups; research on methods of delivery, or clinical procedures. It may relate to ways of delivering nursing care, and may range from 'time-and-motion' studies of specific methods of working to participant/ observer studies on a ward.

Research methods may involve gathering 'hard' quantitative data for statistical analysis and comparison of results from different trials, as in epidemiological studies. Alternatively, research on people's attitudes and psychological reactions to various kinds of treatment, or methods of nursing, may require use of a variety of qualitative methods aimed at gathering and then interpreting a great deal of 'soft' data on individuals or groups of research subjects – e.g. in in-depth case studies, or the use of focus groups, interviews and questionnaires – to investigate doctor/patient, nurse/patient or doctor/nurse communication.

Different kinds of ethical rationale for different kinds of research

One of the key assumptions on which all reputable research is based is that the results of the investigation/s will be published and open to critical examination by other investigators. In contrast to *esoteric knowledge* that is regarded as the confidential private property of individuals, groups or sects, *scientific knowledge in principle must be exoteric*, that is, accessible in the public domain, open to experimental testing and rational public criticism.

In the history of medicine, for many centuries, medical knowledge was passed on exclusively to those who were recognised members of a school such as that of Hippocrates or Galen, or of a Royal College or professional guild. In fact the original form of the Hippocratic Oath makes it clear that medical secrets should not be passed on to lay people, and that access to medical knowledge and expertise should be confined to initiated and trained members of the school. The reason for this emphasis on the secret nature of medical knowledge by doctors was, ostensibly to protect patients on the basis that 'a little knowledge is a dangerous thing'. Also, as has often been pointed out, because 'knowledge is power', exclusive proprietorship of medical knowledge is and has been the secret of a doctor's power over their patients, and the basis of the mystique associated with that most potent of medical drugs: Doctor!

This esoteric approach to medical knowledge, and scientific truth generally, persists in one form in the contemporary concern with 'intellectual property rights', namely the right of innovators or inventors to have their contribution to knowledge and scientific progress recognised, and to protect their patents and rights to profit financially from their publications or inventions. The recognition of 'intellectual property rights' is also the basis for our condemnation of plagiarism, of the dishonest representation of someone else's work or inventions as our own. The conventions of research scholarship require us to fully acknowledge our sources, for not to do so would represent a failure to show gratitude for what we have learned from our teachers or colleagues, and more seriously is a kind of theft, punishable by law in some cases.

However, emphasis on 'patent rights' and 'intellectual property rights' is not driven primarily by the individuals concerned to protect their own entitlements to recognition and remuneration for their efforts and discoveries. Many nurses, scientists and medical researchers recognise that they are only able to achieve what they do because of their reliance on what they have learned from others, their dependence on the use of public facilities or resources, and their need for public or private research funding. The real champions of 'patent rights' and 'intellectual property rights' are the large multinational pharmaceutical companies and other industries who undertake the development and marketing of the products or drugs that are mass produced for sale and often worldwide distribution. In reality, they are less concerned with defending the rights of the originators of the ideas or inventions (who frequently get a bad deal), but rather are they concerned with the rights of their shareholders to benefit from the profits. However, this situation may be changing as many academics or universities have set up their own commercial companies, and are seeking to protect their commercial interests too.

Esotericism has always stood in a relationship of tension with the philosophical and scientific quest for exoteric truth, that is, knowledge that is publicly accessible, open to rational criticism and experimental testing, and which is objective in the sense of being verifiable and thus intersubjectively true. Part of the reason Socrates was put to death was due to the opposition he expressed and showed to the Sophists, the self-appointed experts on a variety of subjects, who claimed a proprietorship of the truth they taught, and the right to charge for their services as teachers or instructors! The power of multinational pharmaceutical companies and cartels, to protect their patents on drugs, and the monopolistic control on prices of some applied medical technology industries, can be seen as a major obstacle to the more universal access of people in poor and developing countries to the benefits of new scientific and medical discoveries. Here the struggle of states in sub-Saharan Africa afflicted by the HIV/AIDS epidemic to get a fair deal for the treatment of victims is a case in point.

In some ways, the central ethical question in all research, including medical research, is the question: Cui bono? For whose benefit is this research? Or, who will benefit from this research?

The other fundamental value that drives, or should drive, scientific, medical and social scientific research is the quest for truth, and the right of all people universally to benefit from new discoveries. In fact, the very word 'university' has its origins in the medieval ideal of 'universitas' or universal truth and a public centre for the study and sharing of exoteric truth, and ongoing research for the benefit of humankind.

The quest for truth, as something that is universally valid and publicly testable, is thus linked to a concern for the public good. Neither should research be undertaken simply for one's own profit, or glory, nor even for the benefit of a particular patient or group, but for the common good. While clinical work and the front-line responsibilities of health practitioners are concerned directly with their own duty of care to their patients or clients, and with the individual rights of their patients or clients, when they move into management, teaching or research, a change of mindset and a change of priorities in values may be required. The change of mindset that may be required

is to move from an approach dominated by reactivity to presenting medical problems and crises, to one that is focused on general assessment, policy and action planning, monitoring of processes and interventions and systematic evaluation of impacts and outcomes. The change in value priorities would involve a shift towards a wider concern with public health and the common good, as well as concern with issues of social justice, inequalities in health status and outcomes, and equity in terms of access to healthcare, and in equal employment opportunities at work.

Research methods and their ethical justification

Quantitative methods

The general ethical requirements for medical and scientific research, based on quantitative methods, is that they should involve the rigorous application of scientific methods in research design, in the meticulous conduct of experiments, the making of careful observations and the accurate recording and publication of results, in the general interests of science and ultimately for the advancement of knowledge and the common good. The researcher also has a duty to their funding body to clarify the terms on which the funds are provided, to ensure that these are ethically and legally acceptable, and ultimately to deliver value for money in terms of the quality of the research work done, if the proposed research is scientifically and ethically acceptable.

Experimental design
- *Methodology*: Planning of a specific research design to test an hypothesis, must be based on pre-testing or pilot study of the method of investigation, and effective control of all factors in the research environment that may influence the outcome, except for the one the programme focuses on. The aim is to generate quantitative data and measurable outcomes. The experimental procedure must be replicable by other investigators.
- *Ethical focus*: Impersonal and detachedly objective investigation aimed at factual truth for general scientific purposes. Results are to be achieved by fidelity to rigorous application of scientific method and commitment to high standards of competence and integrity in research investigators. Outcomes should be generalisable to all countries with similar problems.

Quasi-experimental design
- *Methodology*: This uses a comparator ('control') group to compare with a 'treatment' group, where all factors are the same except for subjects in the

programme of intervention. Here controlled trials, randomised controlled trials and double-blind controlled trials represent efforts to achieve more objective evidence as a basis for comparison of outcomes of similar treatments with different groups, or different treatments with similar groups. Again the main object is to achieve measurable and generalisable results in the interests of 'pure science'.

- *Ethical focus*: Again the rationale for the use of control trials, especially in medicine and scientific research involving human subjects, is a concern for universally valid scientific results, and the various procedural requirements, e.g. to eliminate observer bias or discrimination in selection of research subjects, arise from concerns with achieving this. Further, there are considerations of justice and fairness involved; first, towards research subjects themselves, and, secondly, towards those who may benefit in the long run from the research, or suffer because of inadequate trials and premature release of drugs onto the market.

Population surveys and 'market research'

- *Methodology*: The aim is to obtain information in standard form, from surveying samples large enough to yield statistically significant results, e.g. via pre-coded and pre-tested confidential questionnaires; or market-research style 'clip-board and tick the box' interviews, based on a structured interview schedule. Strict procedures need to be observed to ensure randomised selection of respondents or interviewees, and strict adherence to the interview schedule to eliminate observer bias. The object is to achieve results that are statistically significant and capable of being generalised to large populations.

- *Ethical focus*: While more subjective elements may be involved in the choice of questions to ask and how they are formulated, to avoid bias on the part of the researcher, a number of precautions are necessary: first, that the aims and objectives of the investigations should be made clear to the research subjects in advance of their participation; second, that the interview or questionnaire schedule should be pre-tested for bias and ambiguity by conducting a suitable pilot with a sample of the target group; thirdly, that selection of participants should be on a random basis, ensuring a balanced cross-section of the target group; and fourthly, that arrangements should be made for secure storage and controlled access to the interview data, to protect the anonymity and confidentiality of interviewees.

Qualitative methods

Because qualitative methods of research investigation are employed to gain more in-depth information about individuals and groups, there need to be more specific protections built in to the methods and procedures used, to protect the rights of the individuals and groups involved. Qualitative research may set out to study any of a variety of things: e.g. people's attitudes or responses to various proposed or actual interventions; or to study how systems and processes impact on clients, employees or other stakeholders; or how organisational innovations affect individuals; and the whole policy and practice of human resource management.

In qualitative research, investigators must not only address the same broad ethical concerns applicable to quantitative research studies, but must also consider the issues that relate to the researcher's duty of care towards the research subjects, and to respect for the rights of research subjects. These considerations apply to all the forms of qualitative research described below.

In relation to their duty of care, investigators are obliged to consider the general costs and benefits of the research, the risks to research subjects – to avoid prejudicing their interests, causing them harm, or the consequences of failing to protect their confidences. Out of respect for the rights of research subjects, the researcher must ensure their informed consent to participation, the privacy and secure storage of and access to research data, and the protection of subject anonymity and confidentiality. They also have a duty of care to provide counselling or support, or to refer participants to an appropriate source of support, if participation in a research study engenders distress, e.g. recounting distressing events or personal feelings. The researcher also has a duty to clarify with funding bodies the terms on which research funds are provided, to ensure that these are ethically and legally acceptable, and ultimately to deliver value for money in terms of the quality of the research work done, if the proposed research is scientifically and ethically acceptable; and, to publish the results of the research, whether favourable or not.

In-depth 'case study' of single individual This examines in detail one case, an individual, a group or a specific programme. This is exploratory and seeks to identify themes, patterns, and interrelationships for further study.

Participant/Observer study A suitably qualified practitioner participates in the activities under examination, while implementing a pre-arranged programme negotiated with participants, relating to the investigation of processes, staff performance or client responses to services received.

Focus group discussion Semi-structured group discussion with a number of comparable groups, using a series of prompt questions that have been pre-tested with a control group, to explore professional attitudes, service needs, or to get feedback on the acceptability of proposed innovations – often used in consultative processes and in concept development for management and as an aid to strategic planning.

Semi-structured interviews Used for more in-depth exploration of issues that have been previously identified by other methods (e.g. by focus groups or confidential questionnaires), with groups of individual managers, practitioners or clients. The object is to use a standard set of questions to prompt discussion and to gather detailed qualitative data on the issues in question, to inform analysis and possibly further investigations. Alternatively semi-structured interviews may be used *post hoc* to explore, for example, reactions to changes in practice.

Action research Examination of process and outcome in the course of introducing new methods and approaches – to management, service delivery or practitioner functions – with regular feedback into the process to form the basis of change. Usually used in the developmental stage of an intervention or reform and restructuring process.

Triangulation Use of more than one research method, data source or investigator, in the attempt to get a more comprehensive and 'three-dimensional' picture of the reality being investigated.

Evidence-based practice

'Evidence-based practice' is one of the 'buzz words' of the current management discourse in the health and social services, along with 'clinical audit', 'performance assessment' and 'clinical, staff and organisational governance'. The new jargon is part of the rhetoric of modernising initiatives of government and the reform and restructuring of health and welfare services. The overall objective is to base innovation and change not on speculation or political dogma, but on actual evidence of need and outcomes of current practice, with a view to making health and welfare services more effective and efficient, and to improve the quality of services to clients.

'Evidence-based practice' could be said to be a fancy name for evaluation and research as these are applied to the health and human services. The new rhetoric means in essence the systematic *use of the results of evaluation and research in appraisal* of an organisation, its services and the performance of its

staff. The terms 'evidence-based practice' or 'clinical audit' are not new to the UK NHS. Their origins can be traced back to Cochrane's *Effectiveness and Efficiency: Random Reflections on Health Services* (1971), and to the recommendations of the Chief Medical Officer in the *Independent Inquiry into Inequalities in Health* (Acheson Report 1988), as well as to academic publications on the subject in the early 1990s (Harrison 1998).

Attempts were made by the UK government, in the early 1990s, to introduce clinical audit and to recommend the adoption of evidence-based practice throughout the NHS. However, these 'new approaches' were patchily taken up and not systematically applied. This was partly because the collection of data was patchy and not systematic. It was also because the use of 'clinical audit' and 'evidence-based practice' was associated in the minds of many healthcare practitioners with attempts at imposed reform by the new breed of government-appointed managers (often imported from business and industry). Their controlling form of directive management based on performance appraisal, and evidence-based practice, appeared to threaten the clinical autonomy of health practitioners and expose them to criticism.

By making 'performance management' and 'evidence-based practice' key planks in their proposals for the 'New NHS', the Blair government's attempts to introduce reforms based on 'total quality management' and 'continuous quality improvement' models have faced resistance. While there has been slow acceptance of the need for clinical, staff and organisational governance, it has taken time to get commitment to adopt evidence-based practice and performance management in the NHS. This has been despite the government's attempts to give the new vocabulary a more positive spin; to consult widely and negotiate with management, professional bodies and unions on performance standards; and to emphasise the responsibility for sound record-keeping and data collection at all levels to make possible organisational and professional performance appraisal across the board, and not simply to apply performance appraisal to employees or health practitioners.

As Harrison (2004, pp. 216–217) explains, there was growing recognition that the quality of healthcare cannot be improved without sound evidence and this implies the necessity for adoption of evidence-based practice. There was general acknowledgement that several problems needed to be addressed:

> [F]irst, that clinical practice was not currently informed by accurate and up-to-date research findings; secondly, that ineffective and inappropriate interventions wasted resources that could be used more effectively; thirdly, that variations in the use of effective treatments created

unacceptable inequities, with some people failing to get access to the best care. (see Grayson 1997, Harrison 1998, Muir Gray 2001)

However, the pressure to accept cultural change and a new systematic approach to organisational governance and quality improvement was due to the fact that:

A formidable coalition of support underpinned efforts to improve evidence-based practice. Health professionals saw evidence-based practice as preserving the scientific credibility of health care and enabling them to retain control over their work. Politicians and health service managers believed that it made the health budget go further and gave them greater influence over the allocation of resources. Patients' representatives welcomed it as a means to improve and universalise the quality of care. (Harrison 2004, p. 216)

Harrison points out further that there were several constructive developments arising out of the adoption of 'evidence-based practice' and a basis for the 'New NHS'. These were:

- New funding for research and development had been given following the Culyer Report (DoH 1994) to help determine national and regional research priorities. However, this was consolidated by further funding and policy endorsement by the Blair government (see DoH 2000b, 2001f).
- Other initiatives to strengthen evidence-based practice include continuing professional development and the dissemination of information about effective practice to professionals and managers.
- Those commissioning healthcare are expected to do so on the basis of evidence. Under the Conservative government of the 1990s, guidance was issued to promote investment in effective treatments and disinvestment in those of doubtful effectiveness (NHSE 1996). Under New Labour, increasingly, clinical guidelines and National Service Frameworks are included in the specification of service agreements. This has been reinforced by a duty of quality on NHS organisations, and the introduction of systems of clinical, staff and organisational governance (Harrison 2004, p. 217, Muir Gray 2001).
- Finally, the Blair government established new institutions to oversee clinical effectiveness and service quality: a National Institute for Clinical Excellence (NICE) to produce guidelines on clinical and cost effectiveness of services; and a Commission for Health Improvement (now the Commission for Healthcare Audit and Inspection) to promote improvements in clinical services. In addition, new bodies were established to protect patient safety and improve poor performance among professionals, such as the National Patient Safety Agency (Harrison 2004, p. 217).

Methodological and ethical issues related to evidence-based practice

From the beginning, the introduction of evidence-based practice (EBP) into clinical medicine has been controversial, as well as its introduction into healthcare management (see Muir Gray 2001 and Baggott 2004, p. 218).

At the level of clinical practice, some doctors have objected to the introduction of EBP on several different but related grounds:

- First, that having to base their choice of drugs or treatments on generalised conclusions drawn from large sample surveys fails to recognise that clinical judgements often have to be made in individual cases with reference to their unique features or circumstances.
- Secondly, that use of EBP in the attempt to rationalise the allocation of resources and to reduce costs in healthcare would limit the range of treatment available to NHS patients.
- Thirdly, that resource allocation decisions, based on EBP, would restrict their clinical autonomy and right to choose what they regarded as the best treatment for their patients (Haycox et al 1999).

Both doctors and other health practitioners have questioned the ulterior motives of managers and policy planners for introducing EBP into healthcare. Emphasis on EBP has been seen as having less to do with ultimate benefits for patients, and more to do with 'cuts by stealth'. EPB was seen as a tool to achieve cost cutting under the guise of improving quality (see Hurwitz, 1999, Harrison 1998). Colyer & Karmath (1997) argue from a nursing standpoint that emphasis on EPB has tended to reinforce a medical model of research in healthcare at the cost of ignoring research on patients' emotional and human needs. Others argued that the introduction of EBP would require extra funds for staff training in the use of the new methods, and to meet the costs of research, organisational change, the setting of guidelines and the updating of publications (Jankwoski 2001, Shekelle et al 2001). A similar range of criticisms is reflected in the recent symposium on EBP in the *Journal of Medical Ethics* (Vol. 30 (2), 2004). Saarni & Gylling (2004), for example, question whether EBP is not a solution to rationing or politics disguised as science. This and other papers raise a range of other ethical and methodological questions relating to EBP, to which we now turn.

General methodological criticisms of 'evidence-based practice' have focused on the unexamined use of the term 'evidence' by the advocates of EBP – without either critical discussion of its underlying philosophical assumptions or justification for the kind of epistemology which appears to underlie the whole approach. What we mean by 'evidence' or 'facts' is not self-evident. The uncritical use of these terms begs the question of what interpretative frame of reference and theoretical criteria are being used in decisions as to what is to count as evidence. The terms 'evidence' and 'facts' are systematically ambiguous, unless the proponents of EBP make explicit the underlying theoretical presuppositions and interpretative frame that they are using.

Philosophical criticism of EBP is that its use appears to rest on the methodological assumptions of an unexamined positivistic theory of knowledge, namely, that the meaning of 'evidence' is transparently obvious. The really interesting question, and challenge for those employing EBP to address or negotiate about is what will count as relevant evidence for them, and in relation to what criteria evidence will be interpreted and analysed, or in relation to what targets and what performance indicators evidence will be considered. To ignore these methodological questions is to disregard all we have learned from postmodern criticism of positivism and scientism, namely, that what is critically important, and often controversial, is the theoretical perspective from which we approach scientific method and research. 'Facts' and 'evidence' are not theory-neutral, but only make sense within a specific interpretative frame of reference.

If we do not openly and critically examine the theoretical assumptions underlying the use of EBP, the use of this approach tends to arouse suspicion, because uncritical adoption of EBP may obscure the other pragmatic reasons why EBP has been introduced at this time, and used as part of the restructuring and reform of health and welfare services. Apart from these epistemological questions, the key question as we have said is the question: Cui bono? Whose good or whose interests does EBP serve? Patients? Management? Or government?

Some of the key ethical questions that arise regarding EBP also relate to the methodological issues discussed above. Perhaps the fundamental ethical issue is whether or not those introducing EBP into any organisation, or into the NHS, are open and transparent about their motives and intentions for introducing EBP as a basis for performance management, the rationalising of practice and as a basis for cost-cutting and resource allocation decisions.

Firstly, there are ethical questions to be raised about *how EBP is introduced* – whether by consultation and negotiation, or by managerial edict – as the style in which innovation and change is introduced is critically important to its acceptance and acceptability to all stakeholders in the organisation. Any organisation, if it is to function effectively as a cooperative moral community, must be based on trust and mutual respect. Respect for management cannot be demanded unless management respects the views, expertise and input of staff. Cultural change and innovations in practice cannot be brought about by managerial fiat or even by legislation. High-handed management will generate resentment, distrust and a spirit of non-cooperation. Attempts to enforce change by legislation breed cynicism and passive resistance to change.

Secondly, what is euphemistically called 'change management' cannot be about manipulation of staff, if it is to allay fears and anxiety of staff about restructuring, possible staff cuts, and general job insecurity. If an atmosphere of openness and trust is to be created, then the management of change must be based on developing shared understanding and common agreement about what the strengths and weaknesses of an organisation are. It also requires common agreement about what needs to be done to improve things. Without direct involvement of stakeholders in organisational, staff and clinical appraisal, without their shared contribution to the setting up of arrangements for governance at these different levels, change will be seen as a threat to individuals and established practice, and resisted – rather than seen as an opportunity and supported. Just as there should be joint exploration and acknowledgement of the strengths of an organisation, its systems and practices, there should to be 'full and frank' discussion of its weaknesses at each level of operations. Similarly, there must be open sharing of hopes and fears relating to organisational change and changes to the scope of professional responsibility and practice. Here too there must be open and frank acknowledgement of the threats facing the organisation and individuals, as well as the opportunities that change offers for both, as well as the potential benefits to clients and all concerned from quality improvement.

Research evidence has shown that the chief failure of attempts to introduce total quality management, including performance appraisal based on evidence-based practice, is due to it being imposed from above without proper consultation or negotiation, and without opportunity for all stakeholders to take part in the process of review and planning for the future (George & Weimerskirch 1994, James 1996).

There are other more general ethical considerations to be addressed with the introduction of performance management and evidence-based practice, namely, how the proposed innovation and change is to benefit the organisation's clients or customers, and how they are to be protected from adverse consequences of change as it impacts on the services and treatment that they are entitled to expect. To address these concerns, major organisational and cultural change in healthcare services, in patterns of service delivery, and in redefinition of the roles and responsibilities of staff, all need to be effectively communicated to the general public. Where possible the community should be involved in the process, through consultation and arrangements for critical or positive feedback from patients, clients or customers, as the new systems and services come into operation.

EVIDENCE-BASED PRACTICE AND CONTINUOUS QUALITY IMPROVEMENT

Nutley et al (2004), in their review *Learning from Knowledge Management*, explain that the concern with *evidence-based policy and practice* for public and private sector managers is to ensure that research evidence has a greater impact on the policy-making process, on the organisation of appropriate and effective service delivery, and the patterns of professional formation and practice. In the health and social services this essentially means moving from management, based on anecdotal evidence derived from a reactive individual 'clinical' or case-work approach, to a proactive evidence-based 'epidemiological' approach.

If the goal of a well-administered, properly evaluated, efficient and accountable health service is to be achieved, then the processes, methods and standards that need to be applied in 'performance management' and 'evidence-based' management must be properly understood and applied at all levels in the organisation. In other words, a corporate and strategic approach to evaluation is required. Research evidence (see review of evidence in James 1996) has shown that sound organisational development and staff development depend on one another. This means that all stakeholders in the organisation need to be involved in developing the organisation's strategic plan and ethical policy. In this way, all stakeholders contribute to the development of continuous improvement processes, are encouraged to support its implementation, and become committed to evidence-based practice, by seeing it work in practice – to improve both the quality of services and their own skills and competence.

Performance management is concerned with the efficient and accountable performance of a whole organisation – at strategic, middle management and service delivery levels – and must be based on rigorous evaluation that is responsive to the concerns and needs of all its stakeholders. This must be based on reliable two-way feedback throughout the organisation and at all levels. George & Weimerskirch (1994) stress the need for such an integrated approach to strategic management:

> Management does not mean being controlling, but being in control of oneself and having a grasp of the *raison d'etre* of the organisation. … Leadership and management of organisations small and large, means accepting responsibility for the whole organisation and commitment to its well-being, and that means comprehending in planning, operations and evaluation all the interrelationships between people, processes and things that determine success. It also demands vigilance to recognise those forces that are dysfunctional and deal effectively with them before they become destructive.

Responsibility and accountability are the twin sides of any corporate management that is strategically planned and where performance at all levels can be evaluated and routinely reviewed with a view to continuous improvement of organisational performance, service delivery, competence of staff and client satisfaction.

George & Weimerskirch (1994) set out the following guidance for managers:

- Know exactly what your customers (or clients) require.
- Have well-defined processes to translate requirements into internal actions.
- Align all your tasks and processes along common goals and objectives.
- Use key measures to manage by fact (not fantasy!).
- Involve everyone in continuous improvement processes.
- Understand and improve all your critical processes by regular review.
- Aim to satisfy your customers and be able to prove it.

Reliable evidence of this kind is the only foundation on which sound performance management can be based, for sound performance management requires effective knowledge management. It also requires readily available and intelligible data, usually provided by practitioners as a by-product of casework. Ensuring overall intelligence gathering and sound evaluation in the service as a whole is a challenge in both collaborative development and systems design. It also serves as the foundation for regular organisational review and strategic planning.

Principles required for continuous quality improvement of services and practice

Continuous improvement may sound well as a corporate aspiration, but it remains little more than a pious wish unless there is evidence to back up any claims we make to progress.

It may be self-evident, but not always recognised in practice, that unless we have:

- clear objectives that have been specified in advance
- a baseline against which to measure progress
- agreed standards for appraisal, and
- factual evidence of having attained our declared objectives

then claims that services or practice are good, or have been improved, remain speculative.

Defining our objectives is not a once-for-all activity, but these will have to be constantly reviewed in the light of progress and unscheduled developments. However, objectives do not fall out of the air, nor should they be 'sucked out of someone's thumb'. They need to be generated by a process where representative stakeholders from all levels in the organisation have a direct part.

This process involves a number of important steps for both internal and external stakeholders:

- clarifying the organisation's core business and related mission and setting this down
- developing a vision for the way the mission is to be achieved
- clarifying and formulating a statement of the core values of the service
- developing clear goals and objectives consistent with the service mission and values.

Once these are in place, systems and processes can be introduced to achieve the agreed objectives and then to evaluate their organisational and individual performance in doing so.

Health services, like other public services, face the constant challenge of improving their overall performance *and being able to demonstrate that they are doing so.* They need good evidence that they are responding to clients' needs, meeting community concerns, and constantly improving the service and achieving better outcomes for their clients. This means improving the efficiency of their processes, the effectiveness of their service delivery for patients and

clients, and being able to produce evidence to show the effectiveness of what they have done.

To be able to demonstrate improvement in services and outcomes for clients, managers and practitioners need to have sound data, based on routine record-keeping, which can be aggregated and analysed to produce measurable evidence of their achievements and to identify where further improvements are needed. Once obtained, such evidence can prove a useful lever in negotiations with local health authorities or government for resources, or can serve as a useful weapon to defend the local service from ill-informed public or political criticism.

While local health authorities may wish to develop their own statements of principle, the following *seven guiding principles for continuous improvement* are offered as a starting point for constantly improving service delivery and developing more effective management:

1. Client and community perceptions determine quality.
2. Enhance systems by improving processes.
3. Treat external service providers as partners.
4. Decision-making is based on knowledge and recorded data.
5. Involve everyone creatively in continuous improvement.
6. Strategic planning drives improvement.
7. Managers and practitioners lead by example.

Teamwork, evaluation and continuous improvement

What is said here about the methods needed to ensure continuous improvement is intended to assist local health services to achieve at least the following three desired outcomes as a measure of their future success:

- clients and carers who are satisfied with the service they receive
- enjoyment and fulfilment in work for those in the service
- successful teamwork to achieve agreed objectives within budget.

A major factor in achieving these outcomes will be the development of effective teamwork in the organisation as a whole and at its different levels – corporate executive, middle management, and primary care or hospital teams.

The metaphor of a 'team' is borrowed from sport. While this metaphor, like any analogy, has its limitations, much can be learned from reflection on the requirements for a 'good' team. For example, a sports team requires that a number of people exercise different roles, e.g. as leader, trainer, referee, manager, front-line, mid-field and defensive players and back-up. Some requirements are intangibles like trust and loyalty, commitment and conscientiousness. Others are functional requirements like turning up for joint training, joint planning and willingness to follow the 'game-plan', willingness to share responsibility for the outcomes of the game. Teamwork not only means being willing and able to play effectively together. It also means willingness to contribute to evaluation of team and individual performance, to give and receive feedback on your own performance, to acknowledge and celebrate team and individual achievements and to recognise the need for further skills training.

DIFFERENT ETHICAL RESPONSIBILITIES AT DIFFERENT LEVELS IN MANAGEMENT

In Chapter 2 we introduced what we called the 'Russian dolls model' to represent the different levels of ethical responsibility nested within each other in organisational life, viz:

- micro level – responsibility for direct patient care and delivery of services to patients
- 'macho' level – responsible participation in and leadership of teams of nurses and other staff
- meso level – responsible management of a ward, clinic or institution
- macro level – responsibility for internal and external policy with relevant stakeholders.

We pointed out in that context that different kinds of ethics apply at each of these different levels. The first has to do with the ethics of personal decision-making in dealing with patients or clients. The second has to do with the ethics of leadership and teamwork in both uni-professional and multiprofessional teams. The third relates to ethics in strategic planning, corporate management and administration of financial and other resources. The fourth level concerns the political ethics of dealings with external service providers or with government and funding bodies. When we say that different kinds of ethics apply at these different levels, we are not saying that different principles apply at each of these levels, but rather that the scope of the traditional principles (of beneficence/ non-maleficence, justice and respect for persons) will be wider or narrower, depending on the level at which we are operating. Tensions between these principles, and which principle tends to be given priority, will vary between the different levels.

In Part 3 we concentrated on analysis of the issues that arise directly in clinical practice, both at the level of direct patient care and in management of service delivery at the ground level. Here in Part 4 we will be moving on to examine ethics in nursing management, research and health policy. In other words, in Part 3 we were concerned mainly with the micro and macho levels of nursing practice, and here, in Part 4, we will address the meso and macro levels at which nurses may be expected to exercise professional responsibility.

As we have pointed out earlier, the tensions at the *individual level* of responsibility for patients tend to be between the primary duty of care owed by the nurse to the vulnerable patient (beneficence) and the need to respect the patient's autonomy and individual rights (respect for persons). Clearly individual practitioners have to consider issues of justice and equity when faced with conflicting demands of different individual patients. However, justice and equity issues more commonly arise at the *level of managing groups of patients* on a ward, or a case-load in the community; and, in dealing with the division of labour and resource allocation, in negotiations with other members of the team. At this level, conflicts tend to arise between the demand for equal access to care and treatment for all patients and the need to address the urgent needs of individual patients. The tension here is primarily between justice and equity, on the one hand, and respect for the rights of individuals, on the other. At the *level of corporate management*, the recurrent challenge will be to balance the conflicting demands of all three principles, e.g. justice or fairness for all patients; respect for the rights of both patients and staff; and the statutory requirement that health professionals exercise a duty of care towards the patient (and sometimes impatient) public! Finally at the *policy planning and strategic level*, the principles of equality of access to healthcare (justice and equity) and the state's duty of care and responsibility for its most vulnerable citizens tend to be the primary focus of corporate managers and policy-makers – with less emphasis on individual rights and greater emphasis on the common good.

Nurses, like doctors and other health professionals, have to exercise responsibility at these different levels at different times, at different stages of their careers and in relation to changes in the political climate and public policy on health and social services. It is not surprising therefore that these challenges present some nurses with a kind of 'identity crisis'. This leads us to reflect on the different roles that they are expected to fulfil, and the different possible models in terms of which their identity as nurses in these roles can be appropriately expressed. We proceed to discuss some of these as they apply to the ethics of leadership and management, for nurses and other health professionals.

Early in the last century, Fayol suggested five basic functions of management: *planning, organising, leading, controlling* and *staffing* (Coubrough 1930). In the first place, then, ethics in management is not just about observing a code of ethics, but is about managers' ethical responsibility to develop their knowledge and skills in all these areas, so as to be able to undertake these functions competently and efficiently for the benefit of the organisation, the clients and staff, and for their own professional satisfaction.

- *Competence in planning nursing or health services* would require managers to gain knowledge of government health policy, local strategy, policy and procedures, understanding of the service's general strengths and weaknesses, and reliable evidence of its current standard of performance.
- *Competence in organising nursing or health services* would require not only knowledge of existing systems and procedures, but relevant experience of working in the area and of organising services at a lower level.
- *Competence in leadership* would require a variety of personal qualities or virtues that research has shown are of critical importance, namely courage, dependability, flexibility, integrity, judgement and respect for others (George & Weimerskirch 1994).
- *Competence in controlling systems and processes, resources and employees* would require having had relevant previous experience in similar organisations, ability to see the big picture and to distinguish the relative importance of long-term and short-term goals, and to have proven 'people management' skills.
- *Competence in staffing matters* would require a manager to have knowledge and skills in the legal and ethical aspects of staff selection, their supervision, professional development and performance management, including application of the principles of equal employment opportunity, beneficence, justice and respect for employees' rights.

While in the past, managers might have been able to act as a law unto themselves – especially in private companies, but also where chief executives were government appointees – this is now no longer possible, nor is it culturally acceptable. There has been a growing awareness of the responsibilities of managers, not only to their shareholders, trustees or boards, but also to all their 'stakeholders' – those with an interest or stake in the business or service being delivered (Beauchamp & Bowie 1997, Ch. 2).

It may be obvious to us that the interests of the 'patients', 'clients', 'customers' or 'consumers' should be paramount in the delivery of health services, but this has by no means been the case in the past. Nor have the interests of professional staff and other employees always been considered important. Some regard may have been shown to external stakeholders such as suppliers and partner or competitor organisations, and to local or national government. However, strategic planning is only now beginning to take account of the need for coherent ethical policy in relation to all stakeholders and for methods of evaluation and performance appraisal that can serve as a basis for the public accountability that goes with running a business organisation or providing public services.

The view that ethics is an integral and critically important part of corporate life and management has grown in importance over the past half-century as public and private sector organisations have had to face growing demands for public accountability from various pressure groups representing such stakeholders as 'patients', 'clients', 'customers' and 'consumers', the trades unions representing employees, or legal firms representing these or other shareholders. This movement has been driven partly by public reaction to corruption scandals, and partly by political concern about inefficiency and waste of taxpayers' (or shareholders') money. However, it has also been given impetus by the growing volume of research on the importance of sound corporate ethics to good business and public sector governance (Kitson & Campbell 1996, Grace & Cohen 1998).

We would argue that the primary responsibility of any manager is not simply to manage people and resources effectively and efficiently, but also to help create the kind of moral community at work, which encourages ethical practice. Promoting best practice in the delivery of services and best value for money is itself an ethical enterprise, for critical value-judgements are involved in determining what we mean by 'best practice' and 'best value for money'. These cannot be decided on purely econometric tests, but on agreed criteria of what 'quality' means in terms of standards of performance, efficient and effective service delivery and client satisfaction. Management is therefore critically concerned with the creation of an ethical culture, in which, by good leadership, people will be enabled to deliver client services effectively and efficiently, maintain high standards of professional expertise and competence, and practitioners be enabled to make progress in their careers – because the

Box 9.3 **Taylor's principles of management**

Taylor's worker principles

1. Develop a science for each man's work – the one best way.
2. Scientifically select the one best man for the job and train him in the procedures he is expected to follow.
3. Cooperate with the men to ensure that the work is in fact done in the way prescribed. This should include, but not be limited to, providing for increased earnings by those who follow the prescribed way most closely.
4. Divide the work so that activities such as planning, organising and controlling are the prime responsibility of management rather than the individual worker.

Normative principles of Taylorism

- Always securing the full support of management.

- A complete mental revolution on the part of both management and workers.

- Workers should help management establish scientifically the facts about production.

- Workers should agree to be trained in and follow new methods prescribed.

- Management should set up a suitable organisation which would take all responsibility from the worker except that of actual performance of the jobs.

- Management should agree to be governed by the science developed for each operation and to the facts and in so doing surrender its arbitrary power over the workers.

From James (1996, p. 20).

Box 9.4 **Fayol's principles of management**

1. Division of work: The development of specialised work practices that would enhance the efficiency of the task.

2. Authority and responsibility: Authority is the right to command and expect others to carry them out. However, this may not always occur, for varying reasons. Both authority and responsibility should be balanced.

3. Discipline: This is an expected requirement of adhering to rules and codes. They should be fairly applied and understood by all.

4. Unity of command: Only one superior for each employee because confusing signals and demands may develop.

5. Unity of direction: Each employee, group and department should be working to satisfy the same aims and develop objectives that support these.

6. Organisation: Organisations should have a scalar chain, which is a chain of authority running from top to bottom.

7. Equity: Employees should be treated fairly using published standards and requirements.

8. Initiative: Worker initiative should be encouraged and should carry out plans for improvement.

9. Structure: There should be a balance between centralisation and decentralisation.

From James (1996, p. 23).

working environment encourages staff development, job satisfaction and good working relationships.

Concern with improving the standards and quality of services to patients and their relatives, in hospitals and primary care, has recently become a matter of public interest in the media and in local and national politics in many countries. The media have discovered that coverage of health matters attracts public attention and boosts their sales or viewing figures, and this has impacted on the political agenda. While concern with 'quality control', 'best practice', 'quality assurance', 'continuous quality improvement' and 'total quality management' may have been driven partly by politics and the media, it is from the experience of business and industry that the importance of ethics and an emphasis on standards and quality control has arisen. The use of terms like 'quality assurance' and 'best practice' is not just a matter of rhetoric, or of the use of the latest 'buzz

words' from management consultants. Independent research in health services and other public sector organisations has shown that issues of quality control and performance management are critical both to improving standards and to customer satisfaction (James 1996, Pt 3, Baggott 2004, Ch. 9).

While the rhetoric and business jargon may be new, some of the principles of sound ethical management were articulated at the beginning of the 20th century. Two experienced managers, Frederick Taylor (1856–1915) and Henry Fayol (1841–1925), set out criteria for management that have had an extensive influence on management theory and debate about the role of values and ethics in corporate life and strategic planning. The first looked at the practical and ethical issues of management from the worker's perspective, the latter at the principles of management that apply more universally to corporate life (Boxes 9.3 and 9.4).

Taylor was respected by business and industry,

as an efficiency consultant, and his principles have continued to influence management theory and the quality movement, despite the fact that they relate to a time when the workforce was largely untrained and unskilled. However, even then he was not solely concerned with efficiency and profits, but with empowering workers too.

Henry Fayol was a mining engineer, more broadly concerned with a coherent approach to the management and administration of large organisations with responsibility for large projects. Given his five basic functions of management, discussed earlier, namely planning, organising, leading, controlling and staffing, his principles of management are concerned with the overall strategic direction of organisations, as viewed from the perspective of senior management.

Box 9.5 **Models for management in the delivery of healthcare**

Command management – traditional
(traditional hospital preventive health services)
- *Style*: Directive management based on power of office
- *Paradigm*: Administration of medical or preventive services
- *Main ethic*: Responsible duty to care (protective beneficence)

Critical expertise – research driven
('evidence-based' nursing, intersectoral 'new public health' approach)
- *Style*: Authoritative advice based on scientific evidence and research
- *Paradigm*: Medical or academic health research institute
- *Main ethic*: Rational justice – concern for social equity and the common good

Community development – facilitative leadership
('community health' and positive health promotion)
- *Style*: Facilitative, participative and democratic
- *Paradigm*: Promoting health through community self-help and skills transfer
- *Main ethic*: Respect for personal and community rights – empowering people

Corporate policy planning – strategic management
(free market, consumer-led and economic management approach)
- *Style*: Proactive engagement with politics of healthcare delivery
- *Paradigm*: Business management and quality assurance
- *Main ethic*: Economic justice for taxpayers through cost-efficiency savings

---

FOUR MODELS FOR THE ETHICS OF MANAGEMENT

There is another group of situations in which nurses or other health professionals are involved when they move out of direct patient care into *management*, into *teaching and research*, in the exercise of *community leadership*, and in more 'political' roles in *corporate policy direction*. The models, which are applicable, become more complex and various, but it may be useful to discuss them under four different headings: command management, critical expertise, community development, and corporate planning (Box 9.5).

Command management model (Fig. 9.1)

The exercise of power and responsibility in traditional management roles is tied up with the concept of authority. To exercise authority you must be authorised by some person or body of persons to hold some official post or to carry out some official function. Authority in this sense means legitimate power – power legitimated by election, official promotion, or direct appointment by higher authority, e.g. by a 'matron', 'operations manager' or 'hospital administrator'. To exercise authority also means, as we have said, to exercise power in such a way that you

Command management

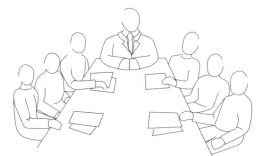

Situation – Institutional Setting

Manager In position of authority	**Staff** In subordinate position
Responsible for:- Implementing policy and strategic plan	**Responsible to:-** Line manager and clients
Accountable to: Higher management/CEO Government/Public	**Accountable to:** Employing authority Public courts

Figure 9.1 Command management model.

work to promote the well-being of those over whom you have authority, and do not act just to promote your own interest or those of the institution. Thus the naked or dictatorial exercise of power offends against the duty to care, the requirements of natural justice and respect for persons under your authority.

Management styles, even within the traditional line-management model, can vary according to the personality and skills (or lack of skills) of the manager. Personal management styles within different systems can vary from a controlling style to a permissive one, from directive to democratic, authoritarian to consensus-based. Organisationally, line management, or a straight 'top-down' chain of command, tends to be the predominant mode of relations within the nursing hierarchy, and it has a long history in traditional hospital organisation. This corresponds to the pattern and requirements of management in large institutions dealing with situations of crisis such as war or disaster, or medical, surgical and psychiatric emergencies. However, some form of team management, with shared authority and responsibility, may be accepted as more appropriate in other areas, as is becoming evident in primary care, rehabilitation, and the care of people who have enduring physical or mental health problems.

The increased emphasis on communication and on working within multidisciplinary teams that is now explicit within the educational curricula of medicine, nursing and allied health professions has directed practitioners towards a more collegiate approach to decision-making.

It is not our purpose to discuss the advantages or disadvantages of the different models or styles of management here, but rather to stress that each embodies certain values and is based on different formal and informal ethical conventions. Roles will be different within each system, as well as the formal and informal rules which obtain, and expectations about who is responsible ('who carries the can') and to whom officers are accountable ('who will blame me if things go wrong?'). From an ethical point of view, each kind of management may be exercised well or badly, and each needs to be assessed in context and on its own terms.

Traditional line management invests considerable power in those at the top, who, it is assumed, will exercise power responsibly in a just and beneficent way, even though they may be employed with a specific mandate to improve efficiency and to make savings. This kind of justification is used in defence of the new managerialism ('Let the managers manage') (Harrison 2004, Baggott, 2004) and their application of economic rationalist criteria in determining priorities.

Thus, for example, if there have to be staff cuts, it is assumed that these will be justifiable on both ethical and economic grounds, that they will not be made capriciously but in a way that is fair, protects the wider interests of the service, does not discriminate against particular groups, and has due regard to the statutory rights of employees.

Alternatively, in a more democratic style of health-care team management, the values of respect for persons tend to have a higher priority. In principle this should be apparent in the respect shown to one another by people of different professional background, in regard for one another's expertise, sharing of work and responsibility, and exchange of information about patients or clients. It should also be reflected in their style of interaction with patients or clients and respect shown for their rights.

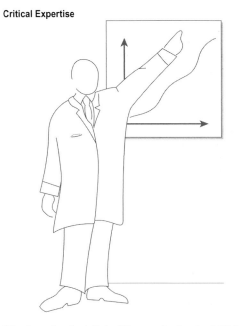

Critical Expertise

Situation – Academic/Scientific or professional establishment

Professional Director	Staff
Identified Expert/ Authority **Responsible to:-** Professional peers and professional body **Accountable to:** Employing authority and the courts	Take orders from expert **Responsible in:-** Dependent executive role and functions **Responsible to:** Director and employers

Key Principle: Rational justice and duty of care

Figure 9.2 Critical expertise model.

Critical expertise model (Fig. 9.2)

All professions base their right to practise, their claim to special status and regard in the eyes of other professions and the public on their mastery of certain knowledge and skills. It is also on the basis of their expertise that they are given responsibility for the disposal and administration of certain public resources (Freidson 1994, Bayles 1989). Therefore, education and training play an important part in the preparation of professionals for their work, serving both as a basis for their claims to special knowledge and expertise, whether in helping others or in performing some other function, and as the means for legitimating their power and authority in the exercise of that service to the public. The responsibility of a profession to maintain the highest possible standards in education and training is not just about maintaining status and power, but it is perhaps more fundamentally a requirement of justice to ensure that they are competent to provide a skilled and efficient service for the benefit of their clients and society as a whole. However, emphasis on professional autonomy often had more to do with protecting the interests of practitioners rather than protecting the public – as several recent enquiries have pointed out in criticising the General Medical Council for its failure to take action when there were allegations of malpractice (Shipman Inquiry 2001).

However, professional education and training are not of much value if they perpetuate bad practice, if they are never properly evaluated. Thus teaching and research must be integrally related, in the interests of ensuring the competence and efficiency of staff, of the service as a whole and effective and cost-efficient care for clients and patients.

This is where 'evidence-based practice' becomes relevant for both ethical and practical reasons. Ability to provide objective evidence and sound research to justify specific interventions or general nursing practice is not only a demand of scientific integrity, but is ultimately also an ethical demand. Incompetence, or the use of ineffective measures, is not only blameworthy in the individual, but is unjust to others who depend on one's expertise, and who may be paying as well. Not only the financial but also the human cost should be considered, thus raising questions of respect for persons and their rights. In comparative evaluation of the cost efficiency of different procedures or management practices, not only considerations of an economic nature are relevant but also the common good of patients.

Specific ethical issues in teaching and research are discussed in Chapter 12 but the point of raising them

here is that critical enquiry and proper evaluation is an important ethical responsibility of any profession. Competent and efficient care is a moral demand of the principle of beneficence, in the protection of clients from incompetence and malpractice, and it is not possible to prevent either without sound education and training, and scientific research to validate professional practice. Truthfulness is not only about honesty and sharing information with individual patients or clients, it is also about scientific integrity, rigour in enquiry, and honesty in the publication of research findings for the benefit of all health services. Use of sound knowledge and skills is essential for the training of professionals in the responsible care and rehabilitation of those who seek help. This is a requirement of beneficence and respect for their rights. It is also a requirement of justice. Skills and knowledge, acquired in training, are meant to be shared with clients, and used to assist them back to health and greater independence.

Community Development

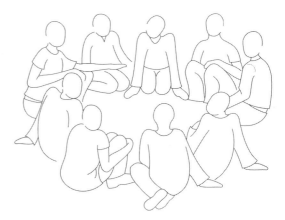

Situation – Community setting

Leader	Community
Appointed to facilitate and empower group	Group of equal members in joint decision-making
Responsible to:	**Responsible to:**
Community and its representatives	One another and to the wider community
Accountable to:	Accountable to:
The group, funding agency, local and state government	Those they represent in the community and grant-giving body

Key Principles: Respect for Communal and Personal Rights

Figure 9.3 Community leadership model.

Community leadership model (Fig. 9.3)

To be a professional, as we have said, means that, by definition, one exercises a public role, a public office. It is therefore impossible for professionals to ignore their duty of accountability to the wider community without ceasing to be responsible professionals. In this sense all professionals have a political role, in addition to the particular function which they perform in the division of labour. Nurses, especially those in senior positions, take on public and 'political' roles in many situations. They may be involved in committees for a variety of purposes: administrative, planning, research and training. They may be involved in professional associations, trade unions, government advisory and policy-making bodies, or interprofessional, inter-agency, or international committees. They may be involved in community nursing and community health in promoting self-help groups, community development projects and community action, or even in direct political action at local, regional or national level.

The skilful, effective and morally sound exercise of community responsibility has to be learned, like anything else. While people are given management training and taught to teach and do research, most skills associated with the exercise of power in these more public and political roles for nurses have to be learned by experience.

Working on committees may be seen to be less 'rewarding' than nursing patients. Campaigning for higher professional standards or better patient care, through professional bodies, unions or pressure groups, may seem remote to those committed to direct patient care. Community development and community action may seem to mix nursing and politics. All these activities are vital to good nursing practice and therefore relevant to a wider view of the scope of nursing ethics.

Ethics and politics in general are never totally separate or separable, but form a continuum, as Aristotle argued more than two thousand years ago. In healthcare, ethics and politics are inextricably mixed, as personal moral responsibility and public accountability, as a professional, overlap in the exercise of our daily work. Even if nurses are not directly involved in healthcare politics, when nurses act as nurses they are not operating in private, but in a public domain and are responsible for the efficient, effective and proper use of public resources.

Healthcare cannot be simply about the alleviation of individual distress. It is also about the meaning of health for society and its place in the good of the commonwealth. Here the World Health Organization (WHO) (UNO 1947) is not so much concerned with a scientific as with a normative definition of health and an aspirational statement of the goals of healthcare, when it affirms that 'health is complete physical, mental and social well-being, and not simply the absence of disease or infirmity'. Here WHO focuses attention on the wider aspirations people have for a good quality of life. Ultimately, health promotion and healthcare services are concerned with human flourishing and, by implication, with the rights and dignity of individuals and the common good. Without health we cannot achieve fulfilment or full realisation of our human potentialities.

Corporate Planning

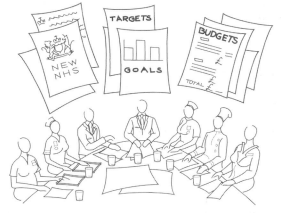

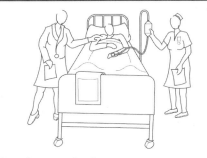

Situation – Corporate planning

Corporate Executive	Professionals and Staff
Direct policy, strategic planning and budgets	Implement policy and strategic plans and keep within budget
Responsible to: Consumers, government stakeholders	**Responsible to:** CEO/ manager to individual clients
Accountable to: Board of directors, and government	**Accountable to:** Line manager and to clients through the courts

Key Principles: Justice and Equity and Duty of care

Figure 9.4 Corporate planning model.

Corporate planning model (Fig. 9.4)

As long as the focus of medicine and nursing is on acute care, the tendency is for styles of management to be driven by presenting need and to fall into a kind of short-termism and crisis management. The strength of the caring ethic is its focus on the individual and the concrete needs of the present. This focus, and the personalist and individualistic values which go with direct involvement in the lives and crises of people, has contributed to the particular character of the 'caring professions'. However, when it comes to managing resources for large hospitals or institutions, conducting scientific research in medicine or nursing, organising preventive and health promotion services, or health service planning, a more long-term and strategic approach is required. Whether traditionally trained health professionals are equipped to take on these responsibilities, without further specialised training, may be doubted. Another consequence of the bias in nursing towards a personalist and privatised ethics of healthcare is reflected in the reluctance of health professionals to engage in what they tend to refer to derogatively as 'politics'.

However, to take on the responsibilities of management is necessarily to have to engage in 'politics' at several levels – internal hospital or institutional 'politics', health board or health authority politics, and perhaps at a wider level in relation to national or local government. However, if the nexus between ethics, power and responsibility is recognised, then perhaps we can be liberated from the kind of 'bleeding heart' view of ethical responsibility and recognise that the ethics of management responsibility and public accountability requires a realistic understanding of power, politics and the relationships between them. The emphasis on corporate planning is a necessary consequence of moving onto the level where objective and transparent processes of accountability for staff and financial resources are required of those exercising management roles on behalf of society.

The emphasis on strategic planning (on models of organisational development based on continuous improvement of the quality and efficiency of services, and of corporate ethical responsibility and accountability) is a relatively recent development in the history of healthcare. It is during the past 20 years, in particular, that the corporate planning model of management took hold. While it is often asserted that this was an import from the world of business and industry, in fact it is within the public sector, in the sphere of government planning and public administration that these concerns first emerged. The history of health services within the various welfare states around the world has been one of attempts to contain public expenditure on health and welfare services by centralised strategic planning and publicly accountable administration. However, before the advent of this kind of 'economic rationalism', there were serious attempts to base the administration of health services on a proactive public health model rather than to allow expenditure to be driven simply by reactive treatment-based services. A focus on epidemiology and scientifically based community medicine has contributed to a more strategic approach to the planning and administration of health and nursing services.

To evaluate any activity, it is necessary to have clear goals and set objectives so that achievements and failures can be measured against these objectives. The watch-cry 'management by objective' which became popular in the 1970s perhaps marked the beginning of a more systematic approach in the UK to strategic planning in healthcare, not simply at the macro level, but encouraged at all levels in the UK NHS. Since then, many philosophies of administration and styles of strategic management have been tried, each enjoying a period of fashionable influence under different government administrations. The 'quality movement' has perhaps been the most influential (see James 1996), including phases associated with 'quality control', 'quality assurance', 'quality improvement' and 'total quality management'. What is significant about the quality movement is that, while earlier approaches to strategic planning and management were essentially bureaucratic, the 'quality movement' sought to introduce values into the process, by emphasising the connection between corporate values and corporate goals and the critical role that values play in decision-making, whether implicitly or explicitly. The purpose of strategic ethical management is to achieve greater effectiveness and efficiency, by applying the methods of strategic planning to corporate administration of human and financial resources for the improvement of productivity and standards in the provision of services. However, it also involves action to develop a more coherent ethical culture and sense of 'moral community' by those in any corporation, by ensuring commitment to the same values.

Corporate planning thus does not simply involve the corporate executive writing a detailed strategic and business plan that is then imposed on the organisation. While strategic planning is often approached in this way, it is largely ineffective and its effects cosmetic rather than real. The objective of strategic planning is to change the behaviour of everyone in an organisation. To achieve this it is necessary to involve the whole organisation in the process. Awareness of and commitment to the same goals and values should result, with associated movement in a direction determined by the whole corporation. Strategic ethical management is essentially about an organisation setting a clear course, with realistic and achievable objectives, and defined milestones to be reached within an agreed timescale. It is a process of clarification of the primary *raison dêtre* ('mission') of the organisation, and assessment of its strengths and weaknesses, of the challenges and opportunities it faces, as well as the threats to its continued existence. In this process, the 'vision' of what it is and where it is going emerges, and it becomes clearer what the whole organisation and its employees most desire to achieve, i.e. what their 'values' and 'goals' are. Values, as we have said before, are important, not only for individuals but also for corporations, for we stake our lives and our decisions on our values. They are the most important instrumental means by which we achieve our short- and long-term goals (see Chapter 1).

Within the framework of this process, if it is conducted thoroughly and well, it becomes clearer what is essential and what is non-essential business of the organisation, what problems need to be addressed, what opportunities there are for improvement and how best to deploy staff and financial resources. By determining clearly the priority values and goals of the organisation, it becomes possible to develop functional strategies to assess the resources required to achieve our goals, to set standards for performance and targets for achievement. Effective and efficient management is thus not driven simply by economic rationalism, important though cost reduction and income generation may be, but also within a framework where wider corporate and community values can be factored in to determine the real human and financial costs and benefits of our strategic plan. This is not possible unless ethical policy is developed alongside each aspect of the strategic plan and its application carefully monitored in practice.

The benefits of sound strategic ethical management do not accrue solely to the organisation itself, because such management also ensures that the organisation is able to be more fully accountable to all of its stakeholders for the administration of corporate and/or public resources.

further reading

Baggott R 2004 Health and healthcare in Britain, 3rd edn. Palgrave Macmillan, Basingstoke

Downie R S, Macnaughton J, Randall F 2000 Clinical judgement: evidence in practice. Oxford University Press, Oxford

Harrison M I 2004 Implementing change in health systems: market reforms in the United Kingdom, Sweden, and the Netherlands. Sage Publications, London

Harrison S, Pollit C 1994 Controlling health professionals: the future of work and organisation in the NHS. Open University Press, Buckingham

James P 1996 Total quality management. Prentice-Hall, London

Kitson A, Campbell R 1996 The ethical organisation: ethical theory and corporate behaviour. Macmillan Business, Basingstoke

Muir Gray J A 2001 Evidence-based health care: how to make health policy and management decisions. Churchill Livingstone, Edinburgh

Nutley S, Davies H, Walter I 2004 Learning from knowledge management (Conceptual Synthesis 2). Research Unit for Research Utilisation, Department of Management, University of St Andrews, Scotland

Rossi P H, Freeman H E, Lipsey M W 1999 Evaluation: a systematic approach, 6th edn. Sage Publications, London

WMA 2000 Declaration of Helsinki – ethical principles for research involving human subjects. World Medical Association, Geneva. Online. Available: http://www.wma.net/e/policy/b3.htm

WMA 2005 Medical ethics manual 2005. World Medical Association, Geneva. Online. Available: http://www.wma.net/e/policy/b3.htm

The political ethics of healthcare: health policies and resource allocation

10

Chapter contents

AIMS

This chapter has the following aims:

1. To demonstrate that ethics is relevant at the personal, team, institutional and state levels of nursing practice
2. To examine the tensions between various types of professional values in the work of nurses, and the way these impact on ethical decision-making in nursing
3. To identify five different theoretical approaches which influence planning and resource allocation decisions in health
4. To use epidemiological and other research data to illustrate the importance of evidence-based decision-making in nursing.

LEARNING OUTCOMES

When you have read and worked through this chapter, you should be able to:

- Give an account of the scope of political ethics in nursing and healthcare and the various levels at which this applies
- Apply the conceptual distinctions between competing values in the work environment of nurses so as to identify areas of conflict and possible consensus
- Demonstrate understanding and ability to apply the different frameworks to the analysis of issues of resource allocation
- Demonstrate knowledge of major trends in morbidity and mortality in your own region and the relevance of this to planning nursing services and training
- Source local and global demographic and health data, relevant to nursing practice.

THE POLITICAL ETHICS OF HEALTHCARE

At the global and national level, the 'political ethics of healthcare' has been characterised by public debate about the scope and limits of the state's responsibility for healthcare, as compared with private healthcare provision on a commercial basis. It has also been concerned with how much the state should intervene to reduce mortality and prevent disease by active programmes of health education, health protection and health promotion, or whether health is the responsibility of the individual. With economic development and changes in the pattern of morbidity and mortality in developed countries, healthcare providers and politicians have also had to address the practical changes in services required by these trends, and how to satisfy the growing public expectations of the responsibilities of governments in this area. Both health and personal social services have become the arena in which debate about personal rights and public policy, and the best means to achieve health for all, has been focused. There are at least four types of issues which have been the particular focus of political debate about the scope of the state's practical responsibility for the health of its citizens in terms of health policy and state-provided healthcare or state-initiated public health programmes (Box 10.1).

Policy decisions taken by governments or local health authorities relating to each of these issues inevitably impact on the work of nurses. Nurses cannot escape from the practical implications of health policy and so should be actively involved in contributing to informed debate about the political ethics of healthcare within their spheres of influence. While nurses may not wish to become involved in party politics, they may become involved by active participation through their unions or professional bodies and as they move into senior positions as managers or policy-makers. Nurses and other health practitioners can hardly avoid becoming involved in the political ethics of healthcare whether as a moral duty in relation to the well-being of their patients, or out of self-interest as employees or as members of their profession. Or again, it may be out of public-spiritedness as taxpayers and citizens, and concern with issues of poverty and health in the developing world, in the interests of justice and peace.

In each of the areas mentioned above, the ethical and political debate for practitioners will be partly about ethical and ideological issues, and partly about practical means, including the implications for their own employment and future careers. For example, in relation to 'quality-of-life' issues: from one point of view, it is arguably the duty of the state to provide

> ### Box 10.1 Some matters of debate in the political ethics of healthcare
>
> - How broad a range of services should state-funded health services provide and what forms of 'treatment' or 'therapy' should be covered by health insurance? (e.g. Organ transplants? Assisted reproduction? Cosmetic surgery?)
>
> - To what extent should the state be responsible for defining 'quality of life' for any group in the population? (e.g. For neglected or abused children? For people with mental health problems or physical disabilities? For frail older adults?)
>
> - How actively should the state be involved in health-related social engineering and social control to promote health? (e.g. By fiscal/legal inducements or controls to reduce smoking and alcohol abuse? By active economic and community development? By legislation for reverse discrimination to overcome inequalities in health?)
>
> - What scope should state-provided preventive services have? What definition should be given to 'health promotion'? (e.g. Initiate proactive screening and preventive programmes? Compulsory immunisation? Health education in schools? By active programmes to bring about lifestyle and behaviour change?)

sheltered housing or age-care homes to protect frail older adults from harm or self-neglect; from another perspective perhaps the state should not interfere in their lives and patronise older people. From the first point of view, the state might be expected to provide specially trained staff and facilities, including specialised hospitals to provide for their needs. From the alternative perspective the state should be encouraged to support older adults to continue to live independent lives for as long as possible, by providing them with money from national insurance (as is the case in Germany), to buy in the services for social care they need, rather than to be dependent on state provision or be institutionalised. The first approach might provide more opportunities for careers in specialist aged-care nursing, the second might involve reduced opportunities for institution-based nursing practice, though it might open up greater scope for community nursing services.

The political ethics of healthcare can range all the way from concern with issues of scarcity on a particular hospital ward to concerns about standards of healthcare provision at local government level, and from debate about general public spending priorities on health, education, housing and welfare, relative say to defence and security, through to global concerns about poverty and international debt and their impact on the health of people in developing countries. All of these raise important ethical considerations. But there are different ethical challenges to be met and discussed at each of these different levels, and ethical discussion of these issues needs to be based on sound evidence and reliable quantitative data, rather than on personal opinions or party dogma.

It is sometimes claimed that these are not matters of real concern or interest to healthcare practitioners: their job is to deal with real people and their problems, and not with abstract discussions of epidemiological and other health statistics, or with examination of economic facts and analyses related to healthcare funding and service delivery. This view is summed up in remarks like: 'Don't blind me with science and statistics' or 'Don't confuse me with the facts!', or cynical repetition of the remark attributed by Mark Twain to Disraeli, namely: 'There are three kinds of lies: lies, damned lies, and statistics!'

Against this view we would argue that nurses and health practitioners have a duty as responsible practitioners both to be informed about the scientific, medical and statistical facts related to their practice, and to be committed to evidence-based practice. To ensure that they are constantly upgrading their skills and improving their standards of care (for the sake of their patients, and their own professional develop-ment) nurses must be not only involved in critical evaluation of their routine practice and specific interventions with individual patients, but also informed about the results of nursing research and possibly involved in doing it themselves.

In order to be adequately informed as responsible professionals, in our day-to-day work, in management and administration, or in influencing policy devel-opment, we need to be aware of research evidence of various kinds: that relevant to our clinical practice, to the effective and efficient delivery of services, to the overall management of a hospital, clinic or health centre. We also need to be aware of the kinds of evidence that shape broader health policy and funding at regional, national and global levels. Here we might refer again to the usefulness of the 'Russian dolls model', introduced earlier in Chapter 2, as it reminds us that there are different kinds of facts relevant to problems at different levels. Ethics and values, it must be emphasised, do not apply in a vacuum, but must relate to facts in the real world and must be applicable to the real needs of patients with their varying health problems.

In this chapter we examine evidence in relation to five kinds of issues with relevance to our health locally, nationally and internationally, to illustrate how ethical and political considerations come into management decisions and policy-making at a number of levels:

- global and local population trends and their ethico-political implications
- *Health for All in the 21st Century* – priorities for health, globally, nationally and locally
- changing perceptions of the HIV/AIDS pandemic in different regions of the world
- costs of health services – can they be controlled?
- the impact on microeconomic health issues of macroeconomic and demographic trends.

THINKING ABOUT HEALTH IN A GLOBAL CONTEXT

Many nurses and health workers – particularly those working, or with experience of voluntary work, in Third World countries – are *concerned both about the inequalities in health* in our own societies and with the huge gap in health status and life expectancy between industrialised countries and the poorer developing countries. Many have taken a lead in campaigning for reappraisal of our social and economic priorities, for ethical and political reasons.

In this context it is sobering to reflect on the escalating costs, at the beginning of the 21st century, of defence, internal security, police and other emergency services. Here, it may be helpful to put the local situa-tion in the UK into a global context. The Stockholm International Peace Research Institute (SIPRI), for example, reported that in 2003 global military expen-diture and the arms trade represented the largest spending in the world at over $950 billion (or £532 billion), and pointed out that military spending in 2003 increased by about 11% in real terms, over the top of an increase of 6.5% in 2002. Some relevant facts are:

- Over two years world military spending increased by 18% in real terms, to reach $956 billion (in current dollars) in 2003.
- High-income countries account for about 75% of world military spending but only 16% of world population.
- The combined military spending of these countries was slightly higher than the aggregate foreign debt of all low-income countries and 10 times higher than their combined levels of official development assistance in 2001.
- There is a large gap between what countries are prepared to allocate for military means to provide security and maintain their global and regional power status, on the one hand, and to alleviate poverty and promote economic development, on the other. (Source: SIPRI Report 2003.)

Both the World Health Organization (WHO), in its *World Health Report* (2005), and the World Bank, in its 2004 *Human Development Report*, have stressed that military conflict is one of the major contributors to social and economic malaise and to deteriorating health status in many countries. The *World Health Report 2005* is subtitled *Make Every Mother and Child Count*, and emphasises that the primary indicators for maternal and child health tend to be missing in countries torn apart by war and revolution. Likewise the World Bank stresses that countries caught up in war and conflict are on a disastrous economic course, and the impact of these on political stability and human rights has been very damaging to the health and well-being of people, restricting the possibilities in these countries for human and economic development. In this context it is illuminating to consider some of our global spending priorities (Table 10.1).

Table 10.1 Global priorities in spending in 1998

Global priority	$US billions
Basic education for everyone in the world	6
Cosmetics in the United States	8
Water and sanitation for everyone in the world	9
Ice cream in Europe	11
Reproductive health for all women in the world	12
Perfumes in Europe and the United States	12
Basic health and nutrition for everyone in the world	13
Pet foods in Europe and the United States	17
Business entertainment in Japan	35
Cigarettes in Europe	50
Alcoholic drinks in Europe	105
Narcotic drugs in the world	400
Military spending in the world	780

Source: Consumerism, Volunteer Now! (undated).

What is most striking about these figures is that when you take military spending, narcotic drugs and alcoholic drinks individually or collectively they dwarf all the other figures. Taken together with the killer infectious diseases, associated with populations made vulnerable by poverty and ignorance, these could be likened to the Four Horses of the Apocalypse. However, unlike these metaphysical beasts we can do something about all four of these major causes of morbidity and mortality around the world. What this requires is not only dedicated work by doctors and nurses in developing countries, but also global cooperation in promoting economic development and sustainable improvements in health education and preventive medicine.

Health for All in the 21st Century, and priorities for health

Clearly we need coherent strategies to deal with these issues and to move towards more rational planning to reorder our priorities and to target our resources more effectively to improve the health and well-being of people, nationally and internationally. Here we might start with consideration of the WHO Health for All programme and its strategic objectives.

The evaluation of outcomes of the global and local HFA2000 strategies and targets subsequently led to the revision of the WHO's *Health for All in the 21st Century* (WHO 1999b), and its latest statement of principles is shown in Box 10.2.

Box 10.2 Key principles of *Health for All for the 21st Century*

1. Health is a fundamental human right and a social goal. Health is defined in a positive sense, in line with the classic WHO definition.

2. There should be an equitable distribution of health resources, both within and between countries.

3. Health is shaped by many factors, social, economic, lifestyle and environmental, and policy-makers must construct 'holistic' and 'intersectoral' policies that take account of other sectors of decision-making which impinge upon health. Governments should adopt 'healthy public policies' which strongly reflect health priorities, coordinate the actions of government agencies, and are based on assessments of their health impact.

4. Health policies must be pre-emptive and precautionary, the aim being to prevent the problems from arising at the earliest possible stage.

5. Health improvements require a community-wide response. This involves partnership between agencies drawn from all relevant sectors and at all levels. Health promotion must include and involve the community, responding to its concerns, while at the same time promoting healthy lifestyles and supportive environments.

6. Health services must be reoriented towards primary healthcare and geared to promoting health rather than simply treating illness.

7. Clear performance targets and review mechanisms must be adopted in order to guide health strategies and achieve their objectives.

The historic 1978 World Health Assembly, which met at Alma Ata in Kazakhstan in the former USSR, reflected on global health needs and epidemiological trends. In response to these needs and changing patterns of morbidity and mortality, the Assembly formulated the 'Health for All by the Year 2000' (HFA2000) policy declaration. Since 1978, the principles underlying HFA2000 have exerted considerable influence worldwide, helping to shape public health strategies nationally and internationally. The original Health for All strategy set global targets for the year 2000 (WHO 1981), and the World Health Organization then charged the leadership in its six global Regions, and all member states of the United Nations, to develop relevant local strategies to achieve HFA2000 policy objectives. The key strategy document for

---

Box 10.3　WHO European Region's general targets for the 21st century

1. By the year 2020, the present gap in health status between member states of the European Region should be reduced by at least one-third.

2. By the year 2020, the health gap between socio-economic groups within countries should be reduced by at least one-quarter in all member states, by substantially improving the level of health of disadvantaged groups.

3. By the year 2020, all newborn babies, infants and preschool children in the Region should have better health, ensuring a healthy start in life.

4. By the year 2020, young people in the Region should be healthier and better able to fulfil their roles in society.

5. By the year 2020, people over 65 years should have the opportunity of enjoying their full health potential and playing an active social role.

6. By the year 2020, people's psychosocial well-being should be improved, and better, comprehensive services should be available to and accessible by people with mental health problems.

7. By the year 2020, the adverse health effects of communicable diseases should be substantially diminished through systematically applied programmes to eradicate, eliminate or control infectious diseases of public health importance.

8. By the year 2020, morbidity, disability and premature mortality due to major chronic diseases should be reduced to the lowest feasible levels throughout the Region.

9. By the year 2020, there should be a significant and sustainable decrease in injuries, disability and death arising from accidents and violence in the Region.

10. By the year 2015, people in the Region should live in a safer physical environment, with exposure to contaminants hazardous to health at levels not exceeding internationally agreed standards.

11. By the year 2015, people across society should have adopted healthier patterns of living.

12. By the year 2015, the adverse health effects from the consumption of addictive substances such as tobacco, alcohol and psychoactive drugs should have been significantly reduced in all member states.

13. By the year 2015, people in the Region should have greater opportunities to live in healthy physical and social environments at home, at school and in the local community.

14. By the year 2020, all sectors should have recognised and accepted their responsibility for health.

15. By the year 2010, people in the Region should have much better access to family- and community-oriented primary healthcare, supported by a flexible and responsive hospital system.

16. By the year 2010, member states should ensure that the management of the health sector, from population-based health programmes to individual patient care at the clinical level, is oriented towards health outcomes.

17. By the year 2010, member states should have sustainable financing and resource allocation mechanisms for healthcare systems based on the principles of equal access, cost-effectiveness, solidarity and optimum quality.

18. By the year 2010, all member states should have ensured that health professionals and professionals in other sectors have acquired appropriate knowledge, attitudes and skills to protect and promote health.

19. By the year 2005, all member states should have health research, information and communication systems that better support the acquisition, effective utilisation and dissemination of knowledge to support Health for All.

20. By the year 2005, implementation of policies for Health for All should engage individuals, groups and organisations throughout the public and private sectors, and civil society, in alliances and partnerships for health.

21. By the year 2010, all member states should have and be implementing policies for Health for All at country, regional and local levels, supported by appropriate institutional infrastructures, managerial processes and innovative leadership.

Source: WHO Regional Office for Europe (1998) Health 21: Health Policy Framework for the WHO European Region.

Europe, Primary Care in Europe (WHO 1979), for example, signalled the need for a major shift in resources from high-technology hospital-based medicine to primary care, and from treatment services to a greater emphasis on health education and health promotion. Health departments of member states were charged with the responsibility to research local needs and to set local priorities and their own HFA2000 targets and to evaluate outcomes at the end of the millennium.

Each of the six global WHO Regions has published targets for the 21st century. Those for the WHO European Region were published in 1998. Based on earlier targets published in 1985 and updated in 1991, they included General Targets for the 21st century (Box 10.3), together with more detailed and specific targets (see WHO website).

These WHO strategies need to be read in conjunction with the complementary World Bank *Human Development Report* and its statement of Key Millennium Goals (Box 10.4). The United Nations through its various global organisations is attempting to achieve better coordination of their various strategies, and

the publication of the World Bank *Investing in Health* report in 1993, alongside the first WHO *World Health Report* in the same year, marked a new era of cooperation between these two agencies. The World Bank has been the target of a great deal of criticism regarding the impact of globalisation in international trade, and its damaging effects on the economies of poorer developing countries. However, the 2005 Gleneagles Agreement gave evidence of positive moves by the G8 countries to take concerted action to cancel the crippling debt burden of 25 of the poorest countries, and to take action to reduce global dependence on use of fossil fuels and other factors causing environmental pollution. Given the emphasis in the WHO definition of health on social and economic determinants of health, it is obvious that cooperation at both international and national levels between governments, non-governmental organisations (NGOs) and multinational business and industrial corporations is necessary if some of the most fundamental determinants of health are to be addressed.

As an example of a Specific Target, Target 12 includes three specific targets to be attained by 2015:

Box 10.4 World Bank's Millennium Development Goals (MDGs)

1. Reducing poverty and improving economic management
- Governance and public sector reform
- Gender and development
- Increased trade
- Economic policy

2. Investing in people
- Education (for development)
- Combating HIV/AIDS
- Health, nutrition and population
- Protecting vulnerable people
- Engaging with children and youth

3. Addressing the challenges of sustainable development
- Agriculture and rural development
- Environment (protection and improvement)
- Social development

4. Revitalising infrastructures
- Poverty alleviation and growth (relative to Millennium Development Goals)

- Development goals
- Access, quality and financing need
- Infrastructure action plan

5. Supporting private sector development
- Research and assessment
- Lending technical assistance
- Private sector dialogue

6. Building strong financial systems
- Knowledge generation and dissemination
- Country diagnostic work
- Lending, policy advice and technical assistance

7. Promoting the modernisation of legal and judicial systems
- Enhancing investment climate by strengthening laws
- Poverty alleviation and the law
- Addressing gender equality
- Countering fraud and corruption

Source: The World Bank Annual Report, 2004 (see World Bank website).

that the proportion of non-smokers should be at least over 80% (and close to 100% in under-15-year-olds); that per capita alcohol consumption should not exceed 6 litres per annum (and should be close to zero in under-15-year-olds); and that the prevalence of illicit psychoactive drug use should be reduced by at least a quarter and mortality by half.

The seven Millennium Development Goals of the World Bank are shown in Box 10.4.

THINKING ABOUT HEALTH IN A NATIONAL CONTEXT

The National Health Service is the largest employer not only in the UK, but also in the whole of Europe. Health policy and the political economy of the NHS are, or should be, matters of great importance to nurses, not only as employees and health professionals, but as citizens and taxpayers. As shareholders,

Table 10.2 Total expenditure on health as % of gross domestic product

Country	1960	1970	1980	1990	2000	2001	2002
United States	5	6.9	8.7	11.9	13.1	13.8	14.6
Switzerland	4.9	5.5	7.4	8.3	10.4	10.9	11.1
Germany		6.2	8.7	8.5	10.6	10.8	10.9
Iceland	3	4.7	6.2	8	9.3	9.3	10.0
Norway	2.9	4.4	7	7.7	7.7	8.9	9.9
Greece		6.1	6.6	7.4	9.9	10.2	9.8
France	3.8	5.4	7.1	8.6	9.3	9.4	9.7e
Canada	5.4	7	7.1	9	8.9	9.4	9.6
Australia	4.1	4.6^{-1}	7	7.8	9	9.1	9.3
Netherlands		6.9^{2}	7.5	8	8.3	8.7	9.3
Portugal		2.6	5.6	6.2	9.2	9.4	9.3
Sweden		6.9	9.1	8.4	8.4	8.8	9.2
Belgium		4	6.4	7.4	8.7	8.8	9.1
Denmark		8.0^{1}	9.1	8.5	8.4	8.6	8.8
Italy				7.9	8.1	8.2	8.4
New Zealand		5.1	5.9	6.9	7.8	7.9	8.2
Japan	3	4.5	6.5	5.9	7.6	7.8	7.9e
Hungary				7.1^{1}	7.1	7.4	7.8
United Kingdom	3.9	4.5	5.6	6	7.3	7.5	7.7
Austria	4.3	5.1	7.4	7	7.6	7.5	7.6
Spain	1.5	3.6	5.4	6.7	7.4	7.5	7.6
Ireland	3.7	5.1	8.4	6.1	6.3	6.9	7.3
Czech Republic				4.7	6.6	6.9	7.2
Finland	3.8	5.6	6.4	7.8	6.7	6.9	7.2
Turkey			3.3	3.6	6.6	6.6^{-1}	6.6^{-2}
Luxembourg		3.6	5.9	6.1	5.5	5.9	6.1
Mexico				4.8	5.6	6	6.0
Poland				4.9	5.7	6	6.0
Slovak Republic					5.5	5.6	5.7
Korea			4.2^{3}	4.5	4.7	5.4	5.3

Copyright OECD Health Data 2005, June.
NOTES: (a) −1, −2, −3, 1, 2, 3 shows that data refers to 1, 2 or 3 previous or following year(s).
(b) For Germany, data prior to 1990 refer to West Germany.
e = estimate.

as it were, in this vast enterprise, citizens and tax-payers have a right to demand a say in what priority is given to health in public expenditure, or what proportion of our gross domestic product (GDP) should be 'invested' in health locally, as compared with defence and security, and what percentage of GDP should be contributed to reducing world poverty and the burden of ill-health in developing countries.

When politicians claim that the cost of health services in the United Kingdom is becoming excessive, there are at least three issues to be considered: First, the proportion of GDP spent on healthcare in the UK compared with other countries (Table 10.2), including the proportion of health services funded by private health insurance compared with state funding; second, the relative priority given to healthcare in local authority and national budgets, in comparison with other public services; and third, the amount we privately spend on tobacco and alcohol products, as major causes of disease and death in our societies.

In relation to these issues it may be useful to consider some global comparisons on expenditure on healthcare in selected OECD countries relative to their GDP, and a few other headline figures relevant to the political ethics of healthcare, so as to establish the position of the UK in the world rankings (Table 10.2).

The matters behind these figures are not only of general public interest, but become matters of ethical and political interest to nurses and health workers, because of their impact on their clients, and because of their implications for health workers themselves. Resources spent elsewhere may result in the lack of resources available for essential improvement and development of health services. These matters may seem remote from the practical day-to-day concerns of nurses, but policy decisions about them will have profound implications for how health services will be provided and determine the context and availability of employment for nurses, including their own pay and working conditions.

In terms of the *proportion of its GDP spent on healthcare*, the UK is not one of the big spenders. On a comparative basis (among countries for which figures were available) in 1980, the UK ranked fourth lowest in terms of the proportion of its GDP spent on healthcare, namely 5.6%. Although this had risen to 7.7% in 2002, it still ranked 12th lowest out of the 30 nations listed in Table 10.2, below Greece, Portugal and Hungary. This amounted to approximately £62 billion out of a total GDP of £796 billion in 2005.

In relation to the *proportion of healthcare privately funded* relative to state funding, in 2005, the United States tops the list with 55.6%, along with Mexico, Korea and Greece, where privately funded healthcare

amounted to more than or about 50%. In Switzerland, Netherlands and Turkey it was about 40% and in Australia, Portugal, Austria, Canada, Hungary, Spain, Poland and Italy the proportion was about 30%. In the UK the proportion of privately funded healthcare amounted to 16.6%. This was among the lowest in the OECD. Here the UK ranks with Germany, New Zealand, Japan and Denmark, where private sector funding accounts for 20% or less of total funding for healthcare, and with Iceland (16.5%), Norway (16.3%), Sweden (14.7%) and Luxembourg (14.6%) at the lower end. Only the two former communist countries, the Slovak Republic (11.7%) and Czech Republic (9.9%), are lower (OECD Health Data June 2005).

When we consider the relative *proportions of the UK budget allocated to health* relative to that of other big spending departments, the Department of Health tops the list (along with the Department of Work and Pensions), with a budget of over £61 billion in 2005/06, that is with 14% of total government spending each. For a summary list of the top spending departments with budgets over £10 billion, see Table 10.3, and for full details refer to the website for the UK Central Government Main Supply Estimates for England and Wales (2005/06).

However, to put these figures into the context of other spending priorities of the public, it should be noted that while the 2005/06 United Kingdom budget

Table 10.3 Westminster Parliamentary Budgets for England and Wales (2005–2006)

Department	Total provision (£000s)
Department of Health	61 323 693
Department for Work & Pensions	61 315 571
Office of the Deputy Prime Minister	55 727 773
Department for Constitutional Affairs	34 993 421
Ministry of Defence	34 611 882
Department for Education & Skills	29 361 288
HM Revenue & Customs	14 602 672
Home Office	13 267 359
Department for Transport	11 429 983
Northern Ireland Office	11 276 103
Department of Trade & Industry	10 161 837
Other Departments of Government	*19 386 203*
(Total Public Sector Pensions)	*78 320 261*
Total Budget	£435 778 046

Extracted from UK Central Government Main Supply Estimates 2005/06.

for the Department of Health amounts to £61.3 billion, the amount spent by the public on tobacco was estimated by researchers for Action on Smoking and Health (ASH) as £31.1 billion and the alcohol market estimated by Alcohol Concern research as £32.5 billion. Given the amount of morbidity and mortality associated with the use of tobacco, alcohol and drugs, it is salutary to reflect that our expenditure on these two non-essential luxury items, or drugs, amounts in total each to more than half of the total budget for healthcare. Clearly the politics of healthcare has to be seen in the context of politics more generally, and what can be done about reducing the dependence of people on alcohol and smoking is not only a health challenge, but a challenge to large vested interests (including in the past the vested interests of ministers of state with investments in British and American Tobacco (BAT) or in major alcohol producing and exporting companies).

Do we allocate health resources nationally on a rational basis?

Alongside pressures on government from business and industry, ideological and political pressures also have a bearing on health policy planning and the allocation of resources for healthcare. A brief review of the history of UK policy on public health from 1975 to 2005 illustrates how the evidence used by successive governments to justify their choice of health priorities and areas of spending on health was subject to interpretation by several different kinds of methodological approach and ideological rationale.

An urgent need to prioritise national public spending, to contain costs and to improve the effectiveness and efficiency of health services was driven by a severe economic recession in the mid-1970s. Labour governments of the period were forced to make cuts in public expenditure at a time when the demands on health and public services were increasing, compounded by high unemployment and economic hardship. It was believed that by improving public health, general morbidity and mortality could be reduced, with general benefits to the economy and ultimate reduction in expenditure on treatment services. Harold Wilson's government adopted a broad socialist and public health approach to health policy planning, setting out as priority areas for action: action on inequalities in health status between the social classes; action to reduce heart disease, road accidents, smoking-related disease, alcoholism and mental illness; and preventive strategies for dealing with drug abuse, inappropriate diet and sexually transmitted diseases. However, the capacity of Wilson's government to deliver on these objectives

was limited by the economic crisis and by his government's vulnerability to political pressure from commercial interests and public resistance to interventionist approaches.

The subsequent Thatcher Conservative government was ideologically opposed to the kind of 'collectivist social engineering' seen by Conservatives to be behind the 'public health approach' advocated by the new breed of 'community medicine specialists'. Conservative ministers of health adopted a more individualistic approach, based on a traditional medical view of factual public health education and elective immunisation, emphasising people's responsibility for their own health choices and their consequences. From the standpoint of those involved in health education and health promotion, this approach was heavily criticised, as failing to take account of social, economic and environmental determinants of health, and as resulting in 'blaming the victim'. The government's approach proved politically unsustainable in the face of media hype and public concern relating to a series of public health crises in the late 1980s: namely, outbreaks of food poisoning and Legionnaire's disease, and later HIV/AIDS, which highlighted its weaknesses. A report by the Chief Medical Officer (Acheson Report 1988) led to attempts to strengthen the leadership role of doctors in the direction of public health. Local authorities were required to appoint directors of public health (a more high-powered version of the traditional medical officer of health or MOH) who were responsible for coordinating the work of health education officers and the local authority treatment services, to meet key targets to reduce morbidity and mortality in the local population.

These developments were also associated with moves to reorientate the healthcare system towards the application of business methods of strategic planning, objective setting and performance measurement. Further, attempts were made to introduce a more competitive environment into the economy of healthcare provision. This was to be effected by encouraging the outsourcing of health and ancillary services to the private sector and the creation of an internal market within the public sector where 'providers', hospital services and related treatment services were supposed to compete for custom from primary care 'purchasers' of their services.

The Conservative government of John Major continued to implement these innovations, which, paradoxically, through attempts to achieve more rational, cost-efficient planning and management of the healthcare system, brought UK health policy back to an emphasis on evidence-based medicine and epidemiologically grounded public health. Pressure from WHO for the UK to implement nationally the policy and strategic objectives of the Health for All programme also meant that the government was increasingly obliged to collect evidence to demonstrate that its performance was not lagging seriously behind other developed countries. The UK government's national health strategy, *Health of the Nation* (DoH 1991), set out a range of targets for the reduction of disease, with priority given in rank order to: coronary heart disease and stroke, cancer, mental health, accidents, HIV/AIDS and sexual health. The watch-words of the new approach were 'intersectoral coordination and collaboration', namely between all levels of government nationally, and locally strategic alliances with local government, the NHS, voluntary organisations, business and industry.

With the arrival of the New Labour government of Tony Blair there was a shift in ideological focus towards a more communitarian approach, exemplified in wide public consultation on voters' views of the strengths and weaknesses of the NHS, and with renewed emphasis on the importance of public health and even the appointment of a Minister for Public Health. The new watch-words were 'a new contract' between the state and the individual, and 'new partnerships' between communities and individuals to improve health, and between the public and private sectors to fund development and innovation in the NHS. This approach was heralded as a 'third way' between the neo-liberal monetarist and socialist economic models, on the one hand, and the 'nanny state' and the 'victim blaming' versions of the welfare state, on the other. However, it also marked a shift back to Labour's traditional concerns with greater social justice in healthcare, the needs for gender equality, for vulnerable dependency groups, including strategies to deal with inequalities in health and to reduce unemployment.

Following countless surveys and focus groups, the original 1998 Green Paper *Our Healthier Nation* was published in the following year as the White Paper: *Saving Lives: Our Healthier Nation* (DoH 1999). This purported to be a comprehensive government-wide public health strategy for England (with separate health policy papers set out for Wales and Scotland, as well as Northern Ireland). Its twin goals were stated simply as:

- to improve health;
- to reduce the health gap (health inequalities).

At national level in the UK the numbers of deaths by cause for England and Wales in 2002 were ranked by the Office for National Statistics (ONS 2004) as follows:

1. Diseases of the circulatory system: 209 433
2. Cancer: 140 174
3. Respiratory disease: 69 600
4. Diseases of the digestive system: 24 214
5. Deaths from accidents and external causes: 16 139
6. Infection/parasitic diseases: 4330
7. Other sundry causes: 69 637.

The strategy aims to prevent up to 300 000 untimely and unnecessary deaths by the year 2010, by adopting the following new targets to reduce the death rate from:

- heart disease and stroke and related illnesses among people under 75 years old by at least two-fifths
- accidents by at least a fifth and reduce the rate of serious injury by at least a tenth
- cancer amongst people aged under 75 years by at least a fifth, and
- suicide and undetermined injury by at least a fifth.

Note: Much of the general information discussed above is summarised from Baggott (2004), *Health and Health Care in Britain.* For more specific information on the detailed targets and statistical data supporting this strategy, see *NHS Plan: Technical supplement on target setting (England & Wales)*, DoH (2005).

It is significant that while the Thatcher and Major Conservative governments were anxious to prove that the NHS was 'safe in their hands', contrary to the claims of the Opposition, the New Labour Blair government went out of its way to consult consumers and various other stakeholder groups, to establish an evidence basis for their claims that they were addressing the public's concerns. The political emphasis in health policy under the Conservative government had been on programmes of screening for breast and cervical cancer to reassure women that they had their interests at heart, on incentives to GPs to engage in immunisation, screening, health checks and other health promotion activities, and massive expenditure media campaigns on smoking, heart disease prevention, and on drug abuse and especially the risks of HIV/AIDS. These high-profile measures were intended to reassure the public that it was concerned about health and doing something about it (Baggott 2004, Chs 12 and 13).

The 'market research' undertaken by the New Labour government was designed not merely to reassure the public about its 'commitment to improving the nation's health', but also to establish what the public's concerns were, and to involve the public and local communities directly as 'partners in working for a healthier nation'. The report *'Shifting Gears' Towards a*

21st Century NHS, prepared by the Office for Public Management (OPM), for the Department of Health, gives details of the results of its public consultations with national fora, focus groups and stakeholder groups, including public opinion surveys (OPM 2000).

The findings of this report helped to shape New Labour's general policy on the NHS. However, since the creation of devolved authorities in Wales and Scotland, in the late 1990s, separate health policies have been developed and published for these regions. In Wales and Scotland there are some differences in the way healthcare services have been organised and delivered, and differences in focus on specific local health problems and priorities (Baggott 2004). However, this is not the place to discuss these in detail, interesting and important though they may be, and readers are encouraged to consult the relevant Welsh and Scottish government and health department websites if they wish to explore these further. For example, the Scottish Executive Health Department has a different budget from the Department of Health in England; and the Scottish equivalent of the National Institute of Clinical Excellence is the Scottish Intercollegiate Guidelines Network (SIGN). Because detailed discussion of the differences between England, Wales and Scotland would require another book, we propose to focus on the developments in England, and to use these to provide examples to illustrate the new focus on NHS consumers' views.

In the light of the prominence given to consumers' rights and opinions; equality of access and equity in terms of outcomes for all groups in society; and to the state's duty of care for vulnerable dependency groups, these developments are of particular interest in a book concerned with the ethics of healthcare. For this reason it may be worth considering briefly the outcomes of this national consultation exercise. For cynics this was just a slick exercise in public relations. For its supporters it was a high-risk strategy, because it raised (unrealistically high) public expectations of what could be done in the short-term. This has brought criticism of the government's performance.

The main themes arising from the OPM's national fora on the NHS were (OPM, June 2000):

- concern about current levels of (under) performance of the NHS
- the need for greater responsiveness to poverty
- poor communication within the NHS and with patients
- the NHS should promote a culture of care that is flexible and adaptable to current needs and lifestyles

- public pride in and valuing of the NHS and concern that it needs support to improve services.

The main themes arising from the *focus groups* were:

- keep the NHS, make it a truly national service with high quality treatment
- treat the patient as well as the symptoms
- bedside manner is crucial and could be improved
- there must be local services for local people
- too much (mis)management and not enough nurses and doctors
- bring back Matron – someone needs to 'take charge' on the wards

Key themes arising from the interviews with patient, carer and *public stakeholder* groups were:

- the need for patient-centred services
- the need for patient-centred policy
- the need for 'root and branch' reform
- the need to support lay involvement
- the need for independent regulation
- The NHS plan needs to 'fit' with other activities – clinical governance, implementation of National Service Frameworks, National Institute of Clinical Excellence
- The plan must be more than the sum of its Modernisation Action Teams.

At the beginning of New Labour's second term in office, the Health Secretary Alan Milburn (DoH 2002) was concerned to produce evidence to reassure the public that real progress had been made across each of the public's priority areas since the publication of the *1999 NHS Plan*, as follows:

- *On cancer*: Over 90% of people with suspected cancer urgently referred by their GP now see a consultant within 2 weeks, compared with 63% in 1997.
- *On heart services*: The maximum wait for heart surgery will be down from 18 months to 12 months by the end of March 2002. There are an extra 10 000 heart operations per year now compared with 1996/97, a 25% increase.
- *On waiting times*: 70% of patients get their operation within 3 months. Average waiting times are lower today than in March 1997. The number of people waiting over 15 months is down by 68% compared with last year.
- *On trolley waits*: The number of over 12-hour trolley waits has fallen by 50% in the last 2 years.
- *On free nursing care*: The Government introduced free nursing care for frail elderly people in October 2001 benefiting over 42 000 extra older people.
- *On cancer screening*: The breast-screening programme has been extended to women aged 65-70 benefiting 50 000 women by March 2002.

- *On nurses' pay*: Nurses have had cash increases of at least 26% since 1997. There has been a net increase of 20 000 qualified NHS nurses and midwives – 16 000 whole time equivalents – in the last two years.
- *On access to a GP within 48 hours*: 60% of GP practices – over 6400 – already achieve this standard. All practices will achieve it by the end of 2004.
- *On the postcode lottery*: The National Institute for Clinical Excellence was set up to tackle the postcode lottery. 19 000 NHS patients each year now benefit from new anti-cancer drugs as a result of NICE guidance.
- *On hospital cleanliness*: We have invested over £60 million in hospital cleaning. Matron is being brought back to make sure the wards are clean, the food is good and the care is there for patients.
- *On research*: The Department of Health now spends £50 million more each year on health-related research than it did five years ago.
- *On mental health services*: The government is spending over £300 million over 3 years to implement the first-ever national standards for mental health services.

These somewhat optimistic claims by the Health Secretary reflect the government's need to persuade the public that the healthcare reforms were working and producing beneficial results. However sceptical one may be about particular claims made, independent investigators confirm that there is real evidence of change and progress being made, albeit at a slower rate than the government might like, or the public and NHS staff might expect (Baggott 2004).

Given our concern in this chapter to highlight issues of importance in the political ethics of healthcare, at its different levels, the *Policy Futures for UK Health 2000 Report*, by the Judge Institute of Management Studies, University of Cambridge (2000) commissioned by the Department of Health, is significant. It begins by emphasising that ethics and politics are inextricably involved in decisions about health policy and spending priorities. The report reminds us that the WHO definition of health, 'A state of complete physical, mental and social wellbeing and not merely the absence of disease or infirmity', not only refers to treatment and care, and the prevention of the causes of ill health in society, but also emphasises that health is both a social 'good'. Health enables us to function within society, and is related to the values and lifestyle choices of individuals.

This means that health policy is necessarily involved 'with resolving tensions between a desire for collective good on the one hand, and moves to bring services closer to individual choice on the other'. In a more classic formulation, the common wealth of the commonwealth should be used for the common good

and to address the common weal, as well as to take account of the human rights of all citizens. The report goes on to say:

> Ethics may help to illuminate the competing values that are played out in modern health debates and the tensions that are evident, … the conflict between individual autonomy and collective welfare characterises many serious ethical challenges in health care illustrated by, among other things, the challenges prompted by emergent technological interventions at the beginning and the end of life and by advances in genetics. The development of medical technology represents a quest for scientific certainty, whilst at the same time the growth of individual consumerism represents a loss of confidence in traditional moral certainties. Developments in human genetics and in technological interventions are challenging our thinking. However, still more important may be the ethical challenges in establishing the place of health care within the wider social context, especially the problem of reconciling individualistic technological interventions with societal health needs, above all the need to reduce inequalities in health. Current trends value autonomy in health, but it is recognised that these are inadequate in dealing with societal issues that require a more 'communitarian' approach.

Given the fact that the authors of this book are all based in Scotland, and are involved in the local scene as consumers of healthcare services, researchers and teachers of health practitioners, we may be excused a few brief remarks on the Scottish scene.

Scotland has set a high standard for the collection of local area health statistics, and these give a good basis for discussion of the political ethics of health services provision and priorities for healthcare and health promotion. Scottish Health Statistics provide an excellent evidential base on which to debate the issues, at both national and local level, for all health practitioners concerned with health policy. The development of excellent small area health statistics has made it possible for health boards to disaggregate factors causing morbidity and mortality on a very specific local basis.

This development was partly the result of moves by successive governments to devolve responsibility down to local health boards, for the management of budgets and resources, and for maintaining and improving performance standards. Scottish local health boards have had to collect relevant data in order to meet these demands for local accountability, namely, to demonstrate evidence of rational planning and delivery of local healthcare services based on assessment and evaluation of actual outcomes. The availability of the data collected, specific to local populations, has made it possible to identify 'hot spots' on a postcode basis, and therefore to target resources more effectively, and to refine strategies accordingly.

The Information Services Division of the Common Services Agency has been responsible for developing the *Scottish Index of Multiple Deprivation* (SIMD). This has six domains at the data zone level (income, employment, education, housing, health and geographical access), which have been combined into an overall index, incorporating data from the earlier *Carstairs and Morris Index*, developed in the 1980s. (For full information see the SIMD 2004 Report, on the Scottish Executive website.) These resources provide a good evidence base from which to identify priorities for local and national healthcare planning, and to assist in the process of rationalising resource allocation.

The development of relevant strategies to deal with the causes of disease and death needs to focus not on universal generalities but on specific facts about matters nearest at hand. Here nurses have played and can play a vital part in recording, collecting and analysing relevant data, both in hospitals and in the community. This is why training in and application of evidence-based practice is so vitally important for a health service committed to continuous improvement and modernisation of its systems and methods of service delivery.

As we stressed at the outcome, sound factual evidence, including economic, epidemiological and demographic statistics, is vital to sound planning and decisions about resource allocation. But as we have seen in the preceding overview of some international and national developments, there are important ethical and political issues and differences in ideological approach to management and allocation of resources, which need to be taken into account in the debate on health policy and priorities. We shall now discuss some of these approaches.

FRAMEWORKS FOR POLICY-MAKING ON RESOURCE ALLOCATION AND MANAGEMENT

At all the different levels of healthcare – international or national levels, at the level of local corporate management of services or healthcare institutions, or at the day-to-day clinical level – it is necessary to determine which areas will be targeted and given priority, and how staff and financial resources are to be allocated to ensure that we attain our targets. Determining priorities may be a contentious matter with conflicting personal and professional interests and different kinds of 'political' pressures. What issues should be given priority will also be based on different *perceptions of the 'problems'* to be addressed and

different assessments of *what counts as 'evidence'*. It is far from evident that the allocation and management of human and financial resources is a rational or exact science, and disagreements are less often about matters of fact than about the interpretation of facts, or how they are to be constellated and about wider political agendas or vested interests!

Clinical decisions, determining day-to-day priorities on a ward and making decisions about how to allocate available staff, for example, might be made by the consultant, based on his perception of clinical priorities, or based on consultation with the ward team. In the latter case assessments made by nursing staff and other health practitioners may be given greater weight in balancing the needs of acutely ill patients with other patients who may require special attention because of their emotional distress or lack of adequate pain control.

Management decisions about the broader allocation of resources in a hospital or health centre, or in the community, will have to balance the competing demands of a number of stakeholders:

- health practitioners concerned with providing high quality medical and nursing care
- staff trade unions concerned with salaries and working conditions of staff
- administrators calling for evidence of increased efficiency and productivity in service provision
- auditors of clinical practice, demanding evidence of high standards of competence from practitioners
- financial auditors concerned with sound and transparent management of human and material resources
- community demands for more accessible and better standards of care, and user-friendly services
- local politicians and special interest groups demanding greater public accountability of healthcare workers.

Corporate planning of local health services will require both the balancing of various local political interests and also consideration of the different kinds of evidence offered in support of claims by various interest groups that their concerns should be given priority. The relative importance of hospital-based clinical services, or primary care and community care services might be one area or controversy. Alternatively, the proportion of budgets to be allocated to preventive and health promotion services in comparison with treatment services might be another. In these debates the evidence that is relevant to the debate will be of a variety of kinds: financial data, clinical data, epidemiological data and socio-economic data.

In relation to *government planning and policy-setting*, it is important to get some idea of where our hospital or health authority stands relative to others. We might need to use comparative data to 'benchmark', i.e. establish a baseline for determining local levels of need or levels of performance, and thus to set appropriate goals and targets for future improvement of services. We might need to compare the performance of different local hospitals, different local authorities, or compare ours with different societies, or more globally, consider comparative data relating to a variety of health indicators from the WHO European or global offices.

In discussing the ethics of resource allocation, the Edinburgh Medical Group put forward in 1979 five kinds of models or frameworks from which decision-making in healthcare has tended to proceed. These were identified as the clinical, epidemiological, ecological, administrative and egalitarian approaches (Boyd 1979). In our view, this early categorisation of frameworks remains a useful way of conceptualising approaches to determining priorities and policy-planning, at all the above levels, as well as helping to clarify options in the course of actual decision-making about the allocation of scarce health resources in our own context. However, given the introduction of the new economic model of the 'internal market' (in the UK and elsewhere), as well as the mixed economy of New Labour, another framework perhaps needs to be added to Boyd's five, namely: the business management model. In what follows we have grouped the ecological and egalitarian models together and introduced the commercial business management model as a fifth.

It must be stressed that these various approaches or frameworks are not mutually exclusive, nor intended as adequate in themselves. In reality many complex decisions about resource allocation will have to take account of all five perspectives and the final outcome of debate about different options and methods of resource allocation will involve negotiated ethical and political compromises between advocates of the various points of view behind the various frameworks.

In discussing the specific ethical and political responsibilities of nurses in both the practical allocation and management of resources, and in their contribution to more theoretical discussion of management policy and political priorities, it will be useful to bear these categories in mind.

Clinical approach (e.g. Murley 1995)

It is sometimes argued that because doctors and nurses are trained to care for people in crisis, and not as administrators, they tend to understand their responsibilities mainly in terms of the rights of individuals and their duty of protective care or beneficence towards 'their' patients. They tend to be more concerned with the clinical needs of individual patients and less concerned with justice for all patients, or equitable outcomes for vulnerable or dependency groups and ensuring adequate access to healthcare for the whole society.

From an ethical point of view, the clinical approach has traditionally emphasised the primacy of the health practitioner's duty of care to the patient, their duty of protective beneficence based on the paradigm of the extreme dependency and vulnerability of the patient. This emphasis on the health practitioner's duty of responsible care has ancient roots in medicine (going back to the Hippocratic Oath), but it is still reflected in the modern post-war Nuremberg Code (1947) and the World Medical Association's Geneva Declaration (1948, amended 1968). This emphasis has endured and, as we have argued in Chapter 4, will endure because of its relevance to the health professional's responsibilities in acute medicine relative to the predicament of the patient who is unconscious or incompetent. However, this approach tends to encourage paternalistic attitudes on the part of health practitioners, to underplay the rights of patients, and, in a broader context to ignore the issues of social justice and equity in healthcare. Further, it tends to be clinically and morally authoritarian, underplaying the expertise of other professionals and, at worst, presuming that health professionals and clinicians have special moral insight denied to others.

From a practical perspective, the strength of the clinical approach lies in the fact that it is rooted in the direct experience of practitioners of the clinical needs of individual patients and the practical problems of managing their acute medical problems. The clinical approach tends to assume that the medical perspective (usually the doctor's or consultant's) should determine and even be responsible for decision-making about resources. It presumes that a doctor's clinical judgement is authoritative and their clinical autonomy is sacrosanct. According to this view, priority should be given to the special knowledge and expertise of health professionals and their right to special authority in decision-making about matters related to healthcare. The limitations of such an approach are that it tends to be individualistic in dealing with clinical and ethical problems which may have complex social origins and consequences. It tends to be crisis-oriented and focused on the short-term crisis management, rather than on long-term strategic planning and wider consideration of research evidence of trends in morbidity and mortality. On the positive side, it emphasises the importance of curative and interventionist medicine and proof of what works, based on rigorous clinical research rather than the more speculative benefits of health promotion, prevention and rehabilitation. Besides, one of the key roles of GPs is to exercise protective beneficence and not only to protect the interests of their individual patients, but to advocate on their behalf in negotiations with other service providers.

In the most recent attempts at reform of the UK National Health Service, including negotiation of the new GP contract, clinical audit has been made mandatory (a recommendation of the 1979 Royal Commission on the NHS that was never properly implemented). This insistence on independent clinical audit in the interests of greater public accountability has given positive weight to the clinical approach. However, these changes were initially resisted by the medical establishment, who chose to see them as a threat to their clinical autonomy, but things have changed and are changing with GPs and consultants having agreed to mandatory audit of their work, and 'significant event analysis' as a condition for the renewal of their contracts (Harrison 2004, pp. 19–20 and 54–55).

Epidemiological approach

The epidemiological approach emphasises the need for objective health data on which to base consideration of health priorities. What is required is the scientific study and statistical analysis of the changing patterns of mortality and morbidity in society, including ability to demonstrate trends in the occurrence and recurrence of epidemics and the relative incidence and prevalence of different types of medical disorders. Typically the epidemiological approach is that favoured by community medicine specialists and health policy advisers. Planning practical public health measures and directions for health policy involves more than individual clinical judgement and requires more objective and universal indicators of both morbidity and health. Their focus tends to be on planning healthcare systems to serve the needs of specific communities, and the common good of those societies. This approach was given classical form in McKeown's study *The Role of Medicine* (1976), where he argues vigorously for the adoption of evidence from medical research and epidemiology rather than anecdotal clinical wisdom as a basis for health planning and resource allocation. The focus of New Labour's strategy for the New NHS has been to refocus attention on public health and primary care,

and the new GP contract makes this emphasis on public health in primary care explicit. The most recent *World Health Report 2005 – Make Every Mother and Child Count* (WHO 2005) attempts to reorientate health priorities globally on the basis of epidemiological evidence.

The main ethical focus of the epidemiological approach is on rational social justice in healthcare, rather than on individual rights or protective beneficence – for its object is to achieve equality of opportunity in access to services and equitable outcomes for different groups within the population. The public health movement of the mid 19th and early 20th century, with the support of WHO after the Second World War, has campaigned to improve the health of the community of nations and to coordinate international efforts to eliminate the worst killer diseases.

The Ottawa Charter (WHO 1986) set out to achieve the following objectives for the 'New Public Health', by a process of enabling, mediation and advocacy with other countries, with the following aims:

- to reorient public health services to better meet actual local needs
- to create supportive environments in which healthy communities can flourish
- to strengthen local community action for health promotion
- to develop the personal skills of people to manage their own health.

The latest global initiative by WHO, namely its proposed programme *Health for All in the 21st Century* (WHO 1999b), purports to provide a framework of principles and targets, based on national and international epidemiological data. These will be useful to member states in developing domestic health planning and cooperation with neighbouring countries. Specifically the WHO's *World Health Report 2005: Make Every Mother and Child Count* focuses attention on maternal and child health as a global priority. Tulchinsky & Varavikova (2000) review progress over a decade in implementing the objectives of the Ottawa Charter and other authors have sought to extend the scope of the new public health to include concern for the environment (Schroeder & Steinzor 2004) and the impact of the new genetics on public health (Petersen & Bunton 2002).

The strength of the epidemiological approach is that it aims to achieve objective and universally valid criteria for planning health services and resource allocation. The limitation of the approach is that it tends to be too abstract and impersonal, too far removed from the emotive reality of individual suffering and the demands of individuals to have their rights respected. In pursuit of rational criteria for decision-making it underestimates the power of medical vested interests and ability to mobilise media interest in 'miraculous' cures to influence public opinion in their favour, while successes in prevention are largely 'invisible' because well people are not noticed. It also tends to be too far removed from such social realities as poverty, deprivation and ignorance which provide the background to ill-health in contemporary society, and to underestimate the countervailing irrational forces which strengthen patterns of unhealthy living, including stress, anxiety, economic insecurity, peer pressure, and the influence of advertisements. Beauchamp & Steinbock (1999) offer a wide-ranging discussion of the ethical basis of and ethical issues in the new public health, which should be of wide interest and importance to health practitioners.

Egalitarian and ecological approach

The egalitarian approach can be identified with a broad concern with human rights and justice and equity in healthcare. It is reflected in the Article 25(1) of the UN Declaration of Human Rights, which states: 'Everyone has the right to a standard of living adequate for the health and well-being of himself and of his family, including food, clothing, housing and medical care and necessary social services, and the right to security in the event of unemployment, sickness, disability, widowhood, old age or other lack of livelihood in circumstances beyond his control.'

The Beveridge Report (Beveridge 1942), which served as the basis for the UK welfare state and informed the planning of the National Health Service, was essentially of this egalitarian nature. As Beveridge expressed it, the welfare state was to serve as a means of organising society to combat the 'Five Giants: Want, Disease, Ignorance, Squalor, and Idleness' in the interests of social justice and more equitable access for all to health, education and welfare.

The same egalitarian approach informed the UK Black Report *Inequality and Health* (DHSS 1980), and *The Health Burden of Inequalities* (Illsley & Svensson 1984) – a survey commissioned by WHO during a period of high unemployment in Europe. More recent studies concerned with the impact of social and economic factors on health include the World Bank's first report on the economics of health *World Development Report – Investing in Health* (1993), the United Nations Development Programme *Human Development Report* (UNO 1993), and WHO's first *World Health Report* 1993 (the fifth published in 2005). The egalitarian approach was given a European scope

and dimension in *Health 21: Health Policy Framework for the WHO European Region* (WHO 1998).

This approach has not been without its critics; for example, in Wilkinson's study *Unhealthy Societies: The Affliction of Inequalities* (Wilkinson 1996), he argues that if one compares the most extreme cases for example in the United States, Hong Kong and eastern European countries, there is no simple correlation between high mortality rates and unemployment or social deprivation. In Hong Kong in the decade before 1996 there had been a marked decline in infant mortality rates as compared with the United States, where levels have remained static. In eastern Europe he argued that the marked increases in infant mortality and in suicide rates among men in heavy industry were associated with rapid social and economic change and loss of hope rather than deprivation. In Hong Kong people saw that there were opportunities and hope and were motivated to value their health and to protect that of their children. Another line of criticism has been that the focus on medical aspects of health has ignored the importance of a good environment to good health, with a degraded environment having the converse effect on people's physical, mental and social well-being (Schroeder & Steinzor 2004).

The strengths of the egalitarian approach are that it encourages us to look at health within a total social, economic and political context. However, it can become so broad and unfocused in its attempt to address all the problems of society and the world that it loses its cutting edge (and to continue the metaphor) to deal surgically and effectively with trauma, physical and mental illness and the more specific problems of health service provision.

Administrative approach

The administrative approach could be described as being based on the traditional model of the welfare state where healthcare and welfare is provided by a largely state-controlled and funded service industry, which has to be managed by rational and accountable processes in the public interest. Those employed in the state public sector are charged with the responsibility to provide cost-efficient health services to the community on behalf of the state, and are accountable to the public only indirectly through government ministers. Health service planners and managers have an implied social contract with the patient public or 'consumers' of health services, to provide the whole range of medical treatment, rehabilitation and preventive services in return for the payment of tax and/or health insurance (Harrison et al 1990, Harrison 2004).

The ethic of public sector administration is one of public service for the common good. While ostensibly governed by consideration of universal fairness and respect for the rights of patients or consumers, the lack of direct accountability to consumers or the public means that the pattern of management and planning tends to be paternalistic and non-consultative – despite the establishment of bodies such as Health Councils or consumer rights groups to represent the concerns, complaints and needs of consumers 'to the authorities'. The administrative model gives particular emphasis to organisational and scientific rationality and to the contractual rights of patients and the duties of health professionals to maintain standards and quality assurance, based on models of public accountability (Beauchamp & Steinbock 1999).

The strengths of this approach are that it encourages centralisation of management, rational planning, data collection and record-keeping to ensure public and financial accountability to Parliament, or to the local health authority, through the health service bureaucracy. Supported by the medical model of applied scientific method, management is set up to monitor services using largely medical indicators of mortality and morbidity as measures of progress. The effectiveness of medical procedures will, according to this model, be based on proper scientific tests, randomised trials and controlled experimentation. While this model has worked fairly well for hospital medicine and the treatment of disease, it is not adaptable enough for the demands of primary care and health promotion services. To improve data collection in primary care the new GP contract offers GPs incentives and financial rewards for doing so. While the administrative approach has provided for systematic collection of statistics to aid strategic planning, rational target-setting, management by objective, sound evaluation and transparent administration, it has been accused of tending to be overly bureaucratic and impersonal and insensitive to the desires and needs of consumers.

Business management approach (e.g. Enthoven 1985, Saltman & von Otter 1995)

This approach has two interconnected forms in the UK, the first being the approach adopted by the Conservative governments of Mrs Thatcher and John Major, arising out of the Griffiths Inquiry into management in the NHS (DHSS 1983) and Enthoven's report for the Nuffield Provincial Hospitals Trust (Enthoven 1985). The second approach, while continuing many of the earlier emphases, adopted a more communitarian approach reflected in the reforms of the Blair Labour government (Honigsbaum 1995, Fairfield et al 1997).

Both approaches were influenced by the advocates of what has been called 'The New Public Management' or 'New Managerialism', who used the slogan 'Let the managers manage!' as a basis for their criticism of the earlier approaches, which were seen as dominated either by conservative medical models or those of public sector bureaucrats. The argument was that by the adoption of a business management approach 'health organizations could be made more efficient and effective by downsizing and applying management techniques that were originally developed by manufacturing firms and mass retailers of goods and services. Introduction of these business techniques would yield tighter managerial control over healthcare practitioners' (Harrison & Pollitt, 1994).

Under the Conservative government, this approach was combined with the adoption of the new model of the 'internal market', which created a new microeconomic framework within which health service planning, decision-making and delivery was to be conducted. The two features of this new economy that are relevant to resource management and resource allocation were the adoption of the business paradigms for the 'purchaser/provider' relationship, and 'customer focus'. The assumptions of this approach are that in the deregulated market for health service provision, there are 'providers' and 'purchasers' of services.

On this model it was argued that individual clients could negotiate their treatment requirements with their doctor and/or other health professionals, who would either provide the service directly themselves or act as brokers in obtaining services from other providers on behalf of their patient. Where not immediately available, service provision could be contracted out to private sector or voluntary service providers. It was further argued that the range and standard of health services provided would be determined not on the basis of *a priori* medical assumptions or the vested interests of established institutions, but by market forces and the laws of supply and demand. The scope of services available would theoretically be determined by their economic viability on the principle of 'user pays' wherever possible, and in the competition for 'customers' the best units would survive and the worse 'go to the wall'. The tests of efficiency, from the health authority or state government point-of-view, would be decided on the relative costs and benefits of alternative procedures. These were to be measured, like levels of productivity or turnover in business or industry, by predetermined 'performance indicators', e.g. the numbers of operations or treatment procedures given, and by bed turnover or discharge rates.

In many respects this approach was a refreshing change from the beneficent paternalism of the clinical model and the directive paternalism of the epidemio-logical model. It emphasised the autonomy of patients and the objectivity of 'consumer' rights. It certainly gave increased impetus to the demand for evidence of what works, based on proven effectiveness, and factual data on cost efficiency of service delivery relative to targeted goals and outcomes, as critical factors in determining priorities for strategic planning and the allocation of resources.

However, the business management paradigm tended to ignore the fact that the provision of medical and nursing care is not just a commercial transaction like that with any other service industry. The relation-ship between the contracting parties is an inherently unequal and asymmetrical one in power terms. The vulnerability and dependence of the patient demands a quality of trustworthy expertise and responsibility on the part of the health professional which is unique to human services – because people's lives and health are at stake. Furthermore, the 'internal economy' was not an example of a free market, because the budgets made available to Health authorities or hospital trusts were limited by government and subject to its regulation, and the relationship between 'purchasers' and 'providers' in the health sector bore little resemblance to that between manufacturers, suppliers and retailers in the wider business economy. The ambiguous status of 'purchasers' and 'providers' has in practice opened the way to abuse. There is growing concern, and evidence from both Australia and the UK, that the system has been subject to corruption and that 'cosy deals' have been done between local insti-tutions, to avoid the inconvenience of going through either strict or transparent tendering processes.

For nurses the mixed economy of healthcare provision has been a mixed blessing. On the one hand, the competitive environment has encouraged the private sector to poach nurses from the state hospitals, and nursing agencies have been able to offer nurses the inducements of improved flexibility, better pay and working conditions (which have been particularly attractive to nurses with family commitments). In primary care, nurses have been given increased responsibility for a lot of work previously done in hospitals, e.g. screening and treatment of diabetes, asthma and cardiovascular disease. This has created opportunities for new career paths for nurses on the primary care team, including the roles of practice nurses, treatment room nurses, nurse practitioners,

besides expansion in the role of district nurses, health visitors and midwives.

However, the contracting out (or contracting in) of nursing services has had the consequence for individuals that they have lost the pension rights and protections of work in the public sector. Furthermore, from a wider social perspective, these developments have resulted in staff shortages in some hospitals and arguably have also depressed the wages and working conditions for nurses in the public sector. Whether these 'reforms' have improved the quality of services is as yet unclear. The 'jury is still out' on whether they should continue.

How individual countries and health districts cooperate with WHO in implementing the global and regional strategic objectives of *Health for All in the 21st Century* (WHO 1999b) will be a matter of intense debate, political disagreement, weighing up of alterna-tives and disputes about competing social values and local priorities. However implemented, the health policies developed locally set new ethical and political challenges for nurses, as they do for other health professionals. In discussing each of the questions posed – regarding funding of the National Health Service, preventive or curative medicine, the relative importance of high technology, acute medicine and advanced medical research versus the provision of better primary and community care – perhaps none of the five models taken by itself is adequate. Discussed against the background of three complementary moral principles, each model has to be qualified. This is the very stuff of ethical and political debate.

Politics, as Aristotle observed, is the art of the possible; or, as he suggested in another context, it is the attempt to find the best means to achieve good ends in the light of both practical constraints and our principles and practical experience. The pleasure of politics lies in the challenge it presents to human creativity of finding new and better solutions to old problems. However, the burden of politics is that of knowing that no solution will be ideal and that our principles may have to be compromised to some degree because of the intractability of human nature, the unpredictable and often tragic nature of events, and global disasters as well as unexpected scientific, technical and medical 'breakthroughs'.

Rodger Neighbour of the Royal College of General Practitioners has remarked that: 'The pattern of reform and changes introduced by successive governments, have tended to create a political climate in which the cycle of promise, pretend and then blame is endlessly repeated.' This pessimistic view reflects the weariness of NHS practitioners with 'restructuring' and being the butt for public and political criticism, when insufficient time is given for the implementation and consolidation of change, before the next round of 'reforms' (see Baggott 2004, pp. 191–192, 'Market reform as policy fashion').

SOME PRACTICAL DILEMMAS OF RESOURCE ALLOCATION IN HEALTHCARE

The dilemmas in resource allocation in healthcare management are of several kinds – practical dilemmas, ethical dilemmas and policy dilemmas. While we can distinguish these formally, it should be remembered, as we said in the Introduction, that because all decisions we make in healthcare impact on people's quality of life this means that no aspect of healthcare is morally 'neutral'.

- Practical dilemmas relate to what can be done in a specific situation if needed equipment or resources at a particular time are not available, e.g. lack of MRI scanners or dialysis machines, or money to pay for locum staff.
- Ethical dilemmas relate to perceived or actual conflicts between different principles or duties in the delivery of quality healthcare, e.g. between the duty of care to patients with acute needs and equitable and fair treatment of all patients, or in continuing to receive patients when a ward is critically understaffed, or between the 'rights' of individuals to 'exotic' treatments and the use of resources for more general needs.
- Policy dilemmas relate to choices of approach to issues of organisation and management at a number of levels, e.g. whether the management style is consultative and democratic or based on strict line management authority; whether ancillary services should be kept 'in-house' or open to tender and contracted out; whether healthcare policy should be directed by medical expertise or consumer preferences.

Here, the ethics of resource allocation is not restricted to debate about issues like the expenditure of money on life-saving medical or surgical procedures for a small number of patients, or about equal rights of access to scarce high-technology equipment such as whole-body scanners or kidney dialysis machines. It refers also to expenditure on staff salaries, to the cost of building and equipping new hospitals or rebuilding and refurbishing old hospitals, to the cost of medical research, expenditure on drugs and disposable medical supplies and on such homely things as furniture, fittings, decor and the quality of hospital food, and how these are to be funded (e.g. by direct local fundraising, by 'public/private funding initiatives', or by the state). They also relate, for example, to the debate about the use of public and teaching hospital resources for private medicine and private patients, and the tendency for the private sector to engage in 'cherry-picking' of areas of work where bed turnover and profits are highest.

The making of public health policy about these issues cannot be the exclusive preserve of doctors or bureaucrats, politicians or any particular class of 'experts'. Nurses not only have the same right to participate in public debate about these issues as any other citizens, but they also have a duty to do so, in view of their own front-line experience and professional expertise. In fact, the objectivity of the judgement of some doctors in these matters may be questioned because they may have a vested interest in defending the prestige and budgets of their units or their related research programmes. Nurses, both as citizens and as professionals with inside knowledge of the working of health services, the practicalities and costs of day-to-day healthcare, have a particular responsibility to speak out on the practical and ethical issues of resource allocation.

As we have already emphasised, sound ethical and political arguments in these areas should not be based simply on ideological dogmatism or unquestioned moral assumptions, but require knowledge of the facts, practical wisdom based on clinical experience, and 'political' judgement in how best to balance emphasis on different values and to reconcile competing interests. Here, in addition to knowledge of the facts, the use of proven methods for analysing the value conflicts involved may be helpful in bringing to light the complexities involved, clarifying the choices to be made and helping to develop consensus (e.g. use of the stakeholder analysis model, Chapter 12).

Responsible decisions, especially by nurses involved as managers and administrators, cannot be simply matters of right/wrong, black or white, decisions, but require ability to make sound value judgements based on proper assessment of the facts. They must be properly informed and their decisions grounded on research into the clinical and epidemiological facts, and on sound financial experience and accounting. To put the 'expense' of controversial new medical procedures or life-saving medical intervention into perspective, it is necessary for nurses in general, and nurse managers in particular, to be well informed about the staffing implications and actual costs of these procedures relative to priority needs of their own region, nationally and internationally. We proceed to outline some examples of issues in relation to which difficult decisions have to be made about rationalising or allocating human, material and economic resources in healthcare.

While less dramatic as resource issues than the challenges of transplants, in vitro fertilisation (IVF) or applications of genetic engineering or cloning to medicine, the issues of shortages of staff and equipment are likely to make a more direct impact on the morale and working conditions of nurses and other health workers. These issues will not only affect the standard of care health practitioners are able to provide for their patients but may also give rise to adverse criticism in the media of particular healthcare staff or the performance of particular hospitals. The trend towards the development of comparative 'league tables' on the performance of different hospitals is claimed to help policy planners and administrators towards more rational service planning, and to meet increasing public demand for public accountability of healthcare staff. However, questions may be raised about the performance indicators that are employed to assess performance; e.g. reduction of waiting lists may not be a fair or adequate measure of the quality of care or effectiveness of treatment given in a particular unit or hospital. The exposure of hospitals and health practitioners to public scrutiny and criticism may in reality leave dedicated staff feeling undervalued rather than having their problems, including shortage of staff or lack of resources to modernise equipment or facilities, dealt with sympathetically, by the media and politicians.

In the past, much of the debate about the reform and restructuring of health services, which has been conducted by health planners, bureaucrats and their technical advisers and consultants, has left nurses' and other health practitioners' views out of account. While the public in the UK have been encouraged by politicians of the right and the left to get involved in the ideological and practical debate about the alleged 'crisis' facing the welfare state, the views of health practitioners on policy and priorities in resource allocation have not been extensively canvassed, nor systematically researched. From the receiving end of politically driven media criticism of the failures of the NHS to meet the exaggerated expectations of the public, professional staff have been left feeling undervalued and made to feel personally responsible for the system's failures. In this context, and 'punch-drunk' from one reorganisation after the next, health professionals have become increasingly cynical about politics and the extent to which health service planning can ever be a rational or exact science. The rhetoric of 'reform', 'modernisation', 'performance management' and 'transparency' has become tiresome to many health practitioners because, despite the demand for evidence-based practice, politicians and bureaucrats do not appear to take into account evidence of the damaging effects on staff of constant reorganisation, when making changes to policy or in restructuring services. In some cases it has not been shortage of evidence that has been the problem, but failure of managers to analyse and interpret the evidence for the benefit of the public administrators and politicians.

The professional bodies and unions representing health workers and practitioners in the UK (e.g. the BMA, Medical Royal Colleges, Faculty of Community Medicine Specialists, and the Royal College of Nursing and staff unions like UNISON) nevertheless have been increasingly prepared to enter the debate about the direction of policy and funding for the NHS, about new contracts and the radical proposals of the *Agenda for Change* (DoH 2003), for example. In reality, health practitioners might be better prepared in their training and professional development to engage with the ethical and political issues involved in these higher-level discussions of policy and resource allocation, many aspects of which are matters not just for healthcare managers, but of direct relevance to front-line workers and clinical practice as well.

Some classic areas of ethical controversy about resource allocation which arise in clinical practice for nurses as well as doctors are, for example: the impact of staff shortages on the standards of care; the shortage of equipment for routine scanning leading to long delays for patients on waiting lists; the limited number of kidney dialysis machines relative to those needing urgent treatment while awaiting transplants; the limited number of organ donors relative to the need for liver, kidney and heart transplants; the ethical problems related to surrogacy or egg donation; the treatment of infertile couples by expensive and risky IVF; the justifiability of life-saving surgery for neonates who have severe disabilities, with possible long-term need for intensive care; and the use of NHS facilities for cosmetic surgery, breast implants and invasive procedures such as liposuction and excision of fat to reduce obesity.

Each and every one of these issues warrants further discussion, and could be the subject of assignments for students. However, we will restrict ourselves to commenting on a few selected examples of important issues that range from local to international concerns. These are:

Example 1: What should be done to reduce the number of unwanted pregnancies?
Example 2: Do we do enough about the impact of alcohol and tobacco on health?

Example 3: Is increased expenditure on organ transplants for preventable health conditions justifiable?

Example 4: Treatment of infertility, by in vitro fertilisation and assisted reproduction.

Example 5: *World Health Report 2005 – Make Every Mother and Child Count*

Example 6: The challenge of the global HIV/AIDS pandemic.

Example 1: What should be done to reduce the number of unwanted pregnancies?

Consider some of the facts summarised and issues raised by the CARE Abortion Statistics Factsheet (based on official statistics from CARE 2003 and ISD 2003):

When the (UK) 1967 Abortion Act was passed, many felt it was a necessary, if regrettable, piece of legislation to deal with a minority of women in desperate situations. The Act has, however, led virtually to abortion on demand by allowing abortions to be performed on certain grounds. Amendments under the Human Fertilisation and Embryology Act 1990 brought in a new upper time limit allowing most abortions to take place only up to 24 weeks, but also allowing certain exceptions with no upper limit set, thus permitting legal abortions up to birth.

In 1968 a total of 23 641 abortions were performed in England and Wales. By 1978 this had increased to 141 558 and in 1988 to 183 798. A peak of 187 402 abortions was reached in 1998. In 2003, the most recent year for available figures, the number of abortions was 190 660. Over 5 million abortions have been performed in England and Wales in the 37 years since the 1967 Abortion Act was passed.

- The total number of abortions in England and Wales for 2003 shows an increase of over 5000 from the previous year, 2002. The overall rate of legal abortions for women resident in England and Wales in 2003 was 17.5 abortions per 1000 women aged 15–44. Between 1968 and 1990 there was a fairly steady rise in abortion rates. Then between 1990 and 1995 this changed to a slight downward trend in the abortion rate until 1996, when rates began to increase again, with fluctuations from year to year. The rate for 2003 is the highest ever recorded.
- Figures for Scotland show a similar steady rise from a total of 1544 abortions in 1968. In 2003 the number of abortions in Scotland was 12 217, compared to 11 772 in 2002. The number of therapeutic abortions has fluctuated around 12 000 per year since 1996. The rate of legal abortions per 1000 women aged 15–44 in Scotland in 2003 increased to 11.5 % compared to 10.9% in 1996.
- The Abortion Act does not apply in Northern Ireland, so women living there who want abortions often travel to England and Wales. A total of 1318 women from Northern Ireland had abortions in England and Wales in 2003, a slight drop from previous years.

Table 10.4 shows that those aged 20–29 years account for half of all abortions.

Table 10.4 Abortions on residents in England and Wales, by age group (2003)

Age	Number	Percentage
Under 15	1 171	1
15–19	37 043	20
20–24	51 124	28
25–29	36 018	20
30–34	28 749	16
35–39	19 868	11
40–44	7 032	4
45 and over	500	–

Specific issues highlighted in this fact sheet are the following:

- The majority of abortions in 2003 in England and Wales took place before 13 weeks gestation (87%).
- Single women make up the largest group having abortions: in 2003 they accounted for three-quarters of abortions on women resident in England and Wales.
- In 2001 9% of all conceptions within marriage resulted in abortion, compared to 36% of conceptions outside marriage.
- Amongst teenagers the rates of abortion are higher: 56% of those who conceived before they were 16 had an abortion in 2003 in England and Wales.

While the mass media and the public express concern from time to time about the rising level of legal abortions in the United Kingdom, there are no signs that the legislation permitting abortion is likely to be abolished, or even radically amended, although there is periodic debate about the legal definition of viability, and the criteria for permitting termination of pregnancy. What remains a live issue in public debate is the ethics of abortion, whether the current legislation is liberal enough to meet the concerns of women's rights pressure groups, or should be made more restrictive to meet the concerns of pro-Life groups. (Here it may be worth observing that in Scotland particularly, where the established Church of Scotland and the Roman Catholic Church are still influential in shaping public policy on sexual health, the issue of deliberate termination of pregnancy is still a highly contentious matter. Throughout the UK, this is also true for some of the evangelical churches, for orthodox Jews and Muslims, and some other religious groups. Government policy-makers have to tread warily not to offend these religious interests, some of which exercise considerable pressure and influence in shaping public policy on issues such as contraception and sex education, and the availability of condoms in schools.)

Whatever a person's moral convictions may be about the ethics of abortion, the above figures should be a cause for concern, mainly because they represent the failure of society and the state to reduce the levels of unwanted pregnancies. Whether this is due to ignorance or failures in social education on sexual health and contraception, or to failures of contraception itself, or to an increasing use of abortion as a substitute for contraception (despite the increasing availability of free or over-the-counter forms of contraception and the 'morning-after pill' on prescription), these are matters for further research. If we are to avoid sterile grandstanding of moral opinions on the subject, policy must be argued on the grounds of evidence and of what preventive measures will be most effective.

Because midwives and health visitors are front-line health educators, they should be particularly concerned that so many unwanted pregnancies occur, that so many women want to terminate their pregnancies, and that there are so many failures of contraception or just failure to use any form of contraception. Individual nurses may also have to make choices, arising out of failures in prevention, about assisting or not assisting at terminations, and hence should be clear about their own views on these matters, and proposed strategies for dealing with them.

Health practitioners also need to be aware that there are many economic and political factors which complicate the whole problem of abortion – relating to the status of women, their working conditions, terms of employment – including socio-economic, environmental and lifestyle factors such as drug abuse. For nurse managers the question is whether they adopt a systematic, strategic and long-term approach to dealing with these issues, or just resort to 'first-aid' and 'crisis management'. Do they confine themselves to their clinical and health education responsibilities with individuals, or take local 'political' action in these areas?

Example 2: Do we do enough about the impact of alcohol and tobacco on health?

Although the government benefits directly from the taxes it levies on the sale of tobacco and excise on alcohol (£8.06 billion from taxes on tobacco and £5.9 billion from alcohol in 2004) (National Audit Office 2004), these amounts together would contribute only about a fifth of what is required to fund the NHS, without taking into account the costs to business and industry, to society itself and the NHS, of smoking and alcohol-related morbidity and mortality.

If we take cigarette-smoking and the use of other tobacco products as an example, there are several kinds of costs to be taken into account when considering its impact on the health and well-being of society. Leaving aside the largely spurious debates about the 'rights' of smokers, the social, economic and health costs of smoking are considerable. Details of these can be obtained from government sources, and in the UK from ASH (Action on Smoking and Health) in particular. These are listed in Factsheet No. 16 (ASH 2004) under the following headings: costs to industry, costs caused by fires, costs to the smoker and to the government.

The costs of smoking to industry

A Scottish study by Parrott et al (1998) estimated the costs of smoking to industry in connection with the following cost factors:

- lost productivity caused by smoking breaks and increased absenteeism amongst smokers: £40 million
- increased absenteeism amongst smokers due to ill-health: £450 million
- fires at work caused by smoking materials: £4 million
- cleaning and building maintenance costs specifically related to smoking: not calculated

The costs of fires caused by smoking materials

According to the *Fire Statistics, United Kingdom, 2002* bulletin, smokers' materials and matches were the most common source of ignition causing accidental fire deaths; although there has been a downward trend, possibly associated with non-smoking policies at work, the total still stood at 4400.

The costs of smoking to the smoker

The financial costs of smoking to the smoker can be considerable; e.g. a 20-a-day smoker will spend about £1650 a year on cigarettes. However, the average proportion of people's income spent on cigarettes has fallen from 3.4% in 1978 to just over 1.3% in 2004 (ONS 2004).

However, it is the health costs that are far more significant for, as the results of a 50-year study show, between a half and two-thirds of lifelong cigarette smokers will eventually be killed by their habit. Death is usually due to one of the three major diseases caused by smoking – lung cancer, chronic obstructive lung disease and coronary heart disease (Doll et al 2004).

The costs to the government (quoted from ASH 2004)

Research by the Centre for Health Economics at the University of York has shown that the cost to the NHS of treating diseases caused by smoking is approximately £1.5 billion a year (Parrott et al 1998). Other costs include the payment of sickness or invalidity benefits to those suffering from diseases caused by smoking and the payment of pensions and other family social security benefits to the dependants of those who die as a result of their smoking. One method of estimating the cost of smoking is to apply the criteria used to estimate the value of the loss of human life. The Department of Transport, for example, put this value at £680 590 in 1997. If this value is applied to the total number of deaths attributable to smoking, the cost of smoking related mortality in the UK in 1997 prices is just under £80 billion (Royal College of Physicians 2000). In December 1998, the Government published its tobacco White Paper in which it pledged £100 million over 3 years on measures to reduce smoking (TSO 1998). Expenditure on tobacco control in the current financial year is around £50m. An analysis of the cost benefits of achieving the government's targets to reduce smoking has shown that £524 million should be saved as a result of a reduction in the number of heart attacks and strokes (Naidoo &Wills 2000).

On the other hand, it has been argued that because smokers die younger they save the NHS and social services expenditure on their care in old age. However, this would hardly be a reason for encouraging people to continue smoking, certainly not an ethical reason!

The health and social costs of alcohol abuse

Figures corresponding to those for smoking are given for the impact of alcohol on health by the Institute of Alcohol Studies in their fact sheets. The following are some of the significant issues covered by these fact sheets:

- alcohol and health
- alcohol and mental health
- alcohol and elderly people
- alcohol and women
- alcohol and young people
- alcohol and road traffic accidents
- alcohol and the workplace safety
- alcohol-related crime and disorder.

Despite the fact that the majority of people in the UK enjoy alcoholic beverages, in social contexts as well as increasingly at home, and despite the evidence that there are some health benefits of moderate consumption (e.g. of red wine as an antioxidant), nevertheless both as concerned citizens, and especially as health practitioners, we should be concerned about the huge impact of alcohol abuse on physical, mental and social pathology, through its contributing to a wide range of types of morbidity and also to a significant proportion of deaths.

Given current legislation in the UK to relax licensing hours (on the basis of the argument that this might 'encourage European-style drinking habits', rather than binge drinking with its associated problems of antisocial behaviour, assaults and public violence on the streets and at football matches), the whole issue of public, ethical and social policy on the control of alcohol supply and regulation of its use has wide implications for the health and well-being of society.

Let us consider a few salient facts and headline figures as summarised in the UK Institute of Alcohol Studies' fact sheet – Alcohol and Health (IAS 2005) (Box 10.5).

Box 10.5 Some facts on alcohol and health

- In developed countries alcohol is one of the ten leading causes of disease and injury. Worldwide, alcohol causes 3.27% of deaths (1.8 million) and 4% of 'disability adjusted life years' lost (DALYs) (58.3 million).

- In developed countries, alcohol is responsible for 9.2% of the disease burden.

- Alcohol causes nearly 1 in 10 of all ill-health and premature deaths in Europe.

- The WHO's Global Burden of Disease study finds that alcohol is the third most important risk factor, after smoking and raised blood pressure, for European ill-health and premature death.

- Alcohol is more important than high cholesterol levels and overweight, three times more important than diabetes and five times more important than asthma.

- This level of alcohol-related death, disease and disability is much higher in men than women and is highest in Europe and the Americas, where it ranges from 8% to 18% for males and 2% to 4% for females.

- Beside the direct effects of intoxication and addiction, worldwide alcohol is estimated to cause 20–30% of cancer of the oesophagus, liver cancer, cirrhosis of the liver, epilepsy, homicide and motor vehicle accidents.

While much more detailed facts and statistics are provided in the same IAS fact sheet, the issues listed above should suffice to remind us personally, as health professionals and as potential contributors to health and social policy, of the significance of alcohol as a major negative factor affecting our health and well-being nationally and globally.

Here the ethical issues to be considered range from our moral responsibility for our own health, and our duty to practise what we preach and to be good role models by responsible drinking, to more public concern and action to both prevent alcohol abuse and to help treat its victims. While nurses and doctors will encounter patients in the casualty department with injuries caused by road traffic and industrial accidents, assaults and domestic violence and even cases of alcohol poisoning caused by over-consumption, they will also have to nurse patients with enduring or even end-state conditions caused by lifelong abuse of alcohol such as: cancers of the oral cavity and pharynx, oesophagus, larynx, breast, liver, colon and rectum; liver cirrhosis; essential hypertension; chronic pancreatitis.

The role of healthcare practitioners

Healthcare practitioners are in the front-line in counselling people about their smoking, alcohol consumption and obesity, whether in clinical nursing settings or in industry. Here they not only have a moral duty to be well informed about the impact of alcohol on physical and mental health, but also skilled in appropriate counselling techniques, to avoid appearing to either patronise or to hector people about their habits. As health professionals become more aware of the risks involved in smoking, alcohol and being overweight, there is also a risk of their being morally censorious and biased towards patients who chronically abuse substances of various kinds, or fail to do anything about their weight. Clearly they are entitled to feel strongly about these issues, and even to campaign publicly on these topics, but they still have a basic duty of care to provide appropriate care, treatment and services to all patients, without discrimination.

For those involved in health education and health promotion, whether in the community or at national level, they should perhaps also be aware of the need for greater resources to be made available for health counselling, health education in the media and general health promotion – given the astronomical sums spent on advertising smoking and alcohol products, compared with the derisory sums made available by governments for health advertising, which has

remained constant at about 0.1% of the total allocation for health services. Consider, by contrast, current figures for expenditure on alcohol and tobacco advertising:

- In 2001 in the UK, the alcohol industry spent £181.3 million on direct advertising of their product and £600–800 million on indirect promotion through sponsorship and marketing (Alcohol Concern 2004).
- During the period September 2001 to August 2002, tobacco advertising expenditure in the UK amounted to £25 million, excluding sponsorship and indirect advertising. The companies spent £11 million on press advertising; £13.2 million on outdoor (billboards); £714 550 on radio advertising; and £106 253 on direct mail (ASH 2004).

One might believe that in a rational world, spending in healthcare would be directly related to the major causes of morbidity and mortality in the community, but for a variety of political reasons this is often not the case, and thus it becomes important to consider the responsibilities of special interest groups and health professionals to lobby government ministers to rationalise health expenditure, just as the smoking, alcohol and fast-food industries employ professional lobbyists to advocate in their interests.

It is important to note that the medical Royal Colleges and Royal College of Nursing and other bodies representing health practitioners have campaigned ceaselessly and with increasing effect in getting the government to restrict tobacco and alcohol advertising and have made a major contribution to shaping current smoking legislation.

Box 10.6 Too old for treatment? The case of 'Mr A' (Report by Darshna Soni)

A judge has ruled that a hospital is able to switch off life support for an 86-year-old man, even though he says he wants to live.

'He's paid his dues – and this is the thanks he gets.' The feelings of a son of and 86-year-old war veteran – whose family lost their fight to make a hospital treat his kidney failure.

He's alive, and has been able to express his wish to live to his family. But the man, known as 'Mr A', is very ill – on life support treatment and in need of dialysis.

A High Court judge has now sided with the healthcare trust, agreeing that the treatment can be withdrawn. His family say it's blatant age-discrimination – and they are appealing the verdict.

Published on Channel 4 News, 26 August 2005.

Example 3: Is increased expenditure on organ transplants for preventable health conditions justifiable?

More accessible perhaps, to some health practitioners, are the issues of the kind highlighted over twenty years ago in recurring media coverage concerning the lack of money and donors to help young people in need of transplants (Box 10.6).

The issues in such cases are never as straightforward or simple as the media would have us believe they are. The hospital consultants dealing with the case gave evidence to the court that 'Mr A' was terminally ill, and unlikely to live for much longer; whereas the defence's medical advice was that 'Mr A' had a reasonable chance of recovery. The pressure on the hospital, to make dialysis equipment available for 'younger and more needy patients', was implied by the defence team as the reason for the position adopted by the hospital team. On the other hand, the hospital questioned whether 'Mr A' was really able to communicate his wishes, given the seriousness of his condition, as reported by nurses and medical staff. Whether or not this was a dilemma of resource allocation, or a matter of different religious and cultural attitudes to the rights of the dying, could be debated. A nurse was reported as saying that she regarded the dialysis as 'treatment for the relative's distress' in the face of the imminent death of Mr A.

Similarly, emotive accounts in the press and on television have dramatically highlighted the life-saving character of heart and liver transplant surgery, in spite of the high costs and relatively poor survival rates of these procedures. These remain experimental procedures despite progress in dealing with problems of immune system rejection of transplanted organs.

More than thirty years ago, Dr Peter Draper from the Unit for the Study of Health Policy, Guy's Hospital, London, argued forcefully that the money spent on heart transplant surgery would be better spent on health education. He argued that because most of the heart conditions being treated by transplant surgery are preventable, and there is disturbing evidence that many recipients of heart transplants fail to change their lifestyles and even continue to smoke, the real problem and challenge is how to change people's attitudes and help them effect changes in their health behaviour (Davey & Popay 1992). Despite their high profile in the media and hospital-based television dramas, evidence that the application of new technologies is cost-effective for either patients or the NHS is weak (Harrison et al 1997) but it is clear that they add over 2% to the cost of the NHS (Wanless 2002).

When we consider the risks to children or adults of inadequate resources for the treatment of victims of kidney disease, we may come to see that difficult decisions have to be made about where to target resources – whether on more dialysis machines, scanners or on prevention (including staff training in health promotion and public health initiatives). The clinical approach will tend to focus attention on individuals in urgent need of treatment, whereas a public health approach will concentrate on epidemiological arguments concerning changes in the pattern of mortality and morbidity in society.

In the UK, the success of immunisation in controlling infectious diseases and the effective use of new medical treatments for many life-threatening conditions has left the vast majority of patients encountered by health practitioners as ones who are affected by disorders which are the result of their lifestyle. These include respiratory disorders and lung cancer caused by smoking, and diseases of the circulatory system caused by poor diet, lack of exercise, smoking and alcohol abuse – all of which may result in damage to organs that need replacing if the patient is to survive. An argument based on considerations of justice and the common good, however, would suggest that priority in the allocation of resources should be given to health education and prevention. On the other hand, heart-rending and tragic cases of individuals requiring exotic and expensive types of therapy are used by the media to emphasise a popular view that the NHS has a duty of care to provide the best possible treatment for anyone who needs it.

It might seem possible to resolve the policy dilemma of how best to deal with coronary heart disease and kidney disease, for example, on the basis that since most cases of both diseases are preventable, priority should therefore be given to allocating resources to prevention rather than treatment. There is an inherent problem in all public health and health promotion in that it is difficult to prove the cost-effectiveness of preventive measures in advance. The fact that more people are healthy or do not suffer from coronary heart disease, liver cirrhosis or kidney failure is not generally regarded as newsworthy or of interest to politicians. Good health is politically invisible, whereas trauma, epidemics and acute medicine make for good media copy and photo-opportunities. The problem in the richer, developed countries is similar to that faced by governments in developing countries, namely, that building 'disease palaces' brings more political kudos than programmes for immunising children. However, this still leaves the unanswered moral and clinical problem of adequate resources for the treatment of patients with renal failure and heart disease.

Similar difficult decisions have to be faced in dealing with fetal abnormalities. It is possible by antenatal diagnosis to determine in some cases that a fetus is abnormal, but what kind of 'therapeutic' choice is abortion as an alternative to bearing a child with Down's syndrome or spina bifida? There are nevertheless still many cases where antenatal tests have not been done or the test refused. Here, faced with the delivery of a spina bifida baby, even one with only a limited hope of survival, nursing staff have to take a position on whether to give the child the necessary care and treatment, or 'cooperate' in withholding treatment. What does the nurse or health practitioner make of the specific demands and rights of the child to treatment, who is owed a duty of care by the doctor and nursing staff, as compared with the abstract considerations of justice in the management of resources and the common good? This is an issue currently being given exposure on the media with parents being encouraged by popular support to challenge medical discretion in the courts on the basis of the child's right to life and right to treatment (even when the consensus of medical opinion would be that this is futile). Perhaps the question here is whose needs are paramount?

Example 4: Treatment of infertility, by in vitro fertilisation and assisted reproduction

In Australia, where human IVF-assisted reproduction was pioneered and much research done by medical entrepreneurs, there are women's pressure groups (often set up by IVF doctors) actively campaigning for IVF as every woman's right. One group has even gone so far as to claim that 'all women have the right to compassionate IVF surrogacy' (Yovich & Grudzinskas 1990). However, research evidence has shown that IVF and intracytoplasmic sperm injection (ICSI) can be a mixed blessing to couples, and in relation to the demands it makes on medical and hospital services. For infertile couples, or individuals, the sheer costs and risks for women associated with hyperstimulation of the ovaries, and the protracted and often unsuccessful nature of the procedures, can also put marital and family relationships under strain.

Dr Fiona Stanley, an eminent Australian specialist in child health research, has argued that state funding for such assisted reproduction is not justified. In the face of other maternal and child health priorities, and in the light of evidence of birth complications among IVF babies, such as premature birth, low birthweight and a high incidence of birth-related cerebral palsy where multiple births occur, scarce health resources should be directed to other health priorities. (Stanley

1992). She was reported in *The West Australian*, 22 July 1992, as saying:

> Australia cannot afford to waste its scarce health dollars on inappropriate technology such as IVF. Money could be better spent researching the causes of infertility or the effectiveness of surgery in treatment of infertility in women. The evidence of the Canadian Royal Commission on *in vitro* fertilisation, is that women who drop out of IVF programmes have the same chance of becoming pregnant as women who stay in the programmes. My major concern is that there has been no randomised control trial, comparing IVF with either doing nothing or doing other things, for example surgery for tubal problems. Without adequate trials we do not know either whether these techniques are really effective, nor do we know what the risks and complications are likely to be. (Stanley 1992)

Some female social scientists have also argued that the commercialisation of assisted reproduction, including IVF, ICSI, egg and sperm donation, and surrogacy arrangements, is driven by the profit motive on the part of doctors and multinational healthcare providers, and is degrading and risky to the health of women. Their ethical objections are of two kinds:

1. That a male chauvinist culture has made reproduction an imperative of sexual 'partnership' and women who may well have had children in earlier partnerships, cooperate with IVF (often to 'treat' male infertility) and are turned in the process into 'baby machines', at the service of men's need to prove their virility.
2. That the process tends to treat children simply as a means to an end, to satisfy parental reproductive ambitions, regardless of the risks to mother and/or child (Grayson 1993).

A recent controversy with particular relevance to the second objection, which has been given much publicity in the media, is the related question of the use of IVF to create 'saviour siblings', for the purpose of obtaining matching donor tissue, bone marrow, or even body organs. This raises critical questions about the fundamental rights of children as persons, relative to their parents and/or siblings, and whether parents have a moral entitlement to use conception of one child as a means to treat the needs of another.

On the other hand, there are dilemmas involving the feelings and opinions of the whole neonatal ward team about commencing and/or terminating assisted life support to infants with severe birth abnormalities. These practical problems raise some of the most difficult medical decisions for obstetricians and very painful problems for nurses involved in their ongoing care. Given the poor prognosis for very premature babies (of less than 24 weeks), if they survive (currently estimated at a 1 in 4 risk of *severe* lifelong disability, and a higher risk of *some* form of disability) this places additional burdens of responsibility on health practitioners, parents (if they are consulted), and on publicly funded health and welfare services. Poor outcomes will certainly add to the financial burden on families or carers, and on society in terms of increased taxation to meet costs.

The pros and cons of decisions about IVF or life support for neonates with severe disabilities are debated, it should be noted, at two different levels – the clinical level, and the policy level – and these involve making quite different kinds of decisions. *Clinical ethical decisions* related to specific cases will be ones that have to be made in the light of the facts of the case, what is permitted by the law, by established policy and precedent, and by direct application of ethical principles. The second type, *ethical policy decisions*, are concerned with proposals for new or changed policy or procedures to deal with recurrent problems of the same type. At the clinical level specific decisions have to be made about particular patients. Here nurses may not have much power to influence medical decision-making, but it is more than likely that they will have to deal with the disappointment of the infertile couple or grief of the parents who have a child with severe disabilities and if the child dies. They also have to cope with their own feelings about the situation. At the policy level, however, where the practice of IVF and neonatal intensive care raise important questions about the responsible allocation of scarce resources, nurses have both a right and a duty to contribute their knowledge and expertise to public debate on these matters of such general public interest.

The 'right' of infertile couples to medical assistance to conceive a child would seem to many people to be a fundamental entitlement. However, a helpless newborn baby with disabilities may be denied life-saving treatment because it is thought to be unjust to burden a family or to make great demands on social resources. In contrast to the infant who is unable to defend his rights, forcefully articulate and determined couples may be able to exert great pressure on health services (and in the UK, on the Human Fertilisation and Embryology Authority (HFEA)) to meet their demands for IVF and assisted reproduction services.

In both cases, difficult decisions may have to be made by health service managers and policy-makers, relating to setting limits to what it is reasonable and just for the public to demand from the health services, in view of other demands on time, manpower and financial resources. The objective assessments of the prospects of the baby with fetal abnormalities, for survival and quality of life, have to be balanced against what burden of responsibility it is reasonable and practicable to expect the medical and nursing staff, the child's parents and society to carry. Justice demands that these other interests should be considered in deciding whether expensive life-saving measures should be taken.

In the case of the childless couple, there may well have to be limits set to what it is fair to expect public health services to provide. Given the low level of risk involved in remaining childless, it might be argued that, in spite of the emotional cost to the young (or elderly!) couple, and 'risk' to their marriage, their 'right' to have a child should not be given priority over other more pressing needs of patients with life-threatening conditions, or to premature babies requiring life support.

Treatment for infertility, on the one hand, is a booming industry, with considerable attractions for doctors and nurses working in obstetrics and neonatal medicine. On the other hand, it may even be regarded as a luxury when the global aim is to limit fertility in the interests of population control and the conservation of diminishing global resources. In many developing countries, moreover, the attempt to set up such services would hardly even be considered, although this may primarily be a measure of the lack of relevant resources in countries where infertility may exist, but fertility is prized. Moreover, it is maintained by some that since the knowledge and technology exists to assist many childless couples to have children (whether by IVF, ICSI or other means such as surrogate parenthood), in a prosperous society, like Britain, this help should be available through the National Health Service. Against this, it is counter-argued that people should be able to get the help privately if they can afford it or can raise the money from charity. Even then would it be reasonable to expect medical and nursing staff to give up time and resources to meet these further demands, which they may not see as important as dealing with life-threatening disease and injury? Or is this a false antithesis, rooted again in lack of resources for healthcare overall?

Critical to this debate is the question: who decides what qualifies as a condition 'requiring medical treatment'. For example, who decides heroic efforts should be made to save the lives of infants with congenital abnormalities or to treat middle-aged or lesbian couples requesting IVF, or gay men seeking help with surrogacy arrangements?

Is this a case where 'money talks' – those that have the financial resources to pay can claim the 'right' to 'treatment' and those who do not have the resources cannot. This clearly raises the question of what is meant by the 'right to healthcare'. What is the scope of this so-called natural right, and who decides whether or not you can exercise this right? How ethical is it for sperm and egg donation to be commercialised by 'off-shore' and internet-based agencies that are not subject to regulation or quality control?

These critical ethical questions will clearly be viewed differently in countries with problems of massive over-population and very limited health resources, as compared with those with negative population growth, declining fertility and generous state funding for health.

Current speculation about the possibilities opened up by genetic engineering and the cloning of the sheep 'Dolly' at the veterinary research establishment at Roslin in Scotland raise questions about the scope and limits of our entitlements to demand assistance from medical science and health services, e.g. for selective breeding of the children of our own choice. Cloning may make possible human tissue regeneration and the development of organs for transplantation, but should one have the right to invest in a spare heart or kidney, just in case one needs it 'further down the track'? Should anyone be entitled to request that a clone, or multiple copies, of themselves be made?

The Human Genome Project has set out to map all human genetic types on the planet. The findings of this project promise to bring huge benefits in the application of genetic science to dealing with hereditary genetic defects. Some of its advocates, moreover (betraying perhaps a naive view of the complexities of genetic inheritance and its interaction with environment), go on to claim that genetic medicine could also mean that in the future parents may be able not only to choose the sex of their child, but to 'order' a child with particular attributes, e.g. with beauty, intelligence and scientific ability, rather than being plain, athletic and sociable!

Discussion of these examples illustrates how in the interests of the survival of the species and of moral communities in which we tolerate diversity; it may be necessary to strike a different balance between the demands of justice, respect for persons and beneficence.

Example 5: *World Health Report 2005 – Make Every Mother and Child Count*

The WHO has sought to focus attention on maternal and child health as priorities in its 2005 *World Health Report – Make Every Mother and Child Count*. In launching the report, the WHO Director General,

Dr Lee, said: 'This approach has the potential to transform the lives of millions of people. Giving mothers, babies and children the care they need is an absolute imperative.' The WHO Press Release summarises the key points:

> According to the 2005 World Health Report, almost 90% of all deaths among children under five years of age are attributable to just six conditions. These are: acute neonatal conditions, mainly preterm birth, birth asphyxia and infections, which account for 37% of the total; lower respiratory infections, mostly pneumonia (19%); diarrhoea (18%); malaria (8%); measles (4%); and HIV/AIDS (3%).
>
> Most of these deaths are avoidable through existing interventions that are simple, affordable and effective. They include oral re-hydration therapy, antibiotics, anti-malarial drugs and insecticide-treated bed nets, vitamin A and other micronutrients, promotion of breastfeeding, immunization, and skilled care during pregnancy and childbirth.
>
> To reduce the death toll, the report calls for much greater use of these interventions, and advocates a 'continuum of care' approach for mother and child that begins before pregnancy and extends through childbirth and into the baby's childhood.
>
> This in turn requires a massive investment in health systems, particularly the deployment of many more health professionals, including doctors, midwives and nurses. 'For optimum safety, every woman, without exception, needs professional skilled care when giving birth,' the report says, adding that continuity of care for the newborn in the following weeks is vital.

According to UNICEF, 1 in every 12 children dies before the age of 5 from preventable disease, and these deaths are concentrated in the developing world (UNICEF 2002). Infant mortality rates in Africa are four times higher than the average in Europe, and average life expectancy at birth in developing countries is two-thirds that of the industrialised nations. The average life expectancy of a European male (69) is twenty years longer than for an African (49) (WHO 1998) (quoted from Baggott 2004).

Here the contrast between the alarming statistics in the 2005 *World Health Report* for maternal and child death in the developing countries as compared with Europe and other industrialised countries is stark. The major causes of death in the developing countries are due to poverty and malnutrition, or as WHO has said: 'Poverty … is the world's deadliest disease.' By contrast, the major causes of death in Europe and other industrialised countries are lifestyle related and connected with diet and lack of exercise, smoking, alcohol and drug abuse, and sexual health.

The question facing WHO, and ourselves as

member states of the United Nations, is how to reorder our priorities to address these challenges. In developing countries the alternatives may be clear, despite the kudos politicians seek from investments in high-technology medicine and 'disease palaces', and the fact that the benefits of public health initiatives on maternal and child health are not politically visible or headline-grabbing. In the richer, developed countries, our responsibility may be to ensure that a greater proportion of our GDP is given to promote economic development of Third World countries, and to relieve the debt burdens that are crippling them and preventing improvements in their people's health.

Example 6: The challenge of the global HIV/AIDS pandemic

To take a problem of rather different proportions, let us consider the implications of resource allocation locally and worldwide for the HIV and AIDS epidemic. Some salient facts about the global situation with respect to HIV/AIDS are provided by WHO/UNAIDS. Table 10.5 shows some selected figures.

Table 10.5 Selected figures for estimated adult and child deaths from HIV/AIDS in 2000

North America	20 000
Caribbean	32 000
Latin America	50 000
Western Europe	7 000
North Africa and the Middle East	24 000
Sub-Saharan Africa	2 400 000
Eastern Europe and Central Asia	470 000
Australia and New Zealand	~500
United Kingdom	~250

Source: UNAIDS.

Significantly, the World Bank *Human Development Report 2004* highlights HIV/AIDS as a major challenge not only to health services worldwide, but especially to the economies of developing countries where, as in sub-Saharan Africa, the working population of countries is being decimated by the epidemic. By way of contrast, it is illuminating to compare some World Bank headline figures for Europe and Central Asia with those for Africa (Table 10.6).

By contrast, according to figures given by the *Hard Facts about AIDS* website, the total AIDS deaths in the UK before 1986 were 562. In 1987 alone the figure

Table 10.6 Some World Bank 'fast facts'

'Fast facts'	Europe and Central Asia	Africa
Total population (billion)	0.5	0.7
Population growth (%)	0.1	2.1
Life expectancy at birth (years)	69	46
Infant mortality (per 1000 births)	31	103
Female youth literacy (%)	99	77
2003 GNI per capita (dollars)	2570	490
Number of people living with AIDS (millions)	1.3	25.2

Database: World Development Indicators.

was 417, this rose to 1719 in 1995, but has fallen since to 310 in 2002 and appeared set to fall further. Their figures for AIDS by country and year are to be found in Table 10.7.

According to the UK Health Protection Agency (HPA 2004), 'since the epidemic began in the early 1980s about 15 750 deaths in HIV infected individuals are known to have occurred in the UK. At the end of 2003 an estimated 53 000 adults aged over 15 were living with HIV in the UK, 14 300 (27%) of whom were unaware of their infection. Currently the number of people living with diagnosed HIV is rising each year due to increased numbers of new diagnoses and decreasing deaths due to anti-retroviral therapies.' Whether the epidemic is running its course in the typical fashion recognised by epidemiologists, or whether the preventive action taken by health professionals and the government has contributed to the decline in deaths and new cases of HIV, could be debated. A matter of concern is that the number of newly diagnosed cases appears to be rising again, but overall the incidence of the disease in the UK appears on the decline. Some key trends are summarised below:

- Cumulatively, the majority of infections reported to the Centre for Infections have occurred through sex between men. This group remains at greatest risk of acquiring HIV infection within the UK. There has been no evidence in recent years of a decline in the numbers of new infections in this group and over 1700 new diagnoses of HIV are currently occurring each year.
- The numbers of heterosexually acquired HIV infections diagnosed in the UK have risen enormously since 1985. The increase since 1996 has been especially marked. As a result since 1999

Table 10.7 UK AIDS cases by country and year (2002)

Year	England	Wales	Northern Ireland	Scotland	Total UK
1986 or earlier	841	16	3	22	882
1987	641	6	1	32	680
1988	844	22	7	32	905
1989	979	16	8	78	1081
1990	1145	18	6	75	1244
1991	1268	16	6	98	1388
1992	1474	15	8	80	1577
1993	1626	28	9	122	1785
1994	1700	30	12	112	1854
1995	1599	30	13	125	1767
1996	1327	20	1	84	1432
1997	985	12	2	70	1069
1998	726	13	2	36	777
1999	668	13	7	51	739
2000	741	6	5	43	795
2001	617	14	8	35	674
2002	450	9	4	47	510
Total	17 631	284	102	1142	19 159

there have been more diagnoses of heterosexually acquired infection than of infections acquired through sex between men.

- Most of those diagnosed in the UK who have acquired infection heterosexually were not infected in this country. Almost 82% are recorded as having acquired infection abroad, with around 70% of the total infected in Africa. In the late 1980s and early 1990s the majority of the African infections were acquired in East Africa but more recently the impact of the HIV epidemics in south-eastern Africa has been greater.
- Cumulatively, around 6% of UK diagnoses have been attributed to injecting drug use (IDU). IDU has played a smaller part in the HIV epidemic in the UK than it has in many other European countries and the numbers of new diagnoses have been around a hundred for the last few years.
- The age at which individuals in this group have been diagnosed rose throughout the 1990s. This suggests that new diagnoses are being made on an ageing population largely infected in the mid-1980s and that new infections have been occurring less frequently than infections are being diagnosed.
- The overall picture masks differences in the geographical distribution in the UK. Eastern

Scotland experienced rapid HIV spread through IDU in the early to mid-1980s.

- HIV-infected injecting drug users are predominantly male. This reflects the pattern in all drug users and has meant that the relatively small heterosexual spread from infected drug users has been predominantly to women, with 75% of those reported infected by this route being female.

WHO has established the International Office of HIV/AIDS and Sexually Transmitted Diseases (ASD), with four main objectives:

- to coordinate global, regional and country-level responses to sexually transmitted diseases (STDs) and HIV/AIDS
- to facilitate integration of activities dealing with STDs and HIV/AIDS through provision of technical and normative support, through WHO regional and local offices
- to ensure liaison between WHO and other non-governmental international and national agencies
- to coordinate within WHO and associated organisations the mobilisation of resources to deal with STDs and HIV/AIDS.

At the most basic level, by cooperation locally in assisting not only with the direct care of patients with STDs and HIV/AIDS, but also in conscientious record-keeping and collection of data, nurses and other health practitioners contribute significantly to the overall strategy for controlling this devastating global pandemic.

WHO has cautioned that the reported global number of HIV/AIDS cases in the various health regions is a relatively crude indicator of trends, for the following reasons (DHH & CS 1993):

- less than complete diagnosis in many cases
- less than complete reporting to public health authorities
- delays in reporting inherent in the passive case surveillance approach
- use of different case surveillance criteria around the world
- limited resources in some developing countries for epidemiological research
- reluctance of some governments to acknowledge the problem or publish data.

The worldwide epidemic of HIV/AIDS has attracted a great deal of attention and concern both from the worried public and from health professionals faced with the fact that there is as yet no cure for the disease. While AZT and more recent anti-retroviral drugs appear to have had some success in delaying the onset of AIDS in those with HIV infection, the major problem is the huge cost of treatment with these drugs. Their use remains completely out of reach of most of those suffering from HIV/AIDS in impoverished Third World countries, where the current cost of one course of treatment with AZT may be more than the per capita funding available for all medical treatment. Concessions negotiated with holders of patents on these drugs, allowing local production of generic forms of the drugs, is helping to bring down the costs. This and increased funding from the World Bank and national governments, including the exemplary donation to Africa from the trust set up by Bill Gates of the Microsoft Corporation, will all help, but the problems of sub-Saharan Africa are currently so acute that these initiatives may be too late to save millions of lives currently affected by HIV/AIDS.

The absence of effective means of immunisation or treatment of HIV/AIDS has left health professionals feeling relatively impotent to do anything effective in the clinical situation, other than to offer victims palliative care. The primary challenge is to address the need for effective primary, secondary and tertiary prevention, and good infection control measures in hospitals and clinics, but initiatives in this area by WHO or other international NGOs are severely hampered by official denial that there is a problem, by governments in affected areas. The South African government of Thabo Mbeki is a case in point, where the fact that HIV infection leads to AIDS was steadfastly questioned. In the face of concerted international pressure, and the pressure of rising AIDS deaths, the position has improved and anti-retroviral drugs are being made available to some.

HIV/AIDS is a good example of an issue where knowledge of the local culture, religious background and health data is critical for the development of appropriate services, training relevant to working with affected and at-risk individuals, and development of sound ethical policies for local HIV/AIDS prevention and patient education.

Because the primary modes of transmission of HIV/AIDS are sexual intercourse and injecting drug use, effective health education and prevention are the most basic measures required to contain the pandemic. However, these behaviours, which can put people at risk of HIV disease, relate to people's intimate sexual behaviour, drug use and personal lifestyles. What kinds of public health measures are taken, or what style of personal health education or wider health promotion is required, and what forms are socially acceptable, raises the question of the limits of personal rights to privacy and autonomy when the health of children and the general public is put at risk. Primary prevention is no 'quick fix' but aims to change people's attitudes and behaviour over time in relation to various forms of high-risk sexual behaviour and substance abuse. Some considerable success has been achieved in the USA and Australia, particularly among those homosexual men who are educated in safe sexual practices and highly motivated to adhere to these. Indeed, the main aim of preventive services has been to encourage the practice of 'safe sex', through use of condoms or other protective measures. The establishment of needle exchanges has helped reduce HIV transmission through sharing injection equipment. Caring by carers for people living with HIV/AIDS, both in the pre-terminal and terminal stages of the disease, has been a model in many countries of how support for the dying and the bereaved can be improved generally. Many nurses have been in the forefront of these efforts to humanise the services dealing with people with AIDS.

These moral quandaries and ethical dilemmas related to working with HIV/AIDS can arise for nurses at two rather different levels – at the more intimate personal level, and at an institutional level in the context of their professional work. At a personal level, the challenge is that before nurses can work effectively with people with HIV/AIDS, either in clinical nursing or in health education roles, they have to confront their own fears and fantasies (including homophobic prejudices), and questions about their own sexuality and lifestyle that have a bearing on how they relate to these patients.

At an institutional level, other kinds of issues arise in the 'management' of people with HIV/AIDS. In the early stages, in the clinical situation (in the clinic, patient's home or hospital) the issues of confidentiality and invasion of privacy are the most important. Nurse managers should be contributing to overall HIV/AIDS policy, but would also be expected to help determine how these policies are implemented at ward- and overall hospital-level; e.g. policies on general infection control, on record-keeping and confidentiality, on segregation of patients and access by relatives and significant others. They also have to decide on relevant in-service and AIDS-awareness training for staff.

In the UK, health authority and health board managers have had to develop AIDS policies on a number of issues: equal employment rights issues relating to affected healthcare staff; workers' compensation for nurses infected through needle-stick injuries or contact with patients' blood or body fluids; training policies; and issues of prioritising the allocation of staff and resources to deal with the often neglected areas of sexual health and sexually transmitted diseases.

The HIV/AIDS pandemic epitomises the themes in nursing ethics that we have attempted to illustrate in this chapter: first, that ethical decisions have to be made in healthcare at a number of different levels, and second, that at each of these levels nurses may be involved and have to accept responsibility for decisions:

- Micro – at the bedside in clinical decisions affecting the direct nursing care of AIDS patients.
- 'Macho' – in multidisciplinary team decisions about the clinical management of people who are HIV positive or with end-stage AIDS, and who on the team takes responsibility for leadership.
- Meso – in hospital or clinic level decisions about policy and procedure for dealing with infection control or prevention, treatment or aftercare.
- Micro – in decision-making and policy-setting at local authority, regional and national level affecting the deployment of nursing services to deal with HIV/AIDS, relative to other needs.

The second theme concerns the competing values in the workplace which shape our priorities and determine choices. These may be relative to the care of individuals, working in teams, management of resources, and shaping healthcare policy as it applies to nursing. HIV/AIDS is just one problem to be addressed among many others, albeit a very important one.

Nurses at a more senior level, managers, and those in positions of power and authority, have a responsibility to be informed about the basics of public administration, the alternative possible frameworks and principles which underlie approaches to policy development. Public panic about the incidence and prevalence of HIV/AIDS may result in poorly informed judgements about the allocation of resources.

Finally, nurses have a fundamental professional responsibility to ensure that their practice is based on sound behavioural and scientific research, and that it conforms to the highest standards of probity and ethics.

further reading

Bowden P 1997 Caring: gender sensitive ethics. Routledge, London

Branmer L M 1993 The helping relationship, processes and skills. Allyn & Bacon, Boston

Campbell A V 1978 Medicine, health and justice: the problem of priorities. Churchill Livingstone, Edinburgh

Davey B, Popay J 1992 Dilemmas in health care. Open University Press, London

Enthoven A 1986 Reflections on the management of the National Health Service. Nuffield Provincial Hospitals Trust, London

Freidson E 2001 Professionalism: the third logic. London Polity Press, London

Hetherington P, Maddern P 1993 Sexuality and gender in history, selected essays. Optima Press, Western Australia

Saltman R, von Otter C 1995 Implementing planned markets in health care. Open University Press, Buckingham

Thompson I E, Harries M 1997 Putting ethics to work. Public Sector Standards Commission, Western Australia

Wilkinson R 1996 Unhealthy societies: the affliction of inequalities. Routledge, London

Corporate ethics in healthcare: strategic planning and ethical policy development

Chapter contents

AIMS

This chapter has the following aims:

1. To introduce nurses to some of the key issues in the political ethics of healthcare which impact on nursing, e.g.
   - how policy decisions are made
   - how to set sound ethical policy
   - when nurses are justified to go on strike
   - whether the welfare state is in terminal crisis
   - whether NHS reforms have worked or not

2. To encourage nurses to be better informed about the ethics of management, policy-making and the administration of healthcare and nursing

3. To encourage nurses to recognise their ethical duty as professionals to contribute to public debate about the political economy of health.

LEARNING OUTCOMES

When you have read and worked through this chapter, you should be able to:

- Give a good account of key current issues in the political ethics of healthcare which impact on nursing and to explain how they do so

- Give an informed account of local health policy and funding of services, and to demonstrate knowledge and practical understanding of how both raise vital ethical questions for nurses

- Demonstrate use of the POLICY model in reference to some matters of direct concern to yourself, and to demonstrate that you know how to apply it to other nursing issues

- Demonstrate ability to debate the pros and cons of nurses going on strike in a way that shows you understand the ethical issues involved and can make informed judgements about different kinds of proposed strikes

- Show evidence of having researched some of the issues related to the funding of services in your hospital, clinic or local authority, and understand the issues at stake in the political debate about the future of welfare states.

ACCOUNTABILITY IN HEALTHCARE – STRATEGIC ETHICAL MANAGEMENT

In this chapter we turn our attention to the question of *responsibility and accountability in the corporate management and public administration of healthcare services* generally. In earlier chapters, we have discussed the responsibility and accountability of nurses in relation to:

- professional responsibility and accountability to the Nursing and Midwifery Council (Chapter 4)
- responsibility and accountability in direct clinical work with patients (Chapter 7)
- responsibility in nursing practice and ward or service management (Chapter 8)
- responsibility for performance management, in strategic management, teaching and research (Chapter 9)
- responsibility and accountability in the local and national allocation of resources (Chapter 10).

In this chapter we will be dealing in more detail with issues that are currently being referred to under the titles of 'corporate governance', 'staff governance' and 'clinical governance'. Again this new rhetoric is interesting because it marks a shift away from individualistic models to an emphasis on corporate responsibility and accountability, or 'total quality management'. It is also significant that while those who use the term 'governance' do so because it has the ring of legal and business-like language about it, it nevertheless incorporates an approach that gives values and ethical policy a central role in standard setting, strategic planning and corporate management. The issues we will discuss are: the steps required to develop sound corporate ethical policy; the process and methods employed in strategic planning; the issues involved in social policy and administration of healthcare services generally; and, the alternatives facing governments in the reform and modernisation of the 'welfare state' and the continuous quality improvement of healthcare services.

STRATEGIC MANAGEMENT OF THE NATIONAL HEALTH SERVICE

The National Health Service (NHS) was set up 56 years ago and since then has grown into the largest organisation in Europe. It also accounts for the single largest slice of public expenditure in the UK. Not surprisingly, the issue of its institutional responsibility and public accountability for administration of public resources has become a recurring theme in public and political debate about the NHS. Some of the issues raised are:

- whether we can afford the escalating cost of healthcare (currently over £62 billion per annum)
- whether the NHS is managed effectively in the most cost-efficient way
- whether existing systems and procedures are effective and efficient in achieving NHS targets
- whether the standards of service provided by doctors, nurses and allied health professionals are of the highest quality
- whether specific clinical methods, types of treatment or chemotherapy, or surgical procedures bring the benefits claimed, in terms of improved health or quality of life.

All these questions relate to issues of professional and institutional responsibility and accountability in the delivery of healthcare. It is perhaps self-evident that health practitioners are responsible for the administration of healthcare resources, because they are entrusted with this responsibility as professionals appointed to perform various functions in the delivery of healthcare services on behalf of the public. Whether as public sector employees or employed in private sector hospitals or service providers, health practitioners are exercising a responsible function in caring for the health needs of the public. It is also perhaps self-evident that as public officers, or public servants, they should also be publicly accountable for the standard of their work and their efficient and effective use of public resources, but the question is: How should institutions be accountable, and by what standards? This brings us to the subject of strategic planning, objective and target setting, and the measurement of performance and outcomes.

In a sense the question of the accountability of the NHS nationally and of health authorities and health boards locally, as well as the accountability of doctors and nurses, has been around for a long time. There have been different emphases in different periods, with different attempts to reform the health system, and in particular, from the mid-1970s onwards because of the economic recession. Three main periods can be identified as these applied in the UK, but also in Sweden, Holland and a number of other countries (Harrison 2004, Ch. 1).

In the *first period*, in the decade from the mid-1970s, reforms in the NHS were mainly concerned with *containing costs and making it more efficient*. The emphasis was on developing an evidence base and objective measures to assess the costs and benefits, effectiveness and efficiency of systems and procedures in the delivery of healthcare. Here the work of Cochrane

(1971) was seminal. He pointed out that much medical practice was based on 'medical pragmatism' and often no more than an appeal to 'common-sense' and anecdotal evidence, or reliance on practices established by custom and practice. In contrast, he emphasised the critical importance of evaluation in healthcare, and four main types of inefficiency to be addressed:

- the use of ineffective therapies
- the inappropriate use of effective therapies
- the inappropriate use of healthcare settings
- the incorrect lengths of stay in treatment facilities.

In the *second period*, from the mid-1980s to the late 1990s, the emphasis moved to making service providers more directly accountable for the quality and costs of their services and more responsive to patients' needs and priorities. With these reforms came greater statutory regulation to contain costs and, in the attempt to make health services more cost-efficient and to improve quality, market-like economic models and competitive processes were introduced into the system. Instead of straightforward privatisation of nationalised systems of healthcare delivery, a kind of mixed economy of service provision was introduced. Here, purchasers of services were to be able to negotiate service agreements with a variety of providers, including private sector and voluntary organisations. Alternatively, in the public sector a range of services had to be put out to tender, and services contracted out on 'best value for money' principles.

In the *third period*, from the late 1990s to the present, while there was a continuation of many aspects of the preceding attempts to achieve market reform, and managed competition, there has been a *renewed emphasis on central planning, strategic planning and target setting, and outcome evaluation, on a foundation of evidence-based practice* (Muir Gray 2001). More attention has been given to *strategies to improve public health and wellness*, to reduce inequalities in health status, to address gender inequalities in employment and to research public needs and expectations of the NHS. In national and local corporate management of the NHS, greater emphasis has been placed on the rights of patients and consumers of health services. This has meant that in the process of strategic planning, *consultation with all relevant 'stakeholder groups' has been encouraged*, rather than simply relying on the views of managers and policy bureaucrats.

Given the convoluted history of healthcare reform, and the different kinds of organisational restructuring that has accompanied these economic and politically driven reforms, there is perhaps understandable cynicism about the continued use of the rhetoric of 'accountability'. In the present situation, where

authority and responsibility for cost management and quality control has been increasingly devolved to local health authorities, there is a tendency for 'accountability' to have negative connotations for staff. This is possibly a hang-over from the period of the 'new managerialism' where accountability primarily meant critical appraisal of staff performance and policing of standards by management (without management being accountable to NHS staff). The attempt within the latest reforms is to emphasise mutual accountability of all stakeholders in the NHS moral community to one another, and to their patients or customers, rather than simply to management or to higher government authority (Day & Klein 1997, Ferlie et al 1996).

Here what is being attempted is a kind of new deal in the relationship of government and people, where each has recognised responsibilities, and they cooperate in an 'open and transparent' kind of 'partnership' of mutual accountability (Day & Klein 1997, Dewar 2003). Whether the new rhetoric of 'partnership' is more than 'public relations spin' remains to be seen. Clearly accountability in 'public/private finance initiatives' is a contentious issue in current politics, and the extent of real partnership between purchasers and providers of services is not only a matter of definition, but needs to be worked out in terms of different types of responsibility and public accountability of public and private sector agencies.

As Baggot (2004, p. 187) points out, 'the NHS has been bedevilled with confusion about different types of accountability in the contexts of health services, and many of these conflict with each other.' He mentions in particular: the clinical accountability of health practitioners to patients; the managerial accountability of the NHS to government; and the political accountability of government to Parliament and to taxpayers.

Part of our aim in this chapter is to tease out these different senses of 'accountability' and, in particular, to clarify the meaning of corporate accountability and the role that sound ethical policy development and strategic planning can play in making this a more constructive process.

First we will discuss the steps involved in policy planning and the vital role of ethics in helping:

- to clarify the values that should direct policy
- to choose appropriate goals, targets and performance indicators
- to set standards for evaluation of the performance of staff and services
- to determine future directions for services in the light of assessment of outcomes.

Then we will proceed to discuss what is involved in strategic planning and will examine how thinking strategically can help at all levels in healthcare, from the delivery of front-line services, to ward or unit management, to corporate management at local and national level. The emphasis here is on the acquisition of relevant skills in thinking, planning and operating strategically, and not on the development of Utopian strategic plans. The object is to improve the standard of management from pragmatism and 'crisis management', to adopt a problem-solving and systematic approach to assessment, planning, implementation and evaluation of all aspects of management and service delivery in healthcare.

Just as strategic planning involves a move away from the trial-and-error pragmatism of crisis management to a more systematic approach based on standardised routines and procedures that allow comparative assessments to be made, so ethical policy development involves a move away from ad hoc ethical decision-making to the adoption of standard rules and policies for dealing with recurrent types of problems. Neither strategic planning and management nor policy-based approaches to recurrent types of ethical problems exclude the possibility of planning for contingencies or recognising the unique nature of some ethical situations or dilemmas in clinical practice. In fact, the kind of rationality in decision-making that strategic planning and ethical policy development requires would be irresponsible and unethical if it failed to take account of the fact that reality does not always conform to generalised strategy or policy. As the Scottish poet Robert Burns famously said, 'The best laid plans o' mice and men gang aft agley!' (Often go awry!)

DEVELOPING ETHICAL POLICY IN HEALTHCARE

Review and reorganisation has been a feature of life in major public sector organisations during the past decade, as governments have sought to reform and corporatise (or privatise) the management and financing of major institutions of the Welfare State. Formulation of 'mission statements', 'values statements' and 'strategic plans' has been the order of the day with the introduction of business models of 'total quality management' (Joss & Kogan 1995).

Corporate statements of an organisation's mission, vision and values are often treated with contempt as being either 'just an exercise in public relations' or 'wishful thinking'. This can certainly be true if they are simply the result of brainstorming on the part of the corporate executive and are not the product of genuine consultation and participation of all significant stakeholders. This can also mean very little in practice if they cannot be 'cashed out' in workable corporate and operational ethical policies, if these are not directly applicable, e.g. to a hospital or clinic's ordinary everyday business.

Values statements are of critical importance here, and need to be modelled by the corporate executive and all managers, to be 'owned' by employees, and endorsed by their patients or clients and main external stakeholders. An organisation's values serve to determine 'the way it does business' and its performance (like that of an individual) will be judged by the congruence or lack of congruence between its practice and the values it professes. Values play a critical role in strategic planning and management because an organisation's choice of values plays a crucial role in defining both its short- and long-term goals. Values also help to give practical meaning to the definition of standards and 'quality' in its service delivery and the products it supplies. Clarifying values also serves to determine what kinds of processes and systems are most appropriate to achieve its objectives, and to monitor and evaluate its performance. This would apply as much to the whole of the NHS, as it would to a local authority health department, to a large hospital, or small health centre or clinic.

Sound strategic ethical management is based on the application to a *whole organisation* of the methods of *continuous quality improvement*. This means that the process of strategic planning and operational management are directed from the start by the values that are fundamental to and endorsed by all stakeholders in the organisation. Where there is collective 'ownership' of an organisation's values, these can play a critical role in defining its leadership and management style, policies for employee development, the way it does business with clients, and the quality of its products or the services it delivers (James 1996).

In the major business corporations on which these forms of organisational development have been modelled, ethical policy and standards development have been found to play an important role in giving direction to cultural change, and quality improvement in organisations that are committed to continuous service improvement. In diagrammatic form this can be set out as illustrated in the RADICALE model for continuous improvement (Fig. 11.1).

What this model serves to illustrate is that ethics is not an optional extra in business or health services management, but is an essential part of sound strategic planning and management.

Ethical policy development is therefore an integral part of both strategic planning and operational management. Setting ethical policy, including policies

(A) Process improvement/Ethical policy development cycle

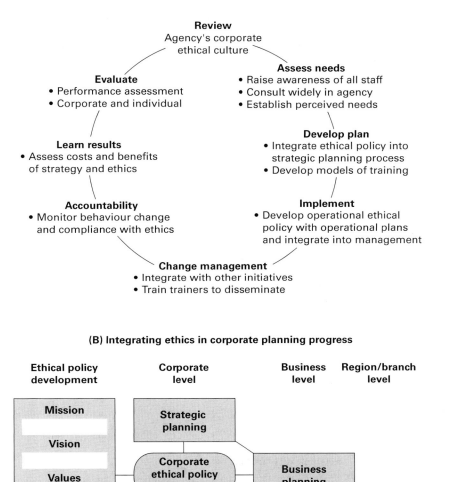

Review
Agency's corporate
ethical culture

Evaluate
- Performance assessment
- Corporate and individual

Assess needs
- Raise awareness of all staff
- Consult widely in agency
- Establish perceived needs

Learn results
- Assess costs and benefits
of strategy and ethics

Develop plan
- Integrate ethical policy into
strategic planning process
- Develop models of training

Accountability
- Monitor behaviour change
and compliance with ethics

Implement
- Develop operational ethical
policy with operational plans
and integrate into management

Change management
- Integrate with other initiatives
- Train trainers to disseminate

(B) Integrating ethics in corporate planning progress

Ethical policy development	Corporate level	Business level	Region/branch level

Mission

Vision

Values

Strategic planning

Corporate ethical policy development

Consolidated business planning

Business planning

Corporate culture

Corporate ethical policy

Operational ethical policy development

Consolidated branch and region planning

Region/branch planning

Figure 11.1 RADICALE model for continuous improvement. Reproduced with the permission of Water Authority of Western Australia from its *Corporate Ethics Training Manual* (WAWA 1994).

on standards and quality, is one of the most basic tasks of management, in consultation with employees and customers. Any policy should give clear expression to the commitment of management to the values of the organisation, and give guidance on how these are to be applied by the whole organisation to identified generic types of problems or recurring processes. The quality of the ethical policy of an organisation is the first important evidence that management is serious about its ethical responsibilities and constant quality improvement of its services and operations.

What James (1996, p. 99) says about quality guidelines and policy applies equally well to corporate and operational ethical policy (including its code of conduct and disciplinary rules). We would paraphrase these in the following way, namely that ethical policy should:

- give clear but generalised guidelines of *what* is to be done, rather than attempt to specify in detail *how* things should be done
- be generic in operation and apply to whole classes of schemes of work or types of problems encountered in organisational life and service delivery
- as actual or implied rules, be prescriptive, but be designed to create an environment conducive to ethical conduct and be helpful to rather than hinder quality-related performance
- apply to the whole organisation, to all levels of staff and be seen to be modelled by all internal stakeholders, both in relation to their clients or customers, and to one another.

More specifically, an ethical policy is an official statement, on behalf of stakeholders (and/or recognised authority within an organisational moral community), which outlines a general ethical approach to deal with recurrent types of problems or difficult situations. An ethical policy must:

- specify the class of problems it is meant to address
- set out the overall ethical approach and objectives adopted
- list standard procedures and the ethical justification for them
- provide a framework for decision-making and conflict resolution
- set criteria for monitoring performance and implementation of the policy
- indicate a clear strategy to achieve endorsement of policy by stakeholders.

In order to develop adequately comprehensive ethical policy it is necessary to get away from a narrow individualistic model of ethics and to recognise the various levels in corporate life where ethical problems arise and ethical policies are required to help us deal with them. Secondly, it is necessary to realise that the task of developing ethical policy is an ongoing one, and should be subject to review in the light of its effectiveness in providing normative guidance. It should certainly not be 'set in concrete' or treated as entirely non-negotiable, and as part of the strategic planning and review cycle, its principles and objectives should be periodically revisited.

The 'Russian dolls model of corporate ethics' introduced earlier, in Chapter 2, is relevant here and should remind us that there are several different levels at which ethical policy needs to be developed and addressed in any organisation, namely:

- External stakeholder level: ethics in strategic planning and inter-agency relations
- Internal stakeholder level: ethics in corporate management of human and financial resources
- Team leadership level: ethics in interdisciplinary cooperation and teamwork
- Individual level: ethics in personal decision-making and service delivery.

In order to engage effectively in the operation of ethical policy development, it is necessary to acknowledge that certain kinds of knowledge and skills are necessary for the task. Too often people 'rely on instinct' or appeal to that 'feeling in the gut that it is right or wrong', whereas those who are to exercise leadership, administrative and management roles in corporate life need to develop knowledge and skills in a number of areas of practical moral competency, viz:

- skills in clarifying and applying values to everyday operations
- skills in making sound and well-justified ethical decisions
- skills in setting organisational standards, ethical policy and rules of conduct.

Developing competence in practical ethics also requires understanding of fundamental ethical principles (e.g. the principles of justice, respect for personal rights and beneficence or responsible care). Sound management practice presupposes that these principles are applied competently with discriminating judgement at individual, team and corporate levels.

Skills in clarifying and applying values to everyday operations

In previous chapters we have discussed the importance of values for ethics and of critical self-assessment of the goals to which one is committed personally and as a health practitioner. Because our choice of values determines the means we adopt to achieve our short- and long-term goals, it is also crucial that in any business or organisation there is clarity about the values that operate within it, at the corporate management, professional and individual levels. It is also important that employers and employees not only have insight into the competing (and sometimes conflicting) values which operate in any business moral community, but also have the necessary skills to deal with and resolve serious conflicts of values. One way this can be achieved is by engaging the key stakeholders (or their representatives) directly in the process of ethical policy development. Codes of ethics or codes of conduct are of little avail if staff are not involved in formulating them, and if there is no evidence of real ownership of them by all the staff in an organisation. This process also enables people to understand how the fundamental principles and values should influence decision-making and policy-setting in the organisation.

Skills in making ethical decisions

In Chapter 2 we pointed out that ethical decision-making is not some kind of mysterious or occult process, but is a type of problem-solving process which requires practice and skill to apply well. We said that whether you are a detective, lawyer, scientist, doctor, counsellor, nurse, accountant or public servant, you follow broadly the same steps in problem-solving:

- collect and assess the evidence and define the problem
- consider what principles and values apply to the case
- review the options and choices available in the situation
- devise an action plan, with clear objectives
- act effectively to implement the plan and observe the process
- analyse and learn from the results.

We will be discussing ethical decision-making in greater depth in the next chapter, and will be examining a number of models which can assist us to understand and apply problem-solving methods to ethical problems more effectively. The main point which needs to be emphasised here, however, is that making ethical decisions must be carefully distinguished from making ethical policy, or setting standards and laying down rules.

- Ethical decisions are always directed to solve particular problems, involving oneself or other

specific individuals, at a particular time and place. Decisions, like incisions, cut into the texture of life and change things, often irrevocably. Choosing one course of action also cuts out the possibility of pursuing some other course of action for the time being, and maybe for ever.
- Policies and rules, however, are general and apply not to single acts, but to classes of acts or problems. They are designed to give us some general guidelines to prevent identified types of problems from recurring; or, if they recur, provide us with rules for dealing with such problems. Because rules are general, they cannot be simply or directly applied to particular situations. To do so requires practical wisdom and life experience, so that we can choose the best available means and methods by which to apply our principles and rules to each problem so as to achieve the best possible outcome. (This is how Aristotle defines prudence.)

Skills in ethical decision-making are not confined to skilled application of problem-solving methods by individuals in making *personal* ethical decisions. In any organisation, hospital, business or government department, most decision-making *is an activity of committees or teams* and requires complex skills in analysis and negotiation to explore the interests of concerned stakeholders. At a corporate level, chief executive officers and senior managers are involved in the complex diplomacy and politics of negotiations with government and in inter-agency consultation and collaboration. Devising means to consult with and involve relevant external stakeholders in the process, and suitable methods for taking account of different agencies' policies and procedures, makes ethical decision-making at these levels even more complex, and we need training and skills to do it properly.

Skills in setting standards and ethical policy – at macro, meso, macho and micro levels

Skills in setting sound ethical policy or determining standards or 'performance indicators' also have to be learned and practised till they become a familiar part of routine management.

Policy development requires: that an organisation has clarified its values, that there are people involved with experience of making responsible ethical decisions, and where management have the skills to work in a genuinely consultative manner with staff, and have wide and relevant experience to develop sound policies. Without these ingredients, policies will be used to wallpaper offices, will not work and will not be 'owned' by all affected by them and consequently 'more honoured in the breach than the observance'.

In this connection, 'management by memorandum', or 'making policy on the hoof' does not demonstrate assertive management, but culpable incompetence. For here, managers mistake government by edict as fulfilling the responsibilities of policy-setting. This is actually the least effective way to manage people, and is frequently unethical in both its demands and methods of implementation. Because 'policy' is often 'handed down from on high' people often think the term 'policy' merely refers to aspirational statements of organisational ideals, or represents simply the arbitrary and autocratic demands of the boss. The former are thought to be vague and as applying to everything in general and nothing in particular, the latter to be unreasonable and arbitrary. Policies are often thought to be impractical because such vague general statements cannot be directly translated into operational rules and procedures that can have measurable impact.

'Management directives' could not be further from what is intended by the term 'policy' in a sound business or public administration environment. Policies are useless unless they are workable, that is, can be operationalised in everyday practice. If they are practical in this sense, then they can result in real benefits to all stakeholders, employees and customers (e.g. better working conditions, increased income and productivity, reduced costs and less inefficiency). Policies are useless unless the effects of their implementation can be measured. Management terms such as 'benchmarking', 'strategic planning', 'target-setting', 'effective implementation' and 'performance management' are all part of the process of applying sound policy to the systems and procedures of any operation.

Sound policy-making can be applied at a personal level to one's own work or family finances; to one's professional performance; or it may relate to the operation of one's team and the operation of a whole corporation. Policies would not be worth the paper they are printed on if they did not 'cash out' in assessable and ethical procedures, improved systems and methods of dealing with conflict, change and the proper monitoring or audit of performance.

Adopting these steps we have been describing, fulfils the requirements of sound policy. In Box 11.1 we set out a type of process and checklist, with proven usefulness, which helps give a practical focus to the steps we must take in setting ethical policy (WA OPSSC 1997).

Some general points need to be made about the value of sound ethical policy development in any

---

Box 11.1 POLICY model for setting ethical standards and policy

P = Problem type that requires standard policy/procedure
- Is the scope of the problem helpfully defined?
- Are the causes of problems of this type known?
- What do you propose to do about it?

O = Outline ethical approach and objectives to be recommended
- Are the relevant ethical principles specified?
- How will you consult about the overall approach?
- Are the objectives of your proposed policy clear?

L = List standard procedures and their ethical rationale
- What practical procedures are to be followed?
- What is your ethical justification for each procedure?
- What incentives and sanctions for compliance / non-compliance?

I = Identify methods to resolve conflict over policy's implementation
- What channels for identifying problems or discontent?
- What measures for negotiation, resolving disagreements?
- What procedures for dealing with appeals and grievance?

C = Check out the effectiveness of policy to achieve its objectives
- What measures for testing effectiveness of policy?
- What means for personal/team performance assessment?
- What measures for audit of corporate performance?

Y = Yes to policy! Strategy to ensure 'ownership' by stakeholders
- How to inform all stakeholders of policy and objectives?
- How to obtain endorsement of policy by stakeholders?
- When should the policy be reviewed and how often?

---

organisation, large or small, and in the NHS, at its various levels of operation, in particular.

Firstly, ethical policy development is a crucial part of the process of organisational review and organisational development. Developing a 'mission statement' and 'values statement' if developed as a whole-corporation community enterprise, with effective consultation and participation at all levels, can be a powerful and invaluable means of building corporate solidarity and commitment to a common vision and goals for the organisation. Staff commitment to and 'ownership' of the ethical policy can give a new sense of purpose and direction to their work and help create a new sense of collective corporate identity and integrity. However, if this is merely a cosmetic and public relations exercise, it is bound to fail, to deepen divisions, and to reinforce workforce cynicism. Properly integrated into organisational development, corporate ethical policy can embrace not only agency–customer relations (including quality assurance and charters of client rights), but also internal policy on human resources management, the ethical accountability of management, staff discipline and fraud control.

Effective ethical review and policy development requires staff with the necessary skills and authority to implement the policies and monitor compliance. The skills required are: 'people management skills', competence in the core skills in applied ethics mentioned above, skills in working out with staff appropriate performance targets and methods of performance assessment (including matters of financial and ethical probity). Applying the now familiar stages of the problem-solving process to corporate ethical review and ethical policy development is necessary – from collective needs assessment, joint planning, teamwork in implementation to meaningful corporate ethical audit and performance assessment. In this way the conditions for the well-being of the whole corporation and improvement of its services can be identified, means found for promoting those ends, and energy and resources committed to achieving them. Ethical policy development is fundamentally about corporate and individual behaviour modification. To work, it requires sincere commitment of management and staff to participate and collaborate in the process, and a major commitment to developing skills in applied ethics, the management of change, conflict resolution and dealing with resistance to change.

Secondly, corporate change can only be effected through fostering a sense of collective or corporate responsibility for that change. Ethical policy development is a key means of building a sense of moral community among those working in an organisation. Here skills in working with groups and experience of power-sharing in groups are essential. Without these there will not be credible ethical direction of the organisation, nor constructive resolution of conflict. Development of a genuinely ethical culture is necessary for mutual trust between management and staff, and commitment to joint action for the common

benefit of the organisation, for all its internal stakeholders and the client population it serves. If real teamwork and collective commitment to common values and standards is achieved, policing of staff performance and behaviour becomes virtually unnecessary. It can be regulated in most instances by informal debriefing or peer review and constructive support and skills training for staff in personal profiling and individual performance review. Disciplinary and grievance procedures will always be necessary. However, these are relegated to a position of much lesser importance if the emphasis in ethical policy development is on meaningful participation. This brings positive benefits to all staff, and to the organisation and its clients, which flow from working by ethical standards, rather than working to rule.

This may sound over-optimistic, for in medicine and nursing there has been a great reluctance to make peer review really work. Too often there has been a 'closing of ranks', out of a misguided sense of loyalty, to defend colleagues from criticism or charges of incompetence (e.g. where the person concerned has a serious alcohol or drug problem, or mental health problem). If peer review is to work there has to be more than token commitment to the policy. It is a prime example where involvement of all stakeholders in developing the policy, and in endorsing its implementation, is necessary if all parties are to 'own' it and apply it in their everyday practice. The Shipman Inquiry (2001) has pointed out that better systems of peer review and clinical audit might have helped prevent the hundreds of deaths for which Dr Shipman was responsible. Although this is an extreme case it is a salutary reminder of the dangers of neglecting systems of audit. However, if peer review is operated on a regular basis and in a constructive and non-threatening environment, these problems are more likely to be prevented and those whose skills need to be improved can be identified and given the necessary help.

Thirdly, the well-being of corporations, the standards of their performance and the quality of their services or products depends critically in practice, as well as ethically, on the corporation's commitment to the personal and professional development of its whole workforce. Justice and equity in access to training and opportunities for self-improvement not only foster a sense of being valued by all staff, but mean that they give value for money in terms of service in return. The 'great discovery' of General Motors, in making its comeback as a giant multinational, from near economic ruin, was summed up by one of its chief executives as 'Train, train, and again I say train your staff' (George & Weimerskirch 1994, Ch. 7). It might be objected that healthcare and manufacturing industry are different; however, in both cases appropriate staff development, education and skills training are essential to quality improvement at all levels. Ethics is fundamentally about human beings, about valuing human beings, and if human resources management is not a priority in any firm, it would be questionable whether it was ethical – however much stress is placed on 'quality assurance' and 'quality improvement'. The time invested in training personnel in interpersonal skills, in group-work and communication skills, in effective support and supervision of others, in skills in developing their potential, pays off not only in better understanding, trust and cooperation, but in effective teamwork and higher productivity. This is not only the boast of multinational companies such as BP and 'caring companies' such as Body Shop, based on their commitment to ethical policy and practice, and consumer audit, but it is also borne out in the experience of large organisations of many different kinds (George & Weimerskirch 1994, Chs 1 and 16, Tricker 1994, Ch. 1).

The process of ethical policy development is more concerned with the definition of the positive values of the corporation, rather than policing poor performance, incompetence or misconduct. Its object is to focus on beliefs held in common in the organisation about what will promote its well-being and productivity and what will benefit its staff, clients and the wider community. In a healthcare setting the ethical goal could be summarised in terms of all NHS institutions becoming health-promoting institutions for all parties involved. There are perhaps obvious contradictions here where hospitals or health centres are or become stressful and unhappy (and unhealthy) places to work. Where little consideration is shown for the physical, mental and social well-being of staff, where working conditions are unsatisfactory, canteen food unhealthy, smoking is permitted and staff relations are poor, these institutions are likely to be illness-inducing rather than health-promoting.

If ethics is about securing the conditions for human flourishing, promoting human well-being, then the 'health-promoting hospital' (health centre or health authority) is not only a requirement for congruence between health policy and practice, but is a necessary ethical ideal as well. However, where the institutional fabric has been neglected, working conditions and pay are poor, where morale is low and absenteeism is high, the malaise may have more to do with the institution's lack of ethical management than with the performance of staff. It may be that the hospital organisation is 'sick' rather than the staff 'malingering'.

Concern about the health of the institution and the environment in which people have to work is a quite proper ethical concern of nurses and other health practitioners. It is just as important as concern for their patients' health and well-being. In fact the health and well-being of patients, and the quality of service they receive, may have more to do with the 'health' of the institution and 'healthy' management/staff relations than strict hygiene and efficient routines. Given serious concern by nurses or other health workers about the poor state of health of an institution, and if management or local government will not negotiate or cooperate in making improvements, then staff and employees may have to contemplate collective action. This might include strike action if necessary, to ensure that attention is drawn to the problems, and something done about them.

Ethics and ethical policy development ought to be an integral part of industrial relations in the management of hospitals and the running of health services. Sound policy should be developed to cover both responsible and publicly accountable service delivery, management of staff and the allocation of resources. Ethics applies to both the management side and the staff side. It is not only about regulating behaviour, disciplining substandard practice or malpractice, eliminating fraud, or resolving industrial disputes. It is also about building an ethical culture in an organisation; promoting cooperation based on real consultation and mutual accountability; encouraging delegation of responsibility to self-directed teams; and building a real sense of community and commitment among staff. Ethics is thus not just about the imposition of management values, corporate ethical policies and standards development on an organisation. It is also about the rights of workers to participation in decision-making, recognition of good service, justice and fair dealing with staff, equal employment opportunities, and good mechanisms for conflict resolution and management.

Adopting a holistic approach to corporate ethics

- Instead of corporate ethics being seen as merely necessary for dealing with discipline, corruption or fraud, it becomes an integral part of the agency's ethos, strategic and operational planning.
- Operational systems, procedures and training programmes are set up in such a way that ethics is introduced to the bloodstream and contributes to the ongoing life of the body corporate, its planning for growth, organisational change and employee development.
- Sound ethical policy is seen to contribute to both corporate and individual well-being, and thus

collective commitment to the new ethos of ethical management and practice is seen to be advantageous to all, to be secured by negotiation rather than edict from above.

- Quality assurance, standards setting, and peer review are seen to be a normal part of ethical management – encouraging development of skills and confidence in self-audit or monitoring, thus reducing dependency on legalistic, authoritarian, 'disciplinary' approaches (Table 11.1).

STRATEGIC ETHICAL MANAGEMENT AND CLINICAL GOVERNANCE IN HEALTHCARE

In Chapter 4 we developed an analysis of different models or approaches to professional ethics, based on *code, contract, covenant* and *charter*, and in Chapter 9, different models for the ethics of management, namely *critical expertise, command management, community development* and *corporate planning*. With the advent of the 'New NHS', with its emphasis on total quality management and continuous improvement of services and clinical standards, a new emphasis has been given to the earlier concept of clinical audit recommended in the 1979 Royal Commission on the NHS, but not widely adopted. The concepts of *corporate and clinical governance* have been introduced as the watchwords of New Labour's policy for the oversight and monitoring of the NHS (Scally & Donaldson 1998, Lugon & Secker-Walker 1998).

However, it is worth noting that whether the talk is about audit of performance, quality improvement or governance, these are all aspects of strategic ethical management. If popular understanding of ethics were not so restricted, privatised and its meaning misunderstood, we could equally well speak of all these aspects of corporate life as aspects of ethics and neces-sary ingredients of professional and corporate ethics. 'Setting and maintaining standards', 'continuous quality improvement', 'striving for excellence', and 'governance' or 'transparency and openness to critical scrutiny, evaluation and audit' – are all fundamental aspects of ethics and the moral life that echo all the way back to the classical virtue ethics of the ancient philosophers. The need to invent new terminology, rather than rehabilitate the meaning of ethics, is made necessary because the meaning of the term 'ethics' has become so debased in popular consciousness by association with censorious moralism, dogmatic fundamentalism, and an over-precious focus on spiritual rather than practical aspects of ethics in everyday life.

In his review of international corporate govern-ance, Tricker (1994) systematically avoids the use of the term 'ethics', and yet much of what he has to say in this comprehensive set of texts, readings and cases, illustrates themes we have referred to in the above discussion of corporate ethical policy development, its implementation and evaluation of outcomes. There are perhaps two issues that are significant about the emphasis on 'governance' from an ethical point of view: first, that it shifts the emphasis from individual to corporate responsibility, and secondly, that it is a term borrowed from corporate law and management which refers in particular to the role of both executive and non-executive members of boards in the manage-ment of corporations. In the second sense, the term 'governance' has particular relevance to the style of partnership between public and private sectors and local communities, in the management and delivery of health services, that the Blair government in the UK is concerned to promote.

The setting up of 'trusts' and 'boards of manage-ment' requires a change of terminology, to encourage

Table 11.1 Corporate ethical policy development – the ethical organisation. Total quality improvement and ethical policy development – focus on 'How?' rather than on 'What?'

Corporate ideals	Opportunities	Monitoring measures
• Corporate values statement	• Professional development	• Ethics discussion document
• Statement of ethical principles	• Quality of life at work	• Staff involvement – aiming for
• Human resources development	• Relevance to promotion	• Self-regulation/peer review
• Communication systems	• Working time and toil	• Structures of support
Ethical review procedures	*Scope for participation*	*Statement of ethics*
• Review corporate culture	• Goals and targets setting	• Ethics in the workplace
• Management styles (managers)	• Skills training	• Business/organisational ethics
• Accounting and accountability	• Planning and audit	• Ethical review procedures
• Specific work procedures	• Enhanced responsibility	• Revisable code of practice
• Individual responsibility	• Debriefing and feedback	• Disciplinary processes
• Performance review	• Rewards and recognition	• 'Fraud-management'

people to get away from the mentality that sees ethics as authoritarian, regulatory and concerned with policing standards, and preventing fraud or incompetence. The approach being recommended, along with increasing devolution of responsibility downwards to local authorities, is governed by the principle of subsidiarity (i.e. that authority and responsibility should not be centralised and concentrated at the top, but should be devolved down to the lowest level at which required functions can be most efficiently and effectively managed and delivered). This not only involves moving away from a top-down legislative and regulatory view of ethics, but also gives local government and management of public sector services the responsibility to develop their own specific ethical policies and strategic plans, with reduced statutory regulation from above and dependence on central government control. While the state would retain responsibility for setting general standards (in consultation with key stakeholders) it would hold local government accountable, on behalf of taxpayers. The object would be for the state to be less directly involved in the affairs of local government (Day & Klein 1997).

As applied to the NHS, clinical governance for local health authorities/boards, would comprise the following processes (Swage 2000, pp. 5–6):

1. determination of clear lines of responsibility and accountability for clinical care
2. development and application of a comprehensive programme of quality improvement
3. specification of procedures for identifying and remedying poor performance
4. development of clear policies for identifying and minimising risk
5. putting in place clinical governance arrangements for the local health authority/board.

Clear lines of responsibility and accountability for clinical care

In England the chief executives of the NHS trusts and primary care trusts have overall responsibility for the quality of services, and are required to appoint appropriate senior officers to ensure that quality standards set nationally in the National Service Frameworks and by the National Institute for Clinical Excellence (NICE) are achieved if possible. They are also required to ensure formal reporting arrangements are in place through clinical governance committees. (Although organisational arrangements in Scotland are different, analogous arrangements have to be made by chairmen of health boards.)

Development and application of a comprehensive programme of quality improvement

To ensure comprehensive and continuous quality improvement, the systematic use of methods of strategic planning is necessary. The strategic planning process or cycle involves at a macro level the familiar stages applicable to most types of problem-solving methods, namely:

- clarification and definition of the problem/s or strategic issues to be addressed
- collection and assessment of relevant evidence, based on present and past performance, and estimates of resource inputs required
- developing relevant action plans to deal with identified problems, with clear and achievable objectives and anticipated outputs
- considering the risks and benefits of various options or alternative courses of action
- managing the implementation of action plans, setting standards for performance assessment and monitoring the overall process
- evaluating the outputs and outcomes of strategic actions in the light of pre-established objectives and performance measures
- feeding back information to the management team to identify areas for quality improvement and for ongoing review.

This process presupposes corporate and individual commitment to evidence-based practice and collection, storage and access to relevant records and aggregated data for the purpose of assessment and review. Methods of strategic planning and corporate governance presuppose a foundation of fact and reliable feedback, and commitment to the idea that an organisation is a 'learning organisation'. This means that organisational and staff development in methods of evidence-based practice and strategic planning is essential too to the improvement of services.

Specification of procedures for identifying and remedying poor performance

This involves negotiating and gaining agreement to methods for performance assessment, including clinical audit, peer review and self-assessment. Together with general data from evidence-based practice, and the specification of standards for performance appraisal, this provides a coherent framework within which to deal with complaints and confidential enquiries.

Development of clear policies for identifying and minimising risk

Methods of risk assessment and risk management have become an essential part of responsible strategic planning and management. These are not simply about trying to eliminate all risks, but to identify what risks there are relative to the benefits to be achieved, and to agree criteria for what will be regarded as acceptable risks. Risk assessment applies as much to clinical procedures and treatments as it does to the implementation of strategic plans for organisational change, and to developments that may generate opposition from trade unions or conflict with individuals.

Putting in place clinical governance arrangements for the local health authority/board

Following an enquiry and consultation, the Commission for Health Improvement (now the Commission for Healthcare Audit and Inspection) set out guidance on standards and arrangements for England and Wales. In Scotland the regulatory body is called NHS Quality Improvement Scotland; both have broadly the same functions:

1. to undertake clinical governance reviews of all NHS provider organisations
2. to monitor all NHS organisations against standards set by NICE and the National Service Frameworks
3. to undertake investigations of serious service failures in the NHS
4. to take the lead in reviewing and assisting in healthcare improvement and the sharing of good practice.

STRATEGIC PLANNING AND STRATEGIC ETHICAL MANAGEMENT

This is not the place to develop a comprehensive account of strategic planning, nor to pretend that a summary account of what is involved, is a substitute for proper training and experience in operating with the processes involved, in consulting with stakeholders, and for practice in strategic ethical management. What we are concerned to emphasise here is the crucial role of values and ethical policy in sound strategic planning and the development of health policy generally.

In a highly centralised welfare state, strategic planning used to be mainly the business of government planners and their advisers. With the adoption in the UK of the principle of subsidiarity in management of the NHS, and with responsibility and accountability for quality having been devolved to local authorities and local trusts, the responsibility for adopting and applying methods of strategic planning and strategic ethical management has become local. In a sense, thinking and working in a systematic and strategic fashion has become everybody's business in the NHS (Box 11.2).

Strategic planning and management based on principles of *continuous quality improvement* (CQI) rely on the application to organisations of the principles of learning theory that apply to individuals, namely the adoption of a problem-solving approach which consists of a factual review of the organisation's needs, problem identification, intelligence-led decision-making, evaluation based on facts, and a built-in feedback loop or learning cycle.

CQI has been used as a model for information or intelligence-led management for several decades, and depends on using evaluative information from a critical appraisal of all aspects of an organisation's performance to improve systems, management and service delivery (George & Weimerskirch 1994, Chs 14 and 15). In outline, the continuous improvement cycle is a 12-stage process, to be repeated at planned, regular intervals in the life of the organisation.

Most forms of strategic planning (or management by objective) begin with application to an organisation of methods such as 'SWOT analysis' (Ernst & Young 1992): a review of the (S)trengths and (W)eaknesses, of the organisation, and, assessment of the internal and external (O)pportunities and (T)hreats it faces.

SWOT analysis as a tool for self-analysis by an organisation, or a process through which an organisation can be taken by a consultant, can be a useful way to identify problems and unmet needs in an organisation, and help those who take part to make realistic assessment of what is possible and so identify possible actions that will help meet those needs. SWOT analysis, or some similar form of systematic critical appraisal, is an essential preliminary to well-informed strategic planning. To be really effective all those with a stake in the improvement of an organisation's performance have a part to play in undertaking such an appraisal.

The other main component in the strategic planning process is the incorporation of a familiar decision-making and problem-solving process illustrated in the simplified seven-stage 'DECIDER' model in Figure 11.2. It represents the process as a cyclical or spiral rather than as a linear one, which involves both information feedback and a learning feedback loop that serves as the basis for on-going review and continuous improvement.

Box 11.2 Summary of key steps in strategic planning

Note: Steps in the strategic planning process follow a problem-solving logic:

1. Clarify the *organisation's mission* – its core business or function – at the level of the corporate executive, with middle management and practitioners, and develop a *common vision* for the organisation – in broad terms *a vision of how*, in practical terms, the organisation might or could achieve its mission.

2. Develop a *common set of organisational values* by the following means:
   - engaging in a process of values clarification with key stakeholder groups
   - recognising the diversity of values and approaches among stakeholders
   - formulating together a common values statement for the organisation
   - clarifying together the practical, operational implications of these values.

3. Formulate clear statements of *organisational goals and objectives* implied in these organisational values, together with health practitioners and other internal stakeholders, and seek endorsement from patients or consumers.

4. Undertake a *comprehensive organisational review* of current performance and quality standards, by engaging with key stakeholder groups, in order to assess both achievements and failures in service provision and to identify issues requiring action at strategic level.

5. Clarify *main problems or strategic issues* to be addressed, and consider the costs and benefits and risks of various methods of dealing with them.

6. Negotiate *agreement on key strategic issues* and priorities among the identified problems, with representatives of both internal and external stakeholder groups.

7. Negotiate *acceptable methods for monitoring performance, and indicators or measures for appraisal*, which are realistic and acceptable to all staff, from the boardroom to the shop floor, viz. executive group, middle managers and practitioners.

8. Develop *agreement on appropriate strategic actions* to be taken to address the identified strategic issues and problems in the organisation.

9. *Implement the strategic plan* and ensure it is put into operation in an effective and efficient manner by responsible managers at the various levels.

10. *Ensure good record-keeping*, to provide a sound evidence base on which to make assessments of performance and service delivery, to enable gaps or failures in services to be identified, and to ensure that areas for improvement can be addressed.

11. *Collect aggregated data on overall service delivery and individual performance* and feed this back through the system to top management to address in the next major review.

12. *Finally, repeat the strategic planning cycle*, after an agreed period and within a reasonable time-scale, alternatively, in a crisis, as and when required.

IDENTIFICATION AND INVOLVEMENT OF STAKEHOLDERS

Research evidence shows that in a *learning organisation*, meaningful participation by all key stakeholders is necessary if this systematic approach is to work – whether it is in the review, planning, assessment or feedback processes, or in undertaking shared responsibility for monitoring and evaluating progress and achieving an organisation's objectives (Nutley et al 2004, George & Weimerskirch 1994).

However, this begs the question what is meant by a 'stakeholder' and to whom the term should apply. While some authorities have argued that in any business, managers are primarily responsible to the organisation's 'stockholders' or 'shareholders', others have argued that many other parties have a real stake in the success or failure of a business or public service organisation, for example employees, customers or clients, suppliers, the community and both local and state government. The list can be almost endless, so it is necessary for practical purposes to establish distinctions between those with immediate interests and more remote interests in the performance of the organisation (Beauchamp & Bowie 1997, Ch. 2).

Assessment of the relative importance of 'stakeholders' (including shareholders) needs to be made if the net for inclusion of people in strategic planning is not to be cast too wide, and if the right people are to be chosen who will make both a constructive and critical contribution to the process. 'Stakeholders' will have a greater or lesser 'stake' in the success or failure of the organisation, in appraisal and improvement of its performance, if they are directly affected by changes in its fortunes. Here the various methods of *stakeholder analysis* can be used:

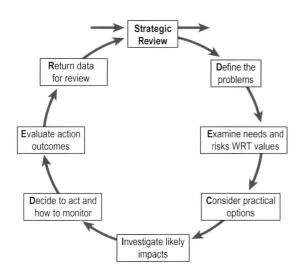

Figure 11.2 The DECIDER model for the strategic review cycle (CJSWDC 2005).

- to brainstorm a comprehensive list of their stakeholders
- to clarify the rights and duties of the various stakeholders in the organisation relative to management and clients
- to rank order these on the basis of objective criteria for their relative importance to the organisation, and finally
- to determine which 'stakeholders' it is essential, or desirable, to involve directly in the process of strategic planning, and, alternatively
- to decide who should be consulted, to ensure understanding of the organisation's mission and objectives, and to gain endorsement and support for implementation of its strategic plan.

Analysing whether 'stakeholders' have an immediate or more remote interest in an organisation's operations and performance is therefore a necessary preliminary to determining (a) the degree to which they should be involved in or consulted in the process of strategic planning, (b) whether they should play a part in defining organisational objectives and related criteria for appraisal of its performance, and (c) whether the organisation and its staff should be accountable to them directly or indirectly.

Real involvement of a wide range of stakeholders, staff and consumers in the processes of strategic planning is costly in terms of time and resources, but it has been repeatedly shown that the investment required is worthwhile if it ensures that representative stakeholders from across the whole organisation are enabled to participate meaningfully in the processes

involved. The evidence is that it more than *pays off in terms of public support, improved staff commitment and organisational productivity and efficiency* (George & Weimerskirch 1994, James 1996).

Involvement in the process of strategic planning *contributes to team-building* and the cultivation of a sense of commitment by all members to the organisation. It contributes to the creation of a moral community in which members recognise that they have both rights and responsibilities. It is an approach where involvement in the process, of learning to think and work strategically, is recognised to be more important than producing some kind of perfect plan which turns out to be Utopian and unrealistic (George & Weimerskirch 1994, James 1996). It is particularly important that all key stakeholders are involved in the initial stages of the strategic planning process, so that they can each contribute meaningfully from their own experience and vantage point in the organisation, and so that they will feel real ownership of the outputs and outcomes of the process, and be willing to work within the performance standards they have mutually agreed.

Strategic planning involves the discipline and requires the skills necessary to manage an organisation's human, financial and material resources, and thus to ensure that:

- the organisation and its stakeholders flourish, as defined by its mission, vision and values
- the organisation achieves both its short- and long-term objectives
- the organisation achieves its optimum potential, in terms of its productivity, customer and staff satisfaction and cost-effective use of resources.

The research that supports 'total quality management' (TQM) indicates that if there is a common understanding and commitment to an organisation's mission and vision, and if these are effectively applied (rather than seen as 'motherhood statements'), then they can make a significant contribution to setting up and operating an organisation that thinks and works strategically at every level. In the process, individuals acquire a greater sense of ownership of the agency's objectives, more control of their work, and pride in and recognition for their achievements. TQM should mean the opposite of the kind of authoritarian or arbitrary management that so many fear. In some places TQM has acquired a bad name because, all too often, it has been imposed without real consultation or participation of either key internal or external stakeholders. *TQM means that the business operations, service delivery and personnel relations of a whole agency or organisation are directed by its values and goals.* To translate strategic planning into effective operation *requires successful communication of and application of the organisation's values and goals to all levels of the organisation* – from the level of corporate management to the level of operational decision-making, from strategic and middle management to practice levels.

ARE THERE LIMITS TO THE STATE'S RESPONSIBILITY FOR HEALTHCARE?

Evolving awareness of the right to health as a fundamental human right

While the preceding discussion may seem to have been rather abstract and theoretical, and far removed from the concerns of practising nurses or front-line health practitioners, the issues discussed have very important implications for practice, and hopefully for improved quality of services and outcomes for patients. Improving the standards of healthcare for the benefit of the whole population requires improvement and reform at the national and corporate planning levels, improvements in management and standards of service delivery, improvements in medical science, pharmacology and applied technology, and improvements in the knowledge and skills of health practitioners of all kinds.

If we consider the situation in the United Kingdom and Europe 150 years ago, for example, the circumstances of people and their health status was not all that different from that which obtains in many developing countries today. Improvements in healthcare and the health of the population have been dramatic, and these are due to the commitment of successive governments to public health reforms, improvements of healthcare services and infrastructure, improvements in standards of available hospital-based and primary care services, and improved access to healthcare for all people regardless of social class or economic standing. For example, a common finding of the 1979 Royal Commission on the NHS (DHSS 1979) and the Black Report on inequalities in health (DHSS 1980) was that in the 1970s there were growing inequalities in health status between people in social class I compared with social class V. Nevertheless, both reports pointed out that for the vast majority of people who fell into the lower social classes at the end of the Second World War, there had been a considerable improvement in their economic status, overall health and life expectancy in the post-war period. The proportion of the population who fell into social classes IV and V in 1945 had fallen dramatically with rising living standards, resulting in the bulk of the population now being in social class III, as their

economic and educational status and opportunities had improved.

It is salutary to be reminded by the Registrar General for Scotland (RGS 2005) in his most recent report, of a few salient statistics on the health of the Scottish people:

> Scotland today is a very different place from Scotland in the mid-1850s. The total population, in 1851 Census, was 2.89 million compared with 5.08 million in 2004. Over 93 000 babies were born in 1855, compared to only 54 000 in 2004. Since 1855, the death rate has fallen from 24 people per 1000 population to 11 people in 2004. This was due, in part, to the ending of the epidemics of smallpox, whooping cough and measles, which were of great concern to the Registrar General in 1855. In 1855, there were only 19 680 marriages compared to 32 154 in 2004. … In the late 1850s, the average Scot would have been called John Smith, with a one in seven chance of dying before his first birthday and a life expectancy of 40. Today, a typical Scot might be called Lewis Brown with only a one in 200 chance of dying before his first birthday and a life expectancy of 74.

Worldwide during the past century, but particularly following the two World Wars, there had been a growing public conviction that everyone is entitled to good health as a matter of right. Good health came to be valued both in itself, as contributing to our general well-being, but also as a necessary means to achieve our life goals as human beings. For this reason the right to health and access to good healthcare was seen as a fundamental human right. In this context health has increasingly been seen not merely in terms of freedom from infection and disabling physical conditions, but in terms of general 'physical, mental and social well-being' (WHO 1947). It was also enshrined in the UN Universal Declaration of Human Rights (UNO 1948) Article 25, which states that every human being has a right to adequate healthcare, and, that all governments have a duty to provide it. Similarly, the preamble to the Constitution of the World Health Organization (WHO) states that: 'Enjoyment of the highest attainable standard of health is one of the fundamental rights of every human being' (WHO 1947). Consequently WHO has actively supported initiatives to promote international awareness of the health rights of individuals and all member states of the United Nations. (For website links related to this topic, please see http://evolve. elsevier.com/Thompson/nursing ethics.)

Global post-war efforts were focused by the United Nations and its various agencies on planning for improvement of the general quality of life of people. It was recognised that this would require action on several fronts, besides reconstruction of social and economic infrastructure, namely: education, health and social services. In this context, the conviction that good health is an attainable ideal and right for all was based on a growing popular faith that medical science and technical innovation would find cures for all our ails, and, together with immunisation and better public health measures, would be able to ensure generally better physical health for the world's population. However, it was recognised that improved education, health and welfare would not be sufficient without concerted action to promote human and economic development and to help prevent the conditions leading to war and social dislocation.

Both within more technologically advanced societies and in developing countries, people came to demand access to healthcare services as a political right. In the optimistic and idealistic environment of the Marshall Plan and post-war reconstruction, a variety of United Nations agencies were set up to promote these ideals – OECD, FAO, UNICEF and the World Bank.

In this context WHO has not only been concerned with coordination and improvement of global health services and medical and nurse education, but has also focused on people's health rights in programmes on Ethics, Trade, Human Rights and Law (ETH) and the programme on Sustainable Development and Healthy Environments (SDE), where WHO seeks to provide technical, intellectual and political leadership in the field of health and human rights. Here WHO's stated objectives are to:

- strengthen WHO's capacity to integrate a human rights-based approach in its work
- support governments to integrate a human rights-based approach in health development
- advance the right to health in international law and international development processes.

The WHO maintains that 'promoting and protecting health and respecting, protecting and fulfilling human rights are inextricably linked', for the following reasons:

- Violations or lack of attention to human rights can have serious health consequences (e.g. harmful traditional practices, slavery, torture and inhuman and degrading treatment, violence against women and children).
- Health policies and programmes can promote or violate human rights in their design or implementation (e.g. freedom from discrimination, individual autonomy, rights to participation, privacy and information).
- Vulnerability to ill-health can be reduced by taking steps to respect, protect and fulfil human rights

(e.g. freedom from discrimination on account of race, sex and gender roles, rights to health, food and nutrition, education, housing). (For website links related to this topic, please see http://evolve. elsevier.com/Thompson/nursing ethics.)

The development of welfare states in Europe and elsewhere

Another feature of post-war reconstruction in Europe, and many other countries, was the establishment of welfare states. Typical perhaps of the thinking which inspired them was the vision of a society organised to tackle what Beveridge (1942) imaginatively called 'the Five Giants': want, disease, ignorance, squalor and idleness. Adoption of the welfare state model required that national governments should take more responsibility for the provision of healthcare, education and social services for all their citizens. This model was adopted by the United Kingdom, Canada, Australia, New Zealand, South Africa, Sweden and the Netherlands, and in modified forms in many other countries (Mishra 1984, Robertson et al 1992).

The welfare state in Britain emerged out of a process which began with the Liberal reforms of the Victorian period and in reaction to the Bismarckian reforms in Germany in the late 19th and early 20th century. These had resulted in piecemeal improvements to welfare rights and services before the First World War. While the Beveridge Report (1942) is often taken to mark the establishment of the British welfare state, a good argument can be made for the fact that Beveridge simply consolidated and rationalised existing welfare provisions begun by the Liberal reformers. These included, for example, labour reforms affecting working hours and old age pensions (1909) and family allowances (1930). The Beveridge Report was not so much a revolutionary as an evolutionary development of ideas that were emerging in Europe. It held out the promise that the 'Five Giants' could be conquered by the development of appropriate public services, such as social security, health and education, and the application of government policies to ensure full employment. The British welfare state thus evolved into five public service divisions: Social Security, Health, Education, Housing, and Personal Social Services.

Beveridge's proposals proved extremely popular, probably because they were in tune with the universalist spirit of the post-war years and also because the scheme's social insurance basis enabled people to regard their benefits as entitlements, thus removing the stigma of the hated 19th century Poor Laws. What he contributed was a good administrative base on which to establish an integrated and universal system of health, education and welfare provision to be funded by a single form of National Insurance. The development of the British welfare state continued post-Beveridge too, e.g. with the provisions of the 1948 Child Protection Act.

After a quarter of a century, it became apparent that with increased public expectations of the welfare state, and with spiralling public expenditure required to meet increased costs and public demand, there was a crisis facing governments over the operation of welfare states. Three broad hypotheses were advanced for the alleged 'crisis' in welfare (Mishra 1984), namely:

- the financial crisis of welfare with politically unacceptable levels of public expenditure
- the crisis brought about by major social and demographic changes in these countries
- the crisis of confidence in the ethical and ideological rationale for the welfare state.

Harrison (2004, pp. 1–7) distinguishes three main periods of reform of healthcare and welfare systems designed to address this alleged crisis facing the welfare state. These are:

1. A mainly administrative focus on containing costs and making health services more efficient, by introducing business-style management practices and increased regulation and control by central government of public sector budgets and expenditure (mid-1970s to mid-1980s).
2. The introduction of the neoliberal economic model of the 'internal market', including competition between public and private sector providers, allowing for wider consumer choice, and with the state making service providers more directly accountable for the quality and costs of their services (mid-1980s to late 1990s).
3. Continued promotion of a mixed economy of public and private sector welfare provision and joint ventures in funding capital developments, but with renewed attention to rational action planning and evaluation of services on the basis of evidence of the actual social and economic determinants of health and the effectiveness of interventions on the basis of empirical outcomes (late 1990s to the present).

Given that public sector costs in general, and healthcare costs in particular, were a matter of growing political concern in 1980s and 1990s, what is interesting and important from the point of view of ethics, as well as social policy, is the different kinds of rationalisations that were used to justify reform and restructuring of national health services. During this period the key argument behind the diagnosis of a 'crisis' in the provision of welfare, and in favour of the private provision of public welfare, was the economic one (cf. Klein 1989, and Papadakis & Taylor-Gooby 1987).

What criticism of the welfare state from the political right did from the mid-1980s onwards was to break the public and cross-party consensus in the UK in support of the welfare state and to make people question the need for a predominantly state-funded NHS. Public and political debate about these issues, however, became increasingly polarised and political, in the sense that it represented a clash of different ideologies and moral convictions, rather than being simply about methods of funding. It was a debate about fundamental political and economic theories and their relative strengths and weaknesses, and about human rights and social justice in healthcare, about the state's duty of care and individual autonomy and choice.

During the past half-century there have been rapid and major cultural and structural changes in the management and delivery of healthcare. Whereas in the early part of the last century, doctors and nurses played key roles in the management of hospitals (e.g. those of the medical superintendent and the hospital matron), there has been a decisive move towards hospitals, health centres and other healthcare institutions being run by professional business managers. While in some cases nurses and doctors have acquired qualifications in management and moved into these new roles, more commonly the new breed of professional managers have tended to be recruited from business, industry and public sector management. With these changes in the style of management have also come changes in the economic models for the management of hospitals, clinics and general practice, and changes in the values that drive these various models, and different forms of public accountability.

Major shifts in health policy and in proposals for reform of health services have generally been driven by or rationalised in terms of different ethical and political philosophies. The relationship between ethical (and political) theory and the formulation of policy in general and in healthcare is the main subject of the final chapter of this book.

DIFFERENT ETHICAL AND POLITICAL RATIONALES FOR REFORM OF HEALTHCARE

Changing social values and forms of healthcare in the past century

The earliest hospitals in the UK and in Europe were either established and run by religious foundations or were parish-based secular 'charitable institutes'. They tended to be driven by an *ethic of care or altruistic service* to others. In both cases funds to cover costs had to be raised either through charitable donations and other kinds of fund-raising, or by charging fees, particularly to those who could afford to pay. These establishments were largely autonomous and self-financing, appointing their own managers to reflect their values and to implement their policy priorities. Despite the supposed protection of the Poor Laws in Britain, growing disparities in health status, life expectancy and ability to access medical services led to widespread discontent and a growing demand that the state should take more responsibility for healthcare.

After the Second World War, 'welfare states' were set up in Britain and several of its dependencies, as well as in several European countries. Health services became 'nationalised' or brought under central government control in some way. Two main factors contributed to the development of the concept of the welfare state: the increasing dependency of private healthcare providers on subsidies from government, and, the quest for *greater justice and equity in access to healthcare* – driven by popular grievances about inadequate healthcare provision as well as idealism. Various forms of national insurance, often supplemented by government funding through taxation, were adopted to ensure that adequate services could be provided for the whole population and that healthcare was not simply a privilege of the rich.

Welfare states were intended to ensure greater social justice and equity in popular access to adequate education, social services and healthcare, and state-regulated improvement in the quality of services delivered. The state was also required to exercise a *quasi-parental role of protective beneficence* towards its citizens, particularly towards those who were most vulnerable and with the greatest need. However, the neoliberal/neoconservative critics of the welfare state argued that it created a culture of paternalism and dependency. They claimed that it did not respect the autonomy or capacity of citizens to make informed choices, nor did it respect their right to have more direct say in how the 'health dollars' or funds raised by health insurance or taxation were spent.

However, with rising standards of living, changes in life expectancy, improved public health, and raised public expectations of what benefits medical science and healthcare could provide, the cost of meeting these expectations began to escalate. The first major reforms were attempted in the late 1970s and early 1980s, but these were aimed at reducing or limiting the costs of health and social services mainly by *attempting to make the management and administration of services* *more efficient and 'business-like'*. This was the era of government-imposed cash limits, budgetary discipline and increasingly centralised governmental regulation of expenditures on health and social services.

After a quarter of a century, it became apparent that the whole concept of the 'welfare state', (as providing 'free' education, health and social services for its citizens) was facing a crisis, driven by ballooning public expenditure (Mishra 1984), and economic recession and rising unemployment. Confidence in Beveridge's vision was shaken as it was predicated on full employment and on intact, traditional family units in which men worked to earn a wage and women did not, and where women took responsibility for childcare and other care, e.g. of older relatives. This situation obviously changed considerably in the interim. In the United Kingdom, the multiparty consensus supporting the welfare state began to break down, and, for better or worse, health expenditure and health administration became a kind of 'political football'.

Positions became polarised around different political ideologies, emphasising different values and offering different kinds of ethical rationale for their positions. The defenders of the welfare state insisted that the government had a *duty of care to protect the needs of the most vulnerable in society* and to *ensure greater social justice and equity in access to healthcare*, and for this reason favoured direct government control and funding of healthcare. The neoliberal or neoconservative critics of what was called the 'nanny state' argued in favour of a *reduced role for central government* in the administration and funding of healthcare and social services, and *more scope for competition*, *respect for professional autonomy and greater consumer choice*.

The Community Care Act in 1990 also emphasised a move of care from institutional settings to those within the community, and this had a fundamental impact on primary care and social welfare and how these services were to work together to support more care in the community.

Finally in the late 1990s, with the advent of New Labour, the Blair government sought to keep up the momentum of the NHS reforms with its own programme of 'modernisation' of government and of the health, education and welfare services generally, but it proposed to do this on the basis of a different set of practical and ethical priorities. What is interesting from an ethico-political point of view is that while the 'New Right' were influenced by neoliberal philosophical and economic theorists, 'New Labour' politicians were clearly influenced by communitarian political philosophers (e.g. Macintyre 1981 and Taylor 1985), both in their criticisms of New Right ideological and economic theories and by communitarian social scientists (e.g. Etzioni 1993, Tam 1998) in setting out their own ideological position and developing their policies on health and human services.

New Labour attempted to transform the culture of the public sector and of the NHS primarily by what Nietzsche might have called a 'trans-valuation of all values' as these applied to both management and practice. To some extent New Labour nodded in the direction of the traditional values of Labour's socialist past, but also sought to give these a new flavour, focus and spin in the 'Third Way', which they recommended. At a national and corporate level this meant steering a middle course between 'Old Labour's' 'command and control' approach to social policy and administration and the Conservative's monetarist internal market approach to the management of the economy and NHS.

On the one hand, there was a return to an emphasis on the responsibility of the state to ensure social justice and equity in healthcare, and a community-based approach to public health. On the other hand, the emphasis in the *New NHS, Modern, Dependable* (DoH 1997) was on assuring quality of care, improving the health and well-being of entire populations and communities, involving patients and citizens in decisions about healthcare funding and service delivery, and reducing socio-economic and regional differences in access to healthcare services.

The New Right and New Labour reforms of the NHS

The alleged 'crisis of the welfare state' was not based on substantial evidence that state-funded welfare was failing or unaffordable, but rather on the 'monetarist' economic and neoliberal political theories adopted by the neoconservative governments of the period. The debate was as much about ideology and ethics as it was about money. Key ideological assumptions of advocates of the 'Reaganomics' or 'Thatcherism' of the period are outlined in Box 11.3.

In the UK (like Sweden and the Netherlands) the Thatcher government recommended the creation of 'an internal market' within the NHS, to open up the nationalised health service to competition and market forces, believing this would drive down costs, improve quality and offer more choice to consumers. In place of a centralised socialist model of the welfare state, the neoliberal model was intended to reduce the direct responsibility of central government in the delivery of health, education and social services. This responsibility was to be devolved down to local health authorities, with a view to reducing public expenditure on

> **Box 11.3** Ideological assumptions behind neoconservative health reforms
>
> - That human beings are necessarily motivated by self-interest rather than altruism, and should be made more directly responsible for their own health, rather than to become dependent on the 'nanny' welfare state.
>
> - That the role of the state in the control of the lives of people should be reduced, and that 'Big Government' was to be replaced by 'Small Government' and responsibility for welfare devolved to local authorities, supposedly better able to interpret the needs of local consumers.
>
> - That the high levels of public expenditure and taxation required to fund the welfare state should be reduced because they exercise a crippling effect on the economy, and by reducing taxes and introducing more competition and private investment, this would stimulate growth in the economy and give more choice to people in how they spend their earnings, rather than be compelled to use public services.
>
> - That the crisis of the welfare state was inevitable once the period of economic growth, which gave credibility to Keynesian economic principles and the Beveridge Plan, gave way to recession, and when state-imposed financial disciplines failed to curb public expenditure, this made the concept of welfare states untenable.
>
> - That the concept of welfare is workable in small communities where face-to-face accountability is possible, but in large, impersonal and bureaucratic states people do not have the same investment in contributing to the commonwealth for the common good.
>
> - That the private sector is always more efficient and cheaper than public sector services can be, that the application of business management to the delivery of healthcare, education and social welfare would be better, and privatising and/or contracting out services would save money and cut public expenditure.

bureaucracy, by operating at arms-length, statutory measures to contain costs and to control and regulate budgets. By encouraging growth in private sector provision, contracting out some administrative and support services (such as cleaning and catering), and by increased use of agency nurses and encouraging families and voluntary agencies to provide more care in the community, it was hoped that costs would be reduced and delivery of local services made more efficient.

Harrison (2004) in his overview of these New Right reforms, particularly with reference to his study of developments in the United Kingdom, Sweden and the Netherlands, points out that:

> Despite important variations (Jacobs, 1998), all the prominent market reforms in Europe sought to foster competition among health care providers, among insurers, or both (Paton, 2000). Both types of government-supervised competition are referred to as managed or regulated competition and as quasi-markets … These terms indicate that governmental regulation was required to foster fair competition. Thus during market reforms, governments explicitly or implicitly set the rules under which competition could occur and continued to regulate emerging market-like relations among health providers and funding agencies. (Harrison 2004, p. 1)

In the UK, under the neoconservative government of Mrs Thatcher, along with other market reforms and attempts to restrict the power of the trade unions, this model of the 'internal market' was introduced. Private healthcare providers were encouraged to enter the market, and business models were imposed on the NHS, in a series of ideologically driven initiatives to restructure the NHS in line with a competitive and commercial ideology. Central government regulation of standards of healthcare delivery was to be reduced, by allowing standards to be set by market forces and the laws of supply and demand. Locally responsibility and accountability was devolved to so-called independent, budget-holding, NHS trusts and to budget-holding primary care trusts and health centres. Behind this move was an attempt to reduce the role of government and public expenditure, by making the various trusts directly accountable, and to reduce the responsibility of central government for the administration of a national health service.

A common assumption made at this time was that private sector management was inherently better and more efficient than public sector management or standards of service delivery. The Griffiths Report (DHSS 1983), on management in the NHS, and other proponents of the New Public Management reinforced these views. Contrary to the findings of the 1979 Royal Commission on the NHS, set up by the Labour government, Thatcher's economic advisers tended to see public bureaucracies generally as overstaffed, subject to institutional inertia, unresponsive to public needs, and lacking accountability. The government advocated the introduction of 'business-style management techniques' and even government-appointed chief executives from the private sector, who were supposed to make public sector organisations more efficient by improved administration, 'downsizing' and 'restructuring', and by tighter control over consultants and other health professionals (Harrison & Pollitt 1994).

It is difficult to evaluate the success of the earlier reforms associated with the Conservative government's introduction of the 'internal market' – including the establishment of hospital trusts, fundholding GP services, and the 'contracting out' of ancillary services. This is because the model was designed to free up health services from the constraints of both 'bureaucratic planning or administration' and the 'conservative medical or public health planning approach', which insist on scientific or epidemiological justification for determining health priorities. Record-keeping during this period was not of the highest standard and the NHS relied on outside consultants to undertake evaluative research, using whatever data they could obtain.

There was growing concern during the decade following these 'reforms' that the determination of health priorities or the regulation of public expenditure could not be simply left to 'market forces'. It was argued that unless a naive faith in Adam Smith's 'hidden hand' guiding the free market could be assumed, it might seem more reasonable to put in place measures to ensure that scientific, epidemiological and administrative rationality could play a more significant role in determining priorities in healthcare. Without research-based planning and policy development, the implementation and monitoring of resource allocation in healthcare tended to be driven by political pragmatism and perhaps even opportunism.

The effectiveness of the 'internal market' will be commented on later in this chapter, along with some evaluative comments on New Labour's NHS innovations, but suffice it to say that a major area of public concern about the introduction of the internal market was the lack of public accountability of the new 'autonomous' hospital trusts and privatised services, and the growing evidence of potential abuse and nepotistic practice in contracting out services.

In response to public concern about abuses in the system, the Nolan Committee was set up to investigate complaints and allegations of impropriety and fraud. The Committee's investigations brought to light some serious problems in the way things were being operated within these supposedly 'reformed' public services. The Commission recommended in its three reports on *Standards in Public Life*, action by the authorities to ensure greater respect for standards of probity and accountability in public life, and more rigorous forms of corporate governance to be put in place to prevent incompetent or corrupt abuse of the system (Nolan 1995, 1996, 1997).

New Labour's reform agenda

There has been considerable change in the pattern of health service funding and management of services in

Britain since 1991, since John Major came into power, and again since New Labour won an overwhelming majority in 1997. The very fact that the public signalled considerable discontent with the way the previous Conservative government had handled the health and social services was taken by the New Labour administration as giving them a mandate to institute yet another round of reforms. What this meant was that the 'reforms' associated with the introduction of the 'internal market' had hardly had time to be bedded in before they were subject to further 'reform' by policy-makers for the New Labour administration. The new administration attempted to retain many 'good features' of the previous government's reforms while attempting to address some of the deepest-felt public grievances about how they were working in their White Papers *The New NHS: Modern, Dependable* (DoH 1997) and *Designed to Care: Renewing the National Health Service in Scotland* (Scottish Office 1998).

In the late 1990s, after two decades of experimentation with these new models, there has been time to evaluate the impact of these developments and their effectiveness in reducing public expenditure, central government control, and improving services for patients and consumers. The findings of researchers are equivocal (Paton 2000, Rice et al 2000, Harrison 2004, Baggott 2004). Most have concluded that ensuring adequate health for all cannot be left to the private sector or to market forces alone (as in the societies in which this course had been followed greater disparities in standards of health and access to healthcare had resulted). The models introduced by New Labour recognised a role for the state in continuing to fund (if not entirely funding) healthcare, to ensure adequate provision for all its citizens and to reassure the public about standards of healthcare by monitoring the quality of healthcare delivery. This meant that despite continued and even extended devolution of responsibility of healthcare to local health authorities, central government remained ultimately responsible and accountable for the NHS – with risky political consequences if New Labour failed to deliver on its promises.

What New Labour attempted was to introduce an element of 'policy directed management' into the supposedly 'free' economy of their predecessors. This was to be achieved by replacing the free 'internal market' with direction of the political economy of health by National Health Service Management Executive Groups to be set up in Scotland and in England, Wales and Northern Ireland. Health service providers, (e.g. hospital trusts and group practices providing primary care services) were to be financially accountable to these Management Executive Groups

through a programme which required them to publish and benchmark their costs on a consistent basis. Regardless of the political rhetoric of the new administration's policy documents, these are interesting moves, because they attempt to factor ethical considerations of care, equity and respect for people's rights into their statement of objectives. See, for example, the implicit reference to these values in the Scottish policy document *Designed to Care (Scotland)* (Scottish Office 1998); for example, the statement of value priorities asserted to be essential to achieving their objectives are, to quote (para 13):

> improving reliability and co-ordination of care through use of new technology;
> improving clinical effectiveness by ensuring that performance meets agreed standards and that these standards are driven upwards;
> promoting the adoption of more effective care based on evidence;
> involving patients to a greater extent in decisions about their own care and treatment;
> providing patients with more information about their health and options for treatment when they are ill.

Significantly, in *The New NHS: Modern, Dependable* (DoH 1997), the move towards a 'One-Nation NHS' involves a 'national drive to improve quality and performance' by providing 'national leadership to support local development', the establishment of a 'National Institute for Clinical Excellence' and a new 'Commission for Health Improvement'. The internal economy of healthcare was to be managed by continuing to apply the principles of quality improvement and total quality management, introduced by the previous government, but with more rigorous accountability to the NHS Management Executive Groups on the basis of sound 'benchmarking' and 'performance management'. The requirements are stated in DoH (1997) as follows:

> **115. Health services should be provided efficiently and effectively. Benchmarking and performance measures have a key role to play in achieving this goal and will help:**
> * inform the process of setting priorities, objectives and targets
> * enable monitoring of progress against objectives and targets
> * promote the use of best practice; and
> * improve the public accountability of the service to patients and the wider public.

In clarifying the rationale for introducing these procedures into the administration of healthcare, the policy-makers have sought to emphasise the ethical justification for the requirements, rather than simply legislate that they are to be followed:

116. The Government believes the main areas in which performance measures are relevant are:

- *the clinical effectiveness of services:*
for instance, the extent to which services achieve reductions in mortality, morbidity and disability;

- *the quality of services:*
for example, waiting times for outpatient appointments and for diagnosis and treatment;

- *the efficiency of services:*
the costs incurred in delivering services, and the use made of staffing, beds and other resources;

- *access to services:*
the availability of services in different areas of the country;

- *inequalities in health:*
differences in morbidity and mortality between socio-economic groups;

- *the appropriateness of services:*
the type of services provided for patients – for example, the use made of day cases.

This is all very fine on paper, but the question is how well this has been implemented in practice. It is too early to assess whether these more ethically and community-medicine based criteria are being implemented and how effectively applied to management of the political economy of Britain as it enters the 21st century. However, it provides us with an interesting model for discussion of the question of how we develop sound ethical policy.

The current emphasis on strategic ethical management, evidence-based practice, corporate governance and clinical audit is important from an ethical point of view, because it represents a serious attempt to ground healthcare-planning and policy development on a more rational and scientific foundation. Given that health practitioners are scientifically trained, and claim to approach their work scientifically, then it can be argued that all health practitioners have a moral duty to be committed to evidence-based practice, and for factually based rather than subjective or politically motivated performance assessment to be applied in the NHS. With appropriate cultural change in the NHS, based on evidence-based practice at all levels, the hope is that professional and corporate accountability should become a matter of routine evaluation of evidence and rational discussion and agreement about action for service improvement, rather than appraisal being personalised or based on politically partisan and media-driven interests. Collective commitment to the same vision for continuous quality improvement and governance, based on transparent audit of clinical, management and corporate performance, would in principle leave no room for nepotism, prevent corrup-

tion and strengthen attempts to reduce sex discrimination and racism in healthcare generally.

EVALUATING THE NEW RIGHT'S AND NEW LABOUR'S REFORMS OF THE NHS

Evaluation has been the watchword of the whole of Part 4 of this book. This is because the demands for increased professional and corporate accountability in the NHS require an evidence base if it is to be either credible or objective. Furthermore the concept of 'evaluation' is linked to our choice of values and standards against which we make assessments of performance and service delivery. In other words, evaluation is centrally connected with ethical practice and ethical management. Rigorous, sound and honest evaluation is a fundamental presupposition of morally accountable practice and transparent corporate accountability. It is important in government, in the sense implied in the Nolan Commission Reports on public standards that is concerned with preventing malpractice, incompetence and fraud. It is also relevant to the wider sense of the government's public responsibility and accountability for the NHS, the adequacy of its services to need, and the quality of care provided. No matter how much responsibility is devolved downwards to local health authorities, trusts and other providers, any government will be held accountable for the standard of healthcare provided to its citizens, especially if the government sets itself up as the guardian of quality in the public interest.

In the 4th edition of *Nursing Ethics*, published at the end of New Labour's first term in office, an attempt was made to give some assessment of the achievements and failures of the Conservative government's various reforms of the NHS. This was based on the available research evidence at the time. Now, nearly 25 years after the Thatcher government instituted its reforms, a lot more research has been done, much of which confirms our earlier summary of their effects and outcomes. It is also possible to begin to evaluate the impact of New Labour's reforms. Since this is not a textbook on social policy but on nursing ethics, we must restrict ourselves to a broad summary and evaluation of trends. For more detailed evaluation two most useful and up-to-date texts are Michael Harrison's *Implementing Change in Health Systems* (Harrison 2004), a comparative study of healthcare reforms and their outcomes in the UK, Sweden and the Netherlands, and Rob Baggott's *Health and Healthcare in Britain* (Baggott 2004), which examines the changes in the NHS, and some of their costs and benefits, in much greater detail. Both books have extensive and useful bibliographies which should be consulted by anyone who wishes to pursue the discussion of healthcare reform in greater depth from either an ethico-political or social policy point of view.

Given the New Right objectives of 'small government' and reduction of public expenditure, the achievements of the Conservative government between 1980 and 1997 were rather modest. While elected on a mandate to strengthen local democracy and to devolve many functions to regional and local level, particularly in this context to reduce by devolution the direct responsibility of central government for the delivery of health, education and welfare services, it is paradoxical that Thatcher's government proved to be the most centralising government ever.

The only area in which real cuts in public spending were achieved were in the area of housing, where the profits and savings were made from selling off half a million homes from public utility housing stock (Taylor-Gooby 1986). Scrutiny of the take-up of such forms of private welfare cover as private health insurance, occupational pensions and sick pay schemes, schooling and commercially rented (as opposed to local authority) housing suggests that the long-term expansion of private welfare has been relatively little influenced by the policies of the Thatcher era. In the health field, for example, take-up of private insurance has been largely linked to occupational schemes. The take-up has tended to be corporate rather than individual. The evidence was that people tend to use private medicine for the treatment of more minor ailments, to avoid the sometimes lengthy waiting times in the public sector. Research showed that where more serious or life-threatening conditions were involved, the public system was still overwhelmingly preferred (Klein 1989).

While on the one hand there is evidence that the 'internal market' model had limited application and relevance to the actual relations between hospitals and their 'clients' (whether individuals or fundholding GP practices), on the other hand there was no substantial evidence that GPs either had the skills or the desire to take on the role of purchasing, or consultants the role of entrepreneurs (Durham 1997). Robertson (1996) summarises the evidence of the strengths of the New Right reforms under the following headings: (a) responsiveness to patients; (b) improved links between different service sectors; (c) increased awareness of quality issues; (d) accountability; (e) improved use of resources. The weaknesses are listed under the following problem areas: (a) adverse selection; (b) administration and transaction costs; (c) 'commercialisation' of NHS values; (d) lack of public account-

ability; (e) problems with contracting; and (f) 'fragmentation' of the NHS. These are set out in Table 11.2 as the first part of a SWOT exercise (examining strengths and weaknesses; opportunities and threats).

We have not completed the SWOT exercise in Table 11.2 as the opportunities/threats are implicit in the identified strengths and weaknesses, and while there was ample evidence that more needed to be done to consolidate achievements, the Major government was inhibited from doing so because of the increase in public expenditure that this would involve. It is possible to argue too that if they had recognised the threat involved they might not have been so vulnerable to attack from the Opposition on their record of reform of the NHS.

Taylor-Gooby's extensive investigation of British attitudes to welfare confirmed a picture of ambivalence towards the welfare state, by highlighting the frustration people felt with the regulations and restrictions of the 'nanny state'. However, he also stressed the importance people attached to what they saw as an 'adequate' level of welfare state provision, and their resulting opposition to real cuts in a system of services which they valued. His conclusions can be summarised as follows (Taylor-Gooby 1986):

- The public by and large appear to wish to retain the welfare state.
- Conservative government attempts to dismantle the welfare state were largely ineffective and regarded with deep ambivalence by the electorate.
- The internal market promoted by the Conservative government fell some way short of New Right ideals of a private market in healthcare, disappointing both the public and potential providers.
- Widespread opposition to the reforms themselves reflected both a popular commitment to the ideal of a public health service and awareness of the electoral peril awaiting parties which attempted to modify that ideal.

Available evidence pointed to a continuing high level of public support for the welfare state (Golding & Middleton 1981, Ranade 1994, Jowell et al 1995). However, these selfsame surveys also indicate that such endorsements of public healthcare provision often coexisted with a degree of acceptance of the private sector.

Here, as Baggott (2004, pp. 113–114) observes, there was an opportunity to promote more rapid and effective implementation of the mixed economy of welfare. However, fiscal restraints put the whole system under too much pressure and the fear of a blow-out in public expenditure to support the

Table 11.2 Strengths and weaknesses of the New Right healthcare reforms

(S) – Strengths	(W) – Weaknesses
On improved responsiveness to patients' needs, he quotes Smee (1995) who claimed there was: '… much evidence that individual trusts are taking advantage of their freedoms to innovate and improve services. These changes cover a very wide range of activities, from patient hotels, through new forms of care for people with learning difficulties, to fuller utilisation of hospital theatres.' He notes that Kennedy & Nichols (1995), a fundholding GP and hospital consultant, argue on the basis of their experience that GP fundholding has brought benefits to patients – in particular, reduction in the numbers of 'long-waiters' and expansion of 'in-house services' to patients; and Glennerster et al (1994) claim that GP fundholders have a greater financial incentive than non-fundholding GPs to engage in health promotion and ensure that their patients are healthy.	**Adverse selection** – Johnson (1990), Hudson (1994), Saltman & von Otter (1995) provided evidence of 'cream-skimming', i.e. that 'providers' and 'purchasers' would be reluctant to take on the type of patients who would require substantial resources for their treatment and ongoing care. Kennedy & Nichols (1995) found that patients were nervous of the implications for themselves if they required expensive treatment or care. Smee (1995) expressed concern about the 'potential perversity' of some of the incentives facing fundholders, and that hospitals might be tempted to concentrate on 'profitable patients'.
Inter-agency liaison – Kennedy & Nichols (1995) claimed that there had been improvement in inter-agency liaison due to regular meetings between key clinicians, hospital managers and community care teams.	**Administration and transaction costs** – Smith (1996), Kennedy & Nichols (1995), Glazer (1995) and Robinson & Le Grand (1995) each produced evidence of increases in administrative and transaction costs of various kinds accruing to purchasers and providers as a result of having to operate under the new internal market requirements: increased management, support and transaction costs; time and resources spent on bidding for and negotiating new contracts each time round; costs of installing appropriate information technology for data-processing and communications to operate the system; the inability of purchasers or providers to rely on long-term contracts to provide stability of service of the kind that are possible in the commercial sphere. Here Glennerster et al (1994) concluded that 'GP contracting seems to be better, but to cost more'.
Improved quality of services – Appleby et al (1992) claimed early on that 81% of district general managers reported that the new contract culture led to improvements in the quality of services. Kennedy & Nichols (1995) claimed that the reforms had led to wider acceptance of medical audit and patient satisfaction surveys.	**'Commercialisation' of NHS values** – Glazer (1995) and Appleby et al (1992) questioned whether the ethos of public service and a caring ethic could be sustained and defended in an environment of increasingly cut-throat competition for contracts, cost-cutting and general economic rationalism.
Standards of accountability – On claims to improvements here, Robertson (1996) observes that democratic accountability in the NHS has always been rather weak, and therefore marginal improvements may appear more significant than they really are.	**Lack of public accountability** – In contrast to the optimistic first reports on accountability in the new contract market system, Glennerster et al (1994) and Collison (1995) observed that so far as accountability to the public was concerned, financial transparency and accountability was sadly lacking, with appeal to 'commercial confidentiality' being used as an excuse not to divulge information of political interest to the public, and Collison pointed out that because CEOs and trustees of the hospital trusts were not elected or democratically accountable, but appointed by the trusts (with the approval of the Secretary of State) there was a risk of cronyism and misuse of public resources, as evidenced by the findings of the Nolan Committee.
On improved use of resources – Glazer (1995) reports that 'in some aspects of care the NHS is better run, wastage is less and patients and GPs are getting a better deal'. Smee (1995) claimed that in the first 2 years of operation, hospital trusts outperformed other hospitals, with increasing numbers of patients receiving treatment. Glennerster et al (1994) review evidence that fundholding GPs were using their purchasing power to pressurise providers into improving services if their custom was not to be withdrawn in favour of others.	**Problems with contracting** – Most serious problems of the internal market related to the fact that it was not (and probably never could be) a truly free market. Munro (1996) conducted a review on behalf of the Scottish Office Health Department, which provided evidence of the fact that purchasers and providers were not really contracting, there was limited 'competition' for contracts, and a tendency to use 'block contracts' and for health boards to award contracts to their own provider units.
	'Fragmentation' of the NHS – This resulted from privatising of services, contracting out and the establishment of a mixed economy of NHS hospital trusts and other hospitals, and was criticised on two grounds: first, that it had complicated access for patients, and second, that it had made overall strategic control, management and public accountability more difficult (Glennerster & Matsaganis 1992, Munro 1996, Durham 1997).

innovations inhibited the whole process, causing disillusionment even among its supporters. He quotes Green (1990, p. 3) as saying that advocates of the New Right reforms saw the way they were implemented as 'a great missed opportunity'. When the Conservative government had the opportunity to implement their strategic blueprint for reform rapidly, because of their large parliamentary majority, they adopted a cautious, pragmatic and tactical approach, fearing a backlash from the public who remained loyal to the NHS and the ideals of justice and equity for the welfare state. As Le Grand et al (1998, p. 30) pointed out, 'the incentives were too weak and the constraints were too strong'. Harrison (2004) suggests a useful set of frames for analysing and evaluating the process and outcomes of policy implementation (Table 11.3).

Baggott concludes (2004, p. 119):

> There is wide agreement that the internal market did make a difference in several respects, notably in promoting managerial, cultural and organisational change. The reforms also enhanced the status of general practice within the British health care system. By giving GPs a key role in the commissioning process, it paved the way for a further series of reforms under the next Government.

Harrison's analysis of the outcomes of the Conservative government reforms is detailed and based on available research. In Table 11.4, we give a very brief summary of his main points, in the form of a partial SWOT analysis, where the opportunities/threats are implicit rather than explicit:

Harrison concludes by saying (2004, p. 62):

> In summary, the reform outcomes reviewed so far raise serious doubts about the feasibility of using market forces to boost provider and health system efficiency in

the UK. So long as the politicians responsible for overseeing the health system remain publicly committed to providing comprehensive health care that is universal, equitable, and affordable, there are limited prospects for market-driven change.

He stresses that the institutional changes and reforms introduced by the Conservatives 'created important precedents for the policies developed by the New Labour party while in opposition and after their election by an overwhelming majority in May, 1997' (Harrison 2004, p. 74).

Appraisal of New Labour's 'New NHS'

Evaluation of the achievements of New Labour is more difficult, partly because of proximity to their reforms in time, partly because these are ongoing, and partly because these are matters of current controversy in political debate. However, there is the same ethical and political responsibility for all concerned with healthcare to make some attempt to assess the impact and outcomes of New Labour's reforms of the NHS.

As Harrison (2004, pp. 74–75) remarks, 'In practice, during its first few years, the new government pursued policies that led in contradictory directions: It sought devolution of authority for commissioning and delivery of NHS services yet continued to centralise control over NHS funding, strategies, and clinical practice standards.' Harrison notes as key emphases:

- In keeping with the policy of a primary-care led NHS, the government planned to devolve budgets and responsibility for primary care, other health services, and some social services, to groups of GPs (Goodwin 2000).

Table 11.3 Four frames for analysing policy implementation

Frame	Processes	Outcomes
Administrative	Top-down transmission through hierarchy; coordination of local actors	Degree of implementation of original policies and programs; fit of outcomes to stated goals of national policy-makers
Bargaining	Bargaining and coalition formation among key national, regional, local actors	Changes in actors' power; new coalitions and political arrangements
Interpretative	Sense-making and valuing by actors; discourse and rhetoric; divergence among actors' orientations (beliefs, norms, preferences, attitudes)	Effects of policies and programs on discourse, beliefs norms, values
Institutional	Structuring of policy-making by social and political institutions; agenda and policy options affected by policy precedents	Policy precedents for future action; changes in institutions, especially those affecting implicitly rules for policy formation and bargaining among actors

Source: Harrison (2004) *Implementing Change in Health Systems*, Sage Publications, London.

Table 11.4 Harrison's appraisal of Conservative government reforms

Strengths	Weaknesses
Administrative	
1. Success in rapidly enacting and diffusing the main structural changes necessary to launch a market for publicly funded healthcare	1. Failure to create vigorous provider competition and rational choice of services by purchasers
2. Success in efforts to privatise some NHS operations, e.g. capital construction and social care for frail elderly patients	2. Failure to provide adequate incentives for providers to improve efficiency and service quality
3. Partial implementation of market-like processes but inhibited by government control of budgets	3. Neither health authority managers nor GP fundholders were assisted to develop competence in the cost-efficient operation and management of healthcare services
Bargaining	
1. *Working for Patients* and *The Patient's Charter* did underline patients' rights and gave patients more flexibility in their choice of GP, and choice of services, through fundholding GPs	1. Emphasis on patients' rights was perceived as a gain, but proved a 'stick to beat the government over the back' when people's expectations of the NHS were not met
2. Introduction of business management methods, organisational and financial accounting disciplines, and scope for service reform were welcomed	2. Instead of curtailing heavy-handed government control over the health system, the reforms led to increased centralisation and control
	3. In their bid to curtail the power of trade unions and professional organisations to engage in negotiation and collective bargaining, the reforms helped to fragment these organisations and undermine their bargaining capacity
Interpretative	
1. The chief achievement of the reforms was to change the culture of the NHS and the rhetoric of management and professional service	1. The risk was that the new rhetoric was seen as lacking substance, as a matter of using new 'buzz words' rather than effecting real change
2. Business philosophy replaced the ethos of the welfare state, and health practitioners came to be viewed as 'public sector employees' rather than as 'public servants' engaged in healthcare	2. With the emphasis on cost-efficiency and on inputs and outputs, the emphasis on serving the commonweal and the role of 'caring professions' changed as well as their motivation for service
3. The style of new public management sought to empower managers to manage, and to focus on the needs of customers, rather than be limited by the power of vested professional interests	3. While some welcomed the opportunity to gain experience (and training) in management, for many health practitioners this meant taking them away from their real clinical work
4. Empowerment of patients or consumers was only partially achieved, mainly by raising public awareness of their rights and choices	4. The gap between rhetoric and reality in relation to the emphasis on patient/client autonomy became increasingly obvious with state control
Institutional	
1. The reforms contributed to improved overall direction of NHS management, but also with increasing centralisation of government control	1. Patients and public representatives lost direct access to NHS decision-making channels
2. The introduction of the internal market made the health system more open to market-like negotiation between healthcare providers and other health-related organisations	2. Healthcare services became more fragmented and subject to the limitations and lack of locally available providers of required services
3. Local NHS managers were supported by government pressures to press for more efficient and higher-quality medical care	3. Pressures on health practitioners to maintain standards and improve productivity, increased the stresses on their work as units were 'down-sized' and bureaucratic controls increased
4. Reforms helped to shift power and resources away from hospitals towards primary care and community services	4. The promised shift of emphasis and resources to health promotion rather than a focus on clinical and treatment services did not occur

- The new government established a National Institute for Clinical Excellence (NICE), with a mandate to develop NHS standards and guidelines for effective practice, derived from evidence-based medicine, and a Commission for Health Improvement (CHI) responsible for assessing the performance standards of NHS trusts and health authorities.
- To promote reform and provide tangible evidence of improvements in NHS performance the government announced a range of modernisation programmes that were to be centrally funded and directed (Appleby 1999), namely, means of scheduling access to primary care and hospital services, the introduction of a 24-hour NHS telephone helpline, and ambitious new hospital construction programmes.
- The government committed itself to increased public sector funding for the NHS, to bring it up to average European levels, and by considerable immediate increases to NHS budgets.

Within the UK government's devolution of responsibility for healthcare to the Welsh Assembly and Scottish Executive, parallel developments took place in Wales and Scotland, which were implemented during the New Labour's second term in office.

Despite attempts by New Labour to give the impression of a radical break with the New Right agenda for reform of the NHS, there were nevertheless strong elements of continuity with the past in Labour's 'New NHS'. Some of the failures of New Right policy and reforms, e.g. to cut public sector expenditure and to promote greater efficiency and improve quality of services by relying on market forces, were cited as reasons for Labour's reforms. New Labour committed itself to greater financial investment in the NHS and to fund the development of supervisory agencies such as NICE and CHI to address the issue of standards and quality improvement. Fundholding in general practice was abolished and larger primary care trusts were to become responsible for commissioning services, with powers to sign 3-year contracts, to ensure better continuity and to cut down on administrative costs, but these would have to be approved by the responsible local health authority. Instead of the emphasis on competition for contracts in the supposed internal market, the new arrangements were intended to improve cooperation in 'partnerships' between purchasers and providers, both in service delivery and in ensuring continuous quality improvement. Some of the main continuities noted by Harrison (2004, pp. 76–77) are:

- The main institutions of contracting and some of the features of the former purchaser–provider split were retained.
- The 'New NHS' continued to deepen central government's commitment to WHO policy, namely by encouraging movement towards a primary-care-led NHS.
- New Labour continued to seek private sector funding and investment in development of NHS services and infrastructure, and continued to encourage private sector providers.
- The move from professional self-regulation to increased public accountability through government-appointed bodies with responsibility for evaluating the impact and outcomes of services continued developments started by the previous government.
- The increasingly centralised and bureaucratic measures used to implement and monitor the reforming agenda closely resembled those of the Conservatives, and for the same reason, namely that they could not escape their overall responsibility for the cost and quality of mainly state-funded healthcare services.

Concerns have been expressed from a number of quarters that the modernisation programme of New Labour is too ambitious given the size and complexity of the NHS, and that the government may well have difficulty sustaining the level of public spending on the NHS, necessary to implement its proposed reforms, and to meet current shortages of doctors, nurses and other allied health professions and to keep pace with public demand (Appleby & Coote 2002, Robinson 2002, Ferriman 2000). And while the rhetoric supports a continuing focus on primary care, most new funding has gone into improving hospital care (King's Fund 2001).

On the positive side, the new structures have been quickly established and legislated for, and with increased funding and extensive consultation, attempts have been made to secure the commitment of local health authorities to the kind of culture change that is required to make their reforms work. In particular, the form of the new primary care groups and primary care trusts was agreed through negotiations with relevant medical bodies. However, despite the spirit of cooperation, these new bodies have struggled to meet the more complex managerial, developmental, strategic planning and accountability standards required, without the allocation of adequate extra funding for staff and organisational development.

The National Institute for Clinical Excellence and Commission for Health Improvement were set up in the face of some resistance from the medical establishment, but through improved consultation have begun to work more effectively with the relevant professional bodies to negotiate more rational policies on the use of generic drugs and alternative medical procedures as means to conserve and use scarce resources more effectively.

At both national and local levels strengthened arrangements for clinical, organisational and staff governance have been put in place with a view to improvement of quality control at the different levels of health service operations, through audit based on evidence, as this becomes available. The previous government's efforts to achieve quality improvement through quality assurance proved only partially successful, because implemented in a fragmentary way and 'because of weaknesses in information systems and the overall knowledge base' (Walshe 2000, Freeman et al 1999). Despite rearguard action by unions representing healthcare workers and the medical profession, progress is being made with the setting up of structures and targets for clinical, corporate and staff governance, and with translating these formal arrangements into quality improvement processes (Wilkin et al 2000, 2001). Combined pressure from government and exposure in the media of failures to maintain adequate standards in clinical governance, which led to high-profile public inquiries, forced the medical establishment to accept the need to support the government's quality initiatives; e.g. the Alder Hey Hospital organ retention scandal (HM Government 2001a), the Bristol Inquiry into high mortality rates of children who underwent cardiac surgery at Bristol Royal Infirmary (Secretary of State for Health 2001), and the Shipman Inquiry into the hundreds of patients Dr Shipman appears to have murdered (Shipman Inquiry 2001). Since these events, the General Medical Council has announced new procedures for revalidating medical practitioners, and the Minister of Health outlined plans for revalidation reviews to cover all doctors by 2005 (Eaton 2002) and one by one the medical Royal Colleges have accepted clinical audit and governance and declared their willingness to cooperate with NICE (and SIGN in Scotland).

Progress towards translation of the rhetoric of 'inter-agency partnership' and 'joined-up services and funding' into practical reality has been slow, particularly between Health, Social Services, Education and Housing. The reasons for this are complex, but it is clearly due in part to the institutional inertia and territoriality of large and long-established public sector departments. Long divided by domains that are not co-terminous, separate structures and budgets,

different occupational biases and interests, and different training and orientation, these ideals have been difficult to realise (Robinson & Paxton 1998).

During its first term in office, the Labour government's 'New NHS' reforms produced very few discernible improvements in service productivity or quality, despite huge injections of additional money into the health system. Harrison (2004, pp. 81–82) remarks:

> So far, an all-too-familiar litany of problems continues to make headlines and worry politicians and policy analysts: incompetent physicians, poor quality, insufficient quality assurance, overcrowding, delays in access to hospital care, unsatisfactory outcome, inadequate information systems and failure to use available performance data. (Feachem et al 2002, Smith 2002b)

Nevertheless, he concludes:

> … the potential long-term impacts of the new policies outweigh their effects so far. Although the official discourse abandoned much of the language of the market-place, the stress on business management techniques continues. Moreover, there is growing use of evidence-based standards as a basis for evaluating and controlling the performance of hospitals and community care (Harrison, Moran & Wood, 2002). Neither hospital physicians nor general practitioners are openly resisting this drift toward increased managerial and governmental supervision and standardisation of their work (Dowswell, 2002). In fact, general practitioners and nurses appear to accept control over their work by the new primary care organisations, and are trying to comply with NHS clinical guidelines (Harrison, Dowswell & Wright, 2002).

Baggott gives a closely parallel evaluation of the achievements and failures of New Labour's reforms since 1997 (Baggot 2004, pp. 361ff.). He summarises these under the following headings: Funding and Efficiency, Private/Public Sector, Quality of Service, the Professions and the Workforce, Access, Fairness and Choice, Accountability, Public Involvement, Primary Care, Public Health and Inequalities, and Devolution and Divergence. Summarising these would duplicate much of what has already been said, but his analysis is to be recommended for being more detailed and in some cases more up-to-date. We propose to conclude by examining only one of his areas of comment, namely 'The Professions and the Workforce'.

One of the most innovative and controversial areas of reform introduced by New Labour is its document *Agenda for Change* (DoH 2003). It proposed a comprehensive review of the NHS workforce and the collective bargaining arrangements and pay structures that have remained virtually unchanged for 50 years. In this context the General Whitley Council has functioned as the overarching joint negotiating body for the NHS public sector, and what the *Agenda for Change* proposed was a fundamental change in the way it has operated. What the *Agenda for Change* proposed was:

- a single job evaluation scheme to cover all jobs in the health service to support a review of pay and all other terms and conditions for health service employees
- three pay spines for (1) doctors and dentists; (2) other professional groups covered by the Pay Review Body; (3) remaining non-Pay Review Body staff
- a wider remit for the Pay Review Body covering the second of these pay spines.

Agenda for Change was, in the words of the Department of Health, 'the most radical shake up of the NHS pay system since the NHS began in 1948. It applies to over one million NHS staff with the exception of doctors, dentists and the most senior managers. Working in partnership UK Health Departments, NHS Employers and NHS trade unions, over a period of four years, negotiated a package worth on average an extra 12.5 per cent on basic pay over three years.'

The increased pay package came with strings attached, namely adoption of a new, modernised pay system for non-medical staff in the NHS. This was implemented from 1 December 2004, with pay backdated to 1 October 2004. Furthermore, the organisation representing NHS employers has worked in partnership with NHS managers and staffside organisations to establish the NHS Staff Council. One of the council's first tasks was to undertake a review of the interim agreement on unsocial hours payments, working toward introduction of a harmonised system of payments from 1 April 2006.

At the same time, the Treasury commissioned Derek Wanless, former Chief Executive of NatWest Bank, to review 'technological, demographic, and medical trends over the next two decades' as they might affect the NHS, and 'to identify the key factors which will determine the financial and other resources required to ensure that the NHS can provide a publicly funded, comprehensive, high quality service available on the basis of clinical need and not ability to pay'.

The second Wanless Report, *Securing Our Future Health: Taking a Long-term View – Final Report* (Wanless 2002), observed, among other things, that employment practice and regulation would in future be subject to Europe-wide legislation. For example, the European Working Time Directives would limit the number of hours healthcare staff, including junior medical staff and nurses, are permitted to work, with a knock-on effect on productivity and staff shortages. What the Wanless Report recommended was a fundamental rethink on the way that the division of labour between doctors, nurses and other allied health professions may need to change in the light of improvements in medical treatment, applied technology and associated work practices. (Here the impact of the use of less invasive forms of 'key-hole' surgery, or laser treatment, which have shortened the times people have to be in hospital, is a case in point.) With a greater emphasis on teamwork in primary care and hospital medicine, and the delegation of an increasing number of traditional 'medical' functions to nurses and other allied health professionals, the traditional boundaries of clinical responsibility between the professions are becoming, and are likely to become more blurred, with the need to renegotiate job descriptions and rates of pay.

What the second edition of the NHS *Job Evaluation Handbook* (NHS 2004) makes clear is that this process is already well in hand, and that much progress has been made in this process.

Other factors that have made this fundamental review of employment practice, job demarcation and pay review necessary are reviews of individual grading structures that have been taking place, e.g. the 1988 clinical grading structure for nurses and midwives, and others for speech and language therapists and hospital pharmacists and others in the 1990s. In addition, the implementation of UK-wide Equal Pay Act 1984 (as amended) and European legislation on equal employment opportunities and non-discrimination in employment have necessitated review of long-established discriminatory practices. However, the *Agenda for Change* tries to make a virtue of necessity by offering incentives for flexibility, adaptability and willingness to change working practices and training in the existing professional groups, including greater emphasis on structured forms of joint interprofessional learning, especially on the job.

What this has required was the setting up of a Job Evaluation Working Party (JEWP1) in the mid-1990s. Its remit was to set criteria for what would make a fair and non-discriminatory scheme for use in the health service. Following the publication of *Agenda for Change* the Job Evaluation Working Party was reconstituted (JEWP2) as one of a number of technical subgroups of the Joint Secretariat Group. This was a subcommittee of the Central Negotiating Group, which comprised, employer, union and Department of Health representatives, set up to negotiate new health service grading and pay structures. The stages in the development of the scheme were as set out in Box 11.4.

Box 11.4 Stages in the development of the NHS Job Evaluation Scheme

(1) *Identification of draft factors*. This part of the exercise drew on the work of JEWP1 in comparing the schemes in use in the health service.

(2) *Testing of draft factors*. This was done using a sample of around 100 jobs for which volunteer jobholders were asked to complete a relatively open-ended questionnaire, providing information under each of the draft factor headings and any other information about their jobs which they felt was not covered by the draft factors. As a result of this exercise the draft factors were refined.

(3) *Development of factor levels*. The information collected during the initial test exercise was used by JEWP, working in small joint teams, to identify and define draft levels of demand for each factor.

(4) *Testing of draft factor plan*. A benchmark sample of around 200 jobs was drawn up, with two or three individuals being selected for each job to complete a more specific factor-based questionnaire, with the assistance of trained job analysts, to ensure that the information provided was accurate and comprehensive.

(5) *Completed questionnaires were evaluated by trained joint panels*. The outcomes were reviewed by JEWP members. The validated results were input to a computer database.

(6) *Scoring and weighting*. The job evaluation results database was used to test various scoring and weighting options considered by a joint JSG/JEWP group.

(7) *Guidance Notes*. Provisional guidance notes to assist evaluators and matching panel members to apply the factor level definitions to jobs consistently were drafted for the benchmark exercise. These were greatly expanded as a result of the benchmark evaluation exercise and have continued to be developed as successive training and profiling have taken place.

(8) *Computerisation*. The scale of the exercise to implement the NHS Job Evaluation Scheme meant that it was essential to consider how it could be assisted by computerisation. Link HR systems were commissioned to adapt their existing computer-aided job evaluation scheme for the purpose and to develop a computerised tool to assist in the process of matching local jobs to the evaluated national benchmark sample.

Of special interest to this book on nursing ethics are the equality features of the scheme, as these changes are likely to impact greatly on the terms and conditions and pay scales applicable to various kinds and grades of nurses. Nurses still account for the overwhelming majority of health practitioners in the NHS (and other healthcare systems worldwide), and changes necessary in their working practices will impact on the whole pattern of service delivery in both hospitals and the community. As primary care 'general practitioners' of a kind, nurses have not only had to specialise more, as the nature and complexity of their work has evolved, but they have also developed new professional subdivisions in relation to nursing. With the rapid developments in medicine and clinical healthcare services, nurses are well equipped to lead the agenda for change, and must take responsibility to do so in their own interest and that of their colleagues in the allied health professions. However, nurses are also the most vulnerable group, as the definition of their role is much less specific than that of radiologists, dieticians, pharmacists etc. The consequences for nurses could be much more far-reaching than those for the other allied health professions.

Harrison (2004) emphasises that the impact of NHS reforms from the beginning has impacted more heavily on nurses than other professional groups. The burden of extra clinical and administrative work that has resulted from these organisational changes fell even more heavily on nurses than physicians (Harrison & Pollitt 1994, Robinson 1993). The same is likely to be the case with the *Agenda for Change*. The issues of justice and equity here are not merely job demarcation and pay issues, but relate to the wider concerns of nurses as one of the main caring professions, who are also involved in the front line in the less visible areas of social deprivation rather than hospital medicine. This is an issue that has yet to be seriously addressed in the otherwise admirable emphasis on equality in the *Job Evaluation Handbook* (NHS 2004) (Box 11.5).

A report by Melia (2005) to the Scottish Executive on the implications of the *Agenda for Change* for nurses emphasises the ambiguous status of nurses in the whole scheme:

One main theme that comes through in the analysis is the shaping of the nursing agenda by medical concerns, the main one being the desire for a consultant-led service. We can add to this shaping of nursing's agenda, the political goals of social inclusion and the existence of targets for the widening of access and participation in higher education for the health professionals.

It is clear that the nursing profession cannot develop in isolation in these modernizing reforms. The focus of attention has been on the opportunities for medicine to devolve some of its work to nursing. This has been

Box 11.5 Equality features of the scheme (NHS 2004)

1 As one of the reasons for NHS pay modernisation was to ensure equal pay for work of equal value, it was crucial that every effort was made to ensure that the NHS Job Evaluation Scheme was fair and non-discriminatory in both design and implementation.

2 The equality criteria drawn up by JEWP1 were developed into a checklist. As the exercise progressed, its stages were compared with the checklist and a compliance report drafted. The final section of the checklist concerned statistical analysis and monitoring of both the benchmark exercise and the final outcomes.

3 The equality features of the NHS Job Evaluation Scheme design include:
   - A sufficiently *large number of factors* to ensure that all significant job features can be fairly measured.
   - Inclusion of *specific factors* to ensure that features of *predominantly female jobs are fairly measured*, for example Communication and Relationship Skills, Physical Skills, Responsibilities for Patients/Clients, Emotional Effort.
   - Avoidance of references in the *factor level definitions* to features which might operate in an indirectly discriminatory manner for example direct references to qualifications under the Knowledge factor, references to tested skills under the Physical Skills factor.
   - *Scoring and weighting* designed in accordance with a set of gender neutral principles, rather than with the aim of achieving a particular outcome, for example all Responsibility factors are equally weighted to avoid one form of responsibility been viewed as more important than others.

Equality features of the implementation procedures include:
   - A detailed matching procedure to ensure that all jobs have been compared to the national benchmark profiles on an analytical basis, in accordance with the Court of Appeal decision in *Bromley v. Quick*.
   - Training in equality issues and the avoidance of bias for all matching panel members, job analysts and evaluators.
   - A detailed Job Analysis Questionnaire to ensure that all relevant information is available for local evaluations.

---

welcomed in part, but there is need for caution, and the professions should not underestimate the consequences. Early evidence from research in primary care suggest that the reactions are mixed where nurse-led services are concerned (Lewis 2001) There was a tendency for nurses to serve vulnerable populations which are often poorly served by general practice. This somewhat missed the point of the Plan and raises the question of a two-tier health service.

In conclusion, we might stress that just as different values drive different programmes for reform and different values are employed in evaluating their impact and outcomes, the task of contributing responsibly to debate about healthcare policy and both its ethical and political implications requires serious study of ethics by all involved in healthcare, as the above chapter should illustrate.

further reading

Role of the state in providing healthcare

Ashford D E 1986 The emergence of the welfare states. Blackwell, Oxford

Harrison M I 2004 Implementing change in health systems: market reforms in the United Kingdom, Sweden, and the Netherlands. Sage Publications, London

Robertson A, Thompson I E, Porter M 1992 Social policy and administration. Health Education Open Learning Project, Keele University, Keele, Staffordshire

Wilkinson R 1996 Unhealthy societies: the affliction of inequalities. Routledge, London

The nature of sound ethical policy

Allsopp J 1996 Health policy and the National Health Service: towards 2000. Longman, London

Harrison S, Hunter D, Pollitt C 1990 The dynamics of British health policy. Unwin Hyman, London

Joss R, Kogan M 1995 Advancing quality: total quality management in the National Health Service. Open University Press, Buckingham

Kitson A 1993 Nursing art and science. Chapman and Hall, London

Deciding priorities for health spending: counting the cost of health

Caplan A H, Callahan D 1981 Ethics in hard times. Hastings Center Series on Ethics, Hastings on Hudson, USA

Mooney G 1992 Economics, medicine and health, 2nd edn. Harvester Wheatsheaf, Hampshire

Wilkinson R 1996 Unhealthy societies: the affliction of inequalities. Routledge, London

The future of health services – socialised or privatised healthcare?

Baggott R 2004 Health and health care in Britain. Macmillan, London

Hudson B 1994 Making sense of markets in health and social care. Business Education Publishers, Sunderland

Mishra R 1984 The welfare state in crisis: social thought and social change. Harvester Wheatsheaf, London

Harrison S, Pollit C 1994 Controlling health professionals: the future of work and organisation in the NHS. Open University Press, Buckingham

PART 5

Ethical decision-making and moral theory

Making moral decisions and being able to justify our actions

12

AIMS

This chapter has the following aims:

1. To clarify what is involved in making a specific decision, as distinct from seeking agreement about general ethical policies
2. To explore the variety of approaches necessary for the effective teaching and learning of competence in practical ethics
3. To explore methods of problem-solving in ethical decision-making and parallels with problem-solving elsewhere
4. To examine the necessary and sufficient conditions for free, purposeful and responsible action as moral agents.

LEARNING OUTCOMES

When you have read and worked through this chapter, you should be able to:

- Describe and analyse typical situations demanding real decisions, rather than agreement about rules and policy
- Discuss critically the role of 'conscience' and 'intuition' in our moral experience
- Demonstrate understanding of different approaches to teaching ethics and skills in ethical decision-making, and ability to apply these in conducting tutorials
- Demonstrate ability to apply the given models of problem-solving to specific cases taken from nursing experience
- Demonstrate ability to make critical appraisals of the extent of a person's responsibility for their actions, by considering specific cases
- Demonstrate understanding of what it means to give a systematic and comprehensive account of the reasons and grounds for a moral decision.

HAVING TO TAKE A MORAL DECISION

It was remarked in Chapter 6 that we tend to focus on the 'big dilemmas' when discussing biomedical and nursing ethics. These are the typical urgent and dramatic situations that are frequently the focus of media attention and the subject matter of hospital-based 'soap-operas' – abortion, euthanasia, resuscitation, compulsory use of ECT, and so on. These 'big issues' are important because they raise questions of *general principle and public policy* in healthcare, but they are not the ones about which rank-and-file nurses have to take routine ethical decisions in everyday practice. However strongly nurses may feel personally about these general and theoretical issues, they are usually bystanders and interested spectators in public debate about ethical policy. In practice, the kinds of ethical competence nurses require for their day-to-day work are skills in applied ethics, and experience of dealing with everyday *practical problems* and how to *apply general ethical principles in actual clinical situations*.

Competence in ethics does undoubtedly require that we gain insight into the relationship between our own moral beliefs and the general ethical policies currently adopted by society and applied in the institutions where we work. However, competence in ethics has much more to do with learning skills in clarifying our own values in relation to those of our profession and social institutions, and gaining experience in the application of ethical principles to everyday practice. To focus too much attention on disputes about general ethical policy, as the media tend to do, tends to distort perceptions of the nature of ethics and to skew approaches to teaching of ethics towards a concern with ethical theory rather than practice. The real question is how do we learn and teach skills in clarifying values, making well-informed and justifiable ethical decisions, and developing ethical policies that are relevant to the workplace.

Both the classical 'big' issues mentioned above, and the challenges presented by application of new medical techniques and genetic engineering (e.g. assisted reproduction, use of IVF, AID and egg donation for genetic research, and withholding life support for severely handicapped infants), all provoke considerable public interest and controversy. This is because they raise general concerns about potential conflicts of principle in the formulation of ethical policy and in the law as applied to healthcare. Reaching public consensus, or agreement on the team, on decisions of principle affecting policy and procedures in working practice is important, but these 'decisions of principle' are not to be confused with practical decisions about specific cases or patients. However, as

nurses gain seniority and acquire greater clinical responsibility they may have to take part in discussions, with colleagues or wider forums, about some of these controversial 'big issues'. If they are to make a useful contribution to such debates, they will need to have reflected on their own ethical standpoint on these disputed topics in the light of their practical nursing experience and knowledge of ethical principles.

However, not all ethical decisions relate to either contested matters of principle or to dramatic clinical situations. Most ethical decisions are as unremarkable as everyday life and routine work on a ward or in the community. Consequently, both clinical and ethical responses to situations presenting in practice become fairly routine. As trained, experienced practitioners, nurses learn to take decisions as a matter of course. They may have little awareness of doing so, and may not stop to reflect particularly deeply on *what* they are doing, *why* they choose a particular course of action, *how* they arrive at a decision or *how they would justify* their decisions and actions to someone else. There is a risk that working to a strict routine may desensitise nurses to the needs of individual patients, or to the unique features of their particular circumstances. However, just as good clinical training puts nurses on their guard against treating everyone in the same way, so too good training in ethics will ensure that nurses address each situation with due attention to the needs of individual patients and their particular circumstances.

It is noteworthy that in Greek the word 'crisis' originally just meant 'decision time', not a time of drama, but a time *when we have to make a judgement about what to do next*. Obviously, when we are faced with life-threatening and urgent problems, we are faced with a crisis in both senses, because we *must take a decision* and *have to do something*. We commonly use the word 'crisis' to refer to major life events, turning points in our lives, or turning points in the course of an illness. Commonly, these events are associated also with making difficult or painful decisions, both for patients and for practitioners caring for them.

However, most decisions we take in life are neither dramatic nor dangerous. In performing routine work, numerous minor decisions are taken every day, including routine moral decisions. It is important to stress again here that not all moral decision-making is associated with drama and crisis. On the contrary, most of us develop remarkable skill at making rapid moral assessments of the problems facing us in the practical situations in our lives and in taking the appropriate decisions. Some decision times will be crises for us, but like the insurance company's advertising slogan, it is important generally 'not to make a drama out of a crisis'!

Our family upbringing and experience of school, work and the wider community usually equip us with adequate knowledge of the moral values and rules applicable in our society, and we develop practical skills in applying them in our daily lives by trial and error. Some of these values and rules we will come to adopt as our own, to others we may simply show the respect that is necessary to get on with people, but there are others we may actively criticise or reject. Whatever we do and whichever lifestyle we choose, our decisions and actions, our moral judgements, will embody and express our value judgements. Like learning to walk or run, where we employ the principles of physiology, mechanics and kinaesthetics without being aware of these, in routine decision-making we are applying scientific knowledge, practical experience, organisational and moral principles in a highly complex process which we would find just as difficult to explain as the man challenged to explain how he manages to walk.

We do not normally reflect critically on what we are doing when we make decisions, particularly those decisions which involve application of our or society's established moral values – unless we are faced with a crisis. In this sense a 'crisis' may be interpreted as a situation which demands a decision, where we are challenged or forced to reflect on what we are doing, and where we are challenged to give a clear explanation of our reasons for deciding and acting as we do or have done.

Several factors may cause us to experience decision time as a crisis.

The *first kind of crisis* is where we are entering unfamiliar territory, for example when the trainee nurse first encounters the practical and moral problems of nursing a dying patient, or when the experienced nurse acquires new responsibility as a ward sister or manager. Here, lack of appropriate knowledge or skills, unfamiliarity with established rules of practice or ignorance of likely outcomes may undermine the confidence of nurses and force them to examine carefully how and what they are doing and why they choose or chose to act in a particular way.

Related to this is a *second kind of crisis*, namely where an individual is suddenly faced with greater-than-usual responsibility, or is obliged to act on his own, without the usual opportunities to check things out with colleagues or friends. Here the urgency of the problem that has to be dealt with and the need to accept personal responsibility may challenge us to seek a clearer justification for what we have done so as to be able to answer criticism if things go wrong, or to give reasons for our actions.

The *third type of crisis* concerns the nature of decisions themselves – namely, that choosing one thing or one course of action forecloses other options. (The word 'decision', coming from the same root as 'incision', has the connotation of 'cutting off' other possibilities.) Deciding to accept one job rather than another or to marry one person rather than another has long-term implications for one's life, and limits one's other decisions – although it may open up new possibilities as well! Choosing a particular treatment option for a patient may mean excluding other options, and following one course of action may mean that one cannot go back later to try another course of action. Confronted with situations where decisions are irreversible or where the consequences will be far-reaching, we are faced with awesome responsibility and these circumstances may also cause us to pause and reflect.

A *fourth type of crisis* is where we are faced with a genuine moral dilemma – an irresolvable conflict of duties or a painful choice between two equally unacceptable moral outcomes. Here we are forced to reflect critically, not on the circumstances in which the decision is demanded, nor on the degree of responsibility demanded of us, nor on the likely consequences, but on the relative priority to be given to our moral principles, on how they are related to one another and how we are to act if we cannot resolve the conflict. Such cases of real dilemmas certainly do arise, and if we are faced with a crisis, namely a situation where a decision *has* to be taken, then we can be in a terrible quandary. We have to face up to the challenge to make a decision and to act as wisely and professionally as we can, without the comfort or security of familiar rules or established procedures to guide us. We also have to be prepared to accept responsibility for the outcomes, particularly if we have misjudged the kind of response required to deal with the crisis. Fortunately such situations are fairly rare. Most moral choices relate to situations that recur in various forms in our routine work. If we deal with moral problems routinely in a responsible, systematic and disciplined way, then we should be able to give a good account of ourselves when we explain why we acted as we did when faced with a moral dilemma. This would simply be to outline the evidence and reasons that we took into account in making our decision. These decisions taken in the face of dilemmas may in turn serve as precedents, and as a guide or basis for future action. Even though there may not be solutions to moral dilemmas, there are still methodical ways we can examine our options, marshal evidence and reasons, clarify the underlying moral principles and act with forethought rather than impulsively or just following blind prejudice.

A *fifth type of moral crisis* arises *when we are forced to re-examine and justify our moral beliefs*. This situation can arise when someone demands that we justify our moral standpoint, or the fundamental moral principles and values that inform our practice, or when some event in our lives causes us to call into question the basis of our whole belief-and-value system. At such times we are forced back to a more basic level where we are obliged to examine the very presuppositions on which our moral beliefs are based and the kind of arguments that we could produce to justify them. While confrontation by another person, or a personal moral crisis, may represent a painful challenge to our moral beliefs, the discipline of philosophy is a systematic way in which we can study these questions and test out our own solutions against those worked out by others over the centuries. This particular aspect of decision-making, namely decisions of principle, relates directly to the concerns of moral theory and the justification of our fundamental moral principles. These topics are the subject matter of the final chapter of this book. At this stage, however, we return to the analysis and description of the more basic characteristics of routine decision-making, and the justification of our practical moral decisions and actions.

CONSCIENCE, FEELING, INTUITION AND MORAL JUDGEMENT

Since we do, in fact, make moral judgements all the time – about what we consider right and wrong in general, what we consider the best course of action in a specific situation – or make judgements about our own or other people's actions and characters, we tend to resist attempts to analyse the process involved (because we do this semi-automatically). We tend to appeal to 'the voice of conscience' or 'intuition', or say that 'it just felt right'. While these expressions have an important and proper place in our moral discourse, they can also represent a 'cop-out', a refusal to look at the underlying reasons why we act or have acted in a certain way.

However, our use of these phrases expresses our sense that moral judgement, decision and action are as natural a part of living and doing as breathing. We all grow up in some sort of moral community. We adopt some of its values, making them our own, while perhaps rejecting others. We form dispositions and learn routine patterns of effective action, by habit and practice, so that they become, as Aristotle said, 'second nature to us' – these are what we have traditionally called 'virtues' and 'vices' (or 'competencies' in modern parlance). We have routine ways of justifying

what we do to others and ourselves, routine ways of making excuses for ourselves if things go wrong. Because our moral experience is coextensive with the rest of our human experience and permeates all we are and do, it seems perhaps rather artificial to try to analyse it and separate out the moral decision-making bit from the rest of our daily living. We often appeal to the 'voice of conscience', 'gut feelings' or 'intuition' in justifying our actions, just because these terms express how much of all this has become second nature to us.

However, appeal to conscience or intuition to justify a moral decision can also be a form of mystification (as we suggested in Chapter 4), suggesting that decision-making is a kind of impalpable and private, even occult, process. The discussion at this point often echoes the school of thought which claims that 'nurses are born not made', that the attributes required of 'good' nurses – empathy and sympathy, sensitivity to the patient's real needs, gentleness, competence, efficiency – cannot be taught. Of course, some people have natural ability to relate to and care for people, and others have not. But if we can rationally understand and describe the nature of the skills required, then in principle we should be able to teach them. Likewise, some people may start with certain advantages of stable family life and moral upbringing, relevant experience and practical wisdom and may therefore appear more competent and confident in making decisions and exercising moral responsibility. However, even the most confident person can be shaken in a crisis, but it is equally true that most people can be trained to exercise or carry responsibility. They can be trained to cope better with routine decisions and crises. They can learn to give an account of what they have done, how and when they did it, and why they did it. However, this all presupposes the need for some awareness of training approaches, methods and management procedures and it is this need which this chapter will address.

Ethical decision-making – occult or rational process?

In ethics, it is important to demystify moral decision-making, both for the sake of clarity and truth and to encourage people to address those forms of knowledge and skill that can be learned and taught to improve competence in this area. Ethical decision-making may be difficult to do well and methodically, but there is nothing occult about the process. Moral decision-making is but one particular form of problem-solving activity among other forms. We can learn a lot in ethics from studying the methods of problem-solving applied in other disciplines, and then apply these to moral problems specifically. But there are also dangers that follow from failure to pay attention to the particular nature and complexity of moral decision-making, or from trying to force ethics to fit the demands of inappropriate methods.

Baruch de Spinoza (1632–1677), in his *Ethics* (Gregory 1955), developed a deductive system in which he sought to reduce ethics to a kind of mathematics. As a mathematician and philosopher Spinoza hoped to achieve the same degree of certainty in moral judgement that we can achieve in mathematics by reasoning about ethics *'more geometrico'*, that is, by attempting to make moral arguments fit the 'procrustean bed' of geometrical reasoning and deduction. The result was either a gross oversimplification of the complexity of moral arguments, or a caricature of them. Other philosophers have tried to apply the methods of the empirical sciences to ethics, to attempt to develop a 'scientific' ethics, based on 'facts' (usually of psychology or sociology), and which they supposed could be proved by scientific experiments (Hobbes and Bentham could be counted among this number). Utilitarians like Jeremy Bentham and John Stuart Mill (1806–1873) envisaged ethics as a kind of empirical science. Bentham tried to develop a 'felicific calculus' to measure the degree of pleasure or pain an act would cause, and Mill suggested that we should be able to find empirical evidence to determine 'the greatest good for the greatest number'. Neither of these approaches has been very successful or very helpful.

We have to recognise the distinctive nature of ethics and the kinds of problem-solving methods that would be appropriate to dealing with moral decision-making. Aristotle (384–322 BC) suggested that 'It is the mark of a civilised man to demand only that degree of certainty in ethics that the subject matter allows.' We could hardly do better than to heed his advice. In his *Nicomachean Ethics*, he developed a system based on prudence or practical wisdom, the ability to integrate two kinds of moral knowledge, through practice of the intellectual and moral virtues. The intellectual virtues involve the acquisition of competence in a variety of methods and approaches to decision-making or problem-solving, while the moral virtues relate to the habits of character required for reliability, effectiveness and efficiency in action. Aristotle's virtue ethics has stood the test of time remarkably well, and there is currently a considerable revival of interest in virtue ethics, and its relevance to personal, professional and business ethics.

There are many different approaches to problem-solving, which we use in different domains of our lives, some, if not all, being relevant to moral decision-making by nurses as well:

- experimental methods in the sciences
- logical analysis in mathematics
- probabilistic methods in statistics
- historical analysis in archaeology, social and personal history
- cultural analysis in anthropology and political science
- the methods of jurisprudence in law
- what Sherlock Holmes called 'deduction' in detective work.

In medicine, doctors take a medical history, examine a patient, seek to elicit signs and symptoms, consult their theoretical and practical knowledge of medicine and allied sciences, and then proceed to make a diagnosis, determine a course of treatment, monitor and evaluate the effectiveness of their interventions, and perhaps venture a prognosis. 'Good' doctors, from the standpoint of their colleagues, will make a general assessment of the success of their treatment of a patient in the light of their original assessment of the evidence and prediction they made of outcomes, taking into account actual results of their intervention. Ideally, doctors should then incorporate what they have learned into their ongoing practice. However, whether a doctor is a 'good' doctor from the standpoint of her patients will depend on her possession of other skills and attributes as well.

The *Nursing Process*, for example, besides being a method of planning nursing care in an intelligent and rational way, also represents a way of demystifying nursing care. This is important to get away from the idea that nursing cannot be taught. However, rigid and unimaginative application of the Nursing Process, will not guarantee either the quality of care or the competence with which it is given. Here feminist critics of rational models of decision-making which ignore feelings and relationships have a point, but caring for individuals alone is not a sufficient basis for making sound nursing decisions either (Bowden 1997). The Nursing Process presupposes that the nurse will apply knowledge and intelligence, as well as skill and sensitivity, to the needs of the individual patient in their particular situation. The knowledge and skills components can perhaps be directly taught, but the common sense and sensitivity are not so much taught as caught – learned by imitation of others with more experience of life and practical wisdom. Just as Aristotle suggests that the intellectual and moral virtues we need to be complete and balanced people are acquired through habit and practice, the same could be said to apply to nursing. The use of the Nursing Process as a problem-solving method in practical nursing is meant to serve as a method to teach and to improve practice.

Whether one is talking about methods in medicine or nursing, religiously following the method does not in itself guarantee that you will be a 'good' doctor or a 'good' nurse. At the very least, however, it should help ensure that you are a 'competent' or 'efficient' doctor or nurse. Similarly, the application of problem-solving models and/or moral theory to decision-making does not guarantee that the decision taken will be either wise or morally sound. Following a method, analysing a decision, or planning a course of action in a systematic way, only ensures that it is done in a more rational manner and enables clearer reasons and coherent justification to be given for what has been done. Acting responsibly means being able to give a response, to give an account, of what you have done, and it means accepting that you are accountable (i.e. liable to have to give sound reasons and evidence for your actions). Following an appropriate problem-solving method for making moral decisions will help considerably in demonstrating intelligent and practical accountability. We would suggest that many of the arguments introduced by Roper et al (1981) to justify the adoption of a problem-solving approach to systematic care planning, in their book *Learning to Use the Nursing Process*, can also be applied to ethical decision-making.

Before continuing with the exploration of methods and requirements for effective moral decision-making and responsible moral action, it is perhaps worth pausing to consider the origin of expressions like 'conscience ', 'intuition' and 'feeling'.

Conscience

While the 'voice of conscience' may mean anything from the echo of parental authority, to Freud's superego or the voice of God, the 'inner voice of conscience' seems to refer, on the one hand, to the sense of conviction we have about our moral beliefs and the internal authority they have for us in deciding what is right and wrong. On the other hand, 'conscience' seems to stand for collected and collective moral wisdom or practical experience which lends weight to our feeling that a course of action, is right. However, it is noteworthy that the original meaning of 'conscience' (from Latin *cum*, with, and *scientia*, knowledge) means 'having comprehensive theoretical and practical knowledge' of a subject. Conscience in the classical sense is that faculty which enables us to integrate awareness of moral values with theoretical knowledge and practical experience, so as to take a circumspect view of things before we take action.

The most influential thinker on the subject of conscience, in the English-speaking world, was the philosopher and theologian Bishop Joseph Butler

(1692–1752). He was a critic of 18th century deism and psychological hedonism, and argued that conscience is both a God-given guide for action instilled in us by the Creator, and the basis for the assurance that God is concerned for us and our ultimate well-being. Conscience gives us a more sure compass to find our way to happiness than the claim of the hedonists that we blindly follow the promptings of pleasure and pain and/or some vague general feeling of benevolence towards others. Conscience is not some irrational impulse, but the capacity to intuit the rational basis for acting in conformity with our God-given nature. Thus he defended the rationality of moral judgements as based on appeal to conscience as a faculty of the mind, or 'principle of reflection' instilled by God in us all. Let us consider a classic passage from his *Sermons* (Butler *Sermons*, 3):

> … man cannot be considered as a creature left by his Maker to act at random, and live at large up to the extent of his natural power, as passion, humour, wilfulness, happen to carry him; which is the condition brute creatures are in; but that, *from his make, constitution, or nature he is, in the strictest and most proper sense, a law unto himself*. He hath the rule of right within: what is wanting is only that he honestly attend to it …
>
> But allowing that mankind hath the rule of right within himself, yet it may be asked, 'What obligations are we under to attend and follow it?' … Your obligation to obey this law, is its being the law of your nature. That your conscience approves of and attests to such a course of action, is itself alone an obligation. Conscience does not only offer itself to show us the way we should walk in, but it likewise carries its own authority with it, that it is our natural guide, the guide assigned us by the Author of our nature.
>
> Conscience and self-love, if we understand our true happiness, always lead the same way. Duty and self-interest are perfectly co-incident; for the most part in this world, but entirely and in every instance if we take in the future, and the whole; this being implied in the notion of the good and perfect administration of all things.

Fundamental to this concept of conscience is that it is not some mysterious 'voice' in our heads, but rather the rational capacity to reflect on our nature and constitution as rational beings, and to intuit or infer what is our duty in a particular situation, if we are to act in harmony or accord with our true nature. For Butler, the fact that our conscience is instilled in us by God is important, because it gives conscience an authority that transcends mere subjective feeling or intuition. However, it can be argued that his account of conscience could be defended even if we did not believe in God, but are merely able to affirm that we share a common and given human nature, and have the capacity to intuit what that is, and judge accordingly.

Intuition and feeling

The same could be said of 'intuitionism'. 'Intuition' literally means 'to look inward' (from the Latin verb *intueri*, to look at intently). In moral philosophy (and the poetry of Coleridge in particular) intuition has been interpreted as an integrative ability of the imagination, i.e. the ability to take the confusing variety of data and phenomena in a situation and make some kind of sense out of them. The faculty of intuition not only helps us to locate our experience in space and time, in relation to preceding and subsequent events and other similar or different situations, but it also enables us to imagine the possible outcomes of alternative courses of action, and assists us in 'making sense' of our experience.

'Feeling things are right' is not necessarily or exclusively a statement about private feelings, (like 'I just had a gut feeling that it was wrong/or the right thing to do'). It can also be taken to refer to the sense of having one's bearings, of being orientated, having a sense of direction about where one is going. It can mean a settled conviction that, in relation to what you know and your past experience, this is the most appropriate thing to do (Campbell 1984b). However, feelings are important in ethics as they are in life. We ignore the feelings of others at our peril, and ignoring our own feelings can lead to our acting in bad faith or hypocritically, as both feminist and existentialist philosophers have emphasised. Much of what existentialist philosophers have sought to correct in the rationalist tradition, which grew up with modern science, concerns the importance of people's feelings as well as their cognitions in the life choices they make.

Augustine (354–430 AD) said, 'If you wish to know what a man is, ask what he loves.' Our interests define who we are, what kind of people we are, what we consider worth striving for or for which we would be willing to die. Because feelings are so personal and ephemeral, taken by themselves they are not a sufficient basis on which to base our judgements, or our moral lives. Clearly we need other evidence, reasons and principles on which to base our moral beliefs and decision-making. However, the logic of our feelings should also be taken into account. As French philosopher Blaise Pascal (1623–1662) said: 'The heart has its reasons, of which reason knows not' (*Pensées*, iv, 277; Stuart 1950). For St Augustine there is a given order (*ordo*) in nature and a corresponding hierarchy in our loves, and it is the 'primary task of the moral life to determine our lives in accord with the proper order

of priority amongst our loves' (*City of God* XIV, 14; Healey 1968).

Exploring what is meant by decision-making in terms of 'conscience', 'intuition' and 'feeling' can only lead so far. Each term, as we have seen, is a metaphor for the possession of some kind of insight – whether self-insight into one's own motives and intentions, or the values one has made one's own, or insight into the demands of the overall moral situation, and one's own feelings about how things are. Obviously all these kinds of insight are important and necessary, but unless we can 'give a reason for the faith that is in us' or give reasons for acting as we do, then we act blindly, and we cannot really expect people to take us seriously – especially if we have to defend ourselves before a disciplinary enquiry or in court. What we need to consider next are the kinds of training or formation which will help us to become more competent and responsible moral agents, and better able to give an account of our decisions and actions.

DOES A GOOD MORAL AGENT NEED SOUND METHODS OR SOUND CHARACTER?

Opinions tend to be divided on which is more important – to teach people decision-making skills, or to teach them virtue (if the latter can be taught!). The debate about this issue is as old as philosophy itself. For example, Socrates (469–399 BC) challenges us with a number of conundrums of the kind posed in the heading above. On the one hand, he suggests that we cannot be responsible moral agents without self-insight ('Know thyself'); on the other hand, he questions 'Can virtue be taught?' Alternatively he suggests that 'Virtue is knowledge', but also suggests 'Wisdom begins in the admission of your own ignorance'. These puzzles take us to the heart of ethics (Rouse 1984). Moral educators through the ages have tended to go for one or other of the two alternatives below, often to the exclusion of the other:

- emphasising knowledge of moral principles and methods of problem-solving, as essential to the competent moral agent as decision-maker
  or
- emphasising the need for self-insight and the cultivation of the personal habits and dispositions which ensure integrity of character, consistency, dependability and responsibility in actions of the moral agent.

Aristotle (384–322 BC), in his *Nicomachean Ethics*, develops a system requiring two kinds of complementary skills or competencies necessary for the balanced moral agent, namely what he calls the 'intellectual and moral virtues'. The intellectual virtues involve the acquisition of knowledge and competence in a variety of methods and approaches to decision-making or problem-solving, while the moral virtues relate to the habits of character required for reliability, effectiveness and efficiency in action. The relationship between the intellectual and moral virtues in the character of a moral agent, and the need for a balance between them, is symbolised in an arch with two legs, one standing on the foundation of wisdom, the other on the foundation of justice, joined by a keystone which is the faculty of prudence (Fig. 12.1).

In what follows, we shall use this model to develop an approach to decision-making, which takes account of methods necessary to develop both types of competencies.

Moral development – can virtue be taught?

Over the centuries philosophers and religious leaders have advanced many theories and advocated a variety of methods to promote the proper moral education and development of individuals, and to shape future society. The very term 'education' has been linked from the earliest times to the 'moral formation', 'indoctrination' and 'moral disciplining' of young people, but also to the drawing out of the natural potential of individuals (from *e-duco*, to lead out) as a means to the creation and sustaining of a moral community.

Both Plato (429–347 BC) and his disciple and critic Aristotle (384–322 BC) believed that the primary function of the state was the moral education of its citizens, as they believed there could be no just state without just citizens, and individuals require a sound moral community in which to flourish. In his *Republic* Plato described a complex process of education through interactive dialectic that was designed to develop and bring out the potential of children as moral and rational beings, so that they might better serve the state. Similarly, Aristotle, at the end of his *Nicomachean Ethics*, addresses the question of how the state can encourage its citizens to develop both the intellectual and moral virtues, to help secure a more genuinely democratic society. He recognises that a person's moral character is partly determined by nature, partly by the acquisition of knowledge, moral persuasion and argument but also by the discipline and habituation of training involving both positive incentives and sanctions or punishments. Here he sees the state as having a responsibility to ensure that education and training is both fair in allowing for the development of individual potential and serves the common good.

In the course of history there is hardly a philosopher worth his salt who has not felt obliged to address the challenge of how best to educate people in virtue and knowledge. The different methods and approaches advocated have resulted in a wide variety of types of schools ranging from the early Greek academies and Jewish rabbinical schools, to the monastic schools and universities set up by the medieval schoolmen. In more modern times Jean Jacques Rousseau criticised the religious indoctrination and methods employed by the Church and set out his own advice on how to bring up non-aggressive children, in his book *Emile – On Education* (1762). Socialist philosophers Karl Marx and Friedrich Engels set out their theories of education as means to liberate people from subservience to religion and the imposed ideologies of the ruling class and to prepare them to take responsibility for radical transformation of capitalist society.

Victorian philosophers and educationalists, such as Matthew Arnold (1822–1888) of Rugby School, were determined through their public school education to shape the minds and bodies of young men and women to be worthy leaders and rulers of the British Empire. American pragmatist philosophers William James

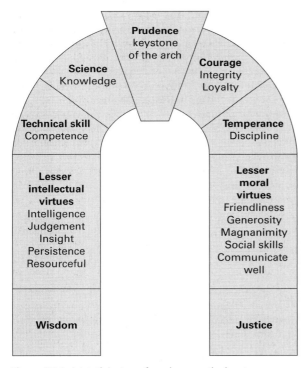

Figure 12.1 Aristotle's view of prudence as the keystone between the intellectual and moral virtues.

(1842–1910) and John Dewey (1859–1952) had a decisive impact on educational theory and experimental practice in education by applying empirical methods to assess the impact of various kinds of educational interventions in achieving desired outcomes. This empirical emphasis continued in the work on developmental psychology of the Swiss psychologist Jean Piaget (1897–1980) and his followers, such as Lawrence Kohlberg. His supposedly empirically grounded account of the stages of moral development and his claim that men and women follow different courses towards moral maturity stirred up a huge amount of controversy (Kohlberg 1973, 1976, 1981, 1984).

Kohlberg commenced a cohort study in the 1950s of 75 boys ranging from 10 to 16 to whom he administered simple tests in which he sought to elicit their ethical responses to the moral dilemmas presented in a series of hypothetical case studies. He monitored their answers and the reasons they gave for their ethical decisions over a 20-year period, and first published his results in 1971. Based on his observations and analyses of the results obtained from this study he identified six developmental stages in the maturing moral attitudes and reasoning of his subjects. He claimed to establish that each stage progressively builds on the previous one/s, and that each of these stages involves a *qualitative* advance from the type of reasoning that preceded it. (Kohlberg assumed that higher on his scale meant better and that although most of his subjects never reached the highest stages, those who did went through the same stages in the same sequence.)

These stages could be broadly characterised as involving progress from an initially immature relativistic and hedonistic philosophy of action, based on the quest for personal pleasure and avoidance of pain or punishment. The next move is to a utilitarian position where rules and laws are regarded as necessary to bring the greatest happiness to the greatest number, then to an ethic based on rationally negotiated contracts, and finally to decisions and conduct based on universal rational principles of justice and duty (Box 12.1).

On the basis of his method of analysing his results, Kohlberg claimed that the average young woman scored a full stage lower than her male counterparts of the same age. His claim that young men and women showed differences in the way they progressed through these different stages led Carol Gilligan, who worked with him at Harvard, to question his findings. Although they co-authored a paper on adolescent development in 1971 (Kohlberg & Gilligan 1971), Gilligan said that the more she used Kohlberg's

---

Box 12.1 **Kohlberg's stages of moral development**
Pre-conventional level: Stage 1: Punishment and obedience orientation Stage 2: Instrumental relativist orientation **Conventional level:** Stage 3: Interpersonal concordance ('good boy'/'good girl') orientation Stage 4: 'Law and order' orientation **Post-conventional, autonomous or principled level:** Stage 5: Negotiated social contract, legalistic orientation Stage 6: Universal ethical principle or rational justice orientation

criteria to judge moral sophistication in young men and women, the more she became uncomfortable with the way women were categorised in his model of development. She argued that Kohlberg's attitudes to women reflected prejudices in male-dominated psychology. She pointed out that Freud had claimed that 'women show less sense of justice than men …, that they are often more influenced in their judgments by feelings of affection or hostility' (Jones 1955). He called women's relationships the 'dark continent' of psychology. Piaget had claimed that 'the most superficial observation is sufficient to show that in the main, the legal sense is far less developed in little girls than in boys' (Piaget 1965).

Gilligan did not challenge Kohlberg's claim that there are differences in approach to moral reasoning between men and women; but she set out in her own research to develop a theory to explain these differences. But she did complain that Kohlberg's influential theory relegated loyalty, compassion and care for the individual to a lower plane than rational arguments about individual rights and justice. To her it is 'an unfair paradox that the very traits that have traditionally defined the "goodness" of women are those that mark them as deficient in moral development'. Against those who sought to defend Kohlberg on the grounds that he was merely reporting the facts of his 20-year study, Gilligan pointed out that his theory was conceived by a man and tested on an all-male sample!

Gilligan (1977) attempted to repeat Kohlberg's research using a sampling method that was controlled for social class and gender bias, and was unable to confirm his findings. However, she did find that there were significant differences between the way women and men respond to moral experience and the responsibilities of moral decision-making. She found that there is empirical evidence that women are more concerned with conflict resolution, acceptance of responsibility to one another and caring for others. She argued that Kohlberg's model fails to do justice to these important social values.

While people still debate the validity of Kohlberg's *Stages of Moral Development*, his original work undoubtedly stimulated a great deal of research, both by those following Gilligan who believed that women speak about moral responsibility 'in a different voice', and also by those who sought to find ways to assess the effectiveness of various forms of moral education in promoting moral development.

With the growing concern with ethics in medicine and nursing, as well as general moral education in schools and professional training, Kohlberg's theory has provided a framework for many experiments in the teaching of ethics and attempts to measure their impact in terms of people's progress through the canonical stages. While the stages as such can be and have been extensively criticised, his work has had the merit of promoting some valuable empirical research on what works and does not work in changing attitudes and developing practical competence in moral reasoning. A quick scan of the contents of the *Journal of Medical Education, Journal of Medical Ethics* and the *Journal of Advanced Nursing* over the past two decades will show the extent and depth of this research, and much of what follows is based on conclusions drawn from this research and practice in the teaching of ethics in healthcare.

However, it should perhaps be pointed out that philosophers have criticised Kohlberg's pre-judgement, made from within the deontological German tradition, that a universalist and rational justice view of ethics must be superior to say a utilitarian or hedonist one. Gillon (1981, 1987) and other philosophers have pointed out that Kohlberg's 'scientific' theory begs the question by making unjustified value judgements about which values we ought to aspire to as human beings. His conclusions conveniently reflect and reinforce his own uncriticised value assumptions based on a (Kantian) view that critical thinking in terms of universal principles is the highest stage of moral development. His approach incidentally also affirms a North American view of personal autonomy as the highest good for the individual (Beauchamp & Childress 1994, Beauchamp & Bowie 1997).

Educationists have criticised Kohlberg's theoretical presuppositions and practical methodology for lack of proper controls in selection of his subjects, hasty generalisation from inadequate empirical evidence and for following Piaget too slavishly – in that his work too was heavily dependent on Kantian rationalism. Feminists have attacked his model for canonising a male stereotype of dominative, competitive and critical intelligence, as the highest and best model for ethics, namely, a type of critical thinking concerned with 'proof' or 'winning arguments'.

It is not our purpose to enter here into the debate about Kohlberg's alleged stages in the moral development of individuals, mainly because we believe that moral character is much more complex, and that the balance achieved in different individuals gives wonderful diversity to the different ways human beings express their growth towards moral maturity. We believe that Aristotle's model of the complex possible interrelationships between and combinations of the intellectual and moral virtues in different individuals, and his virtue ethics, has greater potential to account for the complexity of moral character and the various forms of moral competence in human beings of both genders, including the behaviour of moral recidivists!

Our purpose here is to suggest and to discuss a number of different approaches to the teaching of ethics and the relevance of educational and training methods which are appropriate to the development of the moral and intellectual virtues in people. Discussion of these different approaches has particular relevance to the debate about the form in which ethics education and development of competence in ethical decision-making should be undertaken. But where we agree with Kohlberg, and other researchers, is that educational practice must be subject to rigorous evaluation and research. It is a moral imperative that teaching of ethics, as well as nursing practice, must be evidence-based.

Whatever specific methods may be used, they must ensure acquisition of knowledge about ethics in healthcare, provide opportunities to learn relevant skills and scope to practise them in the exercise of ethical responsibility in the following areas:

- relations between personal and public, professional and corporate ethics
- application to clients, professional colleagues, management of hospitals and inter-agency business
- ethical theory, in practical moral decision-making, setting policy or standards and in ethical audit.

There is a growing literature on moral education and moral development, both in general educational literature and specifically related to the teaching of ethics in business, medicine, nursing, social work, accounting and law.

The Learning and Teaching Support Network (now the Higher Education Academy) at Leeds University provides a substantial range of resources to support those involved in teaching ethics in higher education, and to the healthcare professions in particular. Among their Ethics Resource documents is a most useful review of the research literature on the use of various methods and approaches to the teaching of ethics, and skills in ethical decision-making to students. (For website links related to this topic, please see http://evolve. elsevier.com/Thompson/nursing ethics). However, as we are less concerned here with the empirical research on the effectiveness of different interventions in teaching ethics, but rather with the kinds of rationale adopted for using different methods to teach ethics, we proceed to discuss our own typology for different methods that may be used, their advantages and limitations.

APPROACHES TO TEACHING ETHICS

Approaches to teaching ethics in the professions of nursing, medicine, law and accounting (as well as other professions) could be classified as falling under one of the following four models:

- the moral instruction school
- the ventilatory school
- the critical thinking school
- the situation ethics school.

Each of these approaches is often presented as if it were the only way to approach the pedagogy of ethics, and the others either dismissed as irrelevant or ridiculed. On the basis of our experience we believe each model has something to offer, but we also believe that none of them is adequate taken on its own. Each emphasises a different but valid part of our moral experience and corresponding methods of teaching, but not one of these can be normative for our whole approach. Taken together they are capable of illuminating different aspects of our moral experience and helping us learn the different kinds of insight and skills that are relevant to responsible ethical decision-making. They tend in reality to complement each other.

The moral instruction school

This traditional approach focuses on instruction based on codes of ethics and rules. It reminds us that ethics is not just a private matter, for we are all born into a morally structured environment and a world of rules and regulations. Families have their rules, schools are rule bound, clubs and professions have their rules and partnerships and corporate institutions have their codes of ethics, rules, regulations and well-tried

procedures. Ethics education has to be, among other things, an initiation or induction into the 'rules of the ball game' – whether these are unwritten rules of etiquette, or codes of conduct, formal rules or legal requirements. The 'moral instruction school' focuses on these *deontological* elements in any profession or institution, which serve to define the principles on which we are supposed to act and on our rights and duties. Induction into the values and 'culture' of a profession may also serve to make us more aware of our own moral beliefs and values and the moral baggage we bring with us into adult professional life.

We also need to understand the structure of power and authority within the profession or institution in which we work, to understand the etiquette and 'pecking order' as well as the assumptions on which the ethical culture of the organisation is based. We need instruction in the etiquette and both implicit and explicit values and rules which underlie the ethical culture of institutions. It is just as important as learning the formal rules or disciplinary code of conduct that applies to our profession. These issues are basic to the process of being socialised into a profession, and accommodating oneself to the 'culture' of the hospital, firm, public sector institution or corporation in which one practises (see Chapter 3).

Encouraging familiarity with our own moral beliefs, the ethical culture of the institutions in which we work, and the code of conduct of our profession are all individually important, and help develop insight and confidence that you can 'work the system'. However, this approach, far from exhausting the meaning of ethics also does not help us very much with learning practical skills in moral decision-making in nursing practice, nor does it prepare us to carry the responsibility involved in doing so (Freidson 1994).

Methods of moral instruction: relations between personal, public and professional ethics

The proper concerns of the 'moral instruction school' require implementation of pedagogical approaches that focus in particular on power and authority, roles and rules in social settings. The aim of this approach would be to provide learning opportunities for critical examination of:

- the basis of our personal moral formation – family, school, religious and cultural background
- the process of formal socialisation into the relevant institution or community
- the process of professionalisation and the role of codes of conduct
- our personal commitment to a set of values and applying codes of practice to actual cases

- learning to resolve conflicts between personal, professional and institutional values.

The objectives of moral education in this mode would be to help develop knowledge, insight and skills in individual nurses, to help them deal with the complex and competing demands of personal, professional and institutional values. The kinds of methods for which relevant exercises would need to be developed are:

- personal, professional and institutional values clarification
- social role analysis and definition of responsibilities
- force-field analysis of institutional authority and power structures
- functional analysis of the role of 'codes', 'contracts', 'charters of rights', and 'covenants' between professionals and their clients
- skills in negotiating procedures and boundaries of responsibility at work
- individual and team decision-making and conflict resolution.

The ventilatory school

This approach focuses on how people *feel* about the ethical dilemmas they face or the decisions they have made, and not just on rational considerations or the learning of theory or techniques. It recognises the need for those who will have to make painful decisions in stressful situations to be able to debrief with colleagues and, if necessary, to receive professional counselling. It also recognises that sharing experiences of our successes and failures with more experienced professional colleagues can help us improve our skills and develop insight into our strengths and limitations. Working with feelings can help us confront our prejudices, and clarify in sharing with others the values and moral beliefs which influence our conduct and performance. Individual or group counselling may bring to light for managers what support or further training and supervision staff need. Here the use of structured case conferences and case-based teaching from real-life examples certainly has an important part in training in applied ethics, whether based on simulation, role-play of hypothetical situations, or on actual and current cases. The 'ventilatory' approach gives due importance to the exploration of the practical relations between feelings, attitudes and moral values in practice, and between the psychological and skills-based aspects of health practitioners' work.

By providing scope for regular debriefing, training in counselling skills and group-work, this approach can use 'ventilation' of feelings about one's performance (and perhaps the stress involved) not only to promote catharsis and deepen rational insight, but also as a method of processing experience so that we learn from it in the most successful way. Most importantly it acknowledges that we are not disembodied minds, but also have feelings and experience, anxiety and stress, satisfaction and fulfilment in our work. Finally, it creates opportunities for people to explore the nature and scope of their moral commitments and the extent and limits of their responsibility in practice, in a supportive and non-threatening environment.

Methods of debriefing: ethics in everyday nursing practice and corporate life

The focus of the ventilatory school being on the interrelations of feelings, attitudes and values, in the exercise of personal moral responsibility in practice, training in this area would be aimed at enabling people to explore their feelings, to gain insight into the conflicts which arise in their management of particular cases, and to develop skills relevant to dealing with them and to help others to cope with similar difficulties. The aim here would be to achieve:

- development of insight into personal feelings and attitudes
- understanding of differences between moral problems and dilemmas
- development of models for case analysis, and case conferencing
- understanding of the dynamics of teams and groups
- recognition of the value of experiential and participative learning.

Development of competence in these areas would require the use of a range of methods, which would give nurses practice in the following:

- skills in case analysis and conducting case conferences
- skills in teaching ethical decision-making, using various models
- application of problem identification and problem-solving skills
- skills in counselling, group-work, support and supervision of colleagues
- skills in conducting experiential workshops exploring moral concerns.

The critical thinking school

The critical thinking school has emphasised the importance of teaching moral theory and knowledge of moral principles. It has rightly emphasised the cognitive and rational aspects of ethical decision-making. While this approach can be over-cerebral, its importance lies in offering a different approach to one which simply appeals to authority or to the rules, enacted by authority. It also serves to counteract an over-subjective approach, which the ventilatory approach can encourage. The critical thinking school strives for objectivity in making moral judgements and decisions, based on universal standards and rational problem-solving methods. The critical thinking school emphasises that ethical decision-making is a set of skills that can be learned. It represents a type of problem-solving approach with direct resemblance to other problem-solving activities, and that it is only realistically grounded if it takes serious account of the demands of the specific situation and circumstances surrounding the action in question. It also encourages the setting of clear and assessable objectives. Kohlberg and Gilligan see such a model of 'rational justice' as representing a typically male perspective on ethics – in opposition to an 'ethics of care' with its focus on the impact of decisions on interpersonal relationships, which they identify with the 'different voice' of women in dealing with ethics. Bowden, writing as a philosopher concerned with the moral formation of women in domestic, social, political and professional life, questions the adequacy of a purely rational approach to teaching ethics, taken on its own, and criticises the traditional approach to teaching ethics in philosophy, and emphasises the need to take account of the affective dimensions of our life and their impact on our thinking, whether as men or women (Bowden 1997, Illingworth 2004). Again, the literature review by the Higher Education Academy gives details of a range of studies relevant to this discussion. (For website links related to this topic, please see http://evolve.elsevier.com/Thompson/nursing ethics.)

At its best, the critical thinking school equips students and practitioners with a repertoire of practical skills and insight arising out of supervised practice. Ideally it assists them to integrate moral theory and knowledge of principles, through rehearsed practical experience of choosing and applying different means and methods, action planning and evaluation of their actions. If practised regularly this can lead to the development of competence and reliability in application of standard procedures, but not necessarily the interpersonal skills and moral virtues that make for a caring and empathetic nurse.

Logical and critical thinking approach: ethics in theory and practical decision-making

Generally speaking, the teaching of ethics in most professional courses has tended to be overly theoretical and focused on the academic study of moral philosophy, rather than on the development of practical skills in applied ethics. When we are challenged to justify a moral decision, the proper response is not to appeal to moral theory, but to explain the practical steps we have taken. These would normally involve:

- assessment of the facts and values relevant to the case
- recounting what options we have considered or examples from past experience
- setting out our reasons for our decision or action
- explaining how we would evaluate whether our action was successful or failed.

Moral theory becomes relevant only when we are challenged to provide backing or justification for our underlying moral beliefs and for the very values or principles we employ in everyday moral decision-making. In practice, people tend not to perceive the relevance of moral theory until they are fairly confident about their basic values and principles and have had practical experience of applying them. To address at the outset of training moral theory and the higher-level or meta-ethical questions, which are the concern of moral philosophy, is educationally unsound and generally unproductive. Whereas, dealing with them when people know the rules and are reasonably confident players of the ethical 'ball-game' can be useful in broadening their tolerance of different points of view and deepening their understanding of the roots of ethics.

Developing critical insight and analytical skills in the area of moral decision-making would require a number of different kinds of training. In developing competence in this area the training objective would be to develop understanding of:

- the methods of logical and critical thinking
- the logic of decision-making in general and in ethics in particular
- the types of decision procedures appropriate in different contexts
- the value of role-play, simulation and regular practice of skills in problem-solving methods and their application to values clarification, ethical decision-making and policy setting
- the range of moral theories and what aspects of moral experience these theories address (e.g. intuition, a sense of duty, rule-governed behaviour, consequences, the role of love, etc.).

To facilitate the acquisition of skills and competence in these areas, the kinds of methods for which relevant exercises would need to be developed are the following:

- exercises in the use of different models of problem-solving
- exercises in context or situation analysis to determine the most appropriate decision procedures
- exercises in constructing a sound justification for a decision or action
- simulation exercises to help understand how boundaries of responsibility/accountability shift with context
- exercises to demonstrate how different moral theories are related to different aspects of moral action.

The situation ethics school

In summary, the situation ethics school, at its simplest, suggests that all we need to do is pay attention to the demands of the specific situation and attempt to address it in the most relevant and appropriate way. Its *raison d'être* is to criticise the myth of impartial objectivity and the pretensions and implicit reductionism of universalist grand theories. It is argued that these tend to treat each case as a *specimen of a type*, instead of recognising that each person and situation ethically demands to be addressed on its own terms. The rational justice or duty- and rule-based ethical approaches are seen as trying to force situations to fit preconceived ideal templates.

The situationist approach has its roots in the tradition of Christian agapeistic (love) ethics and in confessional and legal casuistry. Because love is directed to individuals and not to general or universal types, it generates an approach to ethics which focuses on the individual case, and the circumstances of individuals in a particular situation. In existentialism and modern 'situation ethics' we find secular expressions of the same demand that ethics should focus not on general rules and moral laws, but on the demands of genuine encounter or engagement with other people as persons with their own rights and dignity. In this sense situationism is anti-nomian (anti-law). It has recently been appropriated by the advocates of an 'ethics of caring', which can be described as having the following features:

- emphasis on the irreducible specificity of real-life situations in which we have to make moral choices
- willingness to identify the specific character and needs of each 'stakeholder', their personal background and history, the way they interrelate with one another within the fabric of their society
- aiming to achieve insight and understanding of the unique features of the situation for participants

- flexibility in the face of the constantly changing and developing nature of human situations, of action and reaction and mutual adjustment, being willing to live with ambiguity and ambivalence
- sensitivity to gender stereotyping in the rational justice model (seen as predominantly masculine) and encouraging respect for others, avoiding the merely instrumental use of care
- requiring a willingness to look at situations on their own terms (phenomenologically) so as to be open to the unique ethical possibilities of each situation and the type of care each demands
- openness to recognise that one's own self-understanding or sense of identity can change and develop.

The type of pedagogy best adapted to this is perhaps illustrated by the use of traditional casuistry (the study of cases and precedents). Here hypothetical and actual cases have been used as a basis for discussion and to rehearse methods of appraising situations in individual or group training for pastors, counsellors or nurses, and in practical jurisprudence for legal practitioners. Its object is to broaden the capacity of trainees to empathise with other people in their situations, to develop personal insight and skills in caring for the needs of people. The aim is to ensure that the care given should be on the client's terms – rather than practitioners seeking to define clients' problems for them. They should be helping them find their own solutions to their problems, rather than prescribing solutions for them. This approach corresponds to some models of non-directive client-centred counselling; based on 'unconditional regard' for the other person, and a 'non-judgemental' approach, facilitating the client's own self-discovery and problem-solving, resisting the temptation to rush in and give people 'advice' (Campbell & Higgs 1982, Melia 1989).

Situation-based ethics – paying attention to the demands of the specific situation

The critical importance of situation ethics is twofold. First, that it seeks to counteract the tendency of deontological ethics, whether in the form of authority-based codes of conduct or the rational justice model, to be too abstract and general. Its protagonists argue that the other approaches lose the particular in the universal and ignore the role of personal feelings and motives in their attempt to avoid relativism and to achieve universal moral rules. Second, it attacks the 'manipulative', 'managerial' and 'controlling' elements in a teleological or utilitarian ethics that is only concerned with calculating costs and benefits, effectiveness and efficiency. Economic rationalism with its supposedly value-neutral approach would be the object of particular criticism. In contrast, a situationist approach (like virtue ethics, to which it is related) focuses attention on the moral agent, their competence and ability to handle responsibility. It examines the specific conditions and limitations under which they have to operate, and what means and methods are available to them as decision-maker.

The aim of teaching based on the situationist model would be to create a suitable learning environment in which students can gain experientially based knowledge and critical insight into:

- their own strengths and limitations in handling ethical decisions in real-life situations
- what skills training they require to overcome their weaknesses or strengthen their repertoire
- the nature of their own moral prejudices, ethnic and gender biases
- the way institutional structures and practices can be shaped by people's values and prejudices
- the hidden complexity of situations in which there may be a variety of stakeholders.

The kinds of methods which could be used to facilitate experientially based learning in these areas might include some or all of the following:

- self-assessment, as well as peer-group and departmental assessment, using, for example, SWOT exercises (assessment of Strengths, Weaknesses, Opportunities and Threats) as a tool
- group-work to explore issues of prejudice and gender bias in their immediate experience; for example, how they perceive the way the nursing college itself is structured and how it operates
- observation reports in which individual students, or paired groups, are briefed, charged to observe and then report back to the class on their observation of various routine situations, e.g.:
  - admission and history-taking from a patient
  - informing a patient of a bad prognosis
  - dealing with bereaved relatives or a mother who has had a stillbirth
  - a domiciliary visit to a patient in a community setting
  - interviewing student applicants for nurse training
- training through role-play and structured debriefing, with or without use of CCTV, to practise interviewing and listening skills, followed by supervised practice in interviewing clients
- to practise as a group the task of setting practical and workable performance indicators – for their academic performance, and ethical conduct as individuals and as a college.

These are only a selection of a potentially unlimited range of methods that can be employed. We cannot attempt here to be comprehensive, but wish to emphasise that if ethics teaching is to be more than 'chalk and talk' or 'grandstanding of opinions' then it does require some imagination and creativity in designing methods and approaches that will be effective in achieving successful education and formation of nurses. A summary of approaches and methods is given in Box 12.2.

There is no 'quick fix' in teaching ethics

In conclusion, ethics is no 'quick fix' and there are no short-cuts to effective training to ensure the development in people generally, or in nurses in particular, of the necessary skills and competence in ethics or the ability to function as responsible moral agents. The theoretical knowledge which can be taught is, in the case of ethics, perhaps far less important than learning skills that allow people to develop their own character, competencies and critical intelligence in the light of experience of applying moral principles in their professional work. The need for formal instruction in ethics remains, but the place for attention to relevant moral theory will emerge as people wrestle with the actual complexities of life.

The model suggested above for the possible construction of teaching programmes is very complex, and would require a great deal of time if offered as a separate ethics 'module', but that need not be the case. Many of these methods and approaches are already used in nurse training programmes. What is required is not so much the adding on of a new subject to the overcrowded curriculum as raising the awareness of ethics in every dimension of ordinary basic training and in ongoing staff development. The effective use of the kinds of methods and approaches outlined above, to address the moral content of everyday nursing practice and not merely 'hard cases', can be powerfully effective in developing the necessary skills and competencies 'on the job'.

Competence, skills and discrimination in applied ethics can only be learned through a combination of knowledge, practice and experience. The development in us all of a combination of theoretical and practical moral wisdom, and an ability to integrate it and apply it in our lives, (what Aristotle called 'prudence') is probably the crucial kind of competence to be emphasised. In the arch of the virtues, prudence is the keystone linking the moral and intellectual virtues, and is the special type of virtue or competence most relevant to being a wise and responsible moral agent. As we pointed out earlier in Chapter 2, Aristotle

Box 12.2 **Summary of four approaches to teaching applied ethics**

The moral instruction school	**Skills required**
Personal/Professional values clarification	Values clarification skills
Developing an integrated curriculum	Curriculum development in ethics
Promoting a whole-school approach	Awareness of systems theory
Developing community links/involvement	Community building skills
Corporate ethical policy development	Policy negotiation and development
The ventilatory school	**Skills required**
Exploring personal feelings and attitudes	Counselling and helping skills
Building competence in applied ethics	Skills in personal problem-solving
Training in ethical decision-making skills	Case-work and practical experience
Practice in teaching applied ethics	Group-work and interpersonal skills
Professional development for teachers	Training for trainers and teachers
The critical insight school	**Skills required**
Ethics integrated across the curriculum	Cross-curriculum needs assessment
Comprehensive life skills approach	Training in life skills transfer
Familiarisation with values and principles	Critical thinking skills
Practice in ethical problem-solving	Practical experience of work with peers
Developing learner competencies	Support and supervision skills
The situation ethics school	**Skills required**
Assessment of personal strengths and limitations	Practice in self-assessment and peer-group assessment (SWOT)
Skills training and personal development	Interactive group-work and formal debriefing
Insight into moral prejudices and gender bias	Role-play and functional analysis of actual practice
Analysis of corporate ethical 'culture'	Examine dissonance between professed values/practice
Observation of nurse practitioners at work	Practice in applying systematic methods of appraisal
Improvement of interviewing and listening skills	Role-play then supervised practice with feedback
Developing performance indicators	Group project for self-assessment and audit of institution

defines prudence as the knowledge and ability to apply universal principles to the demands of specific situations, in such a way that we choose the best means to achieve a good outcome. Prudence cannot exist, however, without achieving a balance between the scientific or intellectual virtues on the one hand and the practical or moral virtues on the other. The former include critical analytical and logical skills as well as relevant theoretical knowledge and practical life experience. The moral virtues include self-discipline, courage, temperance, honesty and integrity, justice and fairness and a range of social and interpersonal skills. (See Fig. 12.1, and fuller discussion in Chapter 13.)

In developing personal insight and the moral virtues we need all that can be learned from the methods of the 'moral instruction school' and the 'ventilatory school' and the 'situation ethics school'. However, if we are to develop the intellectual virtues, or methods of logical and critical thinking, then we need training in the methods of the 'critical thinking' school as well. All this needs to be subject to critical research and empirical testing of the relative efficacy of the various methods suggested. This is necessary if we are to be sure which methods best facilitate the learning of skills in applied ethics, and the acquisition of the intellectual and moral virtues (McAlpine 1998, Illingworth 2004; for website links related to this topic, please see http://evolve.elsevier.com/Thompson/nursing ethics).

CLASSICAL APPROACHES TO ETHICAL DECISION-MAKING

As we indicated earlier, there are many kinds of problem-solving methods which we employ in different domains of human activity and knowledge. When we come to consider what models to apply to ethical decision-making we have to recognise that there has been a long history of effort to develop and refine appropriate methods to deal with the complexity of moral arguments and judgements. These range from the classical analyses of Plato and Aristotle, through rabbinical and early Christian moral theology, to the sophisticated moral casuistry of the medieval confessors and moral philosophers (Gill 1985). They take in the attempts of rationalists and empiricists to bring moral discourse within the 'logics' of either mathematics or empirical science (Macintyre 1981). They include the attempts of modern philosophers to understand the nature of moral argument by analysing the 'language of morals' (Hare 1952), to consider 'the place of reason in ethics' (Toulmin 1986), or more recent attempts to revive interest in casuistry (Jonsen & Toulmin 1988).

What is specially interesting about the earliest efforts of Plato and Aristotle is that they are concerned to give a three-dimensional account of moral argument and decision-making, as concerned with both living ideals and the practice of living. Plato writes about philosophy in dramatic dialogue form, which enables him to illustrate the point of intersection between theory and practice, between moral theory and life. His great teacher Socrates is shown to be not only a subtle thinker, but a courageous man who was prepared to put his life on the line for what he believed. Plato's *Republic* begins with Socrates asking the question: 'What is justice?'

On the surface this looks a relatively innocent question, but in this dialogue and in several others, Plato demonstrates that by merely asking the question Socrates put his life at risk. Socrates' persistent challenging of people, politicians and self-styled experts, his asking the question with ultimate seriousness was felt to be subversive. Found guilty by the popular court of undermining popular confidence in Athenian justice, because he challenged its institutions in the name of a more ultimate justice, Socrates was condemned to death.

Plato is not only concerned with logical consistency in argument, but with truth of what is said, and the moral consistency or congruence between what people profess and how they act. Thus, in the dialogue *Gorgias* (Hamilton 1960), Socrates and Callicles (a disciple of Gorgias) are shown locked in argument about the nature of rhetoric and truthful communication. The bystanders become frustrated that the argument is not leading to agreement between the two men. Socrates is challenged to agree with Callicles, but retorts that the problem is not to get Callicles to agree with Socrates, but to get Callicles to agree with himself, both in the sense of avoiding contradicting himself and, more importantly, practising what he preaches. Plato is concerned to emphasise that what a man says should square with what he is, and what he does with the fact that he is saying it.

Plato is thus concerned with what we mean by 'agreement' in several related senses of the word, namely, agreement between statements and facts, agreement between different statements, and agreement between different people involved in discussion or argument. All three areas of agreement are of importance when we come to examine ethical arguments and ethical decision-making.

The etymology of the word 'agree' is interesting, for the Latin *ad-gratus* literally means something which contributes *towards pleasing* (someone). Consider the following cognate meanings of the term:

- 'to agree' means to approve or assent to something as correct, to reach consensus about something
- to 'agree to' means to consent to, or hold a similar view or belief about things, to someone else
- to 'agree with' means to be or become in harmony with, or to be compatible with or appropriate to
- to 'be agreed' means to have reached similar conclusions by reasoning together or by negotiation.

The root meaning of 'agreement' is that it contributes to pleasure or harmony between people. Agreement between people is pleasing or agreeable and contributes to cooperation, disagreement is often unpleasant, because it can lead to conflict. Plato was interested in rational agreement between people, for he saw it as the foundation of harmony in political and moral life, and as the basis for scientific and philosophical truth.

Plato's five Cs – correspondence, consistency, coherence, congruence and concord

When Plato approaches the question of truth specifically, it is by way of considering what conditions are both necessary and sufficient to bring about agreement between people. In the dialogues *Gorgias* and *Theaetetus*, Plato distinguishes five different, yet related, kinds of agreement which contribute to achieving mutual understanding and cooperation with other people, or mutual assent to some truth or opinion. We might call these the five Cs: *correspondence, consistency, coherence, congruence* and *consensus* (or *concord*).

What is meant by saying that two people agree or disagree about something? When we agree or disagree it is usually about the truth of opinions or about whether a proposed course of action is good or bad, right or wrong. When we state a belief or make an assertion or judgement, we put forward a truth claim or a value judgement, which we can be challenged to justify. In attempting to justify a truth claim, or to justify a value judgement, we appeal directly or indirectly to the criteria of correspondence, consistency, coherence, congruence and consensus to support the claims we make. Alternatively, when other people criticise or challenge the truth claims or value judgements we make they too tend to test our claims by the same criteria.

These criteria of correspondence, consistency, coherence, congruence and consensus can be construed (as they are in a law court, or in testing scientific claims) as tests of evidence, or tests of truth, as in Case Study 12.1.

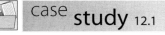

case study 12.1

Smith's wife is found by a woman friend, unconscious and bleeding from a head wound. Mrs Smith is admitted to the accident and emergency department in a comatose state. Her head injuries are consistent with either having fallen and injured her head on the nearby fire-grate, or with her having been assaulted by someone. The hospital staff inform the police. Questioned by the police, Smith states that he was at his local pub at the time of his wife's injury. He says that when called home by the neighbour, he found that there were signs of forced entry and that his wife's handbag containing £500 had been taken. He suggested that his wife's lover, Jones, must have been responsible for he had been told by his wife that Jones had been angry when she told him that she wanted to be reconciled to her husband and had decided to end their affair.

In Case Study 12.1, the five Cs tests might be applied by the police in the following way:

Correspondence: Do the statements of Smith and Jones correspond with the facts?

Smith's claim appears to correspond with the following facts:

- There are signs of forced entry to the house (broken glass on back door, evidence of use of jemmy).
- Smith's wife has bruises and cuts on her face, and there is blood on the grate.
- The missing handbag was found (without the money) in some bushes along the road.
- The barmaid at Smith's local corroborates his alibi, but the police notice he has a plaster on his right hand.
- He explains to the police that he cut his hand on the broken glass when examining the back door.

When interviewed, Jones suggests that Smith was intensely jealous over his wife's affair with him, and

must have assaulted his wife himself, taken her money and thrown away the handbag afterwards to make it appear to be a robbery – in the attempt to implicate him.

- When stopped by the police, Jones had £500 in his purse, which he said he had drawn at the local cashpoint, but was unable to produce a cash-line receipt for it.
- He said he was at the cinema watching the film *Superman II* with a friend at the time of the crime.
- His friend corroborated his alibi and said he was not the kind of man who would ever assault a woman.
- On searching Jones's car, the police find what appears to be a bloodstained shirt in the luggage compartment.

In further investigating the case the police would be seeking first of all to establish whether or not the statements by Smith and Jones *correspond* with facts that could be verified. The test of correspondence with the facts is usually the first and strongest test to be applied.

Consistency: Are Smith's and Jones's statements consistent and free of contradictions?

- Jones's statement does not stand up to critical scrutiny and he contradicts himself in his account of the facts.
- Smith's wife's testimony agrees with his (i.e. does not contradict it). They appear to be on good terms; and she does not appear to be afraid of her husband, as she might have been if he had assaulted her.
- Jones's alibi proves suspect because *Superman II* was not showing at the cinema at the time, despite the testimony of his friend. His claims and those of his friend are not consistent.
- The bloodstains on his shirt match up with Mrs Smith's blood type and his explanation that the blood came from his injured dog was not consistent with the evidence established by the forensic team.

Smith's testimony proves to both correspond with established facts and to be internally consistent, Jones's testimony proves to be full of lies and inconsistencies, his own account is not internally consistent and is inconsistent with the claims made in his defence by his friend. Generally the test of consistency is applied to establish whether different witness statements agree with one another. It is also a strong and important test for truth of evidence.

Coherence: Does the whole 'story' make more sense from Smith's or Jones's evidence?

- Smith's account of the facts 'hangs together', is supported by his wife's testimony, and is further supported by the evidence of neighbours, who saw a man prowling about outside the back of the house and acting suspiciously before they heard Mrs Jones's screams and the voice of her assailant did not sound like that of her husband, and they said they had never heard the couple quarrelling violently before.
- Jones's testimony does not make sense, his alibi appears to be false; he cannot explain why he had £500 on him when he accidentally bumped into a policemen on the beat, why he had blood on his hands and shirt, nor why he was running in the opposite direction from the scene of the assault and robbery.

Coherence is less strong as a test, because it could not be used on its own (as good liars can string a good story) and it is used most effectively in conjunction with the tests of consistency and correspondence with verifiable facts.

Congruence: Do Smith's and Jones's testimony square with what is known of their respective characters and past records?

- Smith is known in the neighbourhood as a friendly neighbour, and, at work, as an honest reliable man.
- His wife's testimony supports this view of his character, as 'almost too good to be true'!
- Jones is known to be a 'ladies man', to have been involved in pub brawls and acts of dishonesty.

Applying the test of congruence we might argue that, on the balance of probability, Smith's testimony is likely to be more trustworthy than Jones's. While not a decisive test of truth or of the veracity of evidence, congruence is 'additive' and strengthens the case, just as obvious incongruities would encourage scepticism and distrust of a witness.

Consensus (or concord): Which interpretation of events would be most likely to be supported by most witnesses or likely to persuade a typical jury?

- Smith's testimony, and that of his wife, is supported by the circumstantial evidence and the consensus of witnesses of events that night,

including the policeman who interviewed Jones and searched his car.
- The majority of the jury hearing the case find Jones guilty on the evidence 'beyond reasonable doubt'.
- Conversely, the court accepts Smith's evidence as reliable and he is exonerated of any blame.

While consensus is not a decisive test of truth, and could be dangerous in some circumstances (e.g. where an accused is already stigmatised by the community, or has been demonised by the media), it is nevertheless important as it expresses the requirement that the test must stand up to public scrutiny and be persuasive to the majority of people 'beyond reasonable doubt'.

These five tests of truth or evidence can be widely applied to the marshalling of evidence in support of a medical diagnosis, a nurse's assessment of a patient's needs or even to the appraisal of all the factors that need to be taken into account in making a well-informed ethical judgement in a complex situation – for example, in a case of sudden infant death syndrome where there is a suspicion of death being caused by non-accidental injury of a child, or respiratory failure where there is no obvious medical explanation for the death.

Aristotle's prudential model for practical moral judgements

Aristotle built on the work of Plato and developed Plato's dialectic, or practical methods of argument and tests for truth, into formal logic and the first systematic account of scientific method. We refer to Aristotle as the 'father of logic' and his contributions to the sciences, ranging from biology to physics, and psychology to treatises on the logic of scientific inference, were ground-breaking, but it is his contributions to the study of ethics and politics that are perhaps of the most enduring value, and of particular relevance here.

In Chapter 2 we used Aristotle's analysis of the structure of moral acts as a basis for the framework in which we developed our account of the different types of ethical theory and how these relate to different aspects of moral action. We pointed out that if we analyse the nature of human action and the structure of moral judgements, this confirms that all human acts have the same basic causes, means, ends structure (Thomson 1976, Bks III and VI).

- *Causes* here refer to the determining forces operating in a situation, the principles and rules applicable in given circumstances and which provide the context and impetus to act.

- *Means* refer to the human and material resources, skills and expertise required to act effectively in the situation to address a given crisis or problem.
- *Ends* refer to both the specific aims and objectives of a plan of action, and to the long-term goal/s of individual or corporate actions.

We pointed out that the key pairs of terms – right and wrong, virtue and vice, good and bad – relate directly to different aspects of the above structure:

- *Right and wrong* relate to the framework of principles and rules, including causal determinants that can direct our actions.
- *Virtue and vice* relate to the competencies we require to act appropriately and effectively and also the means and methods we use to achieve our goals.
- *Good and bad* relate to the actual consequences of our actions as assessed in the light of the aims and objectives we choose at the outset when we set out on a course of action.

On this basis it is logical to suggest that in making an ethical decision, in planning a rational course of action, or acting in a purposeful and responsible way, we should:

- review what determining causes operate in the prevailing circumstances, what the facts of the specific situation are, and what principles and rules apply to the particular 'ball-game' in which we find ourselves
- develop an action plan by considering what practical options are available to us, what expertise, assistance or resources we will require, and what means or methods we need to solve a pressing problem
- clarify our aims, set specific goals and realistic objectives, implement our plan of action and monitor our progress, ensuring that we can evaluate whether our action is successful or not in reaching our goal/s.

These steps are all involved in any action that is intelligently planned, but we may not consider them in the given order, and may in reality move backwards and forwards between these three levels until we have clarified how we decide to act. Further, in situations of crisis we may not have time to reflect and either skip steps, or rely on well-tried courses of action used before.

Aristotle's analysis of what he called the 'practical moral syllogism' should be considered alongside what he says about the practical nature of ethics – as being concerned with the conditions for human well-being and flourishing, and the responsible exercise of power for the good of individuals and community. The 'practical syllogism' is both a form of argument and a statement about the need for congruence between thought and action, between the intellectual and moral virtues. As a form of argument it represents a scheme in which the minor premise is a statement of the case, the major premise a statement of the relevant moral principle under which the case could be said to fall, and the conclusion the judgement of what ought to be done. It is not so much a means of calculating what to do, as a summary of a complex process in which we have to deliberate carefully, weighing up the pros and cons like a judge in a law court, and ultimately have to make a prudent choice, based on the evidence, relevant principles, our past experience and what we believe will be the best means to a good end.

Toulmin, in his influential book *The Uses of Argument* (1958), uses Aristotle's practical syllogism as a basis for developing a much more complex model for the analysis of the structure of practical arguments in ethics and law. Part of his objective is to criticise the tendency to oversimplify the nature of the inferential processes involved in scientific explanation and in ethical and legal arguments. He sets out to clarify the different ingredients in well-formed arguments and the different criteria we need to employ in justifying our decisions or conclusions. The structure he outlines for the layout of arguments includes the following elements:

- data or evidence – including both descriptive and explanatory statements
- warrants – for the claims or assertions we make and criteria for their interpretation
- backing – for the warrants and criteria we employ
- qualifiers – to indicate the degree of certainty or probability we claim for our statements
- conclusions – clear statements of what can be inferred from the argument given the above elements.

PROBLEM-SOLVING MODELS FOR CLINICAL AND ETHICAL DECISIONS

We have referred to both Aristotle and Toulmin because both were concerned with the nature of logic and scientific method, but we are also well aware that ethical arguments, while they share many characteristics in common with other forms of rational discourse, are nevertheless different, in that they are practical in the crucial sense that they issue in decisions and action. What they share in common with other problem-solving activities is the same structures and there are strong analogies between problem-solving approaches in different disciplines. Comparison of how problem-solving processes are applied in different disciplines serves to illustrate the parallels between the different kinds problem-solving models (Table 12.1).

We have stressed that moral decision-making is neither an occult nor an irrational process, but requires complex problem-solving skills. Like the various approaches set out below, moral decisions have to make provision for careful rational deliberation on the available evidence, consideration of relevant moral principles, appraisal of options and possibilities, monitoring of effects and consequences of our actions, and identification of what we can learn for the future from our successes or failures in the past to achieve our goals. This requires skill in using decision-making models which do justice to the complex logic of moral decision-making. These need to take account of the complexity of the situation and the roles of various players in the drama, and make provision for learning and improving our performance in the future.

An obvious difficulty with the naive view that decisions are just either 'right' or 'wrong' is that it fails on all counts to do justice to the various important stages in the decision-making process: viz. assessment, deliberation, action planning, decisive action, progress monitoring and critical reflection on outcomes.

Moral decision-making can be compared with problem-solving approaches to making clinical judgements in both medicine and nursing, both in terms of the stages in the process and the complexity of their problem-solving methods. Clinical decisions in medicine involve taking a medical history, examination of the patient, diagnosis and prognosis, treatment, ongoing observation, further tests and investigations, evaluation and learning from outcomes. In making clinical decisions in nursing, the four stages of the *Nursing Process* have been taught as one means to clarify what is required to assess patients and plan patient care in a systematic way. The four stages are: *assessment* of the problem situation; *planning* what to do about it; *implementation* of the planned decision; and *evaluation* of the success of the action plan. Adopting such a systematic approach enables nurses to act in a responsible way, and to have clear treatment aims in terms of which outcomes can be assessed and as a result of which they can learn from the process on the basis of evidence rather than speculation (Roper et al 1981).

The four-stage Nursing Process problem-solving model has the virtue of being simple and easy to remember. However, it tends to abstract 'the problem' from the context of the existential encounter between individual nurse and patient, and relationships with significant others. If the problem is primarily seen as a clinical one, it can also result in significant socio-economic and cultural variables being overlooked. While the Nursing Process has these limitations it also has features in common with many other models, so it makes for useful comparisons. In what follows we will

Table 12.1 Stages in problem-solving in different disciplines

Legal	Scientific	Medical	Counselling	Nursing
Charge: A crime alleged to have been committed by accused	Definition of problem for investigation	Patient presents with their problem or symptoms	Meeting client who comes for help to deal with crisis	Patient admitted to ward or caseload
Indictment on specific legal charges based on evidence	Formulating alternative theories, hypotheses	Takes medical history and records patient's account of symptoms	Elicits nature of 'problem'	Observation of and communication with patient/family
Prosecution case Defence case	Design of experiment/s to test hypothesis	Examines patient Initial diagnosis	Clarifies nature of problem/s	ASSESSMENT
Cross-examination of witnesses, other forensic evidence	Experimental investigations (Repeated)	Tests, investigations, proposed treatment Prognosis of outcome	Explores options available, transforming problem	PLANNING
Argument on points of law and procedure	Analysis of results and outcomes	Monitoring of patient's progress	Assists client to choose options/ solution	IMPLEMENTATION
Deliberation and judgement	Summary of conclusions	Evaluating final result/ recall for follow-up	Supports client to cope with results	EVALUATION
Sentence: convict or discharge accused	Considering new implications	Discharge patient	Leaves client to get on with their life	Follow-up visit or visits to patient

elaborate a number of models which can be useful in moral decision-making, using the Nursing Process as our starting point, because of its assumed familiarity to nurses (see Johnstone 1991).

Because of the complex nature of the nurse's interaction with the patient (and perhaps the patient's family and community), moral decision-making in nursing has to do justice to several things at once:

- the need to address a particular patient's problem, explore treatment options, give treatment and ongoing care, monitor progress and evaluate outcomes
- the need to be sensitive to the interpersonal encounter and the nurse's ongoing relationship with the patient, based on trust and confidentiality, and the patient's need for support
- the need to attend to the wider social context of the patient's life, family relationships and work situation, and to the various 'players' in both the patient's management and ongoing life.

From an ethical point of view, what is revealing about the Nursing Process is what it leaves out.

Obviously nurses meet patients and have to interact with them at a personal level. They often form significant relationships with patients, and have to face the ending of those relationships, whether the patient recovers or dies. The fact that these features are not 'up front' in the Nursing Process model is revealing. First, it suggests that nurses see their relationship with patients as derived from or secondary to the patient's relationship with the doctors. Second, it suggests a possible concern with the clinical aspects of the contract-to-care, and neglects the interpersonal aspects of the interaction. The beginnings and endings of such relationships may be crucial from an ethical point of view. The psychologist Eric Berne (1966, 1973) (father of transactional analysis) has said that learning to say 'Hello' and 'Goodbye', and to do it properly, are two of the most fundamental skills in life. The way we greet new life and the way we say our farewells in the face of death are two of the most important rituals in every human society. Similarly, calling each other names can be both part of intimate love-play, or verbal abuse. John Bowlby's classical studies of separation anxiety in hospitalised children cut off from contact with their mothers has helped to change policies on admission of mothers in children's hospitals, but he has also taught us to recognise more generally that the pathology of our emotional life and relationships relates to how we cope with 'making and breaking of affectional bonds' (Bowlby 1979). The challenge of beginning and ending relationships, as well as sustaining them, demands not only understanding

and self-insight, but many kinds of skills and coping strategies. Ordinary problem-solving methods have at least to take account of this interpersonal context, if they are to be adapted to help us with ethical problem-solving. Furthermore, they must do justice to the ongoing history of such relationships.

The Nursing Process as a model for ethical decision-making

In the context of nursing care the application of the Nursing Process is not simply a technical method of directing clinical practice in terms of rational care plans, as if moral considerations did not come into them. In any care plan, or application of the Nursing Process, all sorts of moral considerations are both taken for granted and are often explicit. The purpose of pursuing this analogy with the Nursing Process in analysing moral decision-making is not only practical, in seeking to clarify the processes involved, it is also to stress that the nurse's moral experience and nursing experience are one and the same. But what, then, are the practical implications of using this model for the analysis of the moral aspects of decision-making in nursing?

Assessment

Just as a nurse is expected to take a detailed history from each patient, carefully note their general circumstances as well as the specific problems they are experiencing, and apply general knowledge of the principles and practice of nursing to the interpretation and assessment of the situation, so a similar process is involved in making moral decisions.

First, we have to *clarify the facts of the case*, what are the background conditions affecting the life of the patient in question, and what are the immediate causes of the specific crisis demanding a decision, what alternative options and means are available, and what the likely outcomes will be.

Consider, for example, a community nurse visiting a bed-bound elderly patient at home, or a casualty nurse in an ambulance team attending victims of a railway accident in a remote place, or a charge nurse dealing with acutely ill patients in an understaffed ward. In the first case, it may be just as important for the district nurse to have good knowledge of the housing conditions, financial state and family supports (or lack of them) of the bed-bound patient as it would be to know what resources could be called upon to assist in providing good nursing care. In the second case, it is essential to know what effective care can be given, and even what it would be right or wrong to do. Giving emergency first aid to accident victims in a remote place, where only minimal resources are available, will be quite different from doing so in a well-equipped hospital. What can be done and what ought to be done will be determined and limited by the circumstances. In the third case, where a charge nurse is faced with staffing shortages, their moral obligations would be different from those where there is normal cover. A charge nurse would have the same duty to care for all her acutely ill patients, regardless of the circumstances, but what she can or cannot do will be determined by what resources are available. The nurse cannot be held responsible for what she cannot do (for ought implies can). She may feel guilty later that more was not done for some patients in the particular crisis, but her only continuing obligation might be to try to ensure the problem does not arise again.

Secondly, we have to *clarify what kind of knowledge and skills are relevant* in deciding what to do. This will include consideration of the relevant rules and moral principles relating to one's personal and professional duties. Merely to provide nursing care for the bed-bound patient (e.g. to administer a routine bed-bath or pain relief, or to recommend hospitalisation) would be irresponsible if no attempt was made to ensure that family members are provided with what support they need to enable them to manage better on their own. The community nurse might have an obligation to liaise with social services to ensure that the patient's entitlements, e.g. to a home-help, disability allowance and provision of physical aids, is respected. The nurse's duty of care to the patient, interpreted narrowly as simply providing nursing care, would not be sufficient to clarify what should be done. Similarly, in the case of a nurse working at the scene of a railway accident, some painful decisions might have to be taken about who should be given treatment, who can be left to cope and who will have to be left to die. Here the most responsible and caring thing to do would be to recognise first what can and cannot be done, given limited resources, and then giving assistance would mean applying a policy of triage. This would not involve treating all patients equally. Instead it would mean giving what comfort is possible to those who are too far gone to help; reassurance to those who are likely to recover without help; and then to concentrate efforts on those who have a chance of recovery but are unlikely to do so without help. Here the demands of the duty to care may have to take precedence over considerations of justice or respect for the rights of individuals. A nursing officer without sufficient staff to operate an acute ward, by contrast, might have to take political action – for example, threatening to walk

out, or work to rule, unless help is urgently forthcoming. Here a nurse's action might be guided by considerations of justice and respect for the right of all committed into her care.

Planning

Once the problem has been clearly defined (by a careful assessment of the general circumstances, the needs of the specific individuals, available means, and the general nursing and moral principles relevant to the situation), then it may be possible to *plan a course of action.*

Action planning or care planning will involve several stages:

- consideration of the specific knowledge and practical procedures known to be relevant to the defined problem
- retrospective examination of past experience of the success or failure of alternative courses of action for dealing with similar problems
- prospective anticipation of the likely consequences of alternative courses of action in this specific situation
- choice of the best and most appropriate means to achieve the desired goal, including ensuring that adequate resources are available to implement the plan
- formulating a definite plan of action with clear objectives, including possible contingency plans, if things go wrong and circumstances demand a change of plan.

Ability to make sound action plans requires the particular combination of knowledge, skill and practical experience that we call practical wisdom (or what Aristotle and the classical philosophers called the virtue of prudence). Prudence is defined as the 'knowledgeable and skilled ability to apply general principles to particular situations, so as to choose the best and most appropriate means to achieve a good end (outcome or goal)' (Thomson 1976). However, having a good plan and all the experience of a lifetime cannot protect us against the unexpected or chance developments that may throw everything awry. Prudence requires flexibility, resourcefulness and adaptability too, and good planning will allow for contingencies as well (Pieper 1959).

Implementation

How effectively and efficiently decisions are implemented, and plans worked out in practice will have a great deal to do with their success or failure. Aristotle identified a specific virtue or skill (solertia) which is associated with being confident, namely being decisive and courageous in carrying through a decision or action plan. This virtue is something people can learn with experience, enabling them to avoid timorousness and indecisiveness, while nevertheless remaining sensitively responsive to changing situations without being over-rigid in keeping to their plans at all costs (Pieper 1959).

Implementation is the key part of 'action', but it cannot be considered in isolation. From a moral point of view we are concerned with observing and monitoring the soundness of the whole process, against set objectives or targets. Implementation includes ongoing responsible assessment of the prevailing circumstances throughout the process and noting the changing moral demands in the particular situation. Several factors are involved in effective and efficient implementation of practical decisions. These include: responsible monitoring of progress or failure of the action taken to achieve defined objectives, honest evaluation of the actual consequences or outcomes of the action, and noting its general costs and benefits. At each stage, moral deliberation and judgement will require application of relevant knowledge and skills to management of the implementation process.

Evaluation

The term 'evaluation' can be applied generally to the attempt to make responsible judgements at each stage in the process of decision-making, but it is more commonly used in a restricted sense to apply to *assessment of the consequences or outcomes of an action*. Competent evaluation of a decision and its implementation will always involve consideration of whether the actual consequences of an action are the same as the intended consequences. Judging whether the consequences are better or worse than hoped for, and whether the long-term effects of a course of action will be successful, is necessary in order to clarify whether the action taken would justify its becoming standard practice. Evaluation in this sense is part of a learning process. Feedback from experience, if consciously integrated into understanding of what we are doing, should equip us to act more effectively when faced with similar situations in the future.

In this way the feedback in the learning process helps to build in habits (or virtues) which make decision-making potentially easier as we gain in experience and confidence. However, there is a broader aspect of evaluation of importance to moral judgement. This relates to the cost–benefit analysis of alternative courses of action, not merely whether they

are efficient in achieving our desired ends. Evaluation of costs and benefits, like 'quality of life' assessments, is not simply a requirement of sound economics and practical management of professional tasks, it is also a demand of sound moral judgement. This brings us back full circle to the re-examination of the fundamental principles and values we espouse because we believe that they promote human flourishing. In nursing, clinical nursing and promotion of complete physical, mental and social well-being are one and the same activity. Moral considerations are inseparable from proper application of the Nursing Process, and thus by building in the moral dimension not only can we use it to deal with moral problems when they arise, but it will also ensure that nursing work can be undertaken in a way that is both morally responsible and accountable.

Finally, there is the inclusive sense of evaluation, namely review of the whole process. This covers all the steps of the decision-making process (including assessment, planning, implementation and evaluation). Evaluation is concerned both with practical and value judgements about how well individual steps in the process have been completed and with how successfully the whole process has been managed in practical and moral terms.

Ethical disagreements can arise at each of these stages in the process. There can be disputes about facts and values in relation to assessment of what ought to be done, how it should be done, whether the right means have been chosen, how well it is actually done, and whether the specific outcomes or general consequences are good. The words 'ought ','should ','well', 'good' belong to the vocabulary of moral judgement and relate to rules, duties and values for the assessment of performance and general costs and benefits respectively. (As will be seen in the next chapter disputes at the level of moral theory relate to the different ways we justify our moral judgements in each of these contexts (Hare 1952, Nowell Smith 1957)). Box 12.3 illustrates the model.

Social context analysis in ethical decision-making

In the early work of Dorothy Emmet, philosophers and those interested in practical ethics were reminded that we cannot treat human situations abstractly, divorced from the social context in which they occur (Emmet 1966). She suggested that if we are to do justice to the demands of each case we must examine four interrelated factors or variables that are involved in practical decision-making. These are: the demands of the specific situation, the roles of the different

Box 12.3 **Ethics and the Nursing Process**

Initial steps: Clarify and define the nature of the problem
  What is the crisis, (or dilemma) requiring a decision?

Assessment: Identify key facts and values applicable
  What are the crucial facts of the case?
  What *moral principles* are at issue here?
  What decision-procedure is appropriate?

Planning: Explore available and best means to reach our goal
  What is the primary aim or *good* for which we are acting?
  What objectives, *benefits*, moral goals are achievable?
  What previous cases or contingencies should we take into account?

Implementation: Take decisive and effective action to implement plan
  How do we begin, continue, and finish, the process of intervention?
  How do we assess *costs/benefits* of the intervention?
  How do we monitor *success/failure* in the overall process?

Evaluation: Evaluate progress and outcomes with planned objectives
  What means have we set up for debriefing and feedback?
  Have we used the 'right' means to a 'good' end?
  How do we review the pros/cons for the action taken?

Final steps: Retrospect: apply the following tests:
  Could I/we provide a reasonable ethical justification for the course of action taken?
  Can I/we identify what we have learned from applying this model to decision-making?
  How do we integrate this learning into next decision-making cycle?

their vulnerability and dependency, their need for nursing care and medical treatment, their relative lack of privacy, and in a particular ward maybe the same kinds of medical problems. In a patient's home the nurse and patient stand in a different kind of relationship. The district nurse or health visitor is a kind of guest, and the patient, however ill, is more in control. In a health clinic where people come voluntarily for help or screening, and can 'vote with their feet' and leave if they are unhappy with their treatment, the situation is once again different. Further, each individual has a unique medical history, specific identity and social status, a particular set of family or social obligations. Both general and specific factors in the situation, including those relating to the stay and available resources, need to be taken into account. Situational analysis attempts to focus on the specific case and to avoid the tendency to treat every case as simply a specimen of a species or an example of cases of a particular type, and encourages us to address it on its own terms.

Roles and rules

These tend to be interconnected. The *roles* of patient, doctor, nurse, porter, administrator, relative, all tend to be governed by different, implicit and explicit *rules* and conventions relating to permissible and non-permissible behaviour. We also need to consider the general rules governing the institutions in which we work, the more general rules and laws governing society, and the universal moral principles in terms of which we attempt to order and make sense of all these other rules. People in a given situation may play more than one role at a time. A patient, besides being a patient, may be a father, a lawyer, a champion bridge player and a Protestant. The nurse may be a man, a qualified Aikido instructor, union member and Roman Catholic. The doctor may be a young woman, feminist, keen golfer and atheist. In the developing action of a particular case, the rules governing these various roles may appear as more or less important. The value conflicts implied in these different roles may not only complicate the process of decision-making and interaction between the various 'players' in the 'drama', but also set up conflicts within the individuals themselves. Here some effort at clarifying the different value assumptions people bring to their work may be necessary before the various parties can collaborate effectively in dealing with the problem in hand.

  Furthermore, the roles of doctor, nurse, social worker, other health professionals, the patient, friends and relatives may all change as the drama unfolds. For

participants, the variety of rules applicable to the exercise of these roles, and the arbiters to whom we are accountable for our actions – or, simply: *situation, roles* and *rules*, and *arbiters*. In sound ethical decision-making all of these factors must be taken into account (Emmett 1966, Downie 1971).

Situation

The details of a specific moral situation are important. It will involve some general factors common to most human situations and some that are unique to this particular situation. In institutions such as hospitals there are general factors common to most patients:

example, an unconscious and seriously injured victim of a road traffic accident may first be admitted by ambulance to the accident and emergency department for immediate life support or first aid, sent to the X-ray department or elsewhere for tests, transferred to the operating theatre for emergency surgery, be returned to the ward for postoperative care and treatment, sent to a specialist unit for rehabilitation, and discharged home into the care of his family, the local doctor and community nursing services. At each of these stages the value priorities governing interactions between health professionals and the patient may be different. (One of the reasons why the television programme *Casualty* makes compelling viewing on television is not only that life-and-death crises are being portrayed, but also because the situations are inherently dramatic and constantly changing. Also different players occupy central stage at different times, and the roles of nurses change from being part of the crash team to bedside care, from stage management to playing the role of the chorus. Just as acting out a specific role on the stage is governed by the script and the rules of the production, so the varying roles and rules of action in healthcare are dramatically varied and complex.) Downie (1971) points out that all these factors relating to roles and rules are relevant to moral decision-making but to different degrees, depending on what is at issue. Eric Berne has developed a whole school of psychology, namely transactional analysis, based on the various 'transactions' between people interacting with one another while 'acting out' different roles. His analysis of the rich diversity of human interactions in conflictful and cooperative relationships can be helpful for ethical interpretation of complex situations.

Arbiters

When we make moral decisions we also have to consider *to whom we are responsible* and accountable – in other words, those persons to whom we relate as *arbiters* of our actions. Nurses are *responsible for* their patients (though not in quite the same way as the doctor), but they would not normally be *responsible to* the patient (although nurses may feel they are). Nurses are directly *accountable to* their line managers, but also indirectly to their peers and to the doctor responsible for giving instructions relative to the patients in their care. Professionally they are also accountable to their regulatory body (in the UK, this is the Nursing and Midwifery Council). Nurses may be held accountable to, or responsible to, the patient's relatives, and ultimately to society through the courts. The most immediate arbiter of a nurses' professional work and general behaviour would be their charge nurse or line manager. In life we invariably 'look over our shoulder' to consider who is watching our actions, to whom we are expected to be able to give a proper account or justification for our actions.

Because we generally operate in professional life *under authority*, we have to consider whether our actions are appropriate or authorised – given our status, role and responsibilities. Thus, in making moral decisions we are obliged to consider those to whom we are responsible and accountable, those who are arbiters of our actions. Generally nurses must implement care as directed, where the orders given are appropriate and ethical. Normally, they may feel that they should bear in mind what their line manager or the doctor may think of their actions. However, it would not be appropriate for nurses to act simply to please their line manager, or the doctor, if they believed the situation demanded a different response from them. Whether or not a nurse is acting directly under orders they would most likely take the arbiter of their actions into account in deciding what is appropriate for them to do, or they might wish to consult the person concerned before acting on their own responsibility.

Because each situation is different, all these factors are variable. People play different roles, numerous different rules apply, and we are accountable to a variety of people in different ways. Moral decision-making is complex – especially in an institutional setting. Having the ability and confidence to make responsible decisions is a matter of knowledge, and growth in experience and sophistication, sensitivity and wisdom (Emmet 1966, Thompson 1979a). Figure 12.2 suggests a framework for such decision-making. It can be useful in making assessments of one's own decisions and actions, and is also a useful aid to collective moral decision-making in the team management of complex cases, or in deciding moral policy on a committee.

Stakeholder analysis

The process of stakeholder analysis is a useful method for clarifying the nature of the ethical problem (or problems) which need to be tackled, by clarifying what rights and duties apply to the various 'players' in a given situation. Ethical problems frequently arise because the rights of one party or another have been infringed or they have not received their proper entitlements.

In most situations it is sufficient to identify the rights of the patient/client and the duties of the decision maker (nurse or doctor), but in more complex situations it may be helpful to consider both the rights

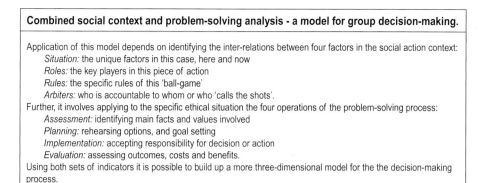

Combined social context and problem-solving analysis - a model for group decision-making.

Application of this model depends on identifying the inter-relations between four factors in the social action context:

Situation: the unique factors in this case, here and now

Roles: the key players in this piece of action

Rules: the specific rules of this 'ball-game'

Arbiters: who is accountable to whom or who 'calls the shots'.

Further, it involves applying to the specific ethical situation the four operations of the problem-solving process:

Assessment: identifying main facts and values involved

Planning: rehearsing options, and goal setting

Implementation: accepting responsibility for decision or action

Evaluation: assessing outcomes, costs and benefits.

Using both sets of indicators it is possible to build up a more three-dimensional model for the the decision-making process.

STEPS	SITUATION	ROLES	RULES	ARBITERS
Assessment				
Planning				
Implementation				
Evaluation				

Figure 12.2 Three-dimensional view of decision-making process.

and responsibilities of the patient/client and the duties and rights of the health professional who has to make the decision about the delivery of the service.

In working through the process it is important to recognise that there will be duties that the decision-maker will have to the wider public and to his or her employing authority, as well as the specific duties owed to the patient or client. The following grid can be a helpful aid to setting out the matrix of rights and duties of the stakeholders, so that a more informed judgement can be made about the real nature of the ethical problem or problems involved (Fig. 12.3).

If the decision is being taken by a team of people, and particularly if the team is made up of people with a variety of kinds of professional expertise, it may be necessary to distinguish carefully their different conceptions of what 'the problem' is, what different kinds of action or 'interventions' are necessary, and what 'outcomes' or 'solutions' they each anticipate (Fig. 12.4).

In a complex situation it is possible that there may be little initial agreement about what the problem is or how it is to be dealt with. If there are serious disagreements at this level, then, it would be necessary to explore how serious the differences are and what scope there is for a negotiated agreement about definition of the problem and the course of action to be adopted.

For example, in dealing with a staff member with a 'drug problem' the doctor may see it as a problem of addiction, needing detoxification; the psychologist may see the problem as a dysfunctional way of coping with life problems, and requiring psychotherapy; the nurse manager may see the problem as one of chaotic behaviour and unreliability, requiring discipline; the chaplain may see the issue as one arising out of his marital problems and financial difficulties, requiring sympathy; while the prosecuting police may see it as a problem of law-breaking and criminal conspiracy, requiring punishment. If all were involved in a 'case

Stakeholders (for example)	Stakeholder's rights	Charge nurse's duties	Charge nurse's rights	Stakeholder's duties
1. Patient				
2. Family				
3. Ward patients				
4. Ward staff				

Figure 12.3 Stakeholders' rights and duties.

Team member (for example)	Value base or expertise	Definition of 'the problem'	Proposed intervention	Expected outcome
1. Head nurse				
2. Medical registrar				
3. Psychologist				
4. Chaplain				

Figure 12.4 Different stakeholder perspectives on a 'problem'.

conference' about how to deal with the person, it might be important to discover first what common ground there was for cooperation in decision-making and management of the problem. Sometimes the complexities that emerge in the course of stakeholder analysis are due to people conflating several problems, each of which needs to be tackled separately and in order of importance or urgency. Sometimes the complexities are due to the different ways in which the same problem is conceptualised and represented by different members of the team of people involved in making the decision.

The DECIDE model for ethical decision-making

In the literature on biomedical and applied ethics there are an increasing number of decision-making models, each of which has certain advantages and limitations (cf. Johnstone 1994, Beauchamp & Childress 1994,

Grace & Cohen 1998, Kerridge et al 1998). This is not the place to evaluate them, but as we have seen there are common features to problem-solving methods as these are applied in a variety of fields. The DECIDE model (Fig. 12.5) which we recommend here is a refinement of the original SPIRAL model.

The usefulness of this model, as will be more fully discussed in the next chapter, is that it provides a practical method of making prudent value judgements and ethical decisions. This is in line with Aristotle's definition of prudence as *the knowledgeable and skilled ability to apply general principles to specific situations, in such a way that we choose the best available means to a good end*. Also, following Aristotle, we recognise the causes – means – ends structure of all intentional acts, and that any sound method of ethical decision-making must take account of all three aspects of purposeful and deliberate acts. What Aristotle means by 'causes', 'means' and 'ends' may need to be clarified.

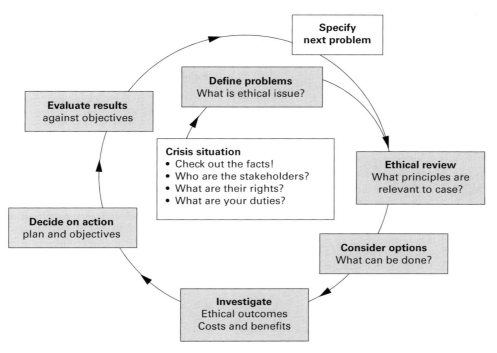

Figure 12.5 The DECIDE model for ethical decision-making.

Causes here refers to the *background conditions* that determine the specific context in which one has to act or make a decision. These include both the external *causes* and psychological conditions which precipitate the 'crisis' (i.e. a time where we must make a decision). However, the term also refers to the 'rules of the ball-game' or principles applicable in the specific situation in which we must act; these may be laws, ethical codes or procedural rules.

Means refers to both the *agent or agents* responsible for implementing the decision or action plan, and also to the choice of *means and methods* required to achieve one's goal. In a sense, the moral agent is the primary means by which principles are applied to specific situations in order to decide what action (or actions) to take, or what changes we wish to effect in the situation by our intervention. However, in any given situation, we may need the help of other people or additional resources in order to act effectively. They too become instrumental means to implement our intended action. Choice of appropriate 'means' may also mean careful consideration of the *best methods* to use, based on our past experience of what works and what does not.

Ends refers to both the purpose, or goal, of the action taken, and the intended consequences or outcomes of the action. Responsible action is not only purposeful, but is also based on realistic and achievable objectives. It is no good having a grand

goal or end in view but one which is impractical or not achievable, either because one lacks the knowledge, skill or power to act effectively, or because one does not have available the resources required to achieve one's goal. So, sound decisions and intended actions must not only have a purpose, but also realistic objectives. If intelligently planned, then the success, or failure, of the action can be measured against the set objectives. Without clear objectives, there can be no proper evaluation and we cannot learn from our experience.

The six steps of the DECIDE model (Box 12.4) relate to the various aspects of the causes – means – ends structure of intentional acts in the following way:

- the first two (D, E) review the background causes and principles applicable in the situation
- the second two (C, I) involve an appraisal of available options, means and methods for action
- the third two (D, E) involve purposeful action and evaluation of results in the light of objectives.

MORAL AGENCY – WHEN ARE WE RESPONSIBLE FOR OUR ACTIONS?

Having discussed systematic methods by which we can make considered and well-justified moral deci-

Box 12.4 **The DECIDE model**

D: Define the problem/s
What are the key facts of the case? Who is involved? What are their rights, your duties? What is the main ethical problem to be addressed?

E: Ethical review
What ethical principles have a bearing on the case and which principle or principles should be given priority in making your decision?

C: Consider the options
What options do you have in the situation? What alternative courses of action? What help, means and methods do you need to use?

I: Investigate outcomes
Given each available option, what consequences are likely to follow from each course of action open to you? Which is the most ethical thing to do?

D: Decide on action
Having chosen the best available option, determine a specific action plan, set clear objectives and then act decisively and effectively.

E: Evaluate results
Having initiated a course of action, monitor how things progress, and when concluded, assess carefully whether or not you achieved your goals.

sions, and having considered the virtues needed in the moral agent, it remains to examine another question: under what conditions can we hold a person responsible for their actions, and what factors would serve to excuse someone from blame?

Aristotle pointed out that we do not apportion praise or blame for actions unless a person is sane and has acted purposely, knowingly and voluntarily. We also assume people must have some sense of the boundaries of permissible action set by the moral community in which they live, and understand what their rights and duties to other people are. People cannot be held responsible for their involuntary behaviour, or when they do not know what they are doing, or when they act in complete ignorance of the likely consequences of their actions, or do not know what the 'rules of the ball-game' are. Although we might want to refine Aristotle's criteria, his common-sense rules are still useful for most practical purposes (Thomson 1976, Bk 3).

However, when we speak thus of people as responsible moral agents we are making a number of assumptions which may be challenged. Perhaps our most fundamental assumption is that human beings are not robots, that they can make independent choices and decisions, that they possess 'free will'. Another assumption we make concerns the nature of moral rules, namely that they are not simply personal, but apply to all human beings, that they are universal. In fact, many people would want to assert that moral principles are absolute, not relative to each person or culture, and that our moral duties are unconditionally binding, not dependent on time, place or circumstances.

To discuss and reflect upon these issues of moral responsibility and the binding nature of moral obligations is to engage in meta-ethics or moral philosophy, that is the higher level activity of critical reflection on the presuppositions of everyday practical ethics and moral action. In moral philosophy we explore what kinds of reasons or evidence can be offered for believing or not believing in moral freedom, or in moral obligation, the universal applicability of moral rules, and fundamental human rights. Some of these theories derive from religious or metaphysical beliefs about the nature of human beings and their relation to God and the universe; others from analysis of what is implied in the concept of human reason or the nature of love and the obligations these impose on us. Other philosophers are more concerned with the logic of the process of moral decision-making and focus on methodological questions. (We will say more about these matters in the next chapter where we explore the nature of moral theory.)

The Enlightenment philosopher Kant (1724–1804) insisted that ethics could not get started without three fundamental beliefs or postulates: God, freedom and immortality (Abbot 1909). He argued that the existence of God, as a transcendent source and point of reference for ethics, is necessary to guarantee that ethics is universal and above individual and cultural differences. He argued that personal immortality is necessary if human life is to have any ultimate meaning, if truth and virtue are to have abiding value and if there is to be any final justice and reward for a life of virtue rather than vice. Finally, he argued that the concept of freedom is logically necessary both as a foundation for ethics as such, and also as the only basis on which we can argue that people are morally responsible for their actions. Given the importance of this concept of human freedom (or 'free will'), we shall undertake a brief examination of the debate about whether human beings are free or determined, before we get into the discussion of specific moral theories.

The determinist argues that while people may think they are free, they are in reality wholly determined in what they do by forces or causes beyond their control.

Determinism can have its roots in religion, in the belief that we are created and controlled by some superior being, an omnipotent God, who wholly predetermines how we will act; or belief that one is bound to the 'wheel of fate' and that one's Karma is determined by forces outside the control of one's will. Alternatively, we may adopt a secular 'scientific' determinism based on the belief that a universal law of causality operates in nature so that causes and effects are necessarily connected in such a way that effects follow inevitably and without exception from their causes. From this point of view, we are so programmed by our genetic constitution, the accidental circumstances of birth and the social conditioning to which we are subject within our culture that everything we do is causally determined, predictable and unavoidable.

The language of law and morality, as well as everyday speech, assumes the distinctions between active and passive moods, assumes that human beings can be both active agents initiating actions, or passive 'patients' at the receiving end of the actions of others or external forces acting upon us. For most ordinary purposes, we describe our actions from the *standpoint of actors or agents* who do things for reasons, and with definite aims or objectives in mind. When asked to justify why we chose to act in a certain way, we rehearse the principles that guide our actions, the reasons and evidence we have taken into account, and what goals or intention we had in acting as we did, and perhaps the beneficial outcomes of our actions.

However, when we explain or justify our actions retrospectively with a view to avoiding blame and/or excusing ourselves from responsibility, we tend to focus attention on the external forces which we claim caused us to act in a particular way. We seek to justify or excuse ourselves by pointing to particular features of our inherited constitution, experience (or ignorance), or limiting factors in our environment that have restricted our freedom of choice. In doing so we adopt a kind of *spectator standpoint* with respect to our actions. As spectators of our actions we attempt to be 'wise after the event', projecting an image of ourselves as determined to a greater or lesser extent by forces or factors beyond our control.

By contrast, from an *actor's standpoint*, and when we seek credit for what we have done, we generally project ourselves as agents who act on the grounds of reason and sound evidence, and with reputable (ethical) purposes or intentions of our own free choosing, and with good ends or goals in mind.

When we attempt to analyse the actions of other people, we are easily persuaded that our causal explanations of how and why they acted as they did are compelling; that, given foreknowledge of the person,

their background and acquired knowledge and attitudes, and the prevailing circumstances, we could actually predict how they would behave. Husbands and wives, lovers and enemies often believe they know one another so well that they can predict exactly what the other will say or do. Strangely, if we really could predict how another person would behave we would have good reason to doubt that the person was really alive and not just a robot. Someone who is alive is always capable of surprising us!

It does not follow from the fact that people can give explanations for their actions that the reasons they give are the direct causes of things happening the way they do, nor that the claimed causes of their actions are the reasons for their doing something. (They may have hidden or unconscious ulterior motives.) Reasons are not to be confused with causes. Anticipatory and subsequent explanations of actions tend to have a different logic. The person who offers reasons for acting in a particular way sees the events in terms of his/her self-determining action as a free agent. Retrospective analysis of the reasons or causes of an action, or analysis of the necessary and sufficient conditions for an action to occur, tends to define the events as determined, the outcome predictable, and the scope of choice limited. It is rather like looking at the world with *Alice Through the Looking Glass*, for determinist arguments see everything retrospectively, in reverse, through the frame of the spectator's mirror. With the 'wisdom of hindsight' things can have a dreadful inevitability.

Similarly predestinarian theology, which argues from the existence of an omnipotent, omniscient God to the conclusion that people cannot in any sense be free or responsible for their actions, follows a similar 'logic'. To argue that because all our actions must be foreknown and therefore predestined by God, the theological determinist adopts the radical spectator point of view. Theological determinists assume that they can personally adopt a God's-eye-view of things, the privileged position from which they can view the universe as a whole, understand what is going on, and declare that moral effort is pointless because everything is predetermined anyway. The argument assumes that:

- if you have complete knowledge of someone (omniscience)
- if you can be constantly present to them (omnipresent)
- if you can comprehend and control all the variables in their lives (omnipotence)
- then you could determine in advance everything they would do.

The argument rests on a number of big 'ifs', but it also makes a dubious logical assumption, namely that foreknowledge is coercive or compelling of future outcomes, and it is for this reason that other theologians, and most notably Augustine (354–430 AD), can argue that God's omnipotence and other divine powers do not necessarily entail that human beings cannot have free will, or that we are predestined to act in a way that we cannot resist (Pontifex 1955).

Arguments for determinism which rest on appeal to the 'law of universal causation' are particularly attractive to those who attempt to offer comprehensive scientific or historical explanations of world events, natural processes and the behaviour of human beings. These arguments rest on the faith that a law of unexceptional causality applies throughout the universe. The law of universal causation is an unverifiable metaphysical belief. It is a methodological presupposition of scientific method and cannot be scientifically proved without circularity of argument. However, it is tempting to extrapolate from causal processes in contained and finite systems to the universe as a whole; but this is not logically justified. Causal inference is a method we apply to the analysis of processes in nature that we can observe under repeatable conditions, and which display predictable regularity. It is a conceptual tool which we freely apply to the ordering of our experience in an attempt to make sense of the finite and observable world, or systems we can control. We cannot argue that our choice, or a scientist's choice, to employ cause-and-effect explanations is itself determined by the law of cause and effect, without getting into a vicious circle or infinite regress (Stebbing 1958).

The types of arguments developed in some forms of determinist psychology (e.g. Freudian or behaviourist) or some forms of sociology (e.g. positivist or Marxist/Leninist) appear to offer very powerful explanations of why people behave in certain ways. For the Freudian, neurotic behaviour in adult life is caused by traumatic emotional disturbances in childhood, or, more generally, human beings are inevitably determined by their particular heredity and environment. For the strict behaviourist like Pavlov, all human and social action is the result of 'conditioning'. It is argued that repeated experience of trial and error, success or failure (or rewards and punishments) builds into our behaviour conditioned reflexes or learned responses. These are not free or spontaneous, but determined by the particular conditioning to which we happen to be subjected by life and experience. Alternatively, Marxist 'social scientists' would explain all human and social processes as the result of external and historical forces, economic and social, acting upon individuals, and over which they have no control. However, the Marxist claims that dialectical materialism gives us privileged insight into these processes and thus ability to direct and control the social and economic forces operating in history, liberating us to some extent from the forces of historical determinism.

The fact is that the terms 'free' and 'compelled', 'active' and 'passive' are correlative terms. We cannot make sense of one term without presupposing its correlative. For this reason, to speak either of 'absolute freedom' or of 'absolute determinism' leads us into nonsense. Similarly, to assert that there is evidence of some logical or empirical connection between factors or events which we label 'cause' and 'effect' does not mean, as Hume (1711–1776) pointed out, that the connection is either logically necessary or that some compulsion operates between 'cause' and 'effect', or that being able to predict (with a high degree of probability) what the result of some action may be forces the outcome (Lindsay 1951).

The freedom required for moral action, is the power of self-determination in a world where in order to act we have to:

- choose between the various causal factors operative in a situation
- understand our own limitations and the constraints placed on us by circumstances
- reflect on the present situation confronting us, in the light of past experience
- deliberate on what resources or means we need to achieve our goal
- calculate the likely outcomes of various alternative courses of action; and
- choose ourselves by acting to become causes or determinants of other effects.

The questions we need to ask of the 'free-willer' or 'determinist' are perhaps those raised by Nietzsche (Cowan 1955), who comments on the irrelevance of the free will/determinism controversy to ethics, though it might have entertainment value in metaphysics and theology:

Why should anyone want to delude themselves that they enjoy absolute freedom? Such a view is literally 'out of this world' and has more to do with individual will-to-power and delusions of grandeur than a responsible view of man's moral and political duty! Why should anyone want to maintain that all men are slaves to economic or material necessity? Unless their ulterior motive is to control people by encouraging them to abrogate their moral responsibility or to persuade oppressed people that they really are slaves and can do nothing to improve the world or their lot! So, we have to choose [sic] whether we are going to believe in our freedom to make decisions, and accept responsibility for the results or outcomes of our actions; or we must pretend that we are victims of circumstance or forces beyond our control and excuse ourselves from moral responsibility! [Paraphrasing Nietzsche]

Aristotle distinguished between voluntary, involuntary and non-voluntary actions. Voluntary acts are those knowingly and purposefully undertaken to achieve a particular goal – for example, forming and executing a plan to go to town to buy some clothes. Involuntary, or reflex, 'actions', such as jumping up with a shout of pain when you sit on a sharp tack, or knocking a cup off the table because you withdrew your hand suddenly on contact with a hot kettle. Both are mechanical reactions, or forms of behaviour, resulting from internal or external causes which are neither purposeful nor subject to conscious control. Non-voluntary actions are actions which are done either through ignorance or in a state of intoxication, when you are not fully aware of what you are doing. Alternatively, you act non-voluntarily when you are compelled to do something against your will – for example at gunpoint or when subjected to forces you cannot control (Aristotle's own example is of the captain forced to jettison his cargo in a storm to avoid his ship being swamped) (Thomson 1976).

In general terms, we cannot be held fully responsible for actions which we were forced to do by external factors or forces beyond our control. Determining the degree to which someone can be held responsible for his/her actions in a particular case will therefore involve careful assessment of the full circumstances in order to establish whether or not the person acted knowingly or in ignorance; voluntarily or involuntarily; or while subject to external (or internal) compulsion.

When a person actively causes things to happen which would not have happened without their intervention, then we normally regard the person as the responsible agent. When a person is the passive object of external forces acting upon them, or simply reacts in a mechanical or reflexive way to external causes, then we do not regard the person as responsible. Obviously there may be difficulty in determining for certain the degree to which a given person acted freely or under duress in a particular situation, or to what extent their ignorance, state of intoxication or inner sense of compulsion could serve as excusing conditions if they were being tried for a serious crime. Making these assessments is part of the day-to-day business of juries and law courts, and also of the assessments of staff performance for disciplinary or promotion purposes. (Aristotle showed some interesting reservations in the treating of ignorance, drunkenness or inner compulsions as excusing conditions – regarding human beings as at least partially responsible for their own ignorance, excessive drinking or tendency to give way to irrational compulsion.) (See Downie 1987, Ch. 3.) (Table 12.2.)

To act responsibly, and therefore to be in a position where one can be held responsible for one's actions, and praised or blamed for the outcomes, one would normally be held to have acted purposefully with knowledge, freedom and the power to achieve the desired outcome. Where these conditions are not met the person might be said to be acting with diminished responsibility. For Aristotle, one's competence as a moral agent increases with one's general growth in intelligence and realisation of one's powers as a human being, but also more specifically as one gains control over oneself through mastery of the intellectual and moral virtues. Because people may vary in their degree of moral maturity (as with physical and psychological development) they may be more or less responsible, depending on the stage of their development. However, he also recognises that a

Table 12.2 Constraints and possibilities in moral choice: factors to be taken into account in planning, executing and evaluating our actions

Reasons and causes	Actions and means	Goals and outcomes
Background circumstances	Options for action	Goals to be set
Causes of the crisis	Precedents to consider	Objectives that can be achieved
Pressures on the agent	Methods to be employed	Monitoring progress along the way
Facts of the case	Stages of process	Trends so far
Rules that apply in the situation	Time frame for action	Short-term results of action
Reasons for acting now	Consequences anticipated	Long-term results of action
Motives for acting in this way	Means available to use	Final outcome
Intentions behind the action	Resources required	Degree of success/failure
Excuses that could be made	Other people involved	Evaluation of costs and benefits

Table 12.3 Conditions for a person to be held responsible for their actions. General assumption: A person must be rational and of sound mind (compos mentis)

Necessary conditions	Elements in the condition specified
KNOWLEDGE As a moral agent you must know what you are doing, that is have understanding of the following elements	Background circumstances The nature of the situation requiring action What alternative courses of action are open to you What the consequences of your actions are likely to be What resources or means are necessary (and available)
VOLUNTARY ACTION You must have the ability to act freely and the power to do so at the time, i.e. be in control of yourself	Act purposefully and in a goal-directed way Control oneself or one's own actions Achieve the type of action required Mobilise the necessary resources to achieve one's goal Control the process and determine the outcome
FREEDOM FROM You must be free from compulsion and not be acting under duress or the effect of intoxicants	Physical compulsion or duress exerted by someone else External restraints on one's ability to act Internal psychological compulsion or irrational prejudice Intoxication or drug-induced confusion or stupor Delusion or ignorance of what one is doing
FREEDOM TO You must have the competence and scope to act in the way you desire or need to do	Choose one's own course of action Determine one's own goals and act on them Appropriate the necessary means to implement the action Exercise decision-making responsibility in the situation Own one's actions and accept responsibility for what one does
GOAL-DIRECTED ACTION As a responsible moral agent you must act purposefully and on the basis of sound evidence and reasons	Need a clear aim or goal in mind at the time of action Have realistic and achievable objectives Have the ability to assess your successes or failures Have the ability to learn from your experience and that of others Have the ability to give a reasonable justification for your actions

person may suffer from 'weakness of will' due to their failure to develop the intellectual and moral virtues. Such a person could be held indirectly responsible (and therefore to blame) for not having cultivated themselves nor having made the effort to develop their potentialities.

The difficulty in assessing the degree to which 'voluntary' acts are actually 'free' acts – given the many factors which limit freedom and predetermine scope for action – may lead us to question more radically whether human beings are free at all. Do human beings have free will or are they wholly determined? It is important to note that both law and social morality rest on the assumption that people are normally responsible for their actions. Those wishing to plead diminished responsibility have to produce strong evidence that they were temporarily insane, incapacitated, acting under duress, or the like. Excusing conditions in law or morality are often offered by way of extenuating circumstances to lessen the degree of guilt or blame for an act, or to reduce the penalties exacted. Moral and legal discourse takes for granted that it is possible to discriminate between voluntary, non-voluntary and reflex behaviour.

Table 12.3 summarises the conditions for an agent's purposeful and rational action to be treated as praiseworthy or blameworthy.

further reading

Considering moral decisions or moral policy
DeBono E 1990 I am right – you are wrong. Penguin Books, Harmondsworth, London

Downie R S, Macnaughton J, Randall F 2000 Clinical judgement: evidence in practice. Oxford University Press, Oxford

Holm S 1997 Ethical problems in clinical practice: the ethical reasoning of health care professionals. Manchester University Press, Manchester

Jonsen A R, Toulmin S 1988 The abuse of casuistry. University of California Press, LA

Are good nurses born, bred or educated?
Crittenden P 1993 Learning to be moral: philosophical thoughts about moral development. Humanities Press International, London

Johnstone M-J 1994 Bioethics: a nursing perspective. WB Saunders/Baillière Tindall, London, Chs 1–6

Melia K 1988 Learning and working: the occupational socialisation of nurses. Tavistock, London

Methods of teaching applied ethics
Illingworth S 2004 Approaches to ethics in higher education: teaching ethics across the curriculum. Learning and Teaching Support Network, University of Leeds

Macintyre A 1990 Three rival versions of moral enquiry. University of Notre Dame Press, Indiana

Thompson I E, Harries M 1997 Putting ethics to work: a training resource pack. Public Sector Standards Commission, Perth Western Australia

What is conscience?
Butler, Bishop Joseph 1970 Sermons, 'On Conscience', iii. In: Roberts T A (ed) Fifteen Sermons preached at the Rolls Chapel. SPCK, London

D'Arcy E 1961 Conscience and its right to freedom. Sheed and Ward, London

Johnstone M-J 1994 Bioethics: a nursing perspective. W B Saunders/Baillière Tindall, London, Ch 13, p 449 ff

How do we make sound ethical decisions?
Jonsen A, Siegler M, Winslade W 1992 Clinical ethics: a practical approach to ethical decisions in clinical medicine. Macmillan, New York

Kerridge I, Lowe M, McPhee J 1998 Ethics and law for the health professions. Social Science Press, Katoomba, NSW, Chs 4 and 5

Thompson J, Thompson H 1985 Bioethical decision-making for nurses. Appleton-Century-Crofts. Norwalk, CT

Assessing moral competence
Hursthouse R 1999 On virtue ethics. Oxford University Press, Oxford

Kohlberg L 1984 Essays on moral development: the psychology of moral development: nature and validity of moral stages, vol 2. Harper & Row, New York

Kurtines W, Gewirtz J (eds) 1984 Morality, moral behaviour and moral development. John Wiley & Sons, New York

The relevance of moral theory: justifying our ethical policies

13

Chapter contents

AIMS

This chapter has the following aims:

1. To assist readers to understand the nature of philosophical disputes about ethical policy and the justification of ethical policies and rules

2. To develop in readers a sympathetic understanding of the variety of ethical theories, what they seek to emphasise about our moral experience, and their strengths and weaknesses

3. To clarify the nature of deontological ethical theories and their attempt to provide a ground for universal principles, rights and duties

4. To clarify the nature of pragmatic theories and their function in drawing attention to the moral agent, personal responsibility for our actions and the choices we make of means and methods

5. To clarify the nature of teleological ethical theories and the importance they give to the values and goals which determine our actions, as well as the consequences of our actions

6. Finally, to emphasise the role of ethical policy and skills in developing rules and standards, in professional life, business and society at large.

LEARNING OUTCOMES

When you have read and worked through this chapter, you should be able to:

- Explain the differences between disputes about policies and rules and disputes about decisions
- Demonstrate understanding of the value and function of deontological theories of ethics
- Demonstrate understanding of the value and function of pragmatic theories of ethics
- Demonstrate understanding of the value and function of teleological theories of ethics
- Demonstrate ability to explain the nature and function of philosophical discourse in both building social consensus and criticising rules.

THE RELEVANCE OF MORAL THEORY

The reputation of ethics for being a subject where everything is contestable is perhaps well deserved, partly because of the nature of the subject, partly because of confusion about the role of moral theory in ethics.

On the first point, Wittgenstein (1971) observed, 'Philosophy is not a theory but an activity.' What he was concerned to emphasise was that philosophy (or ethics) is *not* a body of doctrine or truths that give ready-made answers to the questions of life. Rather, he was concerned to stress that philosophy is concerned with skills in analysis and with rational methods of addressing the various kinds of problems with which life presents us. In ethics, as we have observed before, people often look for moral certainty and simple 'right/wrong' answers to everything. Because life is full of uncertainty and complexity, people do not want to wait to work out rational solutions to problems – hence the appeal of fanatical religious and moral fundamentalisms with their simple certainties. Here we should perhaps remind ourselves of Nietzsche's advice: 'Beware of the dreadful simplifiers!' However, it is also true that there is a lot of confusion about the nature of ethics: first because 'problems' are tackled which are not single problems but complexes of problems, and second because people misunderstand the role of moral theory.

In the previous chapter we were concerned to clarify both what is involved in making ethical decisions and under what conditions a person can be held responsible for their actions. We also considered a number of different approaches to teaching ethics and introduced a number of practical problem-solving methods to assist us in making sound ethical decisions.

In relation to making moral decisions in everyday life, we argued that if our decisions are to be well founded and ethically justifiable, then we normally would be expected to be able to give an informed and intelligent account of the following:

- the background facts of the case and the nature of the problem faced
- the principles and rules which were applicable in the specific situation
- the means and methods we considered and used in making the decision
- what possible consequences of the action taken we took into account beforehand
- what specific objectives we set as the basis for our action plan
- what provision we made to monitor and evaluate the success of our action.

We pointed out that *moral theory plays relatively little or no part in justifying particular actions or decisions in specific situations*, but when we come to consider how we justify our general ethical principles and the policies we develop to deal with general types (or classes) of recurrent problems, then moral theory does become important. In this chapter we proceed to consider the relevance of moral theory and how we both set general ethical standards and policies and how we justify them.

Justifying our moral principles and beliefs

In the previous chapters we discussed practical moral dilemmas in nursing in terms of the rights of patients and the duties of professionals, and discussed also the broader social responsibilities of nurses in terms of the principles of respect for persons, of beneficence and justice. In doing so, we have not questioned the concepts of rights and duties, and have assumed that what was said about respect for persons, beneficence and justice would be commonly understood. In other words we have taken for granted that there is a broad understanding in our society of these fundamental moral concepts and principles. We have argued against a superficial relativism that the principles of beneficence, justice and respect for persons are essential to all human societies – because they relate to the fundamental relationships of power and responsibility that people share in all moral communities. We maintain this is true despite the different weighting these principles may be given in different cultures and the many different forms in which protective care, justice and respect for the rights and dignity of people are expressed in local custom and conventions.

However, it must also be obvious that people may not only challenge the way these principles (of beneficence, justice and respect for persons) are applied in practice, but may also demand adequate theoretical justification for our believing in these principles at all. Some moral disagreements in society, as between conservatives, liberals and socialists, are about the relative weight given to various competing claims, for example of personal rights and liberty versus the state's duty to protect its citizens and maintain law and order, or between personal autonomy and the demand that everyone 'should have a fair go'. Some groups will challenge the established moral consensus about sexual mores or the use of drugs, as when people campaign for gay rights, the legalisation of abortion or the liberalisation of drug laws. Alternatively, we may question the very basis of morality and the moral beliefs we have come to accept as the basis for living. This may occur because of some major personal crisis, social dislocation, experience of war and revolution, exile or imprisonment, or the impact of a different religion or culture on ourselves.

To engage in critical reflection, discussion and analysis of these issues is to engage in the activity that we call moral philosophy. Ethics, as we have said, is the activity of systematic reflection on the principles, moral rules and values on which we act; thoughtful examination and practice of decision-making skills; and learned discrimination in choosing appropriate decision procedures for different action contexts. The systematic study of the means we use to justify moral actions and decisions is what we call ethics. However, the critical study of the theoretical underpinnings of our moral systems, beliefs and principles is what we call meta-ethics, or moral philosophy.

The aim of this book is practical and therefore, as we indicated in the Preface, we have attempted to keep the amount of moral theory or moral philosophy in it to a minimum. In this chapter, however, we will now turn to consider some of the more important and commonly used moral theories, and to discuss both their strengths and weaknesses, to what aspects of moral action they draw our attention, and what they tend to overlook.

Most stable societies have a long tradition of law and custom which embodies the established moral consensus of that society. Obviously, laws and customs do change and develop with the times and may change dramatically in times of war or revolution or rapid social change. Moral rules are not unchanging, neither do we start from scratch and have to invent them anew with each generation. From the time we are born we find ourselves in a morally structured environment, in our family, school, community. Some features of that moral environment we accept or tolerate, some we rebel against and may try to change. Negotiating and renegotiating the boundaries and limits of the moral community is a sign of life in a moral community, as people do not simply accept the imposed social order (say communist or capitalist, democratic or authoritarian) but seek to reinterpret or change society's moral priorities, by appeal to 'higher' moral ideals. Moral communities, even the most traditional and conservative, are not static, but do change and evolve with time – some more dramatically and radically than others, and some, after periods of apparent liberalisation, revert to fanatical and conservative fundamentalism. With the dramatic changes in the geopolitical order in recent decades, the revival of religious and political conservatism may well be an understandable defensive reaction to insecurity and too much change. However, moral and religious bigotry are essentially dysfunctional ways of dealing with moral disagreements and cultural differences in society.

Whether societies can change and adapt to major shifts in moral attitudes will depend on the adaptability of their underlying assumptions about human nature and society. Social institutions cannot function without some stability in laws and customs. Some kind of moral consensus is necessary for the ordered functioning of society. In a relatively stable society we do not constantly question the moral beliefs of our community. For all practical purposes we take these for granted in our day-to-day decision-making, unless and until we are faced with a crisis of some sort. This may be a major social crisis or a personal moral dilemma where our moral convictions are at odds with what we are required to do, or where the majority viewpoint differs from our own. Here we are forced to consider the kinds of reasons and evidence we would advance to defend our moral beliefs.

Subjective, conventional and objectivist accounts of ethics

Birth, copulation and death touch on our private lives most intimately, and these have traditionally been the areas most carefully hedged about with taboos to protect the rights and vulnerability of individuals. These are also the areas where modern society has challenged the traditional taboos most fundamentally and where modern technology has opened up whole new areas of ambiguity in the traditional moral consensus. Fertility control, and assisted reproduction by AID, ovum donation, in vitro fertilisation and embryo transfer, genetic engineering, organ transplants, artificial life support, the possibility of cryo-preservation of human beings – these comprise some of the current issues debated in medical ethics. If we are challenged to say why, as a matter of policy, we think any of these things are wrong and should be prevented, or why we think they are morally justifiable, we may adopt one of a number of different strategies:

- We may say that we just 'feel' it is right or wrong, but do not really know why and would prefer not to discuss it. In so doing we may give expression to the view that moral beliefs are private and subjective, based on our feelings or intuition, and that they cannot be settled by argument or appeal to evidence.
- We may argue that moral beliefs are decided by convention and that these differ from one society to the next. Different societies arrive at a consensus, or some sort of social contract, by

reasoning together and agreeing to certain rules for their mutual protection and benefit. Other societies may have different kinds of conventions based on similar or different reasons and may or may not recognise the validity of one another's conventions.

- We may claim that moral beliefs are grounded in the objective nature of things or the inherent structure of human reason, and must be universally valid. From this point of view, the first approach (subjectivist) leads to arbitrariness and irrationality, the second (conventionalist) to relativism. The 'objectivist' argues that morality is based on the objective 'laws' which govern our given physical and psychological nature as human beings. If morality can be grounded in nature in this way, then it can be argued that ethical principles have interpersonal validity, and a kind of objectivity that the other two approaches do not allow.

Moral principles, however we seek to justify them, are important for our day-to-day living and decision-making. They help in the ordering of moral experience and provide some sort of systematic basis for decision-making. They are both psychologically necessary to help make sense of our lives and moral experience, and practically useful in enabling us to make value judgements in a non-arbitrary manner. In both senses they assist us in our communication with others and in the rationalisation of cooperative action. It is because they perform this primitive ordering function of knowledge and action that we call them principles. They also serve as starting points for reasoning about action and the methods and rules we should adopt to make responsible decisions. It is doubtful whether anyone can do without principles and continue to function in society, or as a member of a moral community.

Agreement about moral principles is obviously highly desirable and makes social life a lot easier and tidier. But how do we arrive at agreement, and what is meant by 'agreement'? The view that moral principles are entirely private and subjective, though commonly held, is an inadequate basis for any kind of social or professional ethics, for ethical decisions would be arbitrary and capricious. Such a view would lead to inconsistency in individual practice, make social cooperation very difficult and ultimately lead to anarchy in society. The fact is that while we may agree to disagree about matters of taste, we do continue to argue about moral principles and try to persuade others to our point of view. That is because we recognise implicitly that for moral rules to have any

validity, to be binding on us and on other people, then they must apply equally and universally to everyone. The legal system and other social institutions could not function without universal rules. In practice we cannot claim our rights as members of any moral community without making a personal commitment to the values and ground rules which operate in that moral community, and without accepting responsibility to uphold and defend the principles we hold in common.

Underlying our moral disagreements and continuing arguments about moral issues is a conviction that moral principles must in some sense be universal and objective. We continue to seek reasons and evidence to establish moral agreement. We could take refuge in irrationality but that does not help either to justify the moral position we adopt, nor defend us against the attempts of others to impose their moral beliefs on us. We have to continue to reason together, in the attempt to find rational grounds for interpersonal agreement and social cooperation. We try to establish some kind of intersubjective validity for moral principles, and by appealing to common sense and universal features of human experience seek to justify and give objectivity to our moral judgements.

In whatever way we attempt to defend our moral principles we are bound to adopt one or other of these three strategies, or a combination of them. The reason is that each strategy emphasises an aspect of moral experience that is important in itself. Ethics does relate in a special way to what it means to be a subject, to be an autonomous moral agent, and to our ownership of a set of values and principles for living. However, it is also concerned with the social conventions which govern the way we relate to one another, and which serve to define our social duties and rights. And, finally, we act out our purposes in the real world, where our actions impact on other people and bring about objective changes in reality, with both desirable and undesirable consequences.

The *subjectivist* is perhaps less concerned to emphasise the private and non-rational nature of moral judgements than to stress that moral principles are something we must choose ourselves and make our own. No-one can decide for you what values you must adopt, or on what principles you must base your life. You have to make your own commitment to them, and try to live your life in accordance with them. In this sense the subjectivist points to the necessary moral autonomy of the mature person. Moral principles and values are always very personal in this sense – insofar as they are believed in and acted upon by persons who may feel very strongly about them and may stake their very lives on them. Because of this very personal identification with a moral point of view we may not like our feelings about moral matters or our commitments to be challenged. However, this personal aspect of moral commitment does open us to accusations of subjective bias or moral prejudice. Part of what the other approaches emphasise is the necessity for external checks.

To the *conventionalist* the most important fact to emphasise is the public and social character of our moral beliefs and their function as necessary conditions for social intercourse and cooperation. Conventionalists do tend to point out the variations in moral conventions between different societies, not primarily to stress the relativity of all values, but rather to emphasise the need for tolerance of other people's values. The universality of moral principles, in this view, is achieved by negotiated rational agreement between people of different cultures and traditions and learning to be tolerant of diversity.

Objectivists are concerned to avoid the dangers of irrational subjectivism and a relativism which they see as threatening to undermine the sense of public moral accountability and the imperative and unconditional character of moral principles. Objectivists seek to anchor the concepts of value and obligation in the real world and not in personal feeling or mere social convention. For them, moral principles must in some sense correspond to the demands of reality, as they believe the universality of moral principles and their objectivity can only be guaranteed in this way. They tend to argue that moral laws are fundamentally laws of our nature, given with the very structure and dynamics of human life in the world. Alternatively, the objectivist argues that the principles of morality are derivable from the given structure and nature of reason, as imperatives which we logically must obey if we are not to contradict our nature as intelligent beings, or which we must follow if we are to achieve fulfilment of our nature as rational beings.

We pointed out in the previous chapter that Plato suggested in his dialogue *Gorgias* that there are five kinds of 'agreement' that are necessary in honest and rational moral discourse and which can serve as a foundation for moral consensus in society (Hamilton 1960).

These kinds of agreement might be called the five Cs:

- *correspondence* – our actions should agree with the factual demands of reality
- *consistency* – our individual statements and actions should agree with one another
- *coherence* – our lives should have unity and integrity, agree with what is good

- *congruence* – our thoughts, actions, profession and practice should agree with one another
- *consensus* – our ethics should be in harmony or agreement with general human values.

Therefore, our moral life and acts should display the above forms of agreement: namely, correspond with the demands of reality, be self-consistent, represent a unified and coherent way of life, be congruent with the rest of our lives, and square with social consensus on what conditions must be satisfied for our life to be fully human. Congruence and consensus relate more to subjective and conventional forms of 'agreement'. The test of congruence is a test of sincerity and agreement between subjective intention and action. Consensus (or agreement in principle with others) is the necessary foundation for social contracts and conventions. Correspondence and consistency relate more directly to the elimination of contradictions in practice between our beliefs, statements, actions, way of life and dealings with other people. We need to consider all five aspects of moral experience when we speak of justification in ethics. These different senses of agreement each emphasise an important aspect of moral experience, but none is adequate by itself to cover the whole complex subject of what it means to lead a moral life in company with other people.

VARIETIES OF MORAL THEORY

Many different kinds of ethical theory have been put forward in the course of history to justify an existing moral consensus, or to justify particular moral principles, and, as we have argued, these can be classified under the headings of 'subjective', 'conventional' and 'objective' theories. Introducing the DECIDE model for ethical problem-solving in the previous chapter, and in Chapter 2, we have suggested an alternative way of classifying types of ethical theories, based on analysis of the causes → means → ends structure of intentional acts, as follows:

- *Causes*: Ethical theories that focus on the antecedent conditions or principles which serve as the foundation for our moral duties and rights, and which we must take into account before we act, relate to the background conditions which serve as causes for action. These theories are called 'deontological' from the Greek *deon*, meaning duty. Typical of these theories would be divine command theory, natural law theory and rational intuitionism.
- *Means*: The second class of theories, which focus on action and the moral agent as the primary

means by which ethical principles are applied to the world of moral experience, can be called pragmatic theories, though traditionally called axiological theories (from the Greek *axios*, meaning value). They include theories that focus on the value we place on achieving our goals as well as criteria for choosing relevant practical means and methods to ensure success. Typical of the first type would be virtue ethics, which focuses on the integrity and competence of the moral agent as key conditions for the achievement of individual excellence and the common good, and of the second type, prudential ethics, pragmatism and situation ethics (including a love ethic such as Christian agapeistic ethics), which all give primary value to the practical demands of the situation and what is needed to deal effectively with presenting problems.

- *Ends*: The third class of ethical theories focus on the intended goals and outcomes of our actions, and are called 'teleological' (from the Greek *telos*, meaning goal or end). Typical of these theories would be: Aristotle's theory that all human action aims at happiness (teleological eudaimonism), utilitarianism, which recommends as a practical criterion that we should strive to achieve 'the greatest happiness for the greatest number', and consequentialism, which seeks to determine whether moral actions are good or bad by assessing their consequences, their social and economic costs and benefits (Box 13.1).

Box 13.1 Classification of types of moral theory

'Causes' – prior conditions and principles

Deontological ethics
- Divine command theories
- Natural law theories
- Duty- or rights-based theories

'Means' – agency, means and methods

Pragmatic or axiological ethics
- Virtue ethics (integrity of agent)
- Prudential or casuistic ethics
- Agapeistic and situation ethics

'Ends' – goals and consequences

Teleological ethics
- Teleological eudaimonism
- Utilitarianism and hedonism
- Consequentialism

DEONTOLOGICAL ETHICAL THEORIES – FOCUS ON PRINCIPLES, RIGHTS AND DUTIES

Divine command theories

In virtually every known society, ethical codes have had their origin in religious traditions and practice. This is not just a matter of anthropological interest but also of philosophical significance, which tells us something important about the nature of ethics. If moral principles and rules are to command our respect and to be equally binding on all members of society, then their authority must be based on something more than personal caprice or the arbitrary edicts of kings or tyrants. The authority of moral principles and rules depends on them being understood to have an authority that transcends the self-interest of individuals, however important or powerful. A divine or supra-personal basis for the authority of moral rules would seem to guarantee their universally binding character, ensuring that they can serve as the foundation for unconditional rights and obligations.

Further, if morality is not to be dictated simply by the edict of the king, high priest or clan leader, and enforced by their authority (as has often been the case), then these powerful figures themselves must be subject to some higher authority, and not allowed to be 'a law unto themselves'. Only submission of king and citizens alike to the same ultimate source of moral authority will ensure that moral rules are respected and obeyed by all. Divine command theories appear to provide such an ultimate and transcendent basis and sanctions for the authority for law and morality.

In Judaism, it is claimed that the Torah – the law of Moses and the Prophets – ultimately came from Jahweh (the God of Abraham, Isaac and Jacob). The Jewish leader Moses, who led his people from oppression and slavery under the Egyptians into the Promised Land, claimed that God gave him the Ten Commandments, on Mount Sinai. The Ten Commandments were to form part of a Covenant between God and His people. According to Moses, God agreed to care for and to protect His people as long as they obeyed His commandments (The Bible: Exodus, Ch. 19). The Jewish law developed over the centuries as a complex body of religious, dietary and social rules as well as basic moral principles. While this law was particularly binding on the people of Israel, the Jews believed these laws were universally applicable to all human beings, and that it was their mission to teach all people to obey the laws of God.

For both the Christian religion and Islam, the Ten Commandments remain the foundation of their ethics.

However, each of these world religions developed an ambivalent attitude to the rest of the Jewish tradition of the law and the Prophets, including the Commentaries by rabbis and legal scholars over the ages. Rejected by orthodox Judaism, both these movements developed in time into independent religions.

Jesus of Nazareth, believed by Christians to be the Son of God, was not only a reforming prophet, proposing a more radical obedience to the spirit rather than the letter of the law, but he also set out in his teaching, and particularly the Sermon on the Mount, a new ethic of love and forgiveness, which was to serve as the foundation for the movement that he started. While Christian ethics is founded on the teaching of Jesus and the two Great Commandments – to love God and to love one's neighbour as oneself – it is also an example of a divine command theory, insofar as Christians believe Jesus spoke with the authority of God Himself. It is on the basis of this claim that Christians maintain that their ethic of love has universal application, and have believed that they are called to preach the gospel of love to all people everywhere.

The followers of Mohammed, and his teachings as recorded in the Koran, make similar claims for the ethical teachings of Islam, namely that they are directly revealed by God to his Prophet, have universal applicability and are binding on all humankind. While Muslims do not believe Mohammed to be divine, they do believe that he was, in a special sense, the primary channel through which Allah has revealed the ultimate principles of human conduct and the truth about human destiny. 'Islam' which means obedience to the will of God, Allah, reasserts a radical monotheism (belief in one God) in opposition to what they see as tri-theism in the Christian belief in Father, Son and Holy Ghost.

These three great world religions emphasise the fundamental importance of ethical living and obedience to the moral law as necessary conditions for salvation and eternal life. However, divine command theories are exemplified not only by these three religious traditions; in many other religious traditions, too, appeal is made to some supernatural source of authority for the moral law. In Aboriginal Dream-time, the ethical and religious traditions of the people are supposedly communicated by the Spirits of the Earth to the ancestors, and by the ancestral spirits to the elders and then to the people, in dreams and re-enactments of the timeless rituals of the people. The authority of ancestral spirits is invoked in African animism and ancestor worship, as the basis for ethical and religious practice, and to reinforce the authority of the moral law and tradition.

Natural law theory

The second form of deontological theory is the type that claims that the moral law is in some sense written into the constitution of things. It is claimed that just as the laws of physics govern the operation of the natural world and serve as the foundation of order in the universe, the moral order is founded on the laws given with the structure of the world and inherent in human nature.

In its classical form natural law theory is difficult to disentangle from traditional religious beliefs, in both the Graeco-Roman and Judaeo-Christian traditions. In the 5th century BC the Greek tragedian Sophocles portrays his heroine Antigone as standing up to the injustice and arbitrary rule of the King Creon in the name of natural justice. Antigone defies the king and gives her brother the proper burial rites, despite Creon's edict forbidding the burial of her brother, because he had raised a rebellion against Creon's tyrannical rule of Thebes. To justify her apparent impiety in opposing the will of the king, Antigone appeals to the divine justice which governs the universe, and which not only the king and all people, but even the Gods must obey (Fagles & Knox 1982).

Plato, commonly regarded as the father of Western philosophy, drew a clear distinction between 'nomos' or conventional law, based on social custom and popular agreement, and 'phusis' or the inherent laws of our own nature as human beings. He argues that 'phusis' or natural justice is more fundamental than 'nomos' or conventional law and morality. He advances two different kinds of reasons for this claim. The first is that unless there is a more fundamental basis for justice than the arbitrary edicts of tyrants and the fickleness of public opinion then there can be no rational basis for objecting on moral grounds to unjust laws or unjust acts. He concludes that because we can conceive of the possibility of rational justice there must be some kind of transcendent standard or form of justice against which unjust actions and laws can be judged and found wanting. Secondly he argues that what makes order and harmony in the cosmos, society and personal life possible is that they are all governed by natural laws inherent in the structures and dynamics of being itself. 'Dikaiosune', the ideal form or standard of justice is, he believes, the principle of order and harmony in things.

His belief in this more fundamental natural justice was inspired by the practical example of the life and death of his master Socrates (469–399 BC). Socrates not only made himself unpopular by interrogating politicians and lawyers, demanding to know the true nature of justice, but was also accused of 'corrupting the youth', because he challenged traditional religion for its lack of moral standards. When condemned to death by poisoning, he voluntarily drank the hemlock, acting as his own executioner. This he said was because he did not wish the city of Athens to commit an even greater injustice by killing an innocent man. By accepting his fate and voluntarily drinking the executioner's cup of poison, Socrates bore witness to his belief in an eternal and incorruptible Justice, which rules the universe and which transcends the corrupt justice of men (Rouse 1961).

Within the biblical tradition we have the figure of Job, in the biblical allegory of that name, who is portrayed as an ideally righteous and innocent man who suffers what Shakespeare called 'the slings and arrows of outrageous fortune'. Despite the injustice and humiliation he suffers at the hands of men, the abuse of his friends, the challenging and questioning of his integrity, and the injustice of the fate which God allows to befall him, Job believes that God, who is ultimate justice, must be consistent with his own nature and will therefore come to his aid and vindicate him. His words have become an expression of hope to many people in despair: 'I know that my redeemer lives, and that he shall stand at the latter day upon the earth … that you may know that there is justice' (The Bible: Book of Job 19: 25–29). In a different vein, the Old Testament prophets rail against the corruption, abuse of power, immorality and injustice of kings and people in the name of the God of Righteousness and Justice. The clear implication of the Judaeo-Christian tradition is that human laws must be subjected to the ultimate test of congruence with this more universal divine justice, in comparison with which the 'justice' of men and their laws are often found wanting.

This belief in a universal cosmic justice, more fundamental than the arbitrary justice of men, is common to many religious and cultural traditions. It has much in common with divine command theories, except that it does not attribute the moral law directly to some kind of divine edict. Instead, this tradition sees the natural moral law as built into the very structure of things in the way an intelligent Creator, in designing things to function in a particular way and to serve a specific purpose, constructs things on the basis of intelligent and therefore intelligible principles. What distinguishes natural law thinking from divine command theories is that while the latter require simple obedience to the will of God, the natural law tradition requires us to use our intelligence or reason to observe and analyse the laws which govern the universe and our own nature. Advocates of this theory claim that we can come to know the principles of natural law without supernatural revelation. All we

require is the ability to learn by trial and error, and from experience and the exercise of reason, to discern what requirements have to be met if we are to fulfil our species being, and to achieve the purposes for which we were made as we are.

The Greek and Roman Stoics argued that the universe is rationally intelligible because it is a cosmos, that is, an ordered whole governed by rational laws. Human reason is just a part of the divine reason, the basis of this rational order in the universe. That is why human reason can grasp and understand the intelligible principles underlying the order and harmony of nature. They argue that as rational beings we must live in accordance with this given rational order in nature if we wish to achieve fulfilment, happiness and a state of harmony with others and to live in harmony with nature. Here again, the appeal is made to a moral law written into nature itself, first, to resist the arbitrariness of personal edicts and the relativism of social conventions and, secondly, to explain the universality and interpersonal validity of moral principles.

When the Roman Empire expanded to include numerous other societies and cultures, Roman jurists found it necessary to develop a distinction between the conventional law of the societies they ruled (e.g. the Mosaic law of the Jewish people) and the universal principles of law which they believed were applicable to all societies and by which the justice of conventional laws might be judged. The former was called the *jus gentium* (law of the people), the latter the *jus naturale* (the natural law). This *jus naturale* became the basis of what in the tradition of Roman-Dutch law was called 'natural law'. Two traditions developed in Roman-Dutch law. The first emphasised the Stoics' view that the rationality of justice derives from it being grounded in the rationality of the order of nature. The second, later tradition sought to ground the rationality of justice in the rationality of human beings and in the social contracts they develop to express that rationality. (See Cowen (1961) on the history of natural law.)

The Roman Catholic tradition of law and morality has traditionally been based on a doctrine of natural law, which tends to be reinforced by arguments taken from revelation. In its classical form, the doctrine is similar to the Stoic one, and rests on a number of connected premises:

- God created the world an ordered harmonious whole, governed by intelligible natural laws
- human beings have the intelligence to deduce these laws of nature from their experience
- they can infer what it is necessary for them to do if they are to fulfil their species nature

- they can choose to live a fully human life in harmony with these natural laws, or live a life of frustration and ultimate self-destruction by acting against the laws of their nature.

Thus natural law theory presupposes that people can arrive at knowledge of the natural law from observation of nature and of their own make-up, and hence deduce what is necessary for them to flourish as human beings, and what to avoid if human life is not to become degrading or subhuman, or if life in society is not to be dehumanising, with people treated in an inhumane way (see D'Entreves 1951, Finnis 1999).

The strength and appeal of the natural law tradition consists partly in the fact that it represents an attempt to ground ethics in something objective and more stable and enduring than individual caprice or changing and culturally determined social conventions. Of course the various interpretations of natural law principles and precepts will have culturally determined features or emphasis, but this tradition has endured for three thousand years, and a lot of its precepts have found their way into the common law, public and international law, declarations of human rights and the constitutions of various states.

However, natural law theory is not without its problems. Perhaps the most hotly debated issue is: what do we mean by 'nature' or 'natural' in the context of ethics and law? Is surgical intervention to prevent a maternal death in the case of ectopic pregnancy a natural, unnatural or non-natural intervention? Further, even if we can agree general and broad guidelines or statements of fundamental rights to be based on natural law, how these are 'cashed out' in terms of operational rules, laws and moral decisions in particular cases may still leave much room for argument and disagreement. Because ethics in this tradition has to be related to the observable features of the world, which we share in common, this helps to give some degree of objectivity to moral debate. It cannot be based on arbitrary subjective opinion, personal or mob feelings, or fickle conventions. This helps provide a framework for agreement as we negotiate democratically with others the mutually acceptable boundaries and rules for a moral community.

In Christian ethics definition of the natural law is often supplemented in practice by appeal to revelation – to the laws given by Moses and the teachings of Christ. When Catholics condemn abortion or contraception as evil, because they claim it is 'unnatural', it is not always clear whether they do so on the basis of natural law or biblical teaching, or a combination of both (Gilson 1994, Gill 2001).

Historically, natural law theory in ethics and legal jurisprudence has had an enormous influence on the development of both our social and legal institutions. Against the view that statutory law enacted by a sovereign parliament has ultimate authority, people have appealed to the concept of natural law and natural justice to challenge unjust laws or what they see to be the tyranny of the majority. When Americans seek to test the validity of laws by their consistency with the Constitution (which embodies a declaration of human rights), or when appeal is made to common law in England, appeal is being made to principles of natural justice, which are considered more universal than statutory law. The United Nations Declaration of Human Rights, and other modern attempts to formulate universal human rights, make implicit or explicit appeal to the idea of rights as grounded in the nature of humans as such, to natural law.

Belief in the absolute sovereignty of parliament (on the basis that it represents 'the will of the people') can be dangerous if it means that enacted laws or statutes can be thought to override any other considerations of justice or morality. Talmon (1966), in *The Origins of Totalitarian Democracy*, traces historically how the appeal to the 'will of the people' and the 'absolute sovereignty of parliament' has led to totalitarianism and tyranny. He also predicts that unless constitutional safeguards are built in, such as the principles of natural law, many modern democracies based on the claimed ultimate sovereignty of parliament can be led down the same road – attempting to define by legislation the scope of social morality, without the possibility of a higher court of appeal against unjust laws (cf. Arendt 1967).

Duty-based or rights-based theories

Although not the first, the German Enlightenment philosopher Kant is the most famous proponent of deontology, or an ethic of duty. He argued that it is not the end result, or consequences of an act, which make it right or wrong, but the good will or intention of the agent. It is the intention to do one's moral duty, above all else, which determines whether an action is morally praiseworthy. To get to this view, Kant developed an argument about the rational nature of moral principles and moral obligation, which has been of the greatest importance for ethics.

He maintained that for a moral principle to be binding as a duty, in other words for a principle to be *moral*, it must be (a) universal, (b) unconditional and (c) imperative. Kant said we can never arrive at the notion of obligation from an empirical study of the tendencies built into nature, or from the study of human psychology, including our feelings of pleasure and pain. The concept of duty, he argues, follows as a logical consequence from our notion of a rational being and rational moral practice. Human actions cannot be consistently rational unless they obey rules, rules which are universal, unconditional and imperative.

In his determination to combat moral scepticism and relativism, Kant set about demonstrating, in his *Groundwork of the Metaphysic of Morals*, that there are universal principles presupposed in, and necessary to, the formulation of any coherent system of ethics (Paton 1969). He argued that any system of ethics based purely on empirical observation of human psychology, of human nature, or study of the practical consequences of actions, cannot lead to certainty. At best such reasoning can lead only to probabilistic conclusions. Similarly, an ethics based on feeling, risks being as arbitrary or fickle as capricious emotion. Unless moral duties are certain and absolute, there is no way to avoid the apparent relativity of all moral values. The way seems open to moral scepticism. Thus it is imperative to ground ethics in principles that are certain and universally true for rational beings.

Kant's confidence in human reason and the rational order in the universe was grounded partly on his religious and metaphysical beliefs, partly on the logical proofs provided in his *Critique of Pure Reason*. In his first *Critique* he demonstrated to his satisfaction that without the *a priori* categories of pure reason we cannot make sense of the jumble of impressions we receive from our senses (Kemp Smith 1973). Furthermore, he adduced that the given order and rationality in the world of our experience must have its origin in a supra-personal cosmic Reason. In his *Critique of Practical Reason* Kant argued that there are three essential and necessary presuppositions of all morality, namely: God, freedom and immortality (Beck 1949). God, he argues, is a necessary postulate for morality. For, without a god it would not be possible to ground the moral law or the absolute duties of the moral life. Neither would it be possible to ensure the universal, categorical and imperative nature of moral obligations. Without freedom or the power of self-determination and choice, we could not speak intelligibly of rational moral action or moral responsibility, for all our behaviour would be automatic, reflex or socially conditioned. Kant considered immortality of the rational soul necessary to guarantee the enduring and universal validity of moral values and rules, and the ultimate significance of the moral life for individual human beings.

In addition to these metaphysical arguments for the existence of God, human freedom of will and the immortality of the soul, Kant developed some powerful formal arguments about the essential logical requirements for an ethical system to be consistent and coherent. What he did was to explore what he called the *constitutive and regulative principles* of ethics as such. In more modern terms he set out to clarify the logical basis of ethics as a universe of discourse in its own right. If ethics is a way of speaking about the world and human actions in it, what are the rules of this 'language game'? Kant adduced several concepts which he claimed are 'constitutive' of ethics as such:

- the concept of a moral law
- the concept of a universal and coherent system of such laws
- the concept of a person
- the concept of a kingdom of ends.

Kant was struck by the fact that moral duties are not conditional (i.e. in the form: if … then …) but rather that they are categorical (Thou shalt … /It is necessary that I must do …), and thus a *moral law* must be imperative in form. The moral 'ought', he argued, is categorical and imperative, but it is also, and must be, universal. Moral duties cannot be accepted as binding unless they are understood to apply universally, in the sense of being equally binding on everyone. The concept of duty and *universally binding moral laws* follow logically, Kant believed, from the concept of a rational agent as such. A rational being is one who knows by introspection that he/she must act rationally in conformity with his/her own rational nature and with the rational structure of the universe, if he/she is to live a life that is rationally self-consistent, moral and thus satisfying to a rational being.

The concepts of 'personhood' and a 'rational kingdom of ends' are more substantive and less purely logical principles of an ethical system. As explained in Chapter 7, Kant argued that ethics cannot get off the ground without the concept of a person, not merely as a rational agent, but as a bearer of rights and responsibilities within a *moral community*. In the *Groundwork of the Metaphysic of Morals* (Paton 1969), the definition of personhood Kant gives is abstract and formal. In order to apply respect for persons as a regulative principle of ethics, this formal definition of 'person' has to be filled out with named human attributes, and the details of specific situations, before it can be 'cashed' in concrete 'moral transactions'. Thus, for example, we will arrive at somewhat different definitions of fundamental human rights depending on whether we define human beings as 'rational animals' (Aristotle), 'having a capacity to love' (Augustine), or as 'capable of creative work' (Marx). There are, however, obvious links and interconnections between these attributes, and differences are mainly about which should be given priority in the definition of human rights or duties.

Similarly, behind his very abstract discussion of the *principle of the universal kingdom of ends* there is something like the ideal of a rational moral community committed to striving for the common good of all rational beings. Behind this is the principle of universalisability, namely the demand that the laws which apply to one person should apply to all for the sake of the common good. Implicit in these two concepts of personhood and a rational moral community is the principle of justice, or universal fairness. Finally, in his concept of doing our duty, based on the principle of reciprocity ('do as you would be done by'), Kant offers a social justification for the principle of beneficence, namely, the demand that we should care for other rational beings in order to assist one another to achieve our common fulfilment as moral and rational beings.

Deontological theories of ethics are often linked to religious beliefs and tend to be absolutist in form. The absolutist character of moral principles or duties can derive, as in Kant's case, from metaphysical and formal arguments about their logically necessary character, or they may be claimed to be absolute because commanded by God or based on sacred scriptures or pronounced by figures representing divine authority. Some kinds of Christian ethics are based on such absolutist deontological principles – exemplified by advocates of total pacifism, or 'pro-life' opponents of abortion or euthanasia under any circumstances – but Marxists and proponents of other secular ideologies may adopt similarly absolutist positions on people's categorical duties to the state or other citizens. Such deontological theories can take two forms: act deontology and rule deontology.

Act deontology is based on the claim that one can directly intuit one's moral duty, what one ought to do in a particular situation, by rational introspection. It represents a personal and subjective view of duty that attempts to determine whether particular actions are right or wrong on the basis of whether one's motives are pure, or intentions good, and conform to what one believes or sees to be one's duty. The appeal by Quakers to the divine light, or the appeal of others to the 'light of conscience', as well as some forms of rationalist belief in the illumination that is possible by rational intuition, are variants of act deontology. As such, they are virtually indistinguishable from intuitionism and do not usually make claims about the universal validity or applicability of moral duties and rules to all rational beings.

Rule deontology, by contrast, is the position outlined earlier which tries to emphasise the universal, un-conditional and imperative character of moral laws or rules, and moral duties. In this sense rule deontology attempts to establish that ethics has an objective, supra-personal character, based on the universal rational structure of the universe that is represented in microcosm in human reason. In rule deontology, actions are right or wrong in so far as they conform to the universal, categorical and imperative demands of moral rules within a coherent and consistent system of ethics. Alternatively, they must satisfy what Kant called the 'principle of universalisability', namely that any general rule by which I act in a given situation can only be said to be moral if it can be universalised. That is, I have to ask myself: 'Could the rule on which I am acting now become the basis of a universal law, and therefore applicable to everyone?'

The value of both forms of deontological ethics is that they draw attention to the fundamental role of the *concept of obligation* in ethics. Other systems of ethics (e.g. teleological and utilitarian, hedonist and subjectivist theories) focus on personal life goals, striving for personal fulfilment, concern with the well-being of the majority and pursuit of personal happiness or pleasure. These theories do not do justice to the reality of duty, or obligation to others, as fundamental to our experience of membership of a rational moral community. They also fail to explain the sense in which duty transcends personal interest or possible pleasure or gain, which is exemplified by selfless service to others or personal sacrifice for a transcendent ideal.

Ethical absolutism has a prophetic quality in offering uncompromising opposition to what is seen as evil. While other more pragmatic approaches may appear to compromise or to be vacillating and indecisive, an absolutist acts confidently and often courageously in the conviction that they are right. However, absolutism may lead to rigidity, intolerance and self-righteousness. In this sense: 'absolutism without prudence is empty and formal, and worldly-wise prudence without principle is blind' (with apologies to Kant).

Deontological theories, and Kant's in particular, are often criticised for empty formalism. This is both the strength and the weakness of this type of theory. The strength of formalism lies in its universality and its emphasis on the supra-personal, supranational character of moral laws. It is thus no accident that there is a direct line of connection between Kant and the later Idealists whose work inspired the first attempts at world government in the League of Nations and the United Nations, including the UN Universal Declaration of Human Rights (UNO 1948). The weakness of deontology, however, is that there is a gap between its high-sounding theoretical principles and their practical application in the real world. This gap is so wide that other lower-level concepts and principles have to be introduced to enable us to work with such a formal system of ethics in practice. A related difficulty is that if we interpret all moral laws as universal and unconditional imperatives, then there is no way we can sensibly decide which rule to obey if we are faced with a conflict of duties (e.g. between telling the truth and lying to protect someone from a person who wishes to kill them). However, the abiding insight of deontological theory is that ultimate (rather than derivative) moral principles must be universal and binding on us all, if they are to serve as a basis for both individual and social life (Maritain 1963.)

Kant's deontological ethics has often been described as a form of *rational intuitionism*. As such, it represents a form of subjective theory of ethics which maintains that we arrive at moral principles by rational introspection. 'Intuition' means looking into our own minds and grasping what we find there, by direct perception and insight. In popular terms, we know what is right by consulting our consciences.

Rational intuitionism

This is the theory that we can know what we ought to do by direct inspection of our own minds. Intuitionism comes in both simple and sophisticated forms, and perhaps there are elements of intuitionism in all ethical theories. For example, how in natural law theory one knows which elements of order are relevant to moral experience is a matter of moral insight. Similarly, knowing what is the most loving thing to do in a particular case means considering all the relevant factors and arriving at a judgement by some kind of intuition, rather than crude calculation. At its crudest, intuitionism may represent a refusal to give reasons or evidence for a moral point of view, and can represent a retreat into inarticulate irrationality. But, more seriously, it is an attempt to draw attention to the activity of the moral subject as an essential factor in moral judgement. Computers cannot make moral judgements; it has to be a human subject, or moral agent, that alone can do so.

Intuitionists have traditionally tried to avoid the charge that moral principles are the products of random, arbitrary and capricious judgement by arguing that there are given structures in the mind or moral experience which we can intuit through rational introspection. For Plato, moral principles are in some sense innate. We are born with certain implicit moral ideas, which it is the function of reason to make explicit in consciousness. For the early Quakers and certain Reformers, we know moral principles by illumination given by the divine light or Holy Spirit. In defending the ultimate authority of personal conscience against the moral authority of the Pope or the Church, Luther and the Reformers appealed to the authority of conscience or our capacity to directly intuit moral principles. For Kant, intuition is the introspective rational activity whereby we grasp the rational principles which alone make logical reasoning and a rational moral life possible. This process gives us insight into the form of the moral law. Intuition of what he called the unconditional and categorical *a priori* forms of reason is, he claims, the ultimate basis on which we justify moral principles. He argued, as we have seen, that moral principles are ultimately grounded in man's rational nature as such, and further that the categorical, or unconditional, nature of moral obligations is guaranteed because finite reason is rooted in the Infinite Reason which is the ground and source of all things.

Intuitionism emphasises two important features of moral experience: first, that our consciences are pre-formed in some way before we come to make moral judgements for ourselves and, second, that to be regarded as responsible moral agents we must have internalised a set of moral values and made them our own. We may explain the pre-formed character of conscience as did Plato, the Quakers or Kant, or we may explain conscience in terms of the process by which we are educated and socialised into the acceptance of a set of values. In practice, it is difficult to separate intuitionism from theories that explain the 'origin' of moral principles in social convention and social conditioning. When someone says, 'That is just not cricket', he appeals implicitly to the moral consensus among Englishmen as to what is acceptable behaviour and what is not. The 'intuition' of what is right or good tends to be filled out in practice by content drawn from religious tradition or social convention. However, as has been said, there is an element of personal judgement or intuition in the way all moral principles are both understood and applied, and it is important that we recognise this.

PRAGMATIC ETHICAL THEORIES – FOCUS ON MEANS AND METHODS

Virtue ethics – an ethics of personal and corporate integrity

Virtue ethics is as old as Aristotle (384–322 BC) and as new as Alastair Macintyre's defence of virtue ethics in his book *After Virtue* (1981). Macintyre's work has stimulated a considerable revival of and continuing interest in virtue ethics. What it does is to focus attention back on the moral agent, rather than focus either on the abstract principles, rights and duties on which we base our judgements or on the practical consequences or outcomes of our actions. Virtue ethics concentrates on the moral agent as the person who is responsible for deciding how to apply general moral principles to specific situations in order to bring about the desired consequences. Among the various means and methods used in effecting change through actions, the moral agent is the primary means or channel through which things get done.

What virtue ethics emphasises is that the quality of the action produced is affected by the integrity and competence of the moral agent. If the agent is corrupt, the action is likely to be corrupt. If the moral agent is incompetent in either a practical or moral sense then the action is likely to be less than satisfactory. If you lack the skill or competence to perform a particular act (e.g. to insert a urinary catheter or intravenous infusion) then it would be morally irresponsible and unjust to the patient to subject them to your incompetence. If you lack any or all of the basic intellectual or moral virtues, then the quality of your action is likely to be compromised. Here we have in mind Aristotle's classification of the forms of intellectual competence (or virtues) which include relevant scientific knowledge, technical skill and experience, intelligence, discriminating judgement and practical wisdom; and his list of moral competencies (or virtues) which include honesty, temperance or self-discipline, courage, justice and fairness, magnanimity and wisdom.

There are close links between virtue ethics and the emphasis on professional competence in modern competency-based training, and the emphasis on striving for excellence in corporate management, business and public administration. The popularity of virtue ethics in current business ethics links with the quality movement in business management (including 'quality assurance', 'performance assessment', 'continuous improvement' and 'total quality management'). Here, the notion of 'quality' is linked directly to striving for excellence at the levels of individual virtue (or competence), corporate virtue (or integrity) and continuous improvement in the quality of services delivered to clients or products manufactured.

In his book *After Virtue*, Alastair Macintyre (1981) challenged the dichotomy which had arisen in contemporary moral philosophy between deontological and teleological or utilitarian theories, and he suggested that virtue ethics represents a bridging third type of ethical theory, which had been neglected in the polarised debates between deontologists and utilitarians.

The way debate about ethical theory had been presented as a choice between deontology and teleology, as mutually exclusive alternatives, led to unproductive adversarial conflict between these two schools of thought and to a misleading focus on this debate as if that was all ethics was about. The polarisation of these two approaches was greatly influenced by Kant, who reformulated the agenda for philosophical ethics by setting up an absolutist ethic of principle and duty against anything else that relativises ethics, in particular pragmatism or utilitarianism.

Kant was concerned above all with the clarification of the logical foundations of ethics, and the defence of ethics as a rational discipline against the psychologising tendency of the Scottish empiricist David Hume. Hume had argued that there can be no necessary connection between facts and values, and that we cannot deduce moral laws from the laws of nature. His most famous sceptical remark about previous attempts to found ethics on 'natural law' was to say that we cannot logically derive 'ought' statements from descriptive or 'is' statements. Instead, in his *Treatise of Human Nature* (Selby-Bigge 1978), Hume fell back on our subjective feelings as the basis for our value judgements, and human sympathy and rational self-interest as the basis for ethical conventions. 'Custom', he said, 'is the great guide of human life'.

For Kant, custom or practical utility cannot be an adequate basis for ethical obligation, nor can it be a sound basis for the universality of rational ethical principles. His attempts to provide rigorous logical proofs for the 'constitutive' and 'regulative' principles of ethics, in his *Groundwork of the Metaphysic of Morals* (Paton 1969), presuppose that reason and logic are the final arbiters of ethics. He argued that we cannot base moral obligation on conditional empirical principles ('*If I do ... then ...* will result'). Considering contingent facts – like whether or not my action is likely to turn out well or badly in reality – he insists is irrelevant. Moral principles have to be universal and unconditionally binding on everyone. Thus Kant emphasises the concept of duty, based on rational rules, to the exclusion of anything else. Utilitarian arguments that attempt to justify moral actions by their outcomes, their costs or benefits either beg the question of what criteria should be applied to determine what will count as 'benefits' or 'costs' or alternatively tend to use the anticipated or actual end to justify the means chosen for our actions. Kant maintains we should always act out of a motive of pure duty for duty's sake. He will have no truck with doing your duty for some kind of personal reward or benefit.

Macintyre believes that by reducing ethics to a choice between deontological and utilitarian ethics modern philosophers have undermined public confidence in ethics. He criticises Kant's ethics for its arid formalism and abstract intellectual approach to our moral experience. He sees Hume's ethic of sympathetic feeling as leading to subjectivism and moral scepticism. The hedonistic utilitarianism of Bentham and Mill he sees as attempting to substitute calculation of the relative importance of various pleasures and pains for oneself and society for the exercise of personal moral responsibility. He argues that contemporary ethics has been reduced either to barren explorations of the logical grammar of the language of morals or to the arbitrary subjectivism of emotivist theories of value. What both schools do is to treat moral judgement abstractly, that is, both traditions ignore the existing historical subject or person who is a member of a particular society or moral community with a defined role, and who, as a good, bad or incompetent moral agent, makes actual decisions and acts in the world for good or ill.

What Macintyre attempts to do is to rehabilitate the concept of virtue, rescuing it, on the one hand, from sanctimonious and pious religious associations, and, on the other, from empty formalism. He encourages us to return to the foundational work of Plato and Aristotle on ethics, where virtue is linked with the striving for excellence and the attainment of knowledge of being. Like them he focuses attention on the key concepts of intellectual and moral competence. He also points out that virtue can only be defined in a social context, in relation to a person's role and duties or responsibilities in a moral community. In focusing on virtue, or those personal qualities of the moral agent that serve as indispensable means for the effective translation of abstract principles into action, bringing about good or bad effects in the world, he is saying in effect: 'a plague on both your houses'! From another point of view he is describing the moral agent as the instrumental means for bridging the divide between principles and practice, and the virtue of prudence as central to moral judgement and achievement of the good life.

The Greek notion of virtue is an 'athletic' concept, both literally and metaphorically, linked with physical and moral strength, and vice with physical and moral weakness. The perfection of bodily development, mastery of skill and balance, and the achievement of outstanding performance, all serve as a model for 'virtue' when applied by Plato and Aristotle in the moral domain. Perhaps the main interest of Macintyre's work here lies not only in its relevance to the notion of professional competence, and the kinds of competencies required for example by the good nurse, but also in its direct relevance to corporate life

and the issues of quality improvement and the achievement of excellence in business and professional practice. His emphasis on virtue as related to the standard of our performance in a given role in society gives importance to the determination of standards for performance appraisal. Thus it has considerable relevance to concern with the qualities of leadership and teamwork in business and to corporate ethics.

Because most modern business is corporate in nature, often involving large national and multinational corporations, a focus on individualistic ethics is likely to miss the mark in terms of what is needed for our times. Here Aristotle's and Plato's emphasis on the moral agent as not being a complete 'law unto themselves' but as needing to cooperate in organisational, political and social life, becomes relevant. Besides, such a non-absolutist approach to ethics, which focuses more on discrimination and judgement and less on simply abiding by the rules, is more appropriate to situations where people have to exercise public leadership and responsibility.

Prudential or casuistic ethics

Prudential ethics (like jurisprudence in law) has its roots in the tradition that goes back to Aristotle, who argues that we cannot solve ethical problems simply by deductive argument from given principles or by simply applying universal principles directly to any and every issue. The process of ethical problem-solving is a complex one, both logically and practically, insofar as it requires knowledge, experience and application of developed skills. While deontologists want to defend the universal and categorical nature of moral principles, Aristotle and the advocates of a prudential and casuistic approach to ethics are concerned to emphasise that decisions always relate to specific individuals acting in particular situations. Further, because no two situations are precisely identical, it requires discrimination and judgement to make appropriate decisions.

Prudential ethics emphasises that ethical decision-making is a problem-solving activity requiring knowledge, skill and experience to do well, and thus has two parts. The first focuses attention on the nature of problem-solving and the logic of decision-making, the second focuses on the types of competencies required in the decision-maker, what Aristotle calls the virtue of practical wisdom. *Casuistic ethics* is related to prudential ethics. It developed within the tradition of prudential ethics and legal practice. What the casuist maintains (as pointed out in Chapter 6) is that ethical issues have to be decided on a case-by-case basis. From this it follows that we cannot simply apply universal rules to each and every case of the same type without considering the specific features of each case. This means, on the one hand, taking account of the specific demands of the situation, identifying who are the affected parties or players in the drama, and the nature of the crisis requiring a decision. On the other hand, the casuist may question the value of universal principles and tends to be sceptical whether we can achieve more than well-founded precedents, based on repeated experience of dealing with similar cases. This means that moral judgements cannot claim to be certain or indubitably right, but rather that they are probably correct, or that a decision based on serious consideration of similar cases is at least likely to be the best practical solution, given our past experience (Beauchamp & Childress 1994, p. 92).

Aristotle's ethics combines the emphasis of virtue ethics on the integrity and competence of the moral agent, with a detailed analysis of the virtues (or competencies) necessary for sound moral judgement and effective moral action. His analysis of the structure of moral problem-solving, which we have already touched on several times, is developed on the foundation of the intellectual and moral virtues. In Figure 12.1 we illustrated by an arch how Aristotle conceives prudence as the keystone of an arch made up, on the one hand, of the intellectual or theoretical virtues and, on the other, of the moral or practical virtues. Aristotle makes it clear that he believes that the fully competent moral agent will possess both types of virtues in a proper balance, held together by the virtue of prudence or practical wisdom, and that ability to exercise these intellectual and moral virtues is a necessary condition for competent decision-making. So what are these virtues?

The intellectual virtues (or competencies)

The intellectual virtues required by the moral agent to make competent decisions are listed and discussed by Aristotle as follows:

- *Science* – theoretical and practical knowledge of the world, human psychology, and of oneself
- *Technical skills* – practical expertise and life skills, acquired through experience
- *Discrimination* – a variety of minor intellectual competencies including: intelligence, judgement, self-insight, persistence and resourcefulness
- *Wisdom* – the ability to integrate all the above and apply them to one's personal life.

For competent nurses, possession of the intellectual virtues necessary to perform their job well and to make sound ethical decisions would include all these virtues. They would need to have a sound grounding in the medical sciences (e.g. anatomy and physiology, genetics, endocrinology and pharmacology), in the behavioural sciences (e.g. social science, psychology and ethics), and in self-understanding gained through participation in training that facilitates personal growth. In addition, nurses would have to have had extensive supervised practice placement experiences in which they had learned to apply their theoretical and practical knowledge in clinical situations and to develop an appropriate level of competence before they are 'let loose' on patients! Finally, a nurse's performance would be subject to regular assessment to establish that they were developing their intelligence, skills and confidence in judgement, self-insight, reliability and resourcefulness. Growth in wisdom would be evident in the extent to which this all becomes 'second nature' to the nurse.

Competence in ethical decision-making within this tradition requires knowledge and skill in a number of different areas, and all these require discrimination and judgement. The knowledge required is knowledge of the world, how things work, knowledge of human nature, and of the basic values and principles that apply to all human societies, as well as those specific to our own moral community. More than mere intellectual knowledge of principles is required. We also require understanding of their scope and application as well. Of the skills required, the following are the most important:

- *Ability to identify the facts of the case, the nature of the problems and their causes*. In reality what may present as one problem may be several entangled problems. Ability to sort these out and identify which is most important to tackle first is the primary task and skill. This may only come with life experience and practice in decision-making.
- *Ability to identify and prioritise the ethical principles relevant to the problem*. Because real-life problems are often complex, several ethical principles may have a bearing on the resolution of a difficult case. Having ability to rank-order the relevant principles aids clarity of thought and responsible decision-making.
- *Ability to consider the variety of available means and possible options for action*. Possession of acquired life and social skills will increase the repertoire of possible and relevant responses we can make to a situation. Life experience will also give us insight into what we can and cannot do ourselves, with or without the help of other people or resources.
- *Ability to appraise the relative value of these options, based on past experience*. In making an assessment

of which is the best option, or the least bad option in a difficult situation, requires that we make competent and informed value judgements. Knowing the rules is not enough, the question is how best to apply them, especially if there is no single rule that conveniently fits the problem at hand.

- *Ability to act with resolution and clear achievable objectives, to execute an action.* Indecisiveness is not only a sign of weakness and lack of competence, but may actually be dangerous. To be decisive means having the courage to take risks and to accept personal responsibility for the outcome. 'Decision' (like the doctor making an *incision*) means having to move out of the area of theorising 'head-talk' and take incisive and decisive action in the real world of real people, by trying to find real solutions to real problems. Provided one has applied appropriate knowledge and skills the risks may be reduced, but are never eliminated. Decisions may be wrong, dreadfully wrong! They may also be the right decisions, and may be rewarding to ourselves and our clients.
- *Ability to review action outcomes against one's objectives and to learn from one's mistakes.* Skilled problem-solving, as Aristotle recognised, is built on learning from experience. It builds the learning 'feedback loop' into the process, as part of all sound decision-making practice, ensuring past experience is put to good use in future decision-making, in improving practice and building in good habits and reliable procedures.

The moral virtues (or competencies)

Moral decisions cannot be taken by robots or puppets, but only by persons who act freely, understanding what they are doing, and who are committed to a clear set of values and principles on which they stake their choices and even perhaps their lives. The person who simply does what they are told, acts either unthinkingly or under the compulsion of an externally imposed rule. Kant regarded this state of dependence on external authority, what he called *heteronomy*, as the enemy of responsible moral action, which he insisted was based on *autonomy* (Abbot 1909). The ideal of moral autonomy is not, as the media would tend to suggest, just being able to do what you want. Autonomy does not mean licence or even just liberty 'to do your own thing'. Autonomous moral choice and action means *acting on a basis of values and principles that you have made your own*. Without moral commitment there is no real personal responsibility.

But what are the personal moral qualities that make the difference to whether my performance is outstanding, mediocre or poor? These *competencies* correspond to what have been called the 'moral virtues', in contrast to the 'intellectual virtues' we have just discussed. What then are the key moral virtues? These classically were defined as temperance, courage, justice and prudence.

Temperance This traditional virtue points to a kind of inner strength of the individual that is expressed in self-mastery, self-discipline and self-control. Like tempered steel it is not brittle but flexible and resilient. It does not mean being a 'teetotaller' but does convey the sense of being a balanced person and one of moderation rather than excess.

Courage This virtue is of particular importance to the person who has to take responsible decisions. It means being able to strike the right balance between timidity and recklessness, based on sound knowledge and experience of life. Courage is linked to loyalty and integrity – in the sense that the courageous person is someone reliable and consistent at work and who is faithful to friends and colleagues. A courageous person is also able to stand up for what he believes is right and good, and stand by his decisions and take responsibility for his actions.

Justice Justice as a personal quality or virtue has to do with the perception that one acts fairly towards others, is even-handed, listens well, respects the rights of other people, and shares power equitably with other people. Justice has to do above all with ability to act always with the good of others in mind, and not to discriminate against or abuse people. However, it also has to do with the need to exercise authority where it is necessary to ensure that the interests of others and the moral community are protected from harm.

Sociability In addition to the four *cardinal virtues* (temperance, courage, justice and wisdom), Aristotle taught us that the morally competent person will also have a range of social skills and that their understanding of human nature is based on ability to get on with other people and to cooperate with them in both work and society. Today we would also recognise that good communication and social skills are essential qualifications for the decisive and responsible person. These skills are necessary for one to be able to think logically and to express one's thoughts clearly. They are also essential if one has to seek help from others or persuade them of the merits of one's plans. These skills are also related to the way we best acquire knowledge of other people, how they think and how they are likely to act normally and in a crisis.

Prudence As the key moral virtue, prudence is the ability to integrate the moral and intellectual aspects of one's life, and to apply one's knowledge and skills with appropriate concern for the good of both oneself and the moral community. As a state of excellence, prudence involves possession of a range of particular skills. These are traditionally described as follows (Pieper 1959):

- clear-sighted objectivity, decisiveness, ability to learn from real experience, and to be flexible
- ability to recollect accurately and record facts, to give reliable testimony, and to check things out
- humility to learn from others, recognising our need for help and for advice from others
- having foresight, a sense of timing and ability to recognise likely outcomes of one's actions
- being cunning or worldly-wise, without being cynical: 'As wily as serpents and harmless as doves.'

The virtue of *prudence* (Thomson 1976) is closely linked in Aristotle's thought with what we would call an *informed conscience*. Conscience for classical philosophy did not mean some 'voice of God' or 'voice of parental authority' echoing in one's head, but rather an intellectual faculty. This *faculty* or *ability* to make sound practical judgements includes both theoretical knowledge of moral principles and practical skill or experience in their application. It also includes the idea that sound moral judgement requires an ability both to assess properly the particular facts of a situation, and also to be able to *see the big picture*, including the past, present and likely future possibilities, which have a bearing on a decision. To describe prudence as a *'faculty for practical judgement'* implies that it is a virtue that has to be developed by habit and practice. It is not an innate ability, nor is it something that can be simply programmed into us. Prudence is described as the measure of the other virtues, in the sense that its role is to maintain a proper balance in life, or sense of proportion between the other virtues. Prudence is also said to inform the other virtues, that is, it provides the knowledge base for the other virtues. It plays a crucial role in moral judgement because it is based in practical life experience, of trial and error, and is concerned with the choice of the best ways and means to achieve our goals. In summary, as we have previously stressed, prudence is the knowledgeable and skilled ability to apply universal principles to the demands of particular situations in such a way that we choose the most effective and appropriate means to achieve a good result or outcome.

For Aristotle, prudence is the key to all the other virtues, determining both the general competence of the moral agent and their specific competence in making effective moral decisions. Failure to develop this capacity or potential, or allowing it to atrophy through lack of practice, results in *weakness of will* (or *akrasia*) and *indecisiveness*. These vices, like the others, relate essentially to a lack of developed competence or a negative state of unfulfilled potential. As the keystone of the arch, prudence is not only the bridge between the intellectual and moral virtues but holds them together, giving strength and resilience to the whole character of the person.

Finally, to return to casuistry, this is really best understood as an adjunct to a prudential ethics, where the existence and importance of universal ethical principles is still recognised, but they have to be adapted and applied in a relevant way to the needs of particular situations. Casuistry without principle has justifiably been the subject of ridicule – for it becomes indistinguishable from an ethic of convenience and compromise. However, it is equally true that an ethic of principle that does not take account of or learn from particular cases can be criticised for being inhumanly rigid, out of touch with reality and abstractly formal (Jonsen & Toulmin 1988).

Agapeistic ethics or an ethics of care

We have encountered the New Testament Greek term *agape*, for caring love of another, in two other contexts in this book already – first in discussing the strengths and limitations of 'caring ethics' in Chapter 6, and then in Chapter 11 in discussing the situationist approach to teaching ethics. In both contexts we emphasised that agapeistic ethics *focuses on the concrete relationships between particular people at a particular time and place*, thus from Chapter 6:

> In the attempt to do justice to the needs of specific people in particular circumstances, the Judaeo-Christian love ethic has emphasised the kinds of obligation that are rooted in caring for others, rather than a more legalistic approach. In fact St Augustine in his commentary on 1 John 7: 8 summed up Christian ethics in the challenging phrase 'love, and do as you like' (Clark 1984). An ethics of caring (or agapeistic ethics), which strives to determine what is the most loving thing to do in the circumstances, serves three different kinds of purposes:
> - First, it offers an alternative to an impersonal rule-based ethics of duty, emphasising that the obligation to care for individuals as we would want to be cared for ourselves, is more important than obedience to formal rules.
> - Secondly, it emphasises that caring love demands that in decision-making we pay attention to the specific individual rather than society in general, to the particular circumstances rather than universal conditions and requirements.

● Thirdly, it underlines the fact that our actions have to be measured by their effects on particular people and situations rather than their conformity to general rules and duties.

Judaeo-Christian ethics has tended to take one of two forms: either to build theistic elements into the doctrine of natural law, making the mind of God the source of the intelligible order in the universe and human life; or to opt for a love ethic (or a combination of both). The tradition of agapeistic ethics is mainly Jewish and Christian, but is not confined to these world religions. Its foundation in the Jewish tradition is summed up in the Shema Israel – the call to the people:

> Listen O Israel: Yahweh our God is the one Yahweh. You shall love Yahweh your God with all your heart, with all your soul, with all your strength. (The Bible: Deuteronomy 6: 4)
>
> You must not exact vengeance, nor must you bear a grudge against the children of your people. You must love your neighbour as yourself. I am Yahweh. (The Bible: Leviticus 19: 18)

In contrast to the natural law tradition, which emphasises the rationality of human beings above everything else, the Judaeo-Christian tradition seeks to define the essential nature of human beings in terms of their capacity to love. In theological terms, the argument is that God is love, and since people are made in the image of God the most important thing about people, the most important value in human life, is love. In terms of this theory, love is not only the essence, the very 'power of being' in human life, but it is also the ultimate test and justification for our moral decisions and actions. Love can also be the specific norm we apply to every situation and on which we base our moral judgements, by deciding what is the most loving thing to do in particular circumstances.

In the theological tradition there has been disagreement about the extent to which we can infer from the essential nature of God as love, that human beings, supposedly made in the image of God, are capable of disinterested and forgiving love of the same kind. Thinkers who have reflected on the evil in the world and human society, and the apparently depraved nature of humankind, have been reluctant to conclude that imperfect human beings are capable of agape love, without supernatural assistance. Anders Nygren in his book *Agape and Eros* (1953) distinguishes radically between 'eros' as natural human love and 'agape' as a form of supernatural caring love only made possible through the action of divine grace in our lives. Martin D'Arcy, because he does not accept the total depravity of human nature, argues in the *Heart and Mind of Love* (1962) that both 'agape' and 'eros' are natural to human beings, although he would agree that the example of Christ and divine grace make it easier for us to practise care and forgiveness towards others. The contemporary Jewish philosopher Levinas, despite his experiences of the Nazi Holocaust, argues passionately in his *Ethics and Infinity* (1985) for the recovery of ethics, not as an intellectual enterprise, but as the actual engagement of person with person, face-to-face: 'Access to the face is straightaway ethical'. In his book *Responsibility for the Other* (1982) Levinas argues that love is an unconditional commitment to the other for their sake, and is made possible by the gift of personhood which the other makes to me face to face – making me self-consciously aware of myself as a person in relation to another person and therefore directly responsible to them as 'the other'.

From a more practical and historical perspective, agapeistic ethics has developed in reaction and opposition to legalistic ethics, within both Judaism and Christianity. Appeal has been made to an ethic of love when ethics has become a matter of fearful obedience to the law, or a matter of empty or superstitious ritual. Agapeistic ethics is a protest against the conception of God as a remote and merciless judge who demands strict justice and ritual purity from adherents, and has insisted that God must be a loving God who cares for us in our frailty. Against moralism, as the morality of false guilt and taboos, and legalism, as the observance of the letter rather than the spirit of the law, agapeistic ethics has demanded authenticity, truthfulness and openness in religious and moral life. Love-based ethics claims that we cannot force concrete human situations, in their everyday variety and uniqueness, to fit the requirements of abstract general laws. Love demands recognition of the particular character of each unique human person, their situation and the painful complexity of the moral choices they make in real life. To live by love rather than by the demands of the law is liberating, it is claimed, while living by law is restricting and guilt-inducing (Pontifex 1955).

The second important emphasis in agapeistic love ethics is on the importance of the affections in our moral life. The emotions are, as the word 'e-motion' suggests, what get us going, and motivate us to act in the first place. St Augustine (354–430 AD), the master psychologist, describes human life as being in the state of *inter-esse*. That is, human life is 'being-in-between'. This means that we are not self-sufficient but contingent beings. We are 'creatures' in his terms. All our interests arise from our state of *inter-esse*. It is because we are incomplete and therefore needy creatures that we have feelings of desire. Our desires relate to our fundamental needs, and these desires drive us to act, to satisfy our desires. Augustine, like Plato, observed that desires are insatiable, they are potentially infinite while realisation is always finite. A particular meal, or experience of sexual delight, may satisfy us temporarily, but sooner or later we seek further satisfaction of our desires. The central challenge, or problem, then becomes how we regulate our desires and loves and do not become slaves to impulse.

The critics of an agapeistic love ethics – which seeks to determine how we should act by simply asking what is the most loving thing to do in the circumstances – argue that one cannot live without rules, and that this anti-nomian, anti-law, form of love ethic leads to anarchy. In response to the charge of anti-nomianism, advocates of agapeistic ethics have adopted two different approaches. The first approach is to say that *there is logic to our loves*, which does provide some guidelines as to how we should act. The second more radical alternative is to say that we do not need rules at all, that rules prejudge human situations and moral experience, that *we must therefore approach each situation as far as possible without preconceptions* and allow love alone to dictate to us what to do.

There are several examples of the first kind of love ethics. The moral philosophy of St Augustine is perhaps the most famous and has been the most historically influential, while the writings of Paul Ramsey (1980) have perhaps been the most important of recent theories. Augustine argued that since God is love and people are made in the image of God, then it is their capacity to love which defines their essential nature. 'If you wish to know what a man is, ask what he loves.' From this it follows that in one's concrete historical existence, the problem is to work out the moral hierarchy of our loves; as Augustine says: 'the primary task of the moral life is to achieve the right order of priority amongst our loves'.

But how do we know what is the right order of human desires, affections and loves? Augustine argues that God has created nature as an ordered hierarchy of beings: from the lowest physical elements to plants, insects, animals and humans, and, he would add, angels at the top of the hierarchy! Corresponding to this order in nature is an order in human life, of the physical, emotional, intellectual and spiritual. Human loves can be ordered in their moral importance accordingly. All lower loves must be subordinated to agape – love of God and love of neighbour. Friendship, the desire for personal fulfilment, erotic love and the basic physical appetites are each important in their own place, but unless each is subordinated to the

other, in the proper order, then chaos is likely to result. Our basic physical appetites must be controlled by and subordinated to the higher loves, or they lead to selfish exploitation of others and to our own harm. The desire for self-fulfilment has to be subordinated to the demands of friendship and the higher duty to care for the well-being of others under God, and so on. Evil for Augustine is but deranged love, giving undue importance to lower loves at the expense of higher, for he says: 'Everything comes forth by love, even evil, for evil is but deranged or inordinate love' (Healey 1968, Frankena 1964, Jaspers 1962).

The second type of love ethics, what has been called 'situation ethics', can also be traced back to another saying of Augustine: 'Dilige et quodvis fac', 'Love and do as you please' (Clark 1984). What Augustine suggests is that love alone is a sufficient 'law' by which to live, and that if we are faithful to the nature of true caring love (agape), then we will always find the most appropriate and loving way to deal with each situation. By emphasising that love is a sufficient criterion by which to judge all other moral rules, St Augustine shows remarkable faith in the ability of human beings to live by the principle of agape-love and to discern how to apply it in each and every situation.

In its 20th century form, situation ethics owes a great deal to existentialist philosophy, in particular to Sören Kierkegaard, Friedrich Nietzsche, Jean-Paul Sartre and Albert Camus. They share a common detestation of hypocritical bourgeois morality, moralism and an ethics of external observance and respectability. In their quest for moral authenticity, they each stress in different ways the need to approach each situation on its own terms, without moral prejudices, and to be open to its possibilities and unique ethical demands. Joseph Fletcher (1979a), in his book *Situation Ethics*, served more than anyone else to popularise a situation-based love ethic. He also attempted, in his book *Humanhood: Essays in Biomedical Ethics* (1979b), to apply this kind of love ethic to medicine. Broadly speaking, he argued that all that doctors and nurses need, by way of moral equipment, is their personal knowledge, skill and expertise as health professionals, a commitment to a love ethic and a sensitivity to what each human situation demands. Deciding what is right to do in each case would then mean simply taking account of the unique circumstances of each patient, the nature of the responsibilities of the caring relationship between the health professional and the needs of each individual patient.

While also advocating a love ethic, Paul Ramsey, in his book *Deeds and Rules in Christian Ethics* (1983), and William Frankena, in his various writings on agapeistic ethics, each criticise Fletcher's position as simplistic and ultimately untenable. Ramsey argues that a love ethic cannot avoid the need for rules, as any case that serves as a precedent, or any general requirement of love is itself a rule of a kind. He goes further to demonstrate that just as Augustine suggests there is an ontological basis for determining a hierarchy of different kinds of love, so in everyday life when we apply the love principle, we have to prioritise our love commitments. As a result of this criticism Fletcher has somewhat qualified his position in his later work. What all three authors wrestle with is the tension between an ethic based on love and the need for rules. We must be faithful to the demands of the situation and the needs of the specific individual, but also operate in ways that are predictable, rule-governed and dependable, and not just arbitrary. Frankena (1964) and Ramsey (1983) both attempted to answer the need for rules in Christian ethics, as well as for caring love, by developing Ramsey's concept of 'covenantal love' as a way of understanding and distinguishing the different kinds of contracts and commitments we make to others in relation to the norm.

David Hume's ethics of sympathy, and the logical positivist emotivist theory of value can each be seen as secularised versions of agapeistic love (Lindsay 1951, Pt 2). For Hume, 'reason is and ought to be the slave of the (sympathetic) passions', by which he means that sympathy is not only what binds society together, but it is also the criterion and norm of what is ethical. For the positivist, moral judgements are but covert expressions of our feelings of approval or disapproval of other people or their actions. While this 'boo–hurrah theory of value' is easy to satirise, it too emphasises the importance of our feelings as motivating our actions, influencing what we value and thus determining our value judgements. However, the limitation of emotivism is that it tends to evacuate ethical discourse of any meaning or rational significance. In *Language, Truth and Logic* (1958), A.J. Ayer puts forward the positivist empirical meaning criterion, namely that 'Every meaningful proposition is either analytic or empirically verifiable', and he argues that according to this criterion the propositions of ethics and theology are literally non-sense. On the positive side, Baier (1995), her book *Moral Prejudices*, has argued that Hume's ethics of sympathy makes his work of particular interest to feminists, where she represents him as 'the women's ethicist' and 'the women's reflective epistemologist'! It is debatable whether Hume would have recognised himself in these descriptions, but one must agree with Baier that Hume's anti-rationalist emphasis on the importance of feelings and the affective side of our personalities is

fundamentally important to our moral lives and to ethics itself (Baier 1995).

What all these pragmatic ethical theories have in common is that they pay primary attention to moral agency. Virtue ethics focuses on the moral agent and the competencies the agent requires to act effectively and ethically. Prudential ethics focuses on the nature of practical, effective and prudent decisions, and the practical means required to implement our decisions. Agapeistic and situation ethics concentrate on the demands of love, the feelings and desires that motivate us to act, and the specific requirements for appropriate and authentic action in each given situation.

TELEOLOGICAL ETHICAL THEORIES – FOCUS ON ENDS, GOALS AND CONSEQUENCES

Teleological theories (from the Greek *telos* = end or purpose) seek to justify moral principles *either* in terms of some overall goal or sense of purpose in nature or human society *or* in terms of the consequences of actions, their results or outcomes relative to goals.

These two approaches relate to two different senses of 'goal' or 'end' in our experience. The latter type of justification relates to *purposeful acts*, which have specific goals. The former is less familiar, though it has been very influential, namely, that of some kind of *built-in purpose, tendency or design in nature*. This is seen as either God-given, or inherent in nature, and perhaps linked to the evolution and development of species.

Teleological eudaimonism – the end of human life is happiness

Aristotle (384–322 BC) was the son of a doctor, and was perhaps first and foremost a biologist. His ethics is described as a form of teleological eudaimonism – 'teleological' because of his belief that we can discern a built-in telos, tendency or purpose in nature and in human beings. It is also called 'eudaimonistic' because he saw human life as fundamentally motivated by the quest for happiness (from Greek *eudaimonia*, meaning happiness or well-being). This system of ethics has been one of the most influential in the history of Western culture, and has greatly influenced Christian ethics, particularly that in the Roman Catholic tradition.

As a biologist, Aristotle was struck by the fact that living things grow and develop, and so he built in to his ethics and philosophy developmental concepts that he derived from his observations of nature. For example, he observed that all living things have a built-in tendency to fulfil the potential they inherit from their parents, to develop from embryonic form to the fulfilled mature form of their species. Plants and animals begin as tiny seeds and grow into what may be large trees or gigantic elephants or whales, progressing through various developmental stages towards the fulfilment of the form of their own species. Acorns do not turn into apple trees nor caterpillars into people. Each species seems to strive toward the fulfilment or perfection of its form and the ongoing reproduction of its kind.

Aristotle observes, in *Nicomachean Ethics* Book 1, that human beings appear to be goal-directed in two senses, first that they are capable of *purposeful and self-directed action*, and second, they have a tendency to *strive towards some ultimate end or telos*, namely, happiness or the fulfilment and perfection of their essential nature as human beings (Thomson 1976). This striving or built-in tendency to fulfil all the potentialities of our species being (to achieve physical, emotional and intellectual well-being) is both innate in us, but also capable of being recognised and then rationally and voluntarily self-directed by each person. The goal which governs this striving is the pursuit of happiness, both in terms of personal well-being and fulfilment, and the happiness of the rest of society, since, as 'political animals', we cannot be happy in isolation.

Aristotle distinguished between 'pleasure' and 'happiness'. Whereas pleasure and pain are physical sensations or psychological states, *happiness is a state of being*. Pleasure and pain may be transitory and may relate to a part of the body, a particular function or to particular feelings. Happiness, however, relates to the state of the whole person, is more enduring, and may persist even if the person is experiencing pain. Happiness relates to purposeful action, and as a disposition or orientation of a person's whole being, is directed towards some ultimate goal or ultimate good. Ethics as a whole is concerned with this goal-directed action and the ordering of life and life's priorities towards the achievement of this ultimate good and personal fulfilment. Virtue and vice are also ultimately defined in terms of whether they promote or frustrate the flourishing of individuals or society, and promote achievement of personal fulfilment and the general health and well-being of society.

According to Aristotle, the quest for pleasure and the avoidance of pain are needs-directed, whereas happiness is goal-directed. Happiness relates to a state of fulfilled being and actions directed towards our self-fulfilment and self-actualisation as human beings. Aristotle recognised that our basic human needs drive us to pursue pleasure and to satisfy our appetites, and that it requires effort to rise above this level to pursue a life of rational reflection and fulfilment. This bears comparison with Maslow's *Hierarchy of Human Needs*. According to Maslow (1970) we can only pursue the higher levels of personal and intellectual self-actualisation when we have successfully met our lower needs. These needs in descending order of importance relative to the necessities for survival are:

- the need for intellectual and personal self-actualisation
- the need for self-esteem and social recognition
- the need for a social role, identity and employment
- the need for personal security – health, emotional and material security
- the need to satisfy our physical needs – for food and water, clothing, shelter etc.

From Maslow's point of view, Aristotle, has a somewhat elitist view of happiness. As a relatively wealthy Greek citizen or freeman, he could afford a view of personal happiness based on the leisured pursuit of the intellectual pleasures of philosophy, whereas his slaves would be prevented from experiencing happiness, to the extent that the practice of philosophy is a necessary means to achieve it. However, this criticism does not completely invalidate what Aristotle says about happiness. For him, all people, including slaves, strive for happiness, even if the conditions of their life frustrate the full realisation of their potential. For happiness is not simply a matter of feeling, but *contentment arising out of fulfilment of one's potentialities as a human being*. Happiness is more enduring than pleasure, because it is concerned not with a part but the whole of one's being, and may thus persist even if the person is an oppressed slave or is experiencing pain. Happiness, as a disposition, consists in the active orientation of one's life towards some ultimate goal or ultimate good. Ethics has as its primary goal the ordering of life and life's priorities towards the achievement of personal and social fulfilment, health, well-being and happiness. Virtues and vices are defined in terms of whether they promote or frustrate the flourishing of individuals or society. Personal growth through the development of the intellectual and moral virtues serves to promote both one's own health and well-being and also that of our whole society, for, according to Aristotle, as 'political animals', we cannot but be concerned about other people, for our fulfilment is involved in theirs, and theirs in ours.

In many respects, this theory has common elements with natural law theories, in emphasising that the tendency to strive for happiness is built into our nature as a law of our very being. It is not just a matter of subjective feeling or personal desire, but a given characteristic or norm of human nature.

Aristotle's theory has been called utilitarian, insofar as his test of the rightness of actions and moral principles is whether they are ultimately conducive to the greater good and happiness of people and society. However, his ethics was more tied to his biology and philosophy of nature, and his view was that the tendency to strive for happiness is inherent in human beings and not a matter of choice by individuals or agreed social policy. He would have agreed that human beings have to understand and strive consciously to achieve fulfilment, but he would have argued that we also have a natural tendency to do so anyway. Whereas the psychological hedonist considers people to be completely determined and unfree, Aristotle believed we are capable of self-determination and thus of moral choice concerning our life and destiny.

Ethical and psychological hedonism

However, happiness can and has been interpreted as a desirable *psychological state* (of pleasure or pain), rather than as a general state of being. And pursuit of a life of pleasure can be seen as a rational goal personally chosen, rather than something built-in by nature. This interpretation of happiness was accepted and promoted by Epicurus (341–270 BC) and his followers in antiquity, and by Jeremy Bentham and John Stuart Mill in the 19th century. These theories, which make the quest for pleasure and the avoidance of pain the basis for making moral choices, have been called *hedonist* (from the Greek *hedone*, meaning pleasure). *Utilitarian* theories seek to base moral judgements or policies on their usefulness or practical value in adding to our pleasure, diminishing our pain, and thus adding to the sum total of human happiness.

The pursuit of pleasure as a principle for living can take both selfish and altruistic forms. The kind of hedonism associated with Epicurus and his followers was not self-indulgent, as common proverbial use of the term 'hedonist' would suggest, but Epicurean hedonism was associated with a disciplined form of community life devoted to pursuit of the higher intellectual pleasures and long-term 'happiness' of the community, rather than indulgence in short-term carnal pleasures. Epicurus believed that people ought to pursue a life of moderation, of pleasurable happiness and avoidance of pain, and that this could only be achieved by subordinating lower pleasures to higher ones, especially choosing pleasures that contribute to the enrichment of friendship. This kind

of hedonism is called moral hedonism to distinguish it from psychological hedonism – the theory that human beings have no choice but are in fact always driven by the instinct to seek pleasure and avoid pain.

Modern utilitarianism is associated with the reforming political movement of 19th century liberalism. It is associated in particular with Jeremy Bentham (1748–1832) and John Stuart Mill (1806–1873), who, as members of the Philosophical Radicals or Whigs (later British Liberal Party), were widely influential in parliamentary reform. In 1832 Bentham played a prominent part in the passage of the Reform Bill, which removed control of the House of Commons from the landed aristocracy and gave more effective political power to the new urban bourgeoisie.

Jeremy Bentham states in *An Introduction to the Principles of Morals and Legislation* (1789):

> Nature has placed mankind under the governance of two sovereign masters, pain and pleasure. It is for them alone to point out what we ought to do, as well as to determine what we shall do. On the one hand the standard of right and wrong, on the other the chain of cause and effects, are fastened to their throne.

He goes on to define the greatest happiness or greatest felicity principle as follows:

> That principle states that the greatest happiness of all those whose interest is in question, as being the right and proper, and only right and proper and universally desirable, end of human action: of human action in every situation, and in particular that of a functionary or set of functionaries exercising the powers of Government.

As a reformer, his main point was to stress that politicians and administrators should not act out of self-interest, nor to their own advantage, but in the interests of their subjects, aiming always to achieve the greatest happiness for the greatest number.

Bentham takes it as self-evident that pleasure is good and pain is bad, and attempts to ground his ethics on this apparently objective fact of human psychology. His initial claim is that the worth of actions can be determined by the degree to which they promote pleasure and prevent or reduce pain. He further assumes that the greater the quantity of pleasure the better things will be. While he enthusiastically promoted the idea of a 'felicific calculus', the problem he faced was how to determine or measure the quantity of pleasure produced or pain avoided by an action or policy. He failed to give specific criteria to define 'pleasure' and 'pain', or to enable us to distinguish them from one another. He uncritically assumed that their meanings were self-evident and that they are intrinsically good and bad respectively, whereas we might want to argue that some forms of pleasure are bad (e.g. associated with cruelty to animals), or that some forms of pain are good (in that they signal warnings to us, or are associated with processes like strenuous exercise or corrective surgery that are meant to do us good).

Thus, his attempt to provide a purely quantitative criterion runs into difficulties as soon as an attempt is made to apply it to actual calculations or discriminations between what are to count as 'pleasures' or 'pains'. In the absence of criteria for making sound value judgements about what pleasures are to count as 'normal' or 'pathological', 'good' or 'bad' we cannot get very far. His utilitarianism seductively suggests that these issues can be decided by reference to facts – falling foul of Hume's argument that an 'ought' statement cannot be logically derived from an 'is' statement. Like other self-styled 'scientific' theories of morality, what Bentham does is to covertly import his own values into his supposedly 'objective calculations' and appraisals of pleasure and happiness. Far from being value-neutral, his 'felicific calculus' begs the question of the real nature of happiness and tends to promote the interests of majority public opinion – even the lowest common denominator in public opinion, rather than the highest common factor. Without qualitative moral criteria his hedonistic calculus proves of little practical worth, and tends to be based on arbitrary interpretations of the pleasure principle.

Bentham, like modern utilitarians, is more concerned to emphasise the psychological than the ontological nature of happiness – identifying it with feelings of pleasure and freedom from pain. He stresses that the pursuit of happiness, whether as an individual goal or social policy, is a matter of rational choice or social contract. At a simple everyday level, the general utilitarian formula – 'choose the course of action which causes the least pain and maximises happiness for the greatest number' – seems to be a useful guide to decision-making and dealing with moral dilemmas. However, when we look at the formula more critically it raises a number of questions:

- What do we mean by 'pleasure' and 'pain'?
- Are pleasures better if more intense or longer-lasting?
- How do we calculate the degree or quantity of 'pain' or 'pleasure'?
- Can we use pleasure alone as a criterion to determine that intellectual interests are preferable to physical pleasures?
- How do we distinguish between normal and abnormal, natural and unnatural pleasures?
- Why should sadomasochistic sex not be better than enjoyment of what we call 'normal' sex?

- How is pleasure related to happiness?
- Do we concern ourselves with the 'happiness' of people like ourselves, or with the whole of society?
- Furthermore, when we attempt to apply the 'general happiness' formula to specific actions, are we talking just about the immediate psychological effects of our actions or their long-term benefits, rather than costs, to us and to society?
- How do we justify adoption of utilitarianism as a policy for action?

John Stuart Mill recognised the obvious defects of Bentham's formulation of the greatest happiness theory, but also recognised its intuitive appeal as a practical test of the rightness of actions. He suggested several modifications which greatly strengthen the theory.

First, he recognised that we need qualitative moral criteria to distinguish between higher and lower pleasures, according to whether they serve short-term or long-term goals contributing to the immediate or the ultimate well-being of the individual. Second, he stressed the complexity of moral decisions, where the choice may not be between pleasure and pain but between different kinds of pains, or different kinds of pleasures: 'The principle of utility does not mean that any given pleasure, as music, for instance, or any given exemption from pain, as for example health, are to be looked upon as means to a collective something called happiness and to be derived on that account. They are desired and desirable in and for themselves; besides being a means, they are part of an end' (Lindsay 1957). Third, Mill stressed that things that count as contributing to the greatest happiness for the greatest number are to be measured by the criterion of the greatest benefit to all, and not simply to the majority. The shift from what Bentham called a 'felicific calculus' to cost–benefit analysis of the likely or actual consequences of actions in promoting the common good is what is definitive of his 'utilitarianism'.

The first modification introduces the principle of totality, the good of the whole rather than the part – to supplement the pleasure principle. The second suggests the need for some kind of hierarchy of pleasures, or qualitative criteria for prioritising pleasures, or for discriminating between desirable and undesirable pleasures. The third introduces covertly the concept of good, or benefit, combining both its positive value for the individual and social justice in terms of promoting the common good of society.

Frankena (1973) and other modern philosophers have introduced a useful distinction between *act utilitarianism* and *rule utilitarianism*.

Bentham's simple formula, insofar as it is applied as a criterion to determine the *rightness or wrongness of particular acts* by considering their effects or consequence, and whether these obtain the maximum amount of happiness for the greatest number, could be taken as an example of act utilitarianism. On the basis of past experience it attempts to predict the likely outcomes of alternative courses of action, or it attempts to assess or evaluate the actual psychological consequences of actions already performed. *Rule utilitarianism* would judge an action right or wrong not according to its consequences in a particular case, but rather would judge an action right if it is based on a general rule, the following of which would be likely to lead to the best consequence for all. Mill's modified version of Bentham's general happiness theory lends itself to interpretation as rule utilitarianism, since actions which serve the principle of totality observe hierarchical distinctions between pleasures and serve the common good, and are not simply determined by attempts to measure degrees of pain or happiness. Rather, what is to count as 'happiness' or 'pain' is determined by one or other or all three of these additional rules.

Utilitarianism has a continuing popular appeal in business with its focus on costs and benefits, and in healthcare because health professionals consider that they are in business to prevent or reduce pain where possible and to promote the health and well-being of patients. Because health professionals are expert at estimating what the likely consequences or side-effects of treatment may be, judging by consequences (act utilitarianism) appears scientific and reinforces their sense of authority in direct one-to-one clinical relationships. They feel less comfortable if asked to define 'health', 'quality of life' or 'happiness' – which would be necessary to apply a form of rule utilitarianism.

However, when the nurse or doctor has to consider wider responsibilities to other patients, to the hospital, to the cause of nursing or medical research, to public health, then rule utilitarianism is the more appealing, for health professionals often believe they know how the greatest benefit for the greatest number is to be achieved. The problem of justifying their conceptions of public health, 'justice in healthcare' or 'the common good' is another matter. This also raises questions about how to justify the connection between their clinical and moral authority. Campbell (1984b) developed a strong argument for an historical link between the utilitarian tradition in Britain and its influence on the development of the welfare state, including the National Health Service. Here, the justification for the socialisation of medical services is to achieve justice by maximising benefits for the majority. Attempts to sustain the welfare state on utilitarian grounds alone (whether measured in terms of the costs and benefits of alternative forms of welfare provision, or the cost-effectiveness of different systems or practical services) raise fundamental questions. For example, how utilitarian administrative policies for rationalising the distribution of health services are to be reconciled with patients' needs and rights, and the demands of beneficence and justice in providing urgently needed clinical treatment.

Despite their limitations, teleological and utilitarian theories appear to be commonsensical because they do emphasise certain important things about moral experience. First, goals are important in human life, both in relation to specific actions and also in relation to society's long-term goals; whether they are conceived as built into our very nature as human beings, or chosen by us individually; and they are determined by social contract or grounded in natural law. Secondly, these theories emphasise that consideration of the demands of the specific situation and the consequences of actions have to be taken into account in determining whether they are right and good. Thirdly, they emphasise that actions must have clear objectives and will only succeed if we choose the most appropriate and efficient means to achieve our objectives, and the outcomes can only be evaluated against the objectives we set in advance.

John Rawls on justice

If we leave aside the growing worldwide influence of socialism and Marxism from the time of the 1917 Russian Revolution onwards, the predominant influence in politics and moral philosophy, at least in the English-speaking world during the 20th century, was that of the great English utilitarians. Against this trend, the work of John Rawls is significant.

While there was a brief revival of natural law thinking after World War II, Rawls turns to social contract theory rather than arguments based on 'human nature' to ground his theory of justice. What he shares in common with the classical tradition, however, is a belief in justice as the most fundamental principle of both ethics and law. In his now famous paper 'Justice as fairness' (Rawls 1970) he argues that classical and modern forms of utilitarianism (including 'economic rationalism') are unable to account adequately for the concept of justice:

> The fundamental idea in the concept of justice is that of fairness. It is this aspect of justice for which utilitarianism, in its classical form, is unable to account, but which is represented, even if misleadingly so, in the idea of the social contract.

He suggests that there are two principles, which he implies are intuitively self-evident, that must serve as the basis for the foundational concept of justice as fairness:

> The **first principle** is that each person participating in a practice, or affected by it, has an equal right to the most extensive liberty compatible with a like liberty for all; and the **second** is that inequalities are arbitrary unless it is reasonable to expect that they will work out for every-one's advantage and unless the offices to which they attach, or from which they may be gained, are open to all.

While utilitarianism would appear, on the surface, to be the ideal moral theory to match the expectations of free market capitalist societies, Rawls argues that utilitarianism is unable to provide a satisfactory basis for a modern theory of rights, or the associated theory of justice as it applies to our life and work within either public sector or private institutions. Throughout he discusses justice as a *virtue of institutions* rather than as relating to particular actions or persons. Against the trend towards 'privatisation' of ethics, Rawls' emphasis on the importance of justice as a virtue of institutions has particular relevance to business ethics. As he points out, justice is not the sole virtue of institutions, for these may have a tradition of inefficiency, or be degrading, but not be unjust. Justice, in his terms, is concerned with how institutions 'define offices and powers, and assign rights and duties'. In this sense he emphasises, as we have done, the importance of the concept of power-sharing as the basis for ethics. He suggests that 'essentially justice is the elimination of arbitrary distinctions and the establishment, within the structure of practice, of a proper balance between competing claims'.

His central concern is to formulate an adequate theory of justice that would be relevant to developing a theory of rights for a modern democratic and capitalist society. His approach shares in common with Kant the idea that certain fundamental ethical principles are intuitively self-evident. Unlike Kant, who suggests one should act on one's duty *because one perceives it to be the rational thing to do*, Rawls suggests that one should do one's duty because one consents to the terms on which rights are cashed out in one's society or place of work. In this sense one must be a party to the process of developing ethical policy and rules for the moral community within which one works. He argues against the utilitarian principle of simply maximising happiness for the greatest number that this may well lead to further disadvantaging of the disadvantaged. Minority group rights cannot be adequately protected within the utilitarian theory, except on the basis of an assumed altruism. He

contends that people intuitively understand when things are unfair, and even when they do not fully understand the structures of power in institutions, or the way authority is exercised in relation to their interests, people will, as a matter of common sense, choose the principles of justice, viz:

- equal liberty, that is, the maximum liberty compatible with the liberty of others
- equality of access, or fair and impartial access to social benefits and resources
- equality of opportunity for employment, status and position in society
- and further, that changes in public policy should benefit those most disadvantaged.

Rawls develops a kind of intuitionist social contract theory, but this differs in significant ways from the traditional social contract theorists. Hobbes (Tuck 1996) and Rousseau (Cole 1973) each postulate an original 'state of nature' without law and government, without ethics. They then proceed to develop their theories of law and morality on the basis of what is required to meet the deficiencies of human nature. Rawls, on the other hand, invites us to engage in a 'thought experiment' in which we have to imagine we are ignorant of our actual circumstances, advantages or disadvantages. Without making assumptions about the depravity of human nature (like Hobbes) or the innocence of man in a state of nature (like Rousseau's 'noble savage'), Rawls asks us to imagine how basically self-interested but reasonable people would set ground rules for their moral community. On the basis of his intuitive notions of fundamental common sense and concepts of justice and fairness, he argues that people will seek equality and the maximum degree of liberty that does not conflict with the liberty of others, nor serve to increase inequalities and disadvantage to others. These notions of fairness he believes are basic to any rational moral community.

Thus he argues there has to be a deontological aspect to every functioning system of ethics. As moral communities address the demand to review their core values, apply principles or existing rules to ethical decision-making, and seek to reach agreement about new policies or rules, they have to address the commonalities that underlie human experience or human nature. Given the common features of the human condition, variations of culture, time and place are perhaps much less important than the common needs and requirements for human flourishing.

While utilitarian theories focus on desirable goals and assessment of ethical value by determining our success or failure in attaining our goals, deontological theories emphasise those universal principles and requirements that are basic to determining ground rules in any moral community. They focus attention on the antecedent conditions, the prevailing circumstances, the underlying causes and principles relating to the situation, the pre-existing rules that apply, and the motives and intentions of the moral agent. No adequate moral theory can afford to ignore these factors and to concentrate exclusively on either means and methods, or ends and consequences. However, by the same token, a deontological theory cannot by itself do justice to the other aspects of moral acts.

MORAL THEORY AND THE STRUCTURE OF MORAL ACTION

If it makes sense to analyse the process of moral and ordinary practical decision-making in terms of the stages of assessment, planning, implementation and evaluation (as in the Nursing Process and many other problem-solving methods), then it is perhaps not surprising that we should suggest that moral actions have a recognisable form or rational structure. In classical and medieval thought, philosophers spoke of human acts having an intentional character, that is, that they have a purpose and direction. This purposeful direction of acts is dictated partly by our own purposes and goals, and partly by the nature of the world in which we act, and in which laws of cause and effect operate. Human acts, whether practical acts of doing and making, or mental acts of judgement, have a structure that reflects this functional interdependence of agent and world, and action as the bridge between them.

This structure was analysed by Aristotle in terms of four kinds of conditions – material and formal conditions, goals or ends, and the efficient cause of something happening. Aquinas analysed the intentional structure of acts in terms of the complex relations between causes, means and ends (Gilson 1961):

- *Causes* in this analysis stood for both the objective conditions (or physical causes) prevailing or operative in a given situation and the subjective conditions (including moral principles and personal aims or motives) introduced by the agent.
- *Means* represented possible options or alternative practical courses of action, the personal skills and physical resources available, and the particular means chosen to execute an action plan.
- *Ends* here covered both the practical objectives or goals of the agent as subject, and the actual consequences or effects of an action.

What this kind of analysis suggests (as we indicated in Chapter 2) is that in considering the nature of human action, we have to take account of all three – causes, means and ends – and in reaching a responsible moral decision we would have to take proper account of the relevant causes, means and ends applying to a particular act in a particular situation.

If called upon to justify a particular action we should be able to do so after having made a proper assessment of the prevailing subjective and objective conditions, having made an informed and realistic plan based on available means and resources, and having anticipated correctly the likely consequences of the action taken to attain a goal. Bearing in mind the causes–means–ends structure of intentional and moral acts may enable us to make more sense of different moral theories, by recognising that they each tend to draw attention to particular features of moral judgement and action. It may be too simplistic to suggest that some of the perennial disputes in moral philosophy could be resolved if only the different protagonists would recognise that they each focus on real but partial aspects of the process, and that from a wider perspective we can recognise that their respective approaches are not irreconcilable but complementary. However, there is some truth and plausibility in this view, and we intend to explore it here.

For example, protagonists of natural law theory (namely that moral laws are somehow grounded in nature) focus attention on the dimension of causes – the prevailing objective conditions in the circumstances of human action generally. Situation ethics (or the theory that we should act spontaneously in the light of the demands of the given situation) also interprets principles for action in terms of given circumstances, subjectively interpreted. Intuitionism (or the theory which seeks to ground moral duty in pre-reflexive apprehension of moral principles) appeals to the given structure of reason and subjective experience as providing motives or causes for action.

By contrast, pragmatism (the theory that something is right because it works) focuses attention on the means required – and rational planning based on the calculation of available means and resources – to achieve our aims. Existentialist ethics (Sartre: 'People make themselves by their decisions') also stresses that in seeking to act morally people should not allow their actions to be predetermined by external causes or principles, nor influenced unduly by unpredictable consequences, but 'should act authentically in the given situation'.

Teleological theories of morals focus on ends. If we make assumptions, as Plato and Aristotle did, that there are inherent tendencies in nature and in human beings to seek their fulfilment or some ultimate goal, then the concept of 'end' is being interpreted at both a physical and a metaphysical level. At a more mundane level, utilitarianism grounds judgements of what is good or bad in terms of an assessment of the consequences or effects of an action in the light of our subjective goals and intentions. Actions are to be judged by their results, that is, by their utility in promoting certain personal goals or the end of general human happiness.

In a sense, what each of these types of theories does is to isolate and draw attention to one aspect of the intentional structure of human acts, and then attempt to make this partial perspective normative and definitive for the interpretation of all human action. The seemingly interminable debates among philosophers about the ultimate basis of moral judgements suggests that each of these theories may be true, in the sense that they emphasise some genuine (if partial) aspect of our moral experience; but also that they are false and distort the reality of moral experience, by failing to take account of other complementary perspectives.

We may need to balance emphasis on one aspect of our moral experience with emphasis on other aspects of the whole causes–means–ends structure of moral acts, in order to get a dynamic and three-dimensional picture of the reality (cf. Downie & Calman 1987, Chs 1–4). Figure 13.1 and Table 13.1 illustrate some of the relationships we have summarised here.

MORAL THEORY AND THE GOAL OF SOCIAL CONSENSUS

The range and variety of theories developed to justify moral principles, the most important and abiding of which have been outlined above, may leave the impression that there can be no real moral agreement or that it is a matter of indifference which theory one chooses. This would be to misunderstand the kind of impulse that has led to the formulation of these theories.

What all these theories have in common is a belief that rational grounds for our moral principles can and must be found, that public agreement and objective decision-making in law and the moral life are important, and cannot be based on whim and arbitrary judgement. Each of the theories produces powerful arguments for the rationality of moral principles, whether we see the principles of respect for persons, justice and beneficence as being based on natural law, the demands of love, intuition, the requirements for the pursuit and achievement of happiness or the concept of duty. Each of these theories marshals certain kinds of evidence taken from our moral experience and attempts to generalise its significance for an understanding of the nature of fundamental principles. It is tempting to say that each of these theories represents a complementary aspect of moral

Prior causes and conditions Principles and obligations	D = DETERMINE PROBLEM the relevant facts, and E = ETHICAL PRINCIPLES	• Divine command theory • Natural law theory • Act or rule deontology • Intuitionist theory
Available means, methods Personnel and resources	C = CONSIDER OPTIONS for decision/action I = IDENTIFY OUTCOMES	• Ethical pragmatism • Virtue ethics • Situation ethics • Agapeistic ethics • Emotivist ethics
Ends or goals of action Outcome or consequences	D = DECIDE ACTION PLAN with clear goals, and E = EVALUATE RESULTS	• Teleological ethics • Eudaimonist ethics • Act/rule utilitarianism • Egoistic hedonism

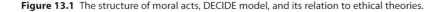

Figure 13.1 The structure of moral acts, DECIDE model, and its relation to ethical theories.

Table 13.1 How ethical theories relate to aspects of the structure of moral acts

Aspect of action	Type of moral theory	Relates to:
Prior conditions Objective conditions	*Deontological and natural law* e.g. natural law theory (Aristotle, Aquinas)	*Principles, rules and duties* Rights derived from reflection on human nature and needs
Subjective conditions	e.g. rational intuitionism (Kant and Rawls)	Principles deduced from the requirements for a rational ethic
Means and methods Objective conditions	*Pragmatic and virtue-based* e.g. pragmatism (Dewey, James, Marx)	*Instruments, action, agent* Trial and error serve to define what is right/wrong, good/bad
Subjective conditions	e.g. virtue ethics (Macintyre, Plato, Aristotle)	The moral character of the agent seen as crucial in ethics
Ends/outcomes Objective conditions	*Teleological and utilitarian* e.g. teleological eudaimonism (Aristotle, Aquinas)	*Costs/benefits, outcomes* The ultimate end of human life is happiness/human fulfilment
Subjective conditions	e.g. utilitarianism and hedonism (Bentham and Mill)	All human action is driven by self-interest or pleasure

experience and that, while each has some value, it is limited to the extent that it is generalised as a basis for the interpretation of all or every aspect of human moral life. However, there are some irreconcilable aspects of these theories and we cannot rest in such an embracing 'ecumenical' view.

We cannot do without rules or principles to organise our lives and moral experience. Society cannot function without some kind of moral consensus on which to base its social institutions. Law and order ultimately rest on government by consent, even under tyranny. No tyrant can succeed in isolation: he has to be able to persuade others to support his cause. Choice between might and right, between government by force and government by consent, if there is to be a choice, has to be based on reasoned argument. If we surrender our faith in reasoned argument, public debate and the possibility of social agreement, then we are lost to the forces of irrationalism, prejudice and anarchy.

The only way to arrive at social consensus is by reasoning together – whether as a whole society or as a medical care team at ward level (Veatch 1981, Boyd et al 1986). While we may be born into already structured moral communities, or take up employment in organisations with a defined ethical culture and their own rules and regulations for professional conduct, nevertheless no such communities are static or cannot be changed. A living, healthy and responsible moral community has to be constantly recreated, by the review, reform or reaffirmation of its values by its members. If the values and rules of a moral community are imposed on people, they do not 'own' them and will almost certainly either disregard them or rebel against them. Negotiating and renegotiating

the scope and nature of the boundaries of the moral community is at the heart of its life, as it is the life-blood of real democracy. There is nothing to be afraid of in this process, or in the need for change. On the contrary, there is more to fear from moral communities that are not real communities, where rules have to be imposed and are not owned by members, communities which are 'stuck in a time warp', dead, unable to either grow or adapt to changing circumstances, or changing roles and responsibilities.

In practice, day-to-day decision-making does not often involve discussion at this level of moral theory. We operate, for the most part, within an existing social consensus in our moral community, whatever it is. We do not generally question the basis of fundamental moral principles – unless challenged to do so.

Perhaps the first time we begin to think critically about our moral beliefs is when we leave home and go to school and encounter people with different cultural or religious backgrounds. Also when we enter training for adult and professional life we are introduced to a complex set of professional and institutional values which may challenge personal and moral beliefs based on family upbringing, education and conviction. When we encounter painful conflicts of duty in professional life (e.g. between the duty to keep secrets and the duty to share information for the benefit of patients, or to choose between the rights of the mother and the father, or to preserve life or to alleviate pain), we are forced to examine the rational basis for our moral beliefs, and other people may demand that we justify them.

When we move from junior to administrative responsibilities in large institutions we have to find criteria in terms of which to choose between the rules we use for dealing with individuals and the rules applicable to large groups of people. When we move out into public life – representing our colleagues in a union or taking part in local government or national politics – we have to begin to think through the connections between morality and law, ethics and politics.

In all these situations, if we think critically and systematically about things, aspects of moral theory become relevant. We do not have to be philosophers to be concerned about these questions. We are drawn to think philosophically if we take seriously the quest for objectivity in ethical and legal debate, and this means adducing the best possible reasons and evidence we can for believing in moral principles at all. The moral theories we have outlined are only a guide to the way some great philosophers have thought about these questions in the past. We may learn a great deal from their wisdom, but we should not be seduced into thinking that they can do our thinking for us, or give us packaged 'answers' to the ultimate questions in life.

Reaching ultimate moral agreement may be an unobtainable goal but it is one of the grandest ambitions and most noble ideals of human beings. If it means agreement in the three senses we discussed earlier, agreement between what we profess and what we do, rational consensus or agreement among people about the ultimate goals and principles of social life, and agreement between our principles and the ultimate demands implicit in the structures and dynamics of being, then moral agreement is a noble goal indeed. It is a symbol of a fully mature, fully human and genuinely humane society.

 ## further reading

Free will and determinism

Augustine St, 354–430 AD (tr Pontifex M) 1955 The problem of free choice. Newman Press, Westminster, MD

Downie R S, Calman K 1987 Healthy respect. Faber, London, Chs 1–4

Hare R M 1963 Freedom and reason. Oxford University Press, Oxford, Ch 4

Montefiore A 1958 A modern introduction to moral philosophy. Routledge & Kegan Paul, London, Ch 12

Justification of our moral principles

Dancy J 1993 Moral reasons. Blackwells, Oxford

Hare R M 1952 The language of morals (reprinted 1964). Clarendon Press, Oxford, Ch 4

Korsgaard C M, Cohen G A 1996 The sources of normativity. Cambridge University Press, Cambridge

Toulmin S 1958 The place of reason in ethics. Cambridge University Press, Cambridge, Chs 11–14

General references on moral philosophy or ethical theory

Foot P 1967 Theories of ethics. Oxford University Press, Oxford

Hare R M 1981 Moral thinking: its levels, methods and point. Oxford University Press, Oxford

Johnson O A (ed) 1994 Ethics: Selections from classical & contemporary writers, 7th edn. Harcourt Brace, New York

Macintyre A 1967 A short history of ethics. Routledge & Kegan Paul, London

Maritain J 1963 Moral philosophy. Bles, London

Rachels J 1993 The elements of moral philosophy, 2nd edn. McGraw Hill, New York

Raphael D D 1980 Moral philosophy. Oxford University Press, Oxford

Deontological theories (and divine command theories)

Frankena W 1973 Ethics, 2nd edn. Prentice Hall, Englewood Cliffs, NJ

Maritain J 1963 Moral philosophy. Geoffrey Bles, London

Paton H J (tr) 1969 The moral law: Kant's groundwork of the metaphysic of morals. Hutchinson, London (reprinted 1991)

Ross D 1969 Kant's ethical theory. Oxford University Press, Oxford

Ross W D 1930 The right and the good. Oxford University Press, Oxford

Natural law theories

D'Entreves A P 1951 Natural law: an introduction to legal philosophy. Hutchinson, London

Finnis J M 1999 Natural law and natural rights. Oxford University Press, Oxford

Gilson E (tr Shook L K) 1994 The Christian philosophy of St Thomas Aquinas. University of Notre Dame Press, Notre Dame, IN

Maritain J 1943 The rights of man and natural law. C Scribner's Sons, New York

Wild J 1953 Plato's modern enemies and the theory of natural law. University of Chicago Press, Chicago

Intuitionist ethics

Broad C D 1930 Five types of ethical theory. Routledge & Kegan Paul, London

Carritt E F 1928 Theory of morals. Oxford University Press, Oxford

Moore G E 1962 Principia ethica, revised edn. Cambridge University Press, Cambridge, Chs 1, 3

Moore G E 1966 Ethics, 2nd edn. Oxford University Press, Oxford

Virtue ethics and ethics of prudence

Crisp R, Slote M 1997 Virtue ethics. Oxford University Press, Oxford

Hursthouse R 1999 On virtue ethics. Oxford University Press, Oxford

Macintyre A 1981 After virtue, 2nd edn. Notre Dame University Press, Notre Dame, IN

Nelson D M 1992 Priority of prudence: virtue and natural law. Pennsylvania State University, University Park, PA

Pieper J 1959 Prudence: the first cardinal virtue. Faber, London

Agapeistic or caring ethics theories

Baier A C 1995 Moral prejudices. Harvard University Press, Cambridge, MA

Bowden P 1997 Caring: gender sensitive ethics. Routledge, London

Brown J, Kitson A, McKnight T J 1992 Challenges in caring: explorations in nursing and ethics. Chapman & Hall, London

Cunningham R L 1970 Situationism and the new morality. Appleton-Century-Crofts, New York

Fletcher J 1979 Situation ethics. SCM Press, London

Frankena W K 1964 Love and principle in Christian ethics. In: Plantinga A (ed) Faith and philosophy. Eerdmans, Grand Rapids, MI

Ramsey P 1983 Deeds and rules in Christian ethics. University of America Press, New York

Teleological or utilitarian theories

Campbell A V, Charlesworth M, Gillett G, Jones D G 1997 Medical ethics. Oxford University Press, Oxford

Foot P 1967 Theories of ethics. Oxford University Press, Oxford

Gillon R 1987 Philosophical medical ethics. Wiley, Chichester, Ch 4

Smart J J C, Williams B 1973 Utilitarianism for and against. Cambridge University Press, Cambridge

References

Abbey R 2000 Charles Taylor. Acumen Publishing, Teddington

Abbot T K (tr) 1909 Kant I (1724–1804): Critique of pure practical reason. Everyman, Dent, London

Acheson Report 1988 Public health in England: Report of the Acheson Committee of Inquiry into the future development of the public health function (Cm 289). HMSO, London

Alcohol Concern 2004 Factsheet: Alcohol advertising. Alcohol Concern, London

Aldridge D 1998 Suicide: the tragedy of hopelessness. Jessica Kingsley, London

Allan P, Jolley M 1982 Nursing, midwifery and health visiting, since 1900. Faber & Faber, London

Allsopp J 1996 Health policy and the National Health Service: towards 2000. Longmans, London

American Accounting Association 1975 Report of the Committee on Accounting for Social Performance. The Accounting Review

American Hospital Association 1973/1992(revised) A patient's bill of rights. American Hospital Association, Chicago

American Nurses Association 2001 Codes of ethics for nurses with interpretive statements. American Nurses Publishing, Washington DC

Anon 2005 Singapore National Healthcare Group Health Professionals' website. Available at: http://www. healthprofessionals.nhg.com.sg/nursing/thoh.html

Appleby J 1999 Government funding of the UK National Health Service: what does the national record reveal? Journal of Health Service Research Policy 4:79–89

Appleby J, Coote A 2002 Five year health check: a review of government health policy, 1997–2002. King's Fund, London

Appleby J, Little B, Tanade W, Robinson R, Smit H P 1992 Implementing the reforms: a second national survey of general managers: project paper 7. National Association of Health Authorities and Trusts, Birmingham

Arendt H 1967 The origins of totalitarianism, 3rd edn. World Publishing, London

Aristotle (384–322 BC) (Thomson J A K, tr) 1976 Nicomachean ethics. In: The ethics of Aristotle, revised edn. Penguin Books, Harmondsworth

Armstrong A H 1957 An introduction to ancient philosophy. Methuen, London, ch XII

ASH 2004 Factsheet no:16. The economics of tobacco. Action on Smoking and Health

Ashford D E 1986 The emergence of the welfare states. Blackwells, Oxford

Atkins S, Murphy K 1994 Reflective practice. Nursing Standard 8(39):49–55

Audi R (ed) 1995 The Cambridge dictionary of philosophy. Cambridge University Press, Cambridge

Augustine (354–430 AD) (Healey J, tr) 1968 The city of God. J M Dent, London

Augustine (354–430 AD) (Pontifex M, tr) 1955 The problem of free choice. Newman Press, Westminster

Augustine (354–430 AD) (Tasker R V G, ed) 1967 The city of God (2 vols). Everyman Library, Dent, London

Augustine (354–430 AD) 1984 Homily on the first epistle of John, 7, viii. In: Clark M (tr) Augustine of Hippo, selected writings. Paulist Press, New York

Australian Nursing Council, Royal College of Nursing, Australia, Australian Nursing Federation 2002 Code of ethics for nurses in Australia. ANC, RCNA, ANF, Canberra

Ayer A J 1958 Language, truth and logic. Gollancz, London

Bacon F (1561–1626) 1996 Meditationes sacrae, 'Of heresies'. Kessinger Publishing, Kila, MT

BACP 2002 Ethical framework for good practice in counselling and psychotherapy. British Association for Counselling and Psychotherapy, London

Baggott R 2004 Health and healthcare in Britain, 3rd edn. Palgrave Macmillan, Basingstoke

Baier A C 1995 Moral prejudices: essays on ethics. Harvard University Press, Cambridge, MA

Baker N, Urquhart J 1987 The balance of care for adults with a mental handicap in Scotland. ISD Publications, Edinburgh

Balzer-Riley J, Smith S 1996 Communication in nursing. Mosby, St Louis, MO

Baric L 1974 Acquisition of the smoking habit and the model of smokers' careers. Journal of the Institute of Health Education 12(1):9–18

Baric L 1982 Measuring family competence in the health maintenance and health education of children. World Health Organization, Copenhagen

Barnhart R K (ed) 1988 Chambers dictionary of etymology. Chambers Harrap, New York

Barr H 2003a Assuring the quality of inter-professional education for health and social care. CAIPE Bulletin No 22

Barr H 2003b Undergraduate inter-professional education. Education Committee Discussion Document, Number 0.1, General Medical Council, London (Includes annotated list of research references)

Barrett R 1998 Liberating the corporate soul: building a visionary organisation. Butterworth-Heinemann, Oxford

BASW 2003 Code of ethics for social work. British Association of Social Workers (BASW), Birmingham

Bayles M D 1989 Professional ethics, 2nd edn. Wadsworth Publishing, Belmont, CA

Beauchamp T, Bowie N E 1997/2003 Ethical theory and business. Prentice Hall, Oxford

Beauchamp T L, Childress J F 1994 Principles of biomedical ethics, 4th edn. Oxford University Press, Oxford

Beauchamp T L, Childress J F 2001/2004 Principles of biomedical ethics, 5th edn (revised edn 2004). Oxford University Press, Oxford

Beauchamp T, Steinbock B 1999 New ethics for the public's health. Oxford University Press, Oxford

Beauchamp T, Veatch R 1996 Ethical issues in death and dying. Prentice Hall, New York

Beck L W (tr) 1949 Kant I (1724–1804) Kant's critique of practical reason and other writings in moral philosophy. Chicago University Press, Chicago

Becker E 1997 The denial of death. Collier Macmillan, London

Becker H S 1963 Outsiders, studies in the sociology of deviance. Free Press of Glencoe, New York

Benner P 1984 From novice to expert: excellence and power in clinical nursing practice. Addison-Wesley, Menlo Park, CA

Benner P, Wrubel J 1989 The primacy of caring: stress and coping in health and illness. Addison Wesley, New York

Bennett A E (ed) 1976 Communication between doctors and patients. Nuffield Provincial Hospitals Trust, London

Benson S, Carr P 1994 The care assistant's guide to working with elderly mentally infirm people. Hawker, London

Bentham J 1830 The principles of morals and legislation, London (see discussion in Smart J J, Williams B 1973 Utilitarianism for and against. Cambridge University Press, Cambridge)

Bentham J (Burns J A, Hart H L A, eds) 1970 An introduction to the principles of morals and legislation (first published in 1789, revised in 1822). Athlone Press, London

Benzeval M, Judge K, Shouls S 2001 Understanding the relationship between income and health: how much can be gleaned from cross-sectional data. Social Policy and Administration 35:376–396

Berlin I 1969 Four essays on liberty. Oxford University Press, Oxford

Berne E 1966 The games people play. Deutsch, London

Berne E 1973 What do you say after hello? The psychology of human destiny. Bantam Books, New York

Beveridge W 1942 Report on the Committee on Social Insurance and Allied Services. Command paper no. 6404. HMSO, London

Bible (The Jerusalem Bible) 1966 Book of Job. Darton, Longman & Todd, London

Bible (The Jerusalem Bible) 1966 Deuteronomy. Darton, Longman & Todd, London

Bible (The Jerusalem Bible) 1966 Leviticus. Darton, Longman & Todd, London

Bolam v. Friern Barnet Hospital Management Committee 1957. Weekly Law Reports 1 WLR 583

Boman T 1960 Hebrew thought compared with Greek. SCM Press, London

Bond J, Bond S 1994 Sociology and health care: an introduction for nurses and other health care professionals, 2nd edn. Churchill Livingstone, Edinburgh

Bonhoeffer D 1955 Ethics. SCM Press, London

Boudreau F, Lambert P 1993 Compulsory community treatment? The collision of views and complexities involved: is it the 'best possible alternative'? Canadian Journal of Mental Health 2(1):79–96

Bowden P 1997 Caring: gender-sensitive ethics. Routledge, London

Bowlby J 1979 The making and breaking of affectional bonds. Tavistock, London

Boyd K M 1979 The ethics of resource allocation in health care. Edinburgh University Press, Edinburgh

Boyd K M, Callaghan B, Shotter E 1986 Introduction. In: Life before death. SPCK, London

Boyd K M, Higgs R, Pinching A J 1997 The new dictionary of medical ethics. BMJ Publishing, London

Bradley J C, Edinberg M A 1990 Communication in a nursing context. Appleton & Lange, California

Brahams D, Brahams M 1983 The Arthur case – a proposal for legislation. Journal of Medical Ethics 9:12–15

Branmer L M 1993 The helping relationship, processes and skills. Allyn & Bacon, Boston

Braun J V, Lipson S 1993 Toward a restraint-free environment. Health Professionals' Press, Baltimore, MD

Bristol Royal Infirmary Inquiry 2001 Learning from Bristol: the report of the public inquiry into children's heart surgery at the Bristol Royal Infirmary 1984–1995. Command Paper: CM 5207. TSO, London

British Association of Social Workers 1971 Discussion Paper No 1: Confidentiality in social work. BASW, London

British Association of Social Workers 1996 The code of ethics for social workers. BASW, London

Broad C D 1930 Five types of ethical theory. Routledge & Kegan Paul, London

Broekmans S, Evers G C M et al 2003 Evidence of negative attitudes of patients, nurses and physicians for preparing a campaign to improve pain treatment with opioids in Belgium. Centre for Health Services and Nursing Research, Catholic University of Leuven, Belgium

Brown J, Kitson A, McKnight T J 1992 Challenges in caring: explorations in nursing and ethics. Chapman & Hall, London

Browne A, Carpenter C, Cooledge C et al 1995 Bridging the professions: an integrated and interdisciplinary approach to teaching health care ethics. Academic Medicine 70(11):1002–1005

Bruce W 1994 Ethical people are productive people. Public Productivity and Management Review 17(3):241–252

Bruyn S T 1987 The field of social investment. Cambridge University Press, Cambridge

Buchanan A E, Brock D W 1989 Deciding for others: the ethics of surrogate decision-making. Cambridge University Press, Cambridge.

Bullough V L, Bullough B 1984 History, trends and politics of nursing. Appleton-Century-Crofts, Norwalk, CT

Bulman S, Schutz S (eds) 2004 Reflective practice on nursing: the growth of the professional practitioner, 3rd edn. Blackwell, Oxford

Burdekin B, Guilfoyle M, Hall D (eds) 1993 Human rights and mental illness, 'Burdekin report'. Report of the National enquiry into the human rights of people with mental illness. Australian Government Publishing Service (AGPS), Canberra, ACT

Burnard P, Morrison P 1994 Nursing research in action: developing basic skills. Macmillan, Basingstoke

Burns N, Grove S K 1999 Understanding nursing research. WB Saunders, Philadelphia

Butler, Bishop J (1970) Sermons, 'On Conscience', iii. In: Roberts T A (ed) Fifteen sermons preached at the Rolls Chapel. SPCK, London

Caleb R 2005 On the effectiveness of student counselling (unpublished dissertation). Brunel University Counselling Service, Brunel University, Uxbridge

Campbell A V 1978 Medicine, health and justice: the problem of priorities. Churchill Livingstone, Edinburgh

Campbell A V 1984a Moderated love: a theology of professional care. SPCK, London

Campbell A V 1984b Moral dilemmas in medicine, 2nd edn. Churchill Livingstone, Edinburgh

Campbell A V 1985 Paid to care. SPCK, London

Campbell A V 1995 Health as liberation. Pilgrim Press, Cleveland, OH

Campbell A V 2004 The wounded healer (Offprint). Nursing Studies, The University of Edinburgh

Campbell A V, Higgs R 1982 In that case. Darton, Longman & Todd, London

Campbell A V, Charlesworth M, Gillet G, Jones G 1997 Medical ethics. Oxford University Press, Oxford

Canadian Nurses Association 2002 Code of ethics for registered nurses. CAN, Ottawa

Caplan A H, Callahan D 1981 Ethics in hard times. Hastings Center Series on Ethics, Hastings on Hudson, USA

CARE 2003 Abortion Statistics Factsheet: Abortion statistics summary, England and Wales. CARE, London

Carmichael S 1969 Stokeley Carmichael's address to the World Council of Churches Consultation on Racism. Notting Hill, London

Carritt E F 1928 Theory of morals. Oxford University Press, Oxford

Carroll L 1954 Alice's Adventures in wonderland, through the looking glass and other writings, Collins, London, ch 6

Chandola T, Bartely M Sacker A, Jenkinson C, Marmot M 2003 Health selection in the Whitehall II Study, UK. Social Science and Medicine 56:2059–2072

Charlesworth M 1993 Bioethics in a liberal society. Cambridge University Press, Cambridge

Chesterton G K 1927 The flag of the world. In: Orthodoxy. John Lane, Bodley Head, London, ch 5

Chesterton G K (1874–1936) 2000 Introduction to the Book of Job. In: The collected works of GK Chesterton. Ignatius Press, San Francisco

CJSWDC (Thompson I) 2005 Youth justice evaluation project resources pack

Clark B 1978 Whose life is it anyway? Amber Lane Press, Oxford

Clark C C 1986 Wellness nursing: concepts, theory, research and practice. Springer, New York

Clark M (tr) 1984 Augustine of Hippo, selected writings. Paulist Press, New York

Clement G 1996 Care, autonomy and justice: feminism and the ethic of care. Westview Press, Boulder, CO

Clough A H 1951 The poems of Arthur Hugh Clough (Lowry H F, Norrington A L P, Mulhauser F L, eds). Clarendon Press, Oxford

Cochrane A L 1971 Effectiveness and efficiency: random reflections on health services. Nuffield Provincial Hospitals Trust, London

COHSE 1977 The management of violent or potentially violent patients. Confederation of Health Service Employees, London

Cole G D H (tr) 1973 Jean Jacques Rousseau (1717–1778) The social contract and other discourses (New edition, revised and augmented by J H Brumfitt & J C Hall). Dent, London

Collins R 1994 Four sociological traditions. Oxford University Press, Oxford

Collison P 1995 The democratic solution. In: Murley R (ed) Patients or customers: are the NHS reforms working? Office for Public Management, London

Colyer H, Karmath P 1997 Evidence-based practice. A philosophical and political analysis: some matters for consideration by professional practitioners. Journal of Advanced Nursing 29:188–193

Commission for Health Improvement 2000 Investigation into: North Lakeland Trust: report to the Secretary of State for Health, November 2000. HMSO, London

Copp L A 1981 Care of the ageing. Churchill Livingstone, Edinburgh

Coubrough A (tr) 1930 Fayol, Industrial and general administration. Geneva International Institute

Cough A H 1974 The latest decalogue. In: Mulhauser F L (ed) Poems. Oxford University Press, Oxford

Couglan P B 1993 Facing Alzheimer's: family care givers speak. Ballantine, New York

Council of Europe 1950/1966 European Convention on Human Rights. Council of Europe, Strasbourg

Council of Europe 1997 Convention for the protection of human rights and dignity of the human being with regard to the application of biology and medicine: Convention on Human Rights and Biomedicine (Oviedo, 4.IV.1997), European Treaty Series – No 164. Council of Europe, Strasbourg

Council of Europe 1999 Report on the protection of the human rights and dignity of the terminally ill or dying. Biomedical Ethics 4(1)

Cowan M (tr) 1955 Nietzsche F (1844–1900) Beyond good and evil. Henry Regnery, Chicago

Cowen D 1961 The foundations of freedom. Oxford University Press, Oxford

Crayford T, Hooper R, Evans S 1997 Death rates of characters in soap operas on British television: is a government health warning required? British Medical Journal 315:1649–1652

Creek J 1997 Occupational therapy and mental health. Churchill Livingstone, Edinburgh

Crisp R, Slote M 1997 Virtue ethics. Oxford University Press, Oxford

Crittenden P 1993 Learning to be moral: philosophical thoughts about moral development. Humanities Press International, London

Cummings J 1994 Care services and priority setting: the New Zealand experience. Health Policy 29:41–60

Curtin L, Flaherty M J 1982 Nursing ethics: theories and pragmatics. Robert J Brady, Bowie, MD

Dancy J 1993 Moral reasons. Blackwells, Oxford

D'Arcy E 1961 Conscience and its right to freedom. Sheed and Ward, London

D'Arcy M 1962 The heart and mind of love. Collins, London

Davey B, Popay J 1992 Dilemmas in health care. Open University Press, London

Davies B 2000 Philosophy of religion. Oxford University Press, Oxford

Davies C M 1995 Competence versus care? Gender and caring work revisited. Acta Sociologica 38:17–31

Davies C M 1995 Gender and the professional predicament in nursing. Open University, Buckingham

Davies C M 2001 Lay involvement in professional regulation: a study of public appointment-holders in the health field. Open University, Milton Keynes

Davis A J, Aroskar M A 1983 Ethical dilemmas and nursing practice, 2nd edn. Appleton-Century-Crofts, Norwalk, CT

Day P, Klein R 1997 Steering but not rowing: the transformation of the NHS. Policy Press, Bristol

De Beauvoir S 1988 The second sex. Picador, London

De Beauvoir S 1991 The ethics of ambiguity. Carol Publishing, New York

DeBono E 1990 I am right – you are wrong. Penguin Books, Harmondsworth, London

D'Entreves A P 1951 Natural law: an introduction to legal philosophy. Hutchinson, London

Dewar S 2003 Government and the NHS: time for a new relationship. King's Fund, London

DFES 2004 Every child matters. Department for Education and Skills, TSO, London

DHEW 1978 (Belmont Report) Protection of human subjects of biomedical and behavioral research. Federal Register 43 (53). US Departments of Health, Education and Welfare, Washington, DC

DHH & CS 1993 Communicable diseases intelligence. Department of Health, Housing and Community Services, Australian Government Publication Services, Canberra

DHSS 1976 Prevention and health – everybody's business. HMSO, London

DHSS 1979 On the best use and management of financial and management resources of the NHS: Royal Commission Report (Cmnd 7615). DHSS, London

DHSS 1980 Inequalities in health: report of a commission of enquiry into the National Health Service (Chairman: Sir Douglas Black). DHSS, London

DHSS 1983 NHS management inquiry (Griffiths Report). HMSO, London

Dingwall R, Rafferty A M, Webster C 1988 An introduction to the social history of nursing. Routledge, London

Dixon A, Mossialos E 2001 Funding healthcare in Europe: recent experiences. King's Fund, London

DoH (Department of Health) 1991 Health of the nation. HMSO, London

DoH (Department of Health) 1994 Supporting research and development in the NHS (Culyer Report). HMSO, London

DoH (Department of Health) 1997 The new NHS: modern, dependable (White Paper; Cm 3807). HMSO, London

DoH (Department of Health) 1999 Saving lives: our healthier nation (White Paper; Cm 4386). DoH, London

DoH (Department of Health) 2000a Caring about carers: a national strategy for carers, 2nd edn. TSO, London

DoH (Department of Health) 2000b Research and development for a first class service: R&D funding for the new NHS. HMSO, London

DoH (Department of Health) 2001a The essence of care: patient-focused bench-marking for healthcare practitioners. Department of Health, London

DoH (Department of Health) 2001b Report of the CFS/ME Working Group: report of the Chief Medical Officer of an Independent Working Group. Department of Health, London

DoH (Department of Health) 2001c Working together, learning together: a framework for lifelong learning in the NHS. Department of Health, London

DoH (Department of Health) 2001d Research governance framework for health and social services. Department of Health, London

DoH (Department of Health) 2001e Treatment choice in psychological therapies and counselling: evidence based clinical practice guideline. Department of Health, London

DoH (Department of Health) 2001f (Milburn) Health priorities for the new government, Ministerial Statement, 13 June 2001. Department of Health, London

DoH (Department of Health) 2002 (Milburn) Public's priorities are NHS plan priorities, Ministerial Statement, 19 February 2002. Department of Health, London (Ref No: 2002/0091)

DoH (Department of Health) 2003 The new NHS pay system: an overview (Agenda for Change). Department of Health, London

DoH (Department of Health) 2005 NHS Plan: technical supplement on target setting (England & Wales). Department of Health. Online. Available: www.dh.gov.uk/PublicationsAndStatistics/

Doll R, Petor R, Boreham J, Sutherland I 2004 Mortality in relation to smoking: 50 years' observations on male British doctors. British Medical Journal 328:1519

Donkin A, Goldblatt P, Lynch K 2002 Inequalities in life expectancy by social class. Health Statistics Quarterly 15:5–15

Donne J (1572–1631) (Sparrow J, ed) 1923 Devotions on emergent occasions. Cambridge University Press, Cambridge

Dorn N, Nortoft B 1982 Health careers. Institute for the Study of Drug Dependence, London

Dostoevsky F (1821–1881) (Garnett C, tr) 1927/1957 The brothers Karamazov. Dent, London

Downie R S 1971/1987 Roles and values: an introduction to social ethics. Methuen, London

Downie R S, Calman K 1987 Healthy respect. Faber, London, chs 1–4

Downie R, Tannahill C, Tannahill A 1996 Health promotion: models and values. Oxford University Press, Oxford

Downie R S, Macnaughton J, Randall F 2000 Clinical judgement: evidence in practice. Oxford University Press, Oxford

Dowswell G, Harrison S, Wright J 2002 The early days of primary care groups: general practitioner perceptions. Health and Social Care in the Community 10:46–54

Doyle D (ed) 1984 Palliative care: the management of far advanced illness. Croom Helm, London, ch 22

Doyle D (ed) 1994 Domiciliary palliative care. Oxford University Press, Oxford

Draper P, Popay J 1980 Medical charities, prevention and the media. British Medical Journal 280:110

Dryden W, Charles-Edwards D, Woolfe R 1989 Handbook of counselling in Britain. Routledge & Kegan Paul, London

Duffy K 2004 Failing students. NMC, London

Durham M 1997 Conjuring trick, no magic pill for the NHS. The Observer, 14 December 1997

Durkheim E 1952 Suicide: a study in sociology. Routledge & Kegan Paul, London

Dworkin R 1977 Taking rights seriously. Harvard University Press, Cambridge, MA

Eadie H A 1975 The helping personality. CONTACT 49(Summer)

Eaton L 2002 Government propose licensing system for doctors. British Medical Journal 324:1235

Eby M 2000 The challenges of being accountable. In: Brechin A, Brown H, Eby M (eds) Critical practice in health and social care. Sage, London

Edward C, Preece E C 1999 Shared teaching in health care ethics: a report on the beginning of an idea. Nursing Ethics 6(4):299–307

Egan G 1986 The skilled helper, 3rd edn. Brooks/Cole, Monterey, CA

Eggland E T, Heineman D S 1994 Nursing documentation: Charting, recording and reporting. JB Lippincott, Philadelphia

Eide A 1992 Universal declaration of human rights: a commentary. Oxford University Press, Oxford

Eliot T S 1944 Four quartets. Faber & Faber, London

Eliot T S 1969 The complete poems and plays of T.S. Eliot. Faber, London

Emmet D 1966 Rules, roles and relations. Macmillan, London

Enthoven A 1978 Consumer-choice health plan: a national health insurance proposal based on regulated competition in the private sector. New England Journal of Medicine 298:709–720

Enthoven A 1985 Reflections on the management of the National Health Service. Nuffield Provincial Hospitals Trust, London

Ernst & Young 1992 The manager's handbook. Ernst & Young, London

Erwin E 1978 Behavior therapy: scientific, philosophical and moral foundations. Cambridge University Press, Cambridge

Etzioni A 1993 The spirit of community. Random House, New York

Ewles L, Simnett I 1985 Promoting health: a practical guide to health education. Wiley, Chichester

Fagles R, Knox B (tr) 1982 Sophocles' Antigone. In: Three Theban plays: Antigone, Oedipus the King and Oedipus at Colonus. Allen Lane, London

Fairfield G, Hunter D, Mechanic D, Rosleff F 1997 Implications of managed care for health systems, clinicians and patients. British Medical Journal 314:1895–1898

Faulkner A 1984 Communication. Churchill Livingstone, Edinburgh

Feacham R, Sekhri N, White K 2002 Getting more for their dollar: a comparison of the NHS with California's Kaiser Permanente. British Medical Journal 321:135–143

Feifel H (ed) 1977 New meanings of death. McGraw Hill, New York

Feifel H, Hanson S, Jones R 1967 Physicians consider death. Proceedings of the American Psychological Association 201–202

Ferlie E, Pettigrew A, Ashburner L, Fitzgerald L 1996 The new public management in action. OUP, Oxford

Ferriman A 2000 Health spending in the UK to rise to 7.6% of GDP. British Medical Journal 320:889

Finnis J M 1980/1999(revised edn) Natural law and natural rights. Oxford University Press, Oxford

Fire Statistics, United Kingdom, 2002 Office of the Deputy Prime Minister, London, April 2004

Fletcher C 1967 Situation ethics: the new morality. SCM Press, London

Fletcher C M 1971 Communication in medicine. Nuffield Provincial Hospitals Trust, London

Fletcher J 1979a Situation ethics. SCM Press, London

Fletcher J 1979b Humanhood: essays in biomedical ethics. Prometheus Books, New York

Foot P 1967 Theories of ethics. Oxford University Press, Oxford

Frankena W K 1964 Love and principle in Christian ethics. In: Plantinga A (ed) Faith and philosophy. Eerdmans, Grand Rapids, MI

Frankena W K 1973 Ethics, 2nd edn. Prentice-Hall, Englewood Cliffs, NJ

Freeman T, Latham L, Walshe K, Spurgeon P, Wallace L 1999 The early development of clinical governance: a survey of NHS trusts in the South West Region. Health Services Management Centre, Birmingham

Freidson E 1970 Profession of medicine. Dodd Mead, New York

Freidson E 1994 Professionalism reborn: theory, prophecy, and policy. Cambridge Polity Press, Cambridge

Freidson E 2001 Professionalism: the third logic. London Polity Press, London

Freud S 1927/1961 Some psychical consequences of the anatomical distinction between the sexes. In: Strachey J (tr and ed) The Standard Edition of the Complete psychological works of Sigmund Freud, vol XIX. Hogarth, London, p 257–258

Gallagher A 1995 Medical and nursing ethics: never the twain? Nursing Ethics 2(2):95–101

George S, Weimerskirch A 1994 Total quality management (The Portable MBA Series). John Wiley, New York

Ghaye T, Lillyman S 2000 Reflection: principles and practice for healthcare professionals. Mark Allen Books, Dinton

Giddens A 1984 The constitution of society. Polity, Oxford

Gilby T 1964 St Thomas Aquinas – philosophical texts. Oxford University Press, London

Gill R 1985 A textbook of Christian ethics. T & T Clark, Edinburgh

Gill R (ed) 2001 The Cambridge companion to Christian ethics. Cambridge University Press, Cambridge

Gilligan C 1977 In a different voice: women's conceptions of self and morality. Harvard Education Review 47:481

Gilligan C 1982/1993 In a different voice: psychological theory and women's development. Harvard University Press, Cambridge, MA

Gillon R 1981 (editorial) Medical ethics and medical education. Journal of Medical Education 7:171–172

Gillon R 1987 Philosophical medical ethics. Wiley, Chichester

Gilson E 1961 The Christian philosophy of St Thomas Aquinas. Victor Gollancz, London

Gilson E 1969 The Christian philosophy of St Augustine. Victor Gollancz, London

Gilson E (Shook L K, tr) 1994 The Christian philosophy of St Thomas Aquinas. University of Notre Dame Press, Notre Dame, IN

Girard R 1986 The scapegoat. Athlone Press, London

Glaser B G, Strauss A L 1965 Awareness of dying. Aldine, Chicago

Glazer G 1995 The impact of NHS reforms on patient care. In: Murley R (ed) Patients or customers: are the NHS reforms working? Office for Public Management, London

Glennerster H, Matsaganis M 1992 The English and the Swedish health care reforms. Welfare state discussion paper WSP/79. London School of Economics, London

Glennerster H, Matsaganis M, Owens S 1994 Implementing GP fundholding: wildcard or willing hand? Open University Press, Buckingham

Glover J 1977 Causing death and saving lives. Penguin, Harmondsworth

GNC 1980 Guidelines on health education. General Nursing Council for Scotland, Edinburgh

Goffman E 1969 The presentation of self in everyday life. Penguin, Harmondsworth

Goffman E 1993 Asylums: essays on the social situation of mental patients and other inmates, 2nd edn. Penguin, Harmondsworth (first published in 1961)

Gold R S, Greenberg J S 1992 The health education ethics book. Wm C Brown, Dubuque, IA

Golding P, Middleton S 1981 Images of welfare. Blackwell, Oxford

Goldman J 1982 Inconsistency and institutional review boards. JAMA 248(2):197–202

Goodare H, Smith R 1995 The rights of patients in medical research. British Medical Journal 310:1227–1278

Goodwin N 2000 The long-term importance of English primary care groups for integration in primary health care and deinstitutionalisation of hospital care. International Journal of Integrated Care 1(1): 1 March

Grace D, Cohen S 1998 Business ethics – Australian problems and cases, 2nd edn. Oxford University Press, Oxford

Graham H 1993 Hardship and health in women's lives. Harvester Wheatsheaf, Brighton

Graham H (ed) 2000 Understanding health inequalities. Open University Press, Buckingham

Granovetter M S 1973 The strength of weak ties. American Journal of Sociology 78(6):1360–1380

Grayson L 1997 Evidence based medicine. The British Library, London

Grayson S 1993 The ideology of fertility. In: Hetherington P, Maddern P (eds) Sexuality and gender in history, selected essays. Optima Press, Western Australia, ch 16

Green D 1990 A missed opportunity. In: Green D, Neuberger J, Lord Young of Darlington, Burstall M (eds) The NHS reforms: what ever happened to consumer choice? Institute for Economic Affairs, Health Unit, London

Green J, Green M 1992 Dealing with death: practices and procedures. Chapman & Hall, London

Gregory T S (ed) 1955 Spinoza B (1632–1677) Ethics. J M Dent, London

Gross P F 1985 Nursing care in the 1980's and beyond: the challenge to be relevant, ethical and accepted, Australian Nurses Journal 15(1):46–48

Growe S 1991 Who cares? The crisis in Canadian nursing. McClelland & Stewart, Toronto

Hallam J 2000 Nursing the image: media, culture and professional identity. Routledge, London

Hamberger L K, Burge S K, Graham A V, Costa A J 1997 Violence issues for health care educators and providers. Haworth Maltreatment and Trauma Press, New York.

Hamilton W (tr) 1960 Plato (427–347 BC) Gorgias. Penguin Books, Harmondsworth

Hanson S 2005 Teaching health care ethics: why we should teach nursing and medical students together. Nursing Ethics 2005 12(2):167–176

Hare R M 1952 (reprinted 1964, 1981) The language of morals. Clarendon Press, Oxford, ch 4

Hare R M 1963 Freedom and reason. Oxford University Press, Oxford, ch 4

Hare R M 1981 Moral thinking: its levels, methods and point. Oxford University Press, Oxford

Häring B 1975 Ethics of manipulation: Issues in medicine, behaviour control and genetics. Seabury Press, New York

Harris J 1981 Ethical problems in the management of some severely handicapped children. Journal of Medical Ethics 7(3):114–117

Harrison M I 2004 implementing change in health systems: market reforms in the United Kingdom, Sweden, and the Netherlands. Sage Publications, London

Harrison S 1998 The politics of evidence based healthcare in the UK. Policy and Politics 26:15–31

Harrison S 2004 Implementing change in health systems. Sage Publications, London

Harrison S, Pollitt C 1994 Controlling health professionals: the future of work and organisation in the NHS. Open University Press, Buckingham

Harrison S, Hunter D, Marnock G, Pollitt C 1992 Just managing: power and culture in the National Health Service. Macmillan, London

Harrison S, Dixon J, New B, Judge K 1997 Can the NHS cope in future? British Medical Journal 314:139–142

Harrison S, Dowswell G, Wright J 2002a Practice nurses and clinical guidelines in a changing primary care context: an empirical study. Journal of Advanced Nursing 39:299–307

Harrison S, Moran M, Wood B 2002b Policy emergence and policy convergence: the case of 'scientific-bureaucratic medicine' in the United States and United Kingdom. British Journal of Politics and International Relations 4:1–24

Hawkins J M (ed) 1986/1996 The Oxford reference dictionary. Clarendon Press, Oxford

Haycox A, Bagust A, Walley T 1999 Clinical guidelines, the hidden costs. British Medical Journal 318:391–393

HDV 1993 Personal communication from State of Victoria Health Department

Healey J (tr) 1968 Augustine (354–430 AD) The city of God. J M Dent, London

Health Department of Western Australia 1997 A clinician's guide to the Mental Health Act 1996. HDWA, Perth, Western Australia

Hellman S 1995 The patient and the public good, Nature Medicine 1(5):400–402

Henderson V 1996 The nature of nursing: a definition of its implications for practice, research and education. Macmillan, New York

Hetherington P, Maddern P 1993 Sexuality and gender in history, selected essays. Optima Press, Western Australia

Hick J H 1990 Philosophy of religion. Prentice-Hall, Upper Saddle River, NJ

Hill L, Smith N 1990 Self-care nursing: promotion of health. Appleton-Century-Crofts, Norwalk, CT

Hill T E 1991 Autonomy and self-respect. Cambridge University Press, Cambridge

Hinton J 1979 Comparison of places and policies for terminal care. Lancet i(6 Jan):29

HM Government 1988 Acheson Report on Public Health in England (Cm 289): Report of the Acheson Committee of Inquiry into the future development of the public health function. HMSO, London

HM Government 1990 The NHS and Community Care Act. HMSO, London

HM Government 1992 Annual abstract of statistics. Central Statistical Office, HMSO, London

HM Government 1995, 1996, 1997 Nolan Committee reports on standards in public life (Vol 1: On standards, 1995, CM2850, Vol 2: Local government, 1996, CM3702-10; Vol 3: Local public spending bodies 1997 CM3270-1). HMSO, London

HM Government 1997 The new NHS: modern, dependable (Cm 3807). TSO, London

HM Government 1998a Our healthier nation (Cm 3852). HMSO, London

HM Government 1998b The Public Interest Disclosure Act. HMSO, London

HM Government 1998c UK Human Rights Act 1998. TSO, London

HM Government 2001a The Report of the Royal Liverpool Children's Inquiry Report 2001. TSO, London

HM Government 2001b The Bristol Royal Infirmary Inquiry 2001. Learning from Bristol: the report of the public inquiry into children's heart surgery at the Bristol Royal Infirmary 1984–1995. Command Paper: CM 5207. TSO, London

HM Government 2005a UK Central Government Main Supply Estimates 2005/06. TSO, London

HM Government 2005b The Shipman Inquiry: final report. TSO, London

Hobbes T (1588–1679) (Tuck R, ed) 1996 Leviathan. Cambridge University Press, Cambridge

Holloway R 1999 Godless morality: keeping religion out of ethics. Canongate, Edinburgh

Holm S 1997 Ethical problems in clinical practice: the ethical reasoning of healthcare professionals. Manchester University Press, Manchester

Honigsbaum F 1995 Priority setting processes for health care in Oregon, USA; New Zealand; The Netherlands, Sweden and the UK. Radcliffe Medical Press, Oxford

Hornblum A H 1997 They were cheap and available: prisoners as research subjects in twentieth century America. British Medical Journal 315: 1437–1441

Horne E M, Cowan T 1992 Effective communication: some nursing perspectives. Wolfe Publishing, London

House of Lords 1997 Bolitho v. City and Hackney Health Authority – House of Lords judgement. TSO, London

HPA 2004 Focus on prevention of HIV and other sexually transmitted infections in the United Kingdom in 2003. An update: November 2004. Health Protection Agency, London

Hudson B 1994 Making sense of markets in health and social care. Business Education Publishers, Sunderland

Hughes E C 1951 Studying the nurse's work. American Journal of Nursing 51(5):294–295

Hume D (1711–1776) (Selby-Bigge L A, ed) 1978 A treatise on human nature (1738). Oxford University Press, Oxford

Hume D (1711–1776) (Beauchamp T L, ed) 1998 An enquiry concerning the principles of morals (1770). Oxford University Press, Oxford

Hunt G 1997 The human condition of the professional: discretion and accountability. Nursing Ethics 4(6):519–526

Hurwitz B 1999 Legal and political considerations of clinical practice guidelines. British Medical Journal 318:661–664

IAS 2005 Alcohol and health: IAS fact sheet. Institute of Alcohol Studies, St Ives, Cambridgeshire

ICAA 1997 Ethics. Institute of Chartered Accountants in Australia, Sydney, Australia

ICN 1998 Nurses and human rights. International Council of Nurses, Geneva

ICN 2000 Code of Ethics. International Council of Nurses, Geneva

Illich I 1977 The limits of medicine. Medical nemesis: the expropriation of health. Penguin Books, Harmondsworth

Illingworth S 2004 Approaches to ethics in higher education: teaching ethics across the curriculum. Learning and Teaching Support Network, University of Leeds, Leeds

Illsley R, Svensson P G 1984 The health burden of social inequalities. World Health Organization (European Office), Copenhagen

ISD 1997 Scottish health statistics. Common Services Agency, Edinburgh

ISD 2003 Scottish health statistics: terminations of pregnancy (abortions). Information Services, NHS National Services Scotland, Edinburgh

Jackson M P 1987 Strikes. St Martin's Press, New York

Jacobs A 1998 Seeing a difference: market health reform in Europe. Journal of Health Politics, Policy and Law 23:1–33

James P 1996 Total quality management – introductory text. Prentice Hall, New York

James W, Nelson M, Ralph A, Leather S 1997 The contribution of nutrition to inequalities in health. British Medical Journal 314:1545–1549

Jankowski R 2001 Implementing national guidelines at local level. British Medical Journal 322:1258–1259

Jaspers K 1962 The great philosophers: the foundations. Rupert Hart-Davis, London

Johns C 2000 Becoming a reflective practitioner. Blackwell, Oxford

Johnson N 1990 Reconstructing the welfare state: a decade of change. Harvester Wheatsheaf, London

Johnson O A (ed) 1994 Ethics: selections from classical and contemporary writers, 7th edn. Harcourt Brace, New York

Johnstone M-J 1991 Ethical issues in nursing research: a broad overview. Faculty of Nursing, RMIT, Bundoora, Victoria

Johnstone M-J 1994 Bioethics: a nursing perspective. WB Saunders/Baillière Tindall, Sydney

Jones E 1955 Freud: Letter to Marie Bonaparte. In: Sigmund Freud: life and work. Basic Books, New York, vol 2, pt 3, ch 16

Jones P 1991 Theory and method in sociology: a guide for the beginner. London, Collins

Jonsen A R, Toulmin S 1988 The abuse of casuistry: a history of moral reasoning. University of California Press, Berkeley, CA

Jonsen A, Siegler M, Winslade W 1992 Clinical ethics: a practical approach to ethical decisions in clinical medicine. Macmillan, New York

Josephson Institute of Ethics 2005 Making ethical decisions. Los Angeles, CA

Joss R, Kogan M 1995 Advancing quality: total quality management in the national health service. Open University Press, Buckingham

Jowell R, Brook L, Taylor B (eds) 1995 British social attitudes: the twelfth report. Dartmouth, Aldershot

Judge Institute of Management Studies, University of Cambridge 2000 Policy futures for UK health 2000 report (Report commissioned by the Department of Health). TSO, London

Juvenal (c60–130 AD) (Braund M, tr) 1996 Satires. Cambridge University Press, Cambridge

Kagan K, Evans J 1995 Professional and inter-personal skills for nurses. Chapman & Hall, London

Kant I (1724–1804) (Abbot T K, tr) 1909 Critique of pure practical reason. Everyman, Dent, London

Kant I (1724–1804) (Paton H J, tr) 1969 The moral law: Kant's groundwork of the metaphysic of morals. Hutchinson, London (reprinted 1991)

Keatings M, Smith O B 2000 Ethical and legal issues in Canadian nursing. WB Saunders, Toronto

Kemp Smith N (tr) 1973 Kant I (1724–1804) Critique of pure reason. Macmillan, London

Kendall L 1998 Local inequalities targets. King's Fund, London

Kennedy R, Nichols J C 1995 The effects of the purchaser/provider split on patient care. In: Murley R (ed) Patients or customers: are the NHS reforms working? Office for Public Management, London

Keown J 1995 Euthanasia examined: ethical, clinical and legal aspects. Cambridge University Press, Cambridge

Kerr Report 2005 National Framework for service change in the NHS in Scotland: building a service fit for the future (Vol 1). Scottish Executive, Edinburgh

Kerr Report 2005 National Framework for service change in the NHS in Scotland: A Guide for the NHS in Scotland (Vol 2). Scottish Executive, Edinburgh

Kerr F 1997 Theology after Wittgenstein, 2nd edn. SPCK, London

Kerridge I, Lowe M, McPhee J 1998 Ethics and law for the health professions. Social Science Press, Katoomba, NSW

Ketefian S, Ormond L 1988 Moral reasoning and ethical practice in nursing: an integrative review. National League for Nursing, New York

Kiersky J H, Caste N J 1995 Thinking critically: techniques for logical reasoning. West, New York

King's Fund 2001 Still no primary care NHS under New Labour, says King's Fund (Information – News). www.kingsfund.org.uk/pr010228.html

Kirby M 1995 Patients' rights – why the Australian courts have rejected Bolam. Journal of Medical Ethics 21:5–8

Kitson A 1993 Nursing art and science. Chapman and Hall, London

Kitson A, Campbell R 1996 The ethical organisation: ethical theory and corporate behaviour. Macmillan Business, Basingstoke

Klein R 1989 The politics of the NHS, 2nd edn. Longman, London

Klein R (ed) 1998 Implementing the White Paper: pitfalls and opportunities. King's Fund, London

Kohlberg L 1973 Continuities in childhood, and adult moral development revisited. In: Bolters P B, Schaie K W (eds) Lifespan developmental psychology, 2nd edn. Academic Press, New York

Kohlberg L 1976 Moral stages and moralization: the cognitive-developmental approach. In: Lickona T (ed) Moral development and behavior: theory, research and social issues. Holt, Rhinehart and Winston, New York

Kohlberg L 1981 The philosophy of moral development. Harper & Row, San Francisco

Kohlberg L 1984 Essays on moral development: the psychology of moral development. Nature and validity of moral stages, Vol 2. Harper & Row, New York

Kohlberg L, Gilligan C 1971 The adolescent as a philosopher: the discovery of the self in a post-conventional world. Daedalus 100:1051–1086

Korsgaard C M, Cohen G A 1996 The sources of normativity. Cambridge University Press, Cambridge

Kurtines W, Gewirtz J (eds) 1984 Morality, moral behaviour and moral development. John Wiley, New York

Laing R D, Esterson A 1970 Sanity, madness and the family. Penguin, Harmondsworth

Lamb M 1987 Nursing ethics and nursing education: past perspectives and recent developments. Perspectives in Nursing, 1985–1987. National League for Nursing, New York, p 3–21

Lapsley I, Melia K M 2001 Clinical actions and financial constraints: the limits to rationing intensive care. Sociology of Health and Illness 23(5):729–746

Larrabee M J (ed) 1993 An ethic of care: feminist and interdisciplinary perspectives. Routledge, London

Laschinger H K, Goldenberg D 1993 Attitudes of practising nurses as predictors of intended care behaviour with persons who are HIV positive. John Wiley, New York

Lawler J 1991 Behind the screens. Churchill Livingstone, Edinburgh

Lebacqz K 1999 A time to die. Biomedical Ethics 4(1):16

Le Grand J, Mays N, Dixon J 1998 The reforms: success or failure or neither? In: Le Grand J, Mays N, Mulligan J A (eds) Learning from the NHS internal market: a review of the evidence. King's Fund, London

Leininger M 1988 History, issues and trends in the discovery and uses of care in nursing. In: Leininger M (ed) Care, discovery and uses in clinical and community nursing. Slack, Thorofare, NJ

Lemert E M 1951 Social pathology. McGraw Hill, New York

Levinas E 1982 Responsibility for the other. Duquesne University Press, USA

Levinas E 1985 Ethics and infinity. Duquesne University Press, USA

Lewis R 2001 Nurse-led primary care: learning from PMS pilots. King's Fund, London

Ley P 1976 Towards better doctor–patient communication. In: Bennett A E (ed) Communication between doctors and patients. Oxford University Press, Oxford

Light D 2001 Comparative institutional response to economic policy: managed competition and governability. Social Science and Medicine 52:1151–1166

Light D, May A (eds) 1993 Britain's health system: from welfare state to managed markets. Faulkner & Gray, New York

Lindley R 1986 Autonomy. Macmillan, Basingstoke

Lindsay A D (ed) 1951 Hume D (1711–1776) A treatise on human nature. J M Dent, London

Lindsay A D (ed) 1957 Mill J S (1806–1873) Utilitarianism, liberty, and representative government. J M Dent, London

Lipson J G, Steiger N J 1996 Self-care nursing in a multi-cultural context. Sage Publications, Thousand Oaks, CA

Lock S 1990 Monitoring research ethics committees. British Medical Journal 300:61–62

Lugon M, Secker-Walker J 1998 Clinical governance: making it happen. Royal Society of Medicine, London

MacAdam A I, Pyke J 1998 Judicial Reasoning and doctrine of precedent in Australia. Butterworths, Sydney

McAlpine H 1996 Critical reflection about professional ethical stances: have we lost sight of the major objectives? Journal of Nursing Education 35(3):119–126

McAlpine H 1998 Ethical reasoning of practising nurses: does ethics education make a difference? Unpublished PhD thesis, Murdoch University, Western Australia

McCall-Smith A 1991 Sexuality and the law. (Occasional Paper) Health Education Board for Scotland, Edinburgh

McClymont A, Thomas S E, Denham M J 1991 Health visiting and elderly people. Churchill Livingstone, Edinburgh

McCormick R 1974 Proxy consent in the experimental situation. Perspectives in Biology and Medicine 18:2–20

McCormick R 1976 Experiments in children: sharing in sociality. Hastings Center Report No 6: 41–46

McCullough L B 2004 Taking the history of medical ethics seriously in teaching medical professionalism. American Journal of Bioethics 4(2):13–14

Macintyre A 1967/1993 A short history of ethics. Routledge & Kegan Paul, London

Macintyre A 1981/1985 After virtue: a study in moral theory, 2nd edn. Notre Dame University Press, Notre Dame, IN/Duckworth, London

Macintyre A 1988 Whose justice? Whose rationality? Notre Dame University Press, Notre Dame, IN

Macintyre A 1990 Three rival versions of moral enquiry. Notre Dame University Press, Notre Dame, IN

Mackay L 1989 Nursing a problem. Open University Press, Milton Keynes

Mackay L, Soothill K, Melia K 1998 Classic texts in health care. Butterworth Heinemann, Oxford

McKeown T 1979 The role of medicine: dream, mirage or nemesis. Blackwell, Oxford

McNeill P 1993 The ethics and politics of human experimentation. Cambridge University Press, Cambridge

McNeill P M, Berglund C A, Webster I W 1990 Reviewing the reviewers: a survey of institutional ethics committees in Australia. Medical Journal of Australia 152:289–296

McNeill P M, Berglund C A, Webster I W 1994 How much influence do various members have within research ethics committees? Cambridge Quarterly of Health Care Ethics 3:522–532

MAFF (Ministry of Agriculture, Fisheries and Food) 1998 National food survey. TSO, London

Maggs C 1987 Nursing history: the state of the art. Croom Helm, London

Marcuse H 1941 Reason and revolution. Routledge & Kegan Paul, London

Maritain J 1944 The rights of man and natural law. C Scribner's Sons, New York

Maritain J 1963 Moral philosophy. Geoffrey Bles, London

Markowitz H M 1992 Markets and morality. Journal of Portfolio Management 18:84–93

Maslow A 1970 Motivation and personality. Harper & Row, New York

Matthies B K, Kreutzer J S, West D D 1997 The behaviour management handbook. Therapy Skill Builders, San Antonio, TX

May W 1975 Code, covenant, contract or philanthropy. Hastings Center Report No 5: 29–38

May W 1983 The physician's covenant. Westminster, Philadelphia

Mead G H 1934 Mind, self and society: from the standpoint of a social behaviourist. University of Chicago Press, Chicago

Mele A R 1995 Autonomous agents: from self-control to autonomy. Oxford University Press, New York

Melia K M 1987 Learning and working: the occupational socialisation of nurses. Tavistock, London

Melia K M 1989 Everyday nursing ethics. Macmillan Education, Basingstoke

Melia K M 1994 The task of nursing ethics. Journal of Medical Ethics 20(4):7–11

Melia K M 2004 Health care ethics: lessons from intensive care. Sage Publications, London

Melia K M 2005 Nursing in the New NHS: a sociological analysis of learning and working (Full Report of research activities and results to the Economic and Social Research Council (ESRC)). School of Health in Social Science, University of Edinburgh

Milburn A 2001 Health priorities for the new government, Ministerial Statement, 13 June 2001. Department of Health, London

Mill J S (Acton H B, ed) 1972 Utilitarianism, liberty, and representative government (1861). Everyman, Dent, London

Mishra R 1984 The welfare state in crisis. Harvester Wheatsheaf, New York

Mishra R 1990 The welfare state in capitalist society. Harvester Wheatsheaf, London

Mitchell B 1970 Morality religious and secular. Oxford University Press, Oxford

Molassiotis A, Margulies A, Fernandez-Ortega P et al 2005 Complementary and alternative medicine use in patients with haematological malignancies in Europe. Complementary Therapy in Clinical Practice 11(2):105–110

Montefiore A 1958 A modern introduction to moral philosophy. Routledge & Kegan Paul, London

Mooney G 1992 Economics, medicine and health, 2nd edn. Harvester Wheatsheaf, Hampshire

Moore G E 1962 Principia ethica, revised edn. Cambridge University Press, Cambridge

Moore G E 1966 Ethics, 2nd edn. Oxford University Press, Oxford

Morse J M, Solberg S M, Neander W L, Bottorf J L, Johnson J L 1990 Concepts of caring and caring as a concept. Advances in Nursing Science 13(1):1–14

Muir Gray J A 2001 Evidence-based healthcare: how to make health policy and management decisions. Churchill Livingstone, Edinburgh

Munro A 1996 Contracting, health care and the internal market. Paper given in the Department of Social Policy, University of Edinburgh, 28/10/1996

Murdoch I 1970 The sovereignty of good. Routledge & Kegan Paul, London

Murley R (ed) 1995 Patients or customers: are the NHS reforms working? Office for Public Management, London

Murray R B, Zilner J P 1989 Nursing concepts for health promotion. Prentice Hall, London

Naidoo J, Wills J 2000 Health promotion: foundations for practice, 2nd edn. Baillière Tindall, London

Naidoo B, Stevens W, McPherson K 2000 Modelling the short term consequences of smoking cessation in England on the hospitalisation rates for acute myocardial infarction and stroke. Tobacco Control ;9:397–400

National Audit Office 2004 HM Customs and Excise: Standard Report 2002–03 Report by the Comptroller and Auditor General. TSO, London

National Health and Medical Research Council (Australia) 1995 Report on the functioning of research ethics committees. Canberra, ACT

National Health and Medical Research Council (Australia) 1999 National statement on ethical conduct in research involving humans, (Cat No 9818566), AusInfo, GPO Box 1920, Canberra, ACT 2601

Nelson D M 1992 Priority of prudence: virtue and natural law. Pennsylvania State University, University Park, PA,

NHS 2003 The new NHS pay system: an overview (Agenda for Change). Department of Health, London

NHS 2004 Job evaluations handbook, 2nd edn. Scottish Executive, Edinburgh

NHS Scotland 2003 Partnership for care (Scotland's Health White Paper). Scottish Executive, Edinburgh. Online. Available: www.scotland.gov.uk

NHS Scotland 2005 Staff governance standard (for NHS employees). Scottish Executive, Edinburgh. Online. Available: www.scotland.gov.uk

NHSE 1995 Priorities and planning guidance for the NHS 1996/7. NHSE, Leeds

NHSE 1996 Promoting clinical effectiveness. NHSE, Leeds

NHSLA (National Health Service Litigation Authority) 2002 Circular 02/2002. Department of Health, London

Nietzsche F (1844–1900) 1954/1982 The gay science. In: Kaufmann W (tr and ed) The portable Nietzsche. Viking Penguin, New York

Nietzsche F 1844–1900 (Cowan M, tr) 1955 Beyond good and evil. Henry Regnery, Chicago

NIMHE 2004 Mental health policy implementation guide – developing positive practice to support the safe and therapeutic management of aggression and violence in mental health in-patient settings. National Institute for Mental Health in England (NIMHE), Redditch, Worcestershire

NMC (Nursing and Midwifery Council) 2002a An NMC guide for students of nursing and midwifery. NMC, London

NMC (Nursing and Midwifery Council) 2002b Accountability never sleeps. NMC News 3:9

NMC (Nursing and Midwifery Council) 2002c Code of professional conduct. NMC, London

NMC (Nursing and Midwifery Council) 2002d Supporting nurses and midwives through lifelong learning. NMC, London

NMC (Nursing and Midwifery Council) 2003 Safe staffing levels. NMC News 6:16

NMC (Nursing and Midwifery Council) 2004 Code of professional conduct: standards for conduct, performance and ethics. NMC, London

NMC (Nursing and Midwifery Council) 2005a Standards of proficiency for pre-registration nursing education. NMC, London

NMC (Nursing and Midwifery Council) 2005b The PREP handbook. NMC, London

NMC (Nursing and Midwifery Council) 2005c Guidelines for records and record keeping. NMC, London

Noddings N 1984 Caring: a feminine approach to ethical and moral education. University of California Press, Berkeley, CA

Nolan 1995, 1996, 1997 Nolan Committee Reports on Standards in Public Life (Vol 1: On standards, 1995, CM2850, Vol 2: Local government, 1996, CM3702-10; Vol 3: Local public spending bodies, 1997, CM3270-1). HMSO, London

Norton D 1975 Research and the problem of pressure sores. Nursing Times 140:65–67

Nowell Smith P 1957 Ethics. Blackwell, Oxford

Nutley S, Davies H, Walter I 2004 Learning from knowledge management (conceptual synthesis 2). Research Unit for Research Utilisation, Department of Management, University of St Andrews, Scotland

Nygren A (Watson P S, tr) 1953 Agape and Eros. Westminster Press, Philadelphia

OECD (Organisation for Economic Cooperation and Development) 2005 Health data 2005, data-base. OECD Health Policy Studies, Paris

O'Keeffe T M 1984 Suicide and self-starvation. Philosophy 59:349–363

Olsson S E 1990 Social policy and welfare state in Sweden. Arkiv förlag, Lund, Sweden

O'Neill O 2002 Autonomy and trust in bioethics. Cambridge University Press, Cambridge

ONS (Office for National Statistics) 2004 Annual Abstract Of Statistics 2004. ONS, London

OPCS 1991 OPCS monitor. Office of Population Censuses and Surveys. HMSO, London

OPM (Office for Public Management) 2000 'Shifting gears': towards a 21st century NHS. Report prepared by the Office for Public Management, for the Department of Health, London

Papadakis E, Taylor-Gooby P 1987 The private provision of public welfare: state, market and community. Wheatsheaf Books, Sussex

Pappworth M H 1967 Human guinea pigs: experimentation in man. Routledge & Kegan Paul, London

Parkes C M 1966 The patient's right to know the truth. Proceedings of the Royal Society of Medicine 66:536

Parkes C M 1972/1996 Bereavement: studies of grief in adult life. Routledge, London

Parkes C M, Markus A 1998 Coping with loss: helping patients and their families. BMJ Books, London

Parrott S, Godfrey C, Raw M et al 1998 Guidance for commissioners on the cost effectiveness of smoking cessation interventions. Thorax 53(Supplement 5, part 2):S1

Parrott S, Godfrey C, Raw M 2000 Costs of employee smoking in the workplace in Scotland. Tobacco Control 9:187–192

Pascal B (1623–1662) (Turnell M, tr) 1962 The pensées. Harvill Press, London

Paton C 2000 Scientific evaluation of the effects of the introduction of market forces in to health systems. European Health Management Association, Dublin

Paton H J (tr) 1969 The moral law: Kant's groundwork of the metaphysic of morals. Hutchinson, London (reprinted 1991)

Pawson R, Tilley N 1997 Realistic evaluation. Sage, London

Pender N 1996 Health promotion in nursing practice. Prentice Hall International, London

Perkin H 1990 The rise of professional society. Routledge, London.

Perkin H 2004 Crisis in the professions: ambiguities, origins and current problems. Royal Society of Arts. Online. Available: http://www.thersa.org/projects/professional_values.asp

Petersen A, Bunton R 2002 The new genetics and the public's health. Routledge, London

Phillips C (ed) 1988 Logic in medicine. British Medical Journal Publications, London

Phillips S S, Benner P 1996 The crisis of care: affirming and restoring caring practices in the helping professions. Georgetown University Press, Washington, DC

Piaget J 1965 The moral judgment of the child. Free Press, New York

Pieper J 1959 Prudence: the first cardinal virtue. Faber & Faber, London

Plato (427–347 BC) (Cornford F M, tr) 1961 The republic of Plato. Clarendon Press, Oxford

Plato (427–347 BC) (Rouse W D, ed and tr) 1984 Great dialogues of Plato. Mentor Books, New York

Plato (427–347 BC) (Hamilton W, tr) 1950 Gorgias. Penguin, Harmondsworth

Pontifex M (tr) 1955 Augustine (354–430 AD): The problem of free choice (de libero arbitrio voluntatis). Newman Press, Westminster

Pope John XXIII 1963 Pacem in terris (Human rights and world peace). Holy See, Vatican City

Porritt L 1990 Interaction strategies: an introduction for health professionals. Churchill Livingstone, Edinburgh

Porter R 1997 The greatest benefit to mankind – a medical history of humanity from antiquity to the present. Harper Collins, London

Preston N (ed) 1994 Ethics for the public sector. The Federation Press, Sydney

Prochaska J L, DiClemente C C 1992 Stages of change in the modification of problem behavior. In: Hersen M, Eisler R, Miller P M (eds) Progress in behavior modification, 28. Sycamore Publishing, Sycamore, IL

Prochaska J O, DiClemente C C, Norcross J C 1992 In search of how people change. Applications to addictive behaviors. American Psychologist 47:1102–1113

Rachels J 1993 The elements of moral philosophy, 2nd edn. McGraw Hill, New York

Ramsey P 1970 The patient as person. Yale University Press, New Haven, CT

Ramsey P 1976 The enforcement of morals: non-therapeutic research on children. Hastings Center Report No 6: 21–39

Ramsey P 1977 Children as research subjects: a reply. Hastings Center Report No 7: 40–42

Ramsey P 1978 Ethics at the edges of life. Yale University Press, New Haven, CT

Ramsey P 1980 Basic Christian ethics. University of Chicago Press, Chicago

Ramsey P 1983 Deeds and rules in Christian ethics. University of America Press, New York

Ranade W 1994 A future for the NHS? Health care in the 1990s. Longman, London

Raphael D D 1980 Moral philosophy. Oxford University Press, Oxford

Rathbone-McCuan E, Fabian D R 1992 Self-neglecting elders: a clinical dilemma. Auburn House, New York

Rawls J 1970 Justice as fairness. Journal of Philosophy 54:653–662

Rawls J 1971 A theory of justice. Harvard University Press, Cambridge, MA

RCN 1977a Ethics related to research in nursing. Royal College of Nursing, London

RCN 1977b Royal College of Nursing (RCN) Code of Professional Conduct: A discussion document by Dawson J D, Altschul A et al. Journal of Medical Ethics 3(3):115–123

RCN 1979 RCN draft code of ethics for nurses. RCN, London. (First published as a discussion document in the Journal of Medical Ethics 3(3))

RCN 2004 Research ethics, RCN guidance for nurses. Royal College of Nursing, London

Reed J, Lomas G 1984 Psychiatric services in the community: developments and innovations. Croom Helm, London

Reuter L 1999 Euthanasia and subjectivity: ethical reflections on the post-modern concept of personhood. Biomedical Ethics 4(1):14–16

Reverby S 1987 Ordered to care: the dilemma of American nursing, 1850–1945. Cambridge University Press, Cambridge

RGS (Registrar General for Scotland) 2005 Registrar General's review of Scotland's population. General Register Office for Scotland, Edinburgh

Rice T, Biles B, Brown E R, Diderichsen F, Kuehn H 2000 Reconsidering the role of competition in health care markets: Introduction. Journal of Health Politics, Policy and Law 25:864–873

Rickinson B, Rutherford D 1996 Increasing undergraduate student rates. British Journal of Guidance and Counselling 24(2):213–225

Roach M S 1992 The human act of caring: a blueprint for health professions. Canadian Hospital Association, Toronto

Robertson A 1996 The internal market reforms of the British NHS. The Italian National Research Council (CNR) conference, Rome, 16–17 December 1996

Robertson A, Thompson I E, Porter M 1992 Social policy and administration. Health Education Open Learning Project, Keele University, Keele

Robertson D C, Schlegelmilch B B 1993 Corporate institutionalisation of ethics in the United States and Great Britain. Journal of Business Ethics 12:301–312

Robinson J 1993 Managed competition and the demise of nursing. In: Light D, May A (eds) Britain's health system: from welfare state to managed markets. Faulkner & Gray, New York

Robinson J, Poxton R 1998 Health and social care partnerships. In: Klein R (ed) Implementing the White Paper: pitfalls and opportunities. King's Fund London, p 56–66

Robinson 2002 The finance and provision of long term care for elderly people in the UK: recent trends, current policy and future prospects. www.ipss.go.jp/English/WebJournal.files/SocialSecurity/2002/02Dec/robinsonpdf

Robinson R, Le Grand J 1995 Contracting and the purchaser/provider split. In: Saltman R B, von Otter C (eds) Implementing planned markets in health care. Open University Press, Buckingham

Rogers C 1961 On becoming a person. Constable, London (first published 1957, Houghton Mifflin, Boston)

Rolfe G, Freshwater D, Jasper M 2001 Critical reflection for nursing and the helping professions. Palgrave, Basingstoke

Roper N, Logan W, Tierney A 1981 Learning to use the Nursing Process. Churchill Livingstone, Edinburgh

Ross T 1981 Thought control. Nursing Mirror: April 23 (see also other articles on psychiatric ethics in the same series)

Ross W D 1930 The right and the good. Clarendon Press, Oxford

Ross W D 1952 The works of Aristotle: the politics. Clarendon Press, Oxford

Ross W D 1969 Kant's ethical theory. Oxford University Press, Oxford

Rossi P H, Freeman H E, Lipsey M W 1999 Evaluation: a systematic approach, 6th edn. Sage Publications, London

Rouse W D (ed & tr) 1960/1961 Plato (427–347 BC) Great dialogues of Plato. Mentor Books, New York

Rousseau, J J (1717–1778) (Cole G D H, tr) 1973 The social contract and other discourses (New edn; revised and augmented by J H Brumfitt and J C Hall). Dent, London

Rousseau J J (1717–1778) (Foxley B, tr) 1974 Émile. Everyman, Dent London

Royal College of Physicians (RCP) 2000 Nicotine addiction in Britain: a report of the Tobacco Advisory Group of the Royal College of Physicians. RCP, London

Royal College of Psychiatrists 1977 Guidelines on the care and treatment of mentally disturbed offenders. British Journal of Psychiatry Bulletin: April

Royal College of Psychiatrists 2003 The mental health of students in higher education (CR112). Royal College of Psychiatrists, London

Royal Liverpool Children's Inquiry Report 2001 HM Government, TSO London

Ruddick S 1989 Maternal thinking: towards a politics of peace. Beacon Press, Boston

Rumbold G 1986/1993 Ethics in nursing practice. Baillière Tindall, London

Rushforth B 2004 Breaking down professional barriers. British Medical Journal 12:309–348

Saltman R B, von Otter C (eds) 1995 Implementing planned markets in health care. Open University Press, Buckingham

Sartre J-P 1948 (Mairet P, tr 1978) Existentialism and humanism. Methuen, London

Sartre J-P 1956 No Exit and three other plays. Vintage Books, London

Sartre J-P 1957/1969/1973 Being and nothingness. Methuen, London

Savage J, Moore L 2004 Interpreting accountability: an ethnographic study of practice nurses, accountability and multidisciplinary team decision making in the context of clinical governance. Royal College of Nursing, London

Scally G, Donaldson L 1998 Clinical governance and the drive for quality improvement in the New NHS in England. British Medical Journal 317:61–65

Schroeder C H, Steinzor R 2004 A new progressive agenda for public health and the environment. Center for Progressive Regulation, Maine, USA. Online. Available: http://www.progressiveregulation.org/index.html

Scottish Office 1998 Designed to care: renewing the National Health Service in Scotland. HMSO, London

Scull A 1992 Museums of madness. St Martin's Press, New York

Seale C 2002 Media and health. Sage, London

Secretary of State for Health 2001 Bristol Royal Infirmary Inquiry: Learning from Bristol: the report of the public inquiry into children's heart surgery at the Bristol Royal Infirmary 1984–1995. HMSO, London

Seedhouse D 1986/2001 Health: the foundations for achievement, 2nd rev edn 2001. John Wiley, London

SEHD (Scottish Executive Health Department) 2000 Our national health: a plan for action, a plan for change. Scottish Executive, Edinburgh

Selby-Bigge L A (ed) 1978 Hume D 1798: A treatise on human nature (1738). Oxford University Press, Oxford

Shaw B 1994 The ragged edge: the disability experience from the first fifteen years of the disability rag. The Avocado Press, Louisville, KY

Shekelle P, Eccles M, Grimshaw J, Woolf S H 2001 When should clinical guidelines be updated? British Medical Journal 322:155

SHHD 1990 Scottish health authorities' revised priorities for the nineties. HMSO, Edinburgh

Shipman Inquiry 2001 First report. TSO, London

Shipman Inquiry 2004 Second report. TSO, London

Sidell M 1997 Debates and dilemmas in promoting health: a reader. Macmillan (Open University), Basingstoke

SIMD 2004 The Scottish Index of Multiple Deprivation. Scottish Executive Health Department, Edinburgh

SIPRI Report 2003, Skons E, Perdomo C, Perlo-Freeman S, Stalenheim P (eds) World military expenditure SIPRI yearbook 2004. Stockholm International Peace Research Unit, Stockholm

Smart J J C, Williams B 1973 Utilitarianism for and against. Cambridge University Press, Cambridge

Smee C H 1995 Self-governing trusts and GP fundholders: the British experience. In: Saltman R B, von Otter C (eds) Implementing planned markets in health care. Open University Press, Buckingham

Smith R 1996 GPs – fundholders or commissioners? In: Bayley H, Jewell T (eds) Health crisis – what crisis? Fabian Society (in conjunction with the Scottish Health Association), London

Smith R 2002a In search of 'non-disease'. British Medical Journal 324:883–885

Smith R 2002b 'Oh NHS, thou art sick'. British Medical Journal 324:127–128

Smithson M, Amato P R, Pearce P 1983 Dimensions of helping behaviour. Pergamon Press, New York

Solomon R C 1994 Above the bottom line: an introduction to business ethics, 2nd edn. Harcourt Brace, London & New York

Sommers T, Shields L 1987 Women take care: the consequences of care-giving in today's society. Triad Publishing, Gainsville, FL

Sophocles (496–406 BC) (Fagles R, Knox B, tr) 1982 Antigone. In: Three Theban plays: Antigone, Oedipus the King and Oedipus at Colonus. Allen Lane, London

Sourial S 1997 An analysis of caring. Journal of Advanced Nursing 26:1189–1192

Spinoza B de (1632–1677) (Gregory T S, ed) 1955 Ethics. J M Dent, London

Stacey M, Homans H 1978 The sociology of health and illness: its present state, future prospects and potential for health research. Sociology 12(2):281–307

Stanley F 1992 New health boss says IVF a waste. The West Australian, 22 July 1992

Staunton P, Whyburn B 1997 Nursing and the law, 4th edn. Harcourt Brace, New York

Stebbing L S 1958 A modern introduction to logic. Methuen, London

Steele S M, Harmon V M 1983 Values clarification in nursing, 2nd edn. Appleton-Century-Crofts, Norwalk, CT

Sternberg E 1994/2000 Just business: business ethics in action. Warner Books, London

Sternberg E 2004 Corporate governance: accountability in the market place. Institute of Economic Affairs, London

Stinson R, Stinson P 1981 On the death of a baby. Journal of Medical Ethics 7(1):5–18

Stuart H F (tr) 1950 Pascal B (1623–1662) Pensées. Routledge, London, IV, p 227

Surtees P, Wainwright N, Pharaoh P 2000 Student mental health, use of services and academic attainment: report to the Review Committee of the University of Cambridge Counselling Service, University of Cambridge

Swage T 2000 Clinical governance in health care practice. Butterworth-Heinemann, Oxford

Szasz T 1974 The myth of mental illness. Harper & Row, New York

Szasz T 1987 Insanity: the idea and its consequences. Wiley, New York

Talmon J L 1966 The origins of totalitarian democracy. Mercury Books, London

Tam H 1998 Communitarianism: a new agenda for politics and citizenship. Macmillan, Basingstoke

Taylor C 1985 Philosophy and the human sciences. Cambridge University Press, Cambridge

Taylor C 1992 Sources of the self – the making of modern identity. Cambridge University Press, Cambridge

Taylor C 2002 Varieties of religion today – William James revisited. Harvard University Press, Cambridge, MA

Taylor C 2004 Modern social imaginaries. Duke University Press, Durham

Taylor-Gooby P 1985 Public opinion, ideology and state welfare. Routledge & Kegan Paul, London

Taylor-Gooby C 1986 Privatisation, power and the welfare state. Sociology 20:228–246

Thompson A 1993 Caring about carers. Research Report for the West Australian Council of Social Service, submitted to the WA Health Department in 1993

Thompson I E 1976 Suicide and philosophy. Contact 54(3):9–23

Thompson I E 1979a Dilemmas of dying – a study in the ethics of terminal care. Edinburgh University Press, Edinburgh

Thompson I E 1979b The nature of confidentiality. Journal of Medical Ethics 5(2):57–64

Thompson I E 1984 Ethical issues in palliative care. In: Doyle D (ed) Palliative care: the management of far advanced illness. Croom Helm, London

Thompson I E 1987a Personal rights and public policy: dilemmas in health education and prevention. In: Proceedings of the Twelfth World Conference on Health Education. International Union for Health Education, Health Education Bureau

Thompson I E 1987b Fundamental ethical principles in health care. British Medical Journal 295:1461–1465. (Reproduced in Phillips C (ed) Logic in medicine, BMJ Publications, London)

Thompson I E, Harries M 1997 Putting ethics to work in the public sector: a training resource pack. Public Sector Standards Commission, Perth, Western Australia

Thompson I E, French K, Melia K M et al 1981 Research ethical committees in Scotland. British Medical Journal 282:718–720

Thompson J, Thompson H 1985 Bioethical decision-making for nurses. Appleton-Century-Crofts, Norwalk, CT

Thomson D 1991 Selfish generations? The ageing of New Zealand's Welfare State. Bridget Williams Books, Wellington

Thomson D 1992 Welfare states and the problem of the common. Social Welfare Research Program, Centre for Independent Studies, Auckland, New Zealand

Thomson J A K (tr) 1976 The ethics of Aristotle, revised edn. Penguin Books, Harmondsworth

Tice C J, Perkins K 1996 Mental health issues and ageing: building on the strengths of older persons. Brookes/Cole, Pacific Grove, CA

Tillich P 1952 The courage to be. Yale University Press, New Haven, CT

Tillich P 1954 Love, power and justice. Oxford University Press, Oxford

Tones K 2001 Health promotion: effectiveness, efficiency and equity, 3rd edn. Nelson Thornes, Cheltenham

Toulmin S, 1958 The uses of argument. Cambridge University Press, Cambridge

Toulmin S 1981 The tyranny of principles. Hastings Center Report 11(6):31–39

Toulmin S 1986 The place of reason in ethics. University of Chicago Press, Chicago (first published 1958, Cambridge University Press)

Townsend P, Davidson N 1982 Inequalities in health: the Black Report. Penguin Books, Harmondsworth

Tricker R I 1994 International corporate governance: text, readings and cases. Prentice-Hall, New York

Tschudin V 1986 Ethics in nursing: the caring relationship. Heinemann Nursing, London

TSO 1998 Smoking kills. A White Paper on tobacco. The Stationery Office, London

Tuck R (ed) 1996 Hobbes, Thomas (1588–1679) Leviathan (revised edn). Cambridge University Press, Cambridge

Tulchinsky T H, Varavikova E A 2000 The new public health: an introduction for the 21st century. Academic Press, London

Tunstall-Pedoe S, Rink E, Hilton S 2003 Student attitude to undergraduate interprofessional education. Journal of Interprofessional Care 17:161–172

UK Central Government Main Supply Estimates 2005/06 HM Government, TSO, London

UNICEF 2002 State of the world's children 2002. UNICEF Headquarters, New York

UNISON 2004 Violence at work: a guide to risk prevention. UNISON, London

United Kingdom Central Council (UKCC) 1984, 1992 Code of professional conduct for the nurse, midwife and health visitor, 3rd edn. United Kingdom Central Council for Nursing, Midwifery and Health Visiting, London

United Kingdom Central Council (UKCC) 1986 Project 2000. United Kingdom Central Council for Nursing, Midwifery and Health Visiting, London

United Kingdom Central Council (UKCC) 1989 Exercising accountability. United Kingdom Central Council for Nursing, Midwifery and Health Visiting, London

UNO 1948 Universal Declaration of Human Rights. United Nations Organization, New York

UNO 1959 Declaration on the rights of the child. United Nations Organization, New York

UNO 1993 United Nations development programme. Human development report 1993. Oxford University Press, Oxford

US Com 1998 The Patient's Bill of Rights of the US Advisory Commission on Consumer Protection and Quality in the Health Care Industry

Van der Ven WP 1990 From regulated cartel to regulated competition in the Dutch health care system. European Economic Review 334:632–645

Veatch R 1981 A theory of medical ethics. Basic Books, New York

WA OPSSC (Western Australian Office of the Public Sector Standards Commissioner) 1997 Putting ethics to work (Thompson I E, Harries M). OPSSC, Perth, Western Australia

Waldron J (ed) 1984 Theories of rights. Oxford University Press, Oxford

Walshe K 2000 NHS trusts make a start on clinical governance. Focus on the NHS. Health Services Management Centre Newsletter 6(1):6

Wanless D 2002 Securing our future health: taking a long term view. HM Treasury, London

Wardhaugh J, Wilding P 1993 Towards an explanation of the corruption of care. Critical Social Policy 37:4–31

Watson J 1988 Nursing: human science and human care. National League for Nursing, New York

Watson J 1990 Caring knowledge and informed moral passion. Advances in Nursing Science 13(1):15–24

WAWA (Water Authority of Western Australia) 1994 Guide to corporate ethics for managers and employees. WAWA, Perth, Western Australian

Webb C 1996 Caring, curing, coping: towards an integrated model. Journal of Advanced Nursing 23:960–968

Webb P 1997 Health promotion and patient education: a professional's guide. Stanley Thornes, Cheltenham

Wellman C 1995 Real rights, Oxford University Press, Oxford

White R 1985 Political issues in nursing, vols 1 and 2. Wiley, Chichester

Whitehead M 1987 The health divide. Health Education Council, London

WHO 1947 Constitution of the World Health Organization. United Nations Organization, New York

WHO 1978 Primary health care. Report of international conference held at Alma Ata, USSR. World Health Organization, Geneva

WHO 1979 Primary health care in Europe (Euro Reports No. 14). WHO, Copenhagen

WHO 1981 Regional programme in health education and lifestyles. Regional Committee for Europe, 31st Session, Berlin, EUR/RIC31/10. World Health Organization, Copenhagen

WHO 1984 Discussion document on health promotion: concepts and principles. World Health Organization, Copenhagen

WHO 1985 Targets for health for all. World Health Organization, Geneva

WHO 1986 The Ottawa Charter. World Health Organization, Geneva

WHO 1990/91 World health statistics annual. World Health Organization, Geneva

WHO 1992 International classification of diseases, 10th revision. World Health Organization, Geneva, Section F

WHO 1994 World health report. World Health Organization, Geneva

WHO 1998, Health 21: the Health Policy Framework for the WHO European Region, World Health Organization, Copenhagen

WHO 1999a World health report. World Health Organization, Geneva

WHO 1999b Health for all in the 21st century. World Health Organization, Geneva

WHO 1999c ASD report on the global HIV/AIDS epidemic. World Health Organization, Geneva

WHO 2005 World health report 2005. Make every mother and child count. World Health Organization, Geneva

Wild J 1953 Plato's modern enemies and the theory of natural law. University of Chicago Press, Chicago

Wilkin D, Gillam S, Leese B 2000 Progress and challenges 1999/2000. National tracker survey of primary care groups and trusts. National Primary Care Research and Development Centre, Manchester

Wilkin D, Gillam S, Coleman A 2001 National tracker survey of primary care groups and trusts 2000/2001. National Primary Care Research and Development Centre, Manchester

Wilkinson R 1996 Unhealthy societies: the affliction of inequalities. Routledge, London

Wilson M 1976 Health is for people. Darton, Longman & Todd, London

Windt P Y, Appleby P C, Battin M P, Francis L P, Landesman B M 1989 Ethical issues in the professions. Prentice Hall, Englewood Cliffs, NJ

Wittgenstein L (Anscombe G E M, tr) 1958 Philosophical investigations. Blackwells, Oxford

Wittgenstein L 1971 Tractatus logico-philosophicus, new edn. Routledge & Kegan Paul, London

WMA 1947 Nuremberg Code. World Medical Association, Ferney-Voltaire

WMA 1948/1968 Declaration of Geneva. World Medical Association, Ferney-Voltaire

WMA 2000 Declaration of Helsinki – ethical principles for research involving human subjects. World Medical Association, Ferney-Voltaire. Online. Available: http://www.wma.net/e/policy/b3.htm

WMA 2005 Medical ethics manual 2005 World Medical Association, Ferney-Voltaire. Online. Available: http://www.wma.net/e/policy/b3.htm

Woozley A D 1981 Law and the legislation of morality. In: Caplan A H, Callahan D (eds) Ethics in hard times. Hastings Center Series on Ethics, Hastings on Hudson, USA

World Bank 1993 Investing in health – 1993. World development report. Oxford University Press, Oxford

World Bank 2004 Human development report 2004. World Bank, Human Development Report Office, New York

Young A, Cooke M 2001 Managing and implementing decisions in healthcare. Baillière Tindall, London

Yovich J, Grudzinskas G 1990 The management of infertility – a manual of gamete handling procedures. Heinemann Medical, London

Glossary

Absolutism (moral)

The moral position adopted by those who claim moral principles are not relative (i.e. dependent on personal bias or differences of culture), but are universally, unconditionally and unquestionably true. The absolutist asserts these moral principles dogmatically as infallible.

Accountability (cf Responsibility)

The terms 'accountable' and 'responsible' are often used interchangeably, because they do in fact mean much the same thing – namely, 'to be able to give an account' and 'to be able to make a response.' However, the terms have acquired more technical meanings in ethics and law. 'Responsibility' is the more inclusive terms as it can be used both to describe being *responsible for* one's own actions, or being *responsible for* the care or protection of someone else, and it can also be used to cover 'being *responsible to* another person' – in the sense that one has a duty to account for one's actions to that person. The term 'accountability' is used in law and ethics to apply to *the duty we have to justify our actions to those with whom we have contractual obligations*, (e.g. to one's line manager, employer, professional colleagues, or to taxpayers, through the courts). This is especially the case when our actions fail to meet legal or professional standards. Whether individual health professionals are directly *accountable to* [or have direct contractual *obligations to*] their patients or clients can be disputed, as this involves an extended use of the term 'contract' to apply to the relationship between practitioner and client. Generally it is the practitioner's employer who would be held accountable, although an individual health professional may be sued by a patient, e.g. where their negligence or incompetence has impacted adversely on the health of the patient.

Act deontology

Moral theory that justifies individual acts by whether they are done in accordance with your duty (Greek *deon*), or based on fundamental principles. (Cf. Rule deontology.)

Act utilitarianism

Moral theory that would justify individual acts by whether they increase your pleasure or reduce the risk of pain. (Cf. Rule utilitarianism.)

Action theory

A philosophical approach which analyses the common features of human acts, that is, conscious, voluntary, intentional and goal-directed actions, and distinguishes these from automatic or reflexive behaviour.

Aesthetics

The theory of beauty, of the philosophical study of the canons and criteria applicable to the appraisal of works of art, architecture or music (from Greek *aisthanomai* for perception).

Affirmative action

Where special efforts are made to ensure equal opportunity for members of groups that have been subject to discrimination (weak sense) or where a definite preference is shown, where candidates have equal qualifications, for members of disadvantaged groups (e.g. women or ethnic minorities) – in order to ensure equality of outcome for such groups where they have traditionally been subject to discrimination (strong sense).

Agapeism

Literally a 'love ethic' (from Greek *agape* for love), or more specifically the type of ethic that applies the criterion of what is the most loving thing to do in a given case, as the basis for all moral decisions.

Agency/Structure

A distinction drawn in the study of society and social organisations, in contemporary sociology, between those aspects of social institutions that are subject to change by the initiative of individuals (agency) and those more enduring features of social institutions which embody traditional practices and systems of organisation (structure). This parallels the distinction between 'interactionism' and 'structuralism' – the emphasis on the scope for interpersonal agency, and the maintenance of social structures and their regulation.

Akrasia/weakness of will

The term was introduced into moral discourse by Aristotle, in his analysis of the moral life. Here, resolution, or strength of will, is essential in making individual decisions, in holding to a course of action and in achieving mastery and excellence in performance. Weakness of will may result either from failure to develop our rational potentialities or to cultivate the virtue of prudence. Alternatively, the will and our moral resolution may be compromised by failure to resolve conflicts between our desires, failure to prioritise our choices or due to intoxication. In the former sense weakness of the will may be inadvertent, due to lack of moral education, but culpable in the latter case, due to our failure to exercise appropriate choices at an earlier stage.

Algorithm

A process or rule for calculation, or rule to be followed in decision-making.

Altruism

A principle for action based on unselfish regard for other people, denying oneself for the sake of others.

Antinomian (from Greek *nomos* for law).

To be antinomian is to be against any kind of law, or formal rules. Historically, antinomians emphasised that to live a moral life is to live by grace and the 'rule' of love, to observe the spirit of the law, rather than to stick to the letter of the law.

A priori

Reasoning from causes to effects or argument from first principles to practical reality.

A posteriori

Reasoning from effects back to their causes, or arguing from evidence to a general theory.

Attitudes

Attitudes are generally 'inherited' dispositions or ways of regarding or reacting to other people, groups, things or ideas. However, they may become 'ingrained' as internalised prejudices or opinions about other people both inside and outside our own group, or towards the external world. Attitudes can include cognitive, affective and behavioural components learned from parents, one's peer group or culture, e.g. racism, sexism, ageism.

Audit/Clinical audit

An audit is a formal hearing or official scrutiny of practice, based on established rules of appraisal. Clinical audit is an appraisal of the clinical performance and competence of a doctor, nurse or member of the paramedical professions, and this may be by the method of peer review, by senior practitioner or manager, by external consultant, or by a regulatory body.

Authority (from the Latin *augere* – to increase, augment or implement).

'Authority' refers to the official power or right to enforce obedience to rules or policy. Those exercising public authority are normally officially appointed or given delegated authority to implement policy so as to augment or promote the well-being of some group or community. The moral basis of authority, as opposed to dictatorship or authoritarian rule, is that it is legitimated by official appointment to promote the common good of the community in which authority is exercised and requires the consent of those subject to authority,

Autonomy

Literally, to be a law unto oneself (from Greek *autos* = self, and *nomos* = law), but while 'being a law unto oneself' usually has derogatory connotations of lawlessness, it was introduced by Kant to emphasise that the responsible moral agent must internalise and make the moral law their own, and not merely act from some duty imposed on them by authority. (Cf. Heteronomy, Theonomy.)

Axiology (from Greek *axia* = value).

Axiology is an approach to ethics based on the theory of value and the study of values. It is linked to virtue ethics in that the rank ordering of the intellectual and moral virtues is based on value judgements about which goals human beings should strive for, given their rational nature and general make-up.

Belief

A belief is a personal judgement for which one makes a truth claim, and which one should be prepared to defend – by producing sound reasons or evidence. While attitudes are generally acquired from others, beliefs comprise the sub-set of attitudes for which we personally make truth claims. To say that we believe something to be true does not mean that we know for certain that it is true, so we do not give beliefs unconditional assent.

Benchmarking

An approach to management and strategic planning which involves setting baseline criteria against which to measure progress.

Beneficence

The principle that we should do good to others (Latin *beneficio* = to do good) rather than harm (Latin *maleficio*). Beneficence means the exercise of responsible care or a duty of care.

Bill of Rights

A statement of human rights claimed to be universally applicable to human beings in virtue of sharing the same 'human nature', however defined.

Binary system

A system of thought or logic that allows two and only two values, e.g. true/false, right/wrong, and does not admit of degrees of comparison.

Bourgeoisie

Term used to describe the new commercial class of upwardly mobile townspeople who, from the 16th century onwards, played an increasing part in the politics of Europe, a term also used by Karl Marx to describe the educated middle class from which the capitalist entrepreneurs emerged in opposition to the aristocracy and working class labourers.

Business ethic

An approach to trade and commercial practice based on a claimed right to seek one's own commercial advantage through free competition and the private accumulation of wealth, based on faith in a self-regulating free market.

Caring ethic

An individualistic approach to ethics based on acceptance of a responsibility for others and the exercise of protective beneficence towards vulnerable people in particular.

Casuistry (cf. Latin *casus* = case).

Casuistry is an approach to ethics based on the study of individual cases and actual precedents, rather than attempting to apply universal rules or laws to all cases of the same type. It corresponds in law to the tradition of jurisprudence based on case law, use and wont, which is the basis of English common law.

Causes/means/ends

These terms refer to three broad aspects of purposeful or intentional acts, namely that acts do not arise in a vacuum, but are due to specific *causal conditions* (background circumstances, contextual rules and specific causes necessitating a decision), where a specific agent needs to choose appropriate *means and methods* to effect their decision, and where an action is given meaning or purpose by the adoption of a predetermined *goal or end* to be achieved by the action.

Clinical audit

see Audit

Code of ethics

(Latin *codex* = a systematic set of laws or rules). A code of ethics (or code of conduct) is a formal statement of the ethical principles and rules by which a group or profession seeks to ensure that members' behaviour conforms to appropriate moral standards and competence in performance of their official duties.

Collective bargaining

In industrial relations, between employers and employees, this term refers generally to collective negotiation over wages, terms and conditions of work, by an organised body of employees or trade union.

Common good

The 'common good' refers to that which can be assumed to promote the general well-being of a given community. In certain circumstances the alleged rights of an individual may conflict with the safety and wider interests of society (the common good), e.g. when a paedophile is deprived of their liberty to protect the public, or when people's movements are restricted to prevent the spread of a contagious disease.

Communitarian/Liberal

A communitarian approach contrasts with that of traditional liberalism, by emphasising that we are members of a community first and only acquire our rights as responsible members of a community, rather than the more individualistic emphasis in liberalism that we should have unrestricted liberty to do what we like so long as we do not harm others.

Competence (legal)

This is a technical term derived from the Latin legal term *compos mentis* meaning that an individual 'has the command of his/her own mind'. An individual may not be regarded as legally competent (to stand as a witness, or plead before a court) if they are mentally disordered, severely intellectually impaired, senile and confused, or too young to know what they are doing.

Competencies

This term refers to the developed skills or abilities which have become established in an individual by training, habit and regular practice. It is roughly equivalent to the classical notion of virtue or personal strength, or state of excellence achieved by habit and practice.

Conscience

A term used to refer to our inner moral sense of what is right and wrong, good or bad, virtuous or vicious. The Greek equivalent *suneidesis* means having a capacity to take a circumspect view of the whole situation in which we have to act, to 'see the big picture'. The English word (from Latin *cum* = with and *scientia* = science) literally means having sound theoretical and practical knowledge of moral principles and their application, and refers to an intellectual faculty of judgement, not to some mysterious 'voice' in our heart or mind.

Consensus

The term refers to a common agreement of opinion on some matter, or common sense among people of what should be done.

Consent – informed

A formal requirement for any medical intervention or invasive nursing procedure is that the patient should give 'informed consent'. While there is a growing body of law to specify what this means in practice, the general requirements for informed consent are that if the patient is of sound mind (a) they should be given adequate and intelligible information in advance, to enable them to understand for what treatment they are giving their permission; (b) they should be able to give their consent to treatment voluntarily and without any kind of pressure or duress.

Consent – proxy

Proxy consent may be required or given where a patient is unable to give their own permission for the treatment proposed for them – because they lack legal capacity (e.g. are too young, mentally disordered or unconscious). This is a difficult area in law and ethics, because there is a risk that the wishes or rights of the patient may be overridden, by

professionals or relatives, supposedly 'in their best interests'. To avoid abuse of proxy consent it has traditionally been the case that parents, or a legal guardian (in the case of a child) or an official *curator bonis* (in the case of an adult) is legally appointed by the state, to advocate for the patient and to give consent to treatment 'in the best interests of the patient', or as some authorities would prefer: 'where it is not against the interests of the patient'. Attempts have been made to clarify the complex issues of proxy consent in the UK in the Adults with Incapacity (Scotland) Act 2000, and the English Mental Capacity Act 2005. Consent for an incapacitated adult's participation in research must also be obtained in Scotland, from 'the patient's guardian or welfare attorney or nearest relative'. In English law the requirement is just that an attorney or someone (not paid for, or professionally) caring for the person (usually a family member), or if all else fails someone nominated by the researcher (but not connected with the research), must be consulted. This is a developing area of case law and on-going ethical debate.

Consequentialism

An approach to ethics in which the outcomes or results of an action are used as the basis for judging whether the action was morally justified. This is a more specific form of utilitarian ethics, where the moral value of an action in achieving a desired goal is determined by reference to its usefulness or utility in achieving that goal.

Constitutive/regulative principles

In any structured and rule-governed activity, from simple games to complex forms of social activity, e.g. in a law court, the conduct of appropriate activity is determined by two kinds of principles, what Kant called 'constitutive' and 'regulative' principles or rules. The former set up (or constitute) the 'game' or activity, by defining the field in which action is to occur, the roles and responsibilities of 'players' and the goals which they must pursue. The latter (regulative rules or principles) set out the operational criteria for judging whether actions 'in the game' are appropriate, conform to the constitutive principles, or whether actions infringe the rules and what penalties should apply.

Continuous quality improvement (CQI)

A systematic approach to the management of organisations in which striving for excellence is based on a process of regular review of performance, in which problems are identified, assessments of needs undertaken, action plans developed with set objectives, interventions are monitored, outcomes recorded and fed back for evaluation and overall performance appraisal.

Conventionalism

An approach to ethics in which social custom and tradition (or conventions) serve as the primary basis for determining what is to be considered right or wrong conduct.

Corporate ethics

An approach to ethics in organisational life in which overall ethical policy development serves as the basis for strategic and operational management and provides the framework within which employees or practitioners exercise their functions.

Counselling

While traditionally 'counselling' has meant giving counsel or advice, and is still used in disciplinary procedures in public sector personnel management for giving cautionary advice, a warning or rebuke, the term has acquired a more specific meaning in psychological counselling, where it refers to skilled listening and helping a client to identify their own problems, what options they have, and to find their own solutions to the difficulties facing them.

Crisis

A decisive moment, or a situation demanding a decision (from Greek *krisis* = decision time).

Critical thinking

While this term has a general meaning, namely to subject our assumptions and the evidence before us to rational criticism, it also refers more specifically to the systematic methods used in informal logic for the examination of argument forms, criteria for the evaluation of evidence and the validity of the conclusions we draw from our premises and given information.

Decision

In making a decision we attempt to resolve difficulties, reach a conclusion about the best course of action to be taken, and commit ourselves to act in a certain way.

Demography

Study of vital statistics related to given populations (Greek *demos* = people), in particular statistics related to births, marriages, diseases, deaths, etc., as illustrating the conditions of life in a community under consideration (or in relation to other communities).

Deontological theory

A general approach to the justification of ethical behaviour, in which priority is given to fundamental principles, rights and duties. (Greek *deon* = duty.)

Determinism

The theory that all our actions are determined by unexceptionable causal laws and that these laws of nature constrain our actions to such a degree that they prevent the possibility of free choice or action. (Cf. Free will.)

Dilemma

In general a situation in which a difficult choice has to be made between two equally attractive or undesirable options. In ethics, a moral dilemma is an apparent or actually irresolvable clash of competing principles or duties. However, genuine or serious dilemmas are rare and most situations which present as dilemmas can be reframed as problems amenable to treatment by problem-solving methods. To describe all moral quandaries as dilemmas often represents an unwillingness to accept responsibility for making decisions.

Divine command theory

(cf. Theonomy from Greek *theos* = god, *nomos* = law). An approach to ethics in which the claim is made that fundamental ethical principles or commandments are God-given, and that human beings are accountable before God for their conduct.

Duties/obligations

What one is bound to do to fulfil one's contractual commitments to clients or one's employer, or what one is required to do by virtue of one's function, for example, to exercise due authority as a parent, leader, manager, etc. Duties usually correlate with the rights or entitlements of others and may be either moral or legal duties, and may or may not be enforceable.

Duty-based theory

see Deontological theory.

Ecological

A study of living organisms (plants, insects, animals and humans) in relation to one another in their surroundings, that is within a specific environment, or changing environment.

Econometric

This refers to the attempt to measure processes or interventions by measurement of their economic impacts. This may take place at a micro or macro level in society.

Economic rationalism

This term is used in Australia for the type of neoconservative economic theory which claims to make value-neutral economic decisions, based on measurable criteria of effectiveness and efficiency, profitability and cost reduction.

Effectiveness

A measure of the impact of a policy in achieving long-term strategic goals.

Efficiency

A measure of productivity by examining operational systems and processes.

Egalitarianism (from French *egal* = equal).

To advocate equal rights for all regardless of specific differences between people.

Emotivism

The theory that a moral judgement is nothing more than an expression of a person's feelings of approval or disapproval of another's actions, sometimes called the 'boo–hurrah theory of value'.

Empiricism

The theory that all knowledge is derived from experience, or more specifically from sense-experience, scientific observation and experiment.

Enlightenment (The)

The period of the 18th and early 19th centuries in European history in which emphasis on reason and scientific method had a great influence on culture.

Epicureanism

The philosophy of life based on the pursuit of pleasure, where the aim is to minimise pain and achieve a positive balance of pleasure over pain by self-control and avoiding excess of any kind. (Cf. Hedonism.)

Epidemiology

Literally epidemiology is that branch of medicine that studies epidemics, but the term has acquired a more specific meaning as referring to the systematic collection of evidence, the aggregation of data, and rigorous statistical analysis of trends in the incidence and prevalence of diseases or lifestyle-related conditions.

Epistemology

(from Greek *episteme* = knowledge). Epistemology is the study of the grounds for knowledge, its different forms, the methods and criteria applied in the systematic expression of it.

Equality/Equity

'Equality' applies to the relationship of individuals and relates to the ideal that every person should have the same opportunities, rights and entitlements to social benefits and the same status as citizens and before the law. 'Equity', on the other hand, refers to the principle of fairness and distributive justice as it applies to groups of people, in the attempt to ensure equality of outcome for different groups in society, particularly those traditionally disadvantaged.

Esoteric/Exoteric

Esoteric knowledge is knowledge that is sometimes secret and often seems obscure, because it is exclusive to members of a group or profession. It refers to knowledge and practices that are unintelligible to those who have not had special training or initiation into the group, sect or profession in question. (Medical knowledge has often appeared esoteric to lay people, and in the past doctors have profited from keeping knowledge of medical secrets to themselves, because it was the basis of their power and right to charge for their services.) *Exoteric knowledge* (and practices) are open to public verification and critical scrutiny and for this reason science and philosophy have traditionally advocated an exoteric approach to truth, where information and new discoveries are shared with the public and for the common good.

Ethics

In general, ethics, from the Greek *ethos*, means the spirit of a community. It refers to the formal cooperative endeavour of a moral community to define its values, the necessary conditions, practical requirements, and protective rules which will ensure its well-being and the flourishing of its members. 'An ethic' refers to the 'belief-and-value system' of any moral community, or to the formal code of practice of a corporate body, or profession. (Cf. Ideology.)

Ethics (applied)

Skill in applied ethics means being able to act responsibly, appropriately and effectively in various situations, and it also means being able to provide a clear, coherent and reasoned justification for one's decisions and actions, with reference to commonly accepted standards. This requires the following skills:

- knowledge of the basic principles which express our fundamental values and from which we derive practical moral rules
- competence in practical problem-solving and decision-making skills required for dealing with moral problems
- discretion in formulating sound ethical policies and choosing relevant decision procedures for use in different types of situations
- sound habits and stable dispositions (competencies) to ensure that one acts effectively as a responsible moral agent.

Etiquette/social mores

These terms refer to the traditions or social customs that define one's social comportment or acceptable ways of relating to others, e.g. rules of dress; manners; culture-specific practices in a society, sect, club or group; court ceremonial and procedure; business and professional courtesies. All social groups have such rules, whether written down or simply taken for granted, and modern professional groups and business corporations are no exception. (From French *tiquette* = ticket of entry, and Latin *mores* = manners or fashion.)

Eudaimonism

Eudaimonism refers to a type of philosophy in which the pursuit of happiness, rather than mere pleasure, is the highest goal (from Greek *eudaimonia* = happiness or well-being). Aristotle's ethics is called teleological eudaimonism because he believed all things, and especially living things, have a built-in tendency, or drive, to fulfil their potentialities, which, in the case of human beings, is striving for happiness, well-being or fulfilment.

Euthanasia (from Greek *eu* = good, and *thanatos* = death).

Euthanasia is literally the facilitation of a gentle and easy death, particularly in the case of incurable and chronically painful disease. 'Passive euthanasia' is generally applied to action to terminate treatment and 'let nature take its course'. 'Active euthanasia' by contrast applies to direct action to terminate life, e.g. by fatal injection or other means, or by assisting the patient to commit suicide.

Evaluation – formative, summative

'Formative evaluation' relates to the assessment of an individual's progress in training, their level of skills development and practical competence. 'Summative evaluation' relates to the assessment of an individual

at the end of a process of training or education and the attempt to measure or assess their overall performance by the application of various tests and correlation of various results and outcomes of these. (These terms correspond roughly to 'process' and 'outcome' evaluation as applied to interventions with patients or clients, or to the evaluation of organisational changes and their impact on systems and professional practice affecting outcomes for clients.)

Evidence-based practice

Evidence-based practice refers to the conscientious, explicit and judicious use of current best evidence in making decisions about the care of individual patients or the effectiveness of procedures used in managing patients' needs.

Existentialism/Essentialism

Existentialism is a movement in philosophy which began in the 19th century but was at its most influential following World War II. It represented a critical reaction to idealist philosophy with its concentration on abstract principles, universal ideas or essences. Existentialist philosophers sought to refocus the attention of ethics and political philosophy on the uniqueness of each human individual and the often lonely and painful choices which we must make in actual existence in the exercise of our individual freedom. The slogan: 'existence is prior to essence' makes this point equally for religious and atheist thinkers. Kierkegaard, Buber, Tillich, Marcel, Maritain and Levinas emphasise the ultimate concern of each unique person (or existing historical subject) with the meaning of being, which drives them in their quest for faith and authentic existence. Proclaiming the death of God, Nietzsche, Camus, Heidegger and Sartre argue that human beings 'create their own values' and must 'make themselves by their decisions', and as there is no God-given 'essence' to human nature to direct us or constrain our freedom, we are 'condemned to be free'. Essentialist philosophy by contrast has sought to ground universal moral principles and rules on the given structure and dynamics of being, whether this is God-given or is the universal and intelligible nature of things disclosed to reason in its investigation of our world.

Feeling/Emotion

'Feeling' literally means the receptive and passive response of our senses to the world around us, including people and things, animals and plants. Whereas 'emotion' usually refers to our reaction to or response to what we feel. (Feeling the pain of sitting on a tack may give rise to the emotion of anger, as we seek to find the person who put the tack on our chair!) 'Emotions' can and do motivate us to action, e-motions set us in motion and move us to act.

Felicific calculus

Literally, a calculus for measuring the degree of happiness produced by an action or policy. A concept introduced by Bentham in his version of utilitarianism – sometimes referred to as psychological hedonism because it is concerned with attainment of sustained feelings of pleasure. Attempts by modern economists to measure the 'quality of life' owe something to Bentham.

Fiduciary duties/responsibility

A protective duty of care owed to a client by someone in a consulting role as a result of a person entrusting themselves, their affairs or their secrets to you. (From Latin *fiducia* = trust.)

Force-field analysis

Method for clarifying the forces that are operating on a situation or giving rise to a problem, by systematically examining four related fields: the present reality, the hoped for ideal, forces resistant to change and forces promoting change. The object is to identify and prioritise those resistant forces that need to be addressed and the supportive forces that should be exploited to achieve desired change.

Free will

The belief that despite the influences on us of heredity and environment, human beings have the capacity for free choice or self-determinism, because we have the ability to gain insight into the operation of causal laws, and therefore can direct the course of events by becoming causes ourselves.

Fundamentalism

Strict maintenance of the letter of the law of traditional religious beliefs, often associated with belief in the infallibility of religious authority or the authority of sacred Scriptures. In ethics, fundamentalism is associated with unquestioning acceptance of traditional systems of moral rules.

Globalisation

Generally 'globalisation' means the worldwide spread of cultural ideas and practices. However, the term is most commonly used in the media today to refer to worldwide trends in economics, whether these be the development of international trade and competition, or the role of hugely powerful multinational business corporations in promoting the spread of international capitalism. However, there are other aspects of globalisation which relate to the global influence of 'catholic' or universal religious faiths or political ideologies, the development of international institutions (e.g. the International Court of Human Rights), the worldwide spread of scientific knowledge and technology, the international sharing of medical expertise and new technology, including international travel and the risks of rapid transmission of global pandemics.

Golden Rule

Variously expressed in different religious and cultural traditions around the world, but generally expressed as 'Do to others as you would wish that they should do to you' or in negative and stronger terms as 'Never do to others what you would not wish them to do to you in similar circumstances'.

Good/bad

The terms 'good' and 'bad' belong to our vocabulary of value judgements, and are the most general terms of appraisal which we apply to things that we value or of which we disapprove.

Ground rules

The foundational rules (or constitution) of a group, sports club, society or moral community, which are agreed to and observed by members.

Health/Disease

There is a vast literature in the sociology of health and disease, but it is perhaps worth remarking that 'health' comes from the Old English word *hal* meaning 'whole', whereas 'disease' comes from disease or discomfort. When the WHO defined health as 'complete mental, physical and social well-being, and not merely the absence of disease or infirmity', it echoed this ancient tradition, linking health with happiness or optimum well-being of body, mind and soul. More technically traditional medical definitions have been given in terms of the maintenance of an optimum balance or homeostasis in the operation of the various body systems, and disease with disturbances in this balance caused by either injury or pathogens.

Healthist/Healthism

A healthist is someone who makes health their ultimate value and thus ignores other competing human values, including those things which might be valued by someone who was suffering chronic pain and/or an incurable disease, for example love or religious faith. Healthism is a term used to apply to the ideology of health as the ultimate value and to those who seek by aggressive health promotion to pressurise other people to adopt the same ideology. Applied to government policy it means the use of mass media health promotion or statutory means used as instruments of social engineering to bring about changes in social behaviour.

Hedonism

A philosophy in which the pursuit of pleasure (and avoidance of pain) are the primary objectives. (From Greek *hedone* = pleasure.)

Heteronomy

Submission to the rule of an externally imposed authority, or to laws imposed by some outside power. (From Greek *hetero* = alien or other, and *nomos* = law.)

Hippocratic Oath

This Oath is the first known code of medical ethics, attributed to Hippocrates (422 BC) and which served as the basis for the Hippocratic school or esoteric brotherhood of physicians which he established, on the Greek island of Cos. It is believed that the code is of Pythagorean origin, as Hippocrates' school appears to have been modelled on earlier Pythagorean ones.

Hobson's choice

This is a choice that is not a real choice, or the option of taking what is offered or nothing at all. It refers to T. Hobson (d. 1831) who when hiring out his horses required clients to take the horse nearest the stable door or none at all.

Honesty and truth-telling

Honesty refers to the giving of reliable and trustworthy testimony. From the Latin *honestus* = honour, honesty is a requirement of respect for persons, dishonesty being the most contemptible way to treat another person. 'Truth-telling' likewise has a wider meaning than merely recounting the facts, because it has to take account of the context and to have regard to the intelligence, maturity and mental state of the hearer.

Iatrogenic (from Greek *iatros* = doctor, *genea* = birth). This is a term applied to diseases, injury or harmful side-effects caused by medical neglect, malpractice or incompetence, or inadvertently caused by ignorance of the long-term effects of drugs, chemotherapy or other surgical or medical interventions.

Ideologue

Advocate or proponent of some ideology.

Ideology

A comprehensive world-view, framework of meaning, or belief-and-value system that enables people to organise, make sense of, and change their world, both social and physical.

Imperatives/indicatives

Imperatives are 'ought' statements, or statements of duties and obligations. Indicatives are 'is' statements or statements of facts, evidence or truth claims.

Inalienable right

A right claimed to be intrinsic to one's nature as a human being and therefore not able to be removed (though it may be subject to restriction by others).

Individualism

Belief that individual rights should not be restricted in any way, and which correspondingly underplays the importance of society and societal duties.

In loco parentis

The legal or moral responsibility to act on behalf of an (absent) parent.

Innate knowledge

Knowledge claimed to be inborn in us and accessible by either introspection or direct intuition. Some advocates of deontology claim we can directly intuit our rational duty, because the notion is innate in rational beings.

Institutionalisation

This is a term popularised in E. Goffman's *Asylums*, a study of the dehumanising effects on both patients and healthcare staff, or inmates and their warders, and others who are subject to living or working in long-term confinement in what he called a 'total institution' (e.g. in a hospital, asylum, prison, boarding school, army barracks, or aged-care home).

Integrity

A virtue that implies sound character or the wholeness of the moral person, combining consistency, reliability, honesty and fairness. (From Latin *integer* = whole, undivided, uncontaminated.)

Intellectual virtues

Traditionally, according to Aristotle, these comprise theoretical and practical knowledge (of a discipline), acquired skill and practical expertise, judgement, intelligence, self-insight, resourcefulness, persistence and wisdom.

Intentional acts

Purposeful actions that have a clear goal or objective.

Intentionality

The characteristic of all conscious acts, namely that they refer to (intend) some object independent of consciousness – that 'object' may be some thing or person or an 'object' in the sense of a goal or objective.

Interactionism/Structuralism

Micro-social theories (e.g. those of Mead (1934) and Goffman (1969)) deal with the interactions people have with one another on an individual level (interactionism). Macro-social perspectives deal with the formation and maintenance of social structures, such as health services and regulatory bodies (structuralism). Giddens's (1984) theory of structuration proposes that neither interactionism nor structuralism is adequate by itself, and that a more comprehensive sociological explanation of human behaviour should combine elements of both.

Internal market

A microeconomic theory that large bureaucratic public sector organisations (e.g. health services, education and social services) can be made more cost-effective if an element of competition between public and private sector providers is introduced into the system so that the procurement and commissioning of services is based on competitive tendering, or contracting out of traditionally public sector services to private sector providers.

Intuition/Intuitionism (rational) (from Latin *in – tueri* = to look inwards).

'Intuition' describes the introspective process of making sense of what is given in our experience. It is traditionally the faculty that complements and integrates the information derived from sense perception. 'Intuitionism' or 'rational intuitionism' in ethics is the theory that we can grasp moral principles by introspection or by direct inspection of the contents of our minds or consciences.

Justice (distributive, restorative and retributive)

(from Latin *jus* = law or right).

In general terms, 'justice' means fairness in the distribution of goods, in attempting to make good the harm done by people's actions, and in imposing sanctions on those who infringe the rights of others. *Distributive justice* is fairness in the sharing out of social benefits and responsibilities, in ensuring equality of opportunity for all individuals, and equality of outcomes for different groups in society. *Restorative justice* refers to the variety of ways in which attempts are made to compensate the victims of crime or those who suffer discrimination of one kind or another. More recently it has been associated with attempts to bring perpetrator and victim together to help the perpetrator understand the impact of their actions on the victim, and to mediate between them in agreeing ways in which the perpetrator can repay their debt to society and their victim/s. *Retributive justice* refers to the various sanctions or forms of punishment that are applied to those guilty of crimes, misdemeanours and antisocial behaviour, and whether the intent of these is reformative and educative of the guilty party, deterrent or simply punishment as such.

Justification

To provide an argued and rational defence of a person, a decision, action or theory.

Kingdom of ends (moral community)

Introduced by Immanuel Kant, the phrase 'kingdom of ends' was used to refer to the community of interest of those who share the same rational goals and agree to be governed by the same obligations and rules. A modern equivalent is the term 'moral community' referring to any community of interest that shares the same values and goals.

Labelling, stereotyping

Generally, a 'label' is a mark identifying some object or class of objects. The theory of labelling originated within sociological perspectives of deviance (Lemert 1951, Becker 1963) and refers to attitudes towards people who have attributes that society considers abnormal. These attributes may relate, for example, to an individual's physical or mental health problems, their physical appearance, personality type or sexual orientation. A 'stereotype' is literally an unalterable cast of printing type, and 'to stereotype', by extension of the metaphor, is to employ an unduly fixed mental image or impression of a person or group of persons.

Legalism

An attitude to ethics and social behaviour which places undue emphasis on laws and rules and living in accordance with these, rather than making allowance for individual differences between people, their circumstances and the requirement of mercy as well as justice.

Liberalism

Belief in achievement of the autonomy of the individual as the ultimate objective of moral and political action; alternatively in the economic sphere it refers to the *laissez faire* doctrine of unrestricted free trade and unregulated open competition.

Liberty/liberties (cf. Rights).

'Liberty' means freedom in the sense of *freedom from* restraint or the risk of punishment, rather than referring to our positive *freedom to* do something, or entitlement to act. Liberties are distinguished from rights in that liberties are simply permissive – to have the liberty to do something means that I am permitted to do something (without moral or legal sanctions on my behaviour) provided that my action does not harm anyone else, or infringe their rights or restrict their liberty. (Cf. Rights, Duties.)

Litigious (from Latin *litigare* = to contest a matter in a law court).

To be litigious is to be fond of litigation or engaging in law suits.

Logic

The intellectual discipline that studies the forms of consistent and coherent thought and the rules that ensure that this is possible.

Managerialism

An approach to the management of organisations which places the emphasis on the directive power and authority of the 'boss', rather than adopting a participative and consultative approach to employees and industrial relations. ('Let the managers manage!')

Medicalisation

A term used to describe the tendency of those involved in healthcare, and particularly doctors, to treat all human problems as medical problems and as legitimate areas in which to expand the influence and control of medicine and health services.

Mentor/mentoring

Where an experienced and trusted adviser is appointed to assist trainees, to encourage them to share the problems they are encountering in their work, to debrief on their successes and failures, and to provide them with encouragement and support.

Meta-ethics *see* Moral philosophy.

Metaphysics

(Literally 'beyond physics'). Metaphysics is that branch of philosophical inquiry in which the most general categories and concepts applicable to our knowledge of the world and ourselves are examined and their systematic connections explored, e.g. being, existence and essence, substance, matter and form, act and potency, causality, time and space, relations and modality. 'Metaphysics' is also often applied to rational debate on the existence of God, of the foundations of freedom or determinism, mortality and immortality, and the origin of the universe.

Mission

The given task or reason for the existence of a group or organisation. The term has been adopted to encourage business organisations to identify the primary nature of their business, who are its primary customers and what goals should direct its strategic and operational planning. (From Latin *missio* = sending off.)

Modernity

Generally we refer to the 'modern world' as the new social, political and scientific order that emerged in the Renaissance, due to the secularisation of society and the triumph of rationalism and empiricism over 'religious superstition'. The three pillars of 'modernity' are generally agreed to be a combination of the scientifico-technical world-view, the emergence of capitalist economy and the emphasis on the self-sufficiency or autonomy of human beings. (Cf. Postmodernism.)

Moral autonomy *see* Autonomy.

Moral community

Term used to refer to any group of people who are united in their commitment to a set of common ground rules for action and dealing with other people.

Moral majority

Term used in the media to refer to those conservative religious or moral pressure groups that claim to represent the 'silent majority'.

Moral philosophy/meta-ethics

For many who have studied philosophy, their introduction to ethics has not been to ethics as a practical discipline, but to moral philosophy, or meta-ethics. Both refer to the critical and academic study of different moral theories or different 'belief and value systems' ('the science of morals'). Moral philosophy is not so much concerned with practical moral decision-making or the justification of actual decisions and actions. It is concerned rather with equipping us to understand the general philosophical grounds on which we can justify our principles and belief-and-value systems, both on theoretical grounds, and when faced with practical challenges from sceptics. In this sense 'meta-ethics' is a higher level or 'second-order' study of the theoretical underpinnings of our moral systems (e.g. deontology, virtue ethics or utilitarianism).

Moral scepticism

The philosophical attitude that moral truth is unattainable and that there are no moral certainties, or moral principles that can be said to have universal applicability.

Moral theory *see* Moral philosophy.

Moral virtues

Traditionally, following Plato and Aristotle and the Christian tradition, the most important or 'cardinal' moral virtues have been regarded as temperance (self-control or self-mastery), courage, justice (or fairness) and prudence (or practical wisdom).

Moralism

Moralism is in many ways the enemy of authentic morality. It is the morality of mere conformity to moral rules for the sake of appearances and respectability. It is associated with hypocritical self-righteousness, the morality of taboos, false guilt and inauthentic being. It is the object of criticism and satire in the writings and plays of many existentialist philosophers.

Morals/morality

The terms 'morals' and 'morality' generally refer in English to the goodness or badness of a person's character or dispositions, or to their personal conduct. 'Moral'/'immoral' have thus come to refer to a person's private standards, values and lifestyle as well. For this reason the paired terms 'morality'/'immorality' are commonly applied to people's sexual behaviour, or personal standards (or lack of standards) of behaviour. However, the terms are not restricted to the private sphere, for in any family or community, morality tends to be grounded in more universal cultural, ethnic, religious or ideological beliefs. (From Latin *moralis* = custom or convention.)

Nanotechnology (from Greek *nanos* = dwarf).

In scientific terms 'nano' means a fraction of 'one thousand millionth'. Nanotechnology is therefore the study of the techniques for manipulating micro particles or sub-atomic processes for various purposes, including medical ones.

Natural justice

Generally refers to the requirements of due process and fair and public trial in court, but can be applied more generally to the entitlement to be treated fairly and equitably, based on the assumption of universal human rights.

Natural law

The theory that there are intelligible structures and dynamic principles in nature, and in the nature of human beings, which can help us determine the conditions that promote or frustrate the development and well-being of things generally and human life in particular. For religious thought, theistic and pantheistic, this rational and intelligible order is God-given and can be discerned, understood and applied by us as rational beings in our conduct and ordering of the world. For non-theists, the rational and intelligible order of reality is simply taken for granted as a starting point for the development of law and morality to reflect the demands of living according to nature.

Nepotism (cf. Latin *nepos* = nephew).

The term originally meant 'favouritism shown to relatives in conferring titles, offices or benefits'. However the meaning of the term has been extended to apply to corrupt practices in public life, where preferment is shown to personal friends, members of one's own political party or religious community. Colloquially expressed, this is sometimes referred to as 'cronyism' or 'jobs for pals'.

Norm

A standard or scale by which we check, compare or measure things, or assess people's performance and the consistency of their actions. A norm or standard allows degrees of comparison to be made (e.g. 'bad', 'worse', 'worst', 'good', 'better', 'best') on a continuum where terms like 'good' and 'bad' mark the limits of the scale at either end. Norms point to a scale of performance indicators by which we make qualitative or quantitative assessments based on the available evidence. (From Latin *norma* = carpenter's square.)

Normalisation

A term coined for policies and practices aimed to combat the alienating, de-powering and dehumanising effects of institutionalisation on people with mental health problems or learning difficulties, by seeking to support their reintegration into normal society and to 'valorise' or empower them to achieve their optimum potential by living as normally as possible.

Normative (from Latin *norma* = a rule or carpenter's square).

A norm is a rule or standard against which we measure performance or achievements. 'Normative' discourse relates to the determination of standards, their application in practice, or judgements made with reference to accepted norms.

Objectivism/absolutism *see* Absolutism.

Objectivity

The claim to achieve a detached and independent point of view. Whether this ideal is attainable can be debated, and the term is often used tendentiously to recommend one's opinions as superior, e.g. in debate with someone else.

Obligation

Being required to do something by law, moral duty or contract. (The term 'obligation' is often used interchangeably with the term 'duty', except that the former suggests that those imposing and fulfilling an obligation should be obliging to one another!)

Openness (cf. transparency)

'Openness' has acquired currency in current usage (in 'management speak') as a substitute for 'honesty' and 'truthfulness'; however, it carries the additional connotation in business and public life of being candid about how one feels as well.

Operational plan

In the strategic planning process, broad objectives are clarified and goals set. Operational plans are then determined as the means by which we make sure our strategic objectives are met within a determined time-frame, budget, etc. Integrating ethics into the process of operationalising a strategic plan results in the formulation of operational ethical policy.

Option appraisal

The process of considering a variety of possible options, assessing their likely costs and benefits and determining which options are given priority.

Pandemic

An epidemic disease that spreads, or threatens to spread, rapidly throughout the world.

Paradigm (from Greek *para* = beside, *deiknumi* = to show).

A paradigm is a standard example, typical model or established pattern to be adopted for thought or practice.

Pedagogy

A technical term for the science or theory of teaching or education (from Greek *pais* = child and *agogos* = a guide).

Peer review

A form of performance appraisal where instead of the manager, members of a team, or of the profession, appraise one another's performance – giving both positive feedback and constructive criticism.

Performance appraisal

Assessment of your professional performance against previously negotiated targets and predetermined criteria or 'performance indicators'. 'Benchmarking' is a process in which such performance indicators are set, so that you know what standard is expected of you in your work.

Performance indicators

These are agreed standards or measures for the assessment of people's working practice, relative to the achievement of agreed goals or targets, where individual and staff input is measured in terms of the outcomes or actual results of their actions or interventions.

Performance management

This refers to evidence-based practice and management in a context of strategic and operational planning to set mutually agreed objectives and performance indicators (see above) for all functions of the organisation. Performance management involves regular appraisal against agreed performance measures. It is applicable at all levels of an organisation, from senior executives and middle managers to front-line practitioners, and is motivated by a drive for continuous quality improvement in service provision and its delivery.

Person, personality, personhood

The term 'person' comes from the Latin *persona* for a mask (or more fundamentally from *per-sono* = to sound through, as a mask is that through which we speak and express ourselves, especially on stage). An individual's personality refers to the identity and role that they adopt in society, to the 'mask' they wear in performing a particular role or function on the stage of life (or in their professional work). What the concept of personhood expresses is the fact that we do not have a fixed identity, and that we can 'make ourselves by our decisions' and have personal responsibility for what we make of our lives and opportunities.

Personal autonomy *see* Autonomy.

Personalist ethic

An approach to ethics in which a primary emphasis is given to personal considerations and maintaining caring relationships. (Cf. Individualism.)

Phenomenology

The term refers to that school of philosophy that recommends attention to the given phenomena of consciousness, rather than abstract speculation about being itself. The term was coined by Edmund Husserl, whose work greatly influenced the existentialist philosophers, as it focuses attention on our direct experience of existence, of consciousness and its objects, and of the nature of our intentional acts and their reality-related or oriented nature.

Philosophy

Literally (from the Greek), philosophy is the love of wisdom. It is not a body of theory but an activity in which we reflect on our ordinary life experience from a 'higher level'. For example, philosophy is not just another science, but seeks to understand the fundamental presuppositions common to all sciences. It is reflective knowledge of knowledge, or reflective consideration of the theoretical foundations of ethics as such, and so on. It seeks to clarify the nature of the answers we give to ultimate questions about the nature of the Self, the Good Life and the Good Society. Philosophy demands the courage to subject all theories given in the past to critical scrutiny in the quest for ultimate truth.

Plagiarism

From the Latin word for a kidnapper, plagiarism involves appropriating the ideas or inventions of other people, and dishonestly passing these off as our own without due acknowledgement of or recognition given to their author.

Policy

An official statement, on behalf of stakeholders in any organisation (or developed by a recognised authority within the organisation), which outlines a general or standard approach to deal with recurrent types of problems or difficult situations. By analogy an ethical policy must:

- specify the class of problems it is meant to address
- set out the overall ethical approach and objectives adopted
- list standard procedures and the ethical justification for them
- provide a framework for decision-making and conflict resolution
- set criteria for monitoring performance and implementation of the policy
- indicate a clear strategy to achieve endorsement of policy by stakeholders.

Positive discrimination (cf. Affirmative action)

This refers to a demand of restorative justice in which the attempt is made to redress past injustices or discrimination against individuals by discriminating in their favour in appointments or improvement of wages and conditions of work, to compensate for the injustices they have previously suffered.

Postmodernism

This refers to both a movement in philosophy and an attitude to modernism (see above). In general post-modernism involves a critique of the preoccupation in modern philosophy with the generalising and 'totalising' tendencies of scientific and technical thought. Like existentialism, to which it is related, it seeks to emphasise the fact that what we mean by truth and values is relative to a variety of perspectives and differing standpoints which are culturally determined, as well as matters of personal preference.

Pragmatism

A theory of truth and value that maintains that all truth and valuations are necessarily provisional and should be subject to revision in the light of experience, trial and error. If they work and prove useful, then we may be more confident that they are true or valuable, but we can never be certain.

Precedent

Generally a precedent is a previous case taken as an example for subsequent cases, but in law and morality, precedents are cases to which appeal is made in the justification of action in relation to another different and present case.

Principle (moral)

A statement of a basic and universal moral truth, or general moral requirement that serves as the starting point for moral reasoning. Alternatively, it may be a fundamental belief that is the source of inspiration or direction for moral action, and basis for reasoning about moral priorities. (From Latin *principium* = beginning or starting point from which to proceed.)

Principlism

The standpoint in ethics that emphasises the primacy of principles in judgements of what is right and wrong, good and bad, virtuous or vicious. It tends to be critical of utilitarian arguments in particular, or attempts to make the end justify the means employed in any action.

Privatisation (ethics)

The tendency to treat all ethical matters as personal and private to the individual, something that contradicts our moral tradition which has emphasised that ethics is about power and power-sharing among people and responsibility and public accountability within a moral community.

Probity

Uprightness and honesty in one's dealings with others.

Problem

A doubtful or difficult matter requiring solution, something hard to understand or to deal with, an exercise, test or challenge set for us, or 'thrown up' by life or experience. However, 'problems' in principle have 'solutions'. Problems may be difficult, but we make the assumption that they are soluble. (Greek *problema* from *pro-ballo* = throw towards.)

Process improvement

A systematic approach to the review of management systems within an organisation in which opportunities for improvement are identified, support from colleagues obtained, data collected and needs investigated, the problems identified and analysed, planned intervention undertaken and its impact evaluated and then standardised if appropriate. The whole 'continuous improvement cycle' can be repeated as frequently as necessary.

Professional indemnity

An indemnity is an official exemption from a penalty, which may be given by law for certain functionaries, or may be accepted by the employing organisation on behalf of its employees. 'Professional indemnity' generally refers to a form of corporate protection or insurance that professionals are advised to take out to protect themselves or to meet claims against them, in the event of legal action – where claims of

incompetence or allegations of malpractice are made against a practitioner.

Protective beneficence *see* Beneficence and Duty of care.

Prudential ethics

The standpoint in ethics that emphasises the crucial role of the virtue of prudence or practical wisdom in the moral agent, as a basis for sound discrimination regarding the demand for action in given circumstances, the principles that should be applied and how these may need to be adapted to meet the needs of a specific situation and specific individuals.

Purchaser/provider *see* Internal market.

Quality assurance

This refers to a systematic and planned approach to overall management based on a comprehensive audit of the processes, actions and outputs in a service industry. The object of the audit of quality is to establish baseline data on what is required to improve performance and to achieve consistent quality, by setting and maintaining standards so as to ensure the best possible service or product, and thus to give customers or clients a guarantee of quality.

Quandary

A perplexed state, a state of practical uncertainty or puzzlement over alternative choices, a practical difficulty, which may be resolved with help or access to additional resources. (Origin unknown.)

Randomised control trial

A 'control trial', in contrast to a simple trial of treatment, involves a comparative study of a 'treatment group' and a 'control group' where the former group are given some new experimental treatment while the control group are given either the traditional treatment or a placebo. In a 'randomised control trial' the allocation of patients or research subjects to the 'treatment group' or the 'control group' is on a random basis, to avoid investigator bias and to avoid any form of discrimination against patients on the basis of their condition, gender, race or other factors. Or the trial may be randomised on the basis of who gets the new, standard or placebo treatment. A 'double-blind' control trial is set up so that the investigator does not know to which group the patient or subject belongs, and who is receiving which treatment.

Rationalism

A type of philosophy which emphasises the role of reason rather than sense experience as the ultimate arbiter of truth and value, and one which assumes that we can know certain self-evident (innate) truths by introspection.

Reciprocity

To be in a relationship of mutual giving and receiving from one another, of mutual recognition of one another's rights and duties and in the exchange of privileges.

Reductionism

The attempt to explain everything in terms of one simple hypothesis, or to reduce all theories to one basic theory.

Reflective practice

A general term applied to systematic higher-level critical appraisal of one's own practice, adopting the standpoint of an imaginary observer and reviewing one's performance in the light of one's objectives, achievements and failures.

Regulative criteria

Those rules which regulate an activity, in contrast to constitutive criteria which set up the framework for the activity in question. In tennis, for example, the constitutive criteria define the size and shape of the court, the nature of the ball, rackets used and height of the net. Regulative criteria determine how you score points and what actions result in penalties. In ethics the concepts of freedom, responsibility and the existence of a moral community would be constitutive. Regulative criteria determine what actions are considered good/bad or right/wrong.

Relativism

The philosophical position that no objective truth or values can exist for these are relative to the unique experience of each individual (interpersonal relativism) or are distinctive to each society or culture (cultural relativism), or are bound up with the ideology that you adopt (philosophical relativism). (Cf. Absolutism.)

Respect for persons

The fundamental moral principle that embodies the demand that we show due regard to the rights and dignity of other human beings and seek to empower them to achieve their full human potential – to our mutual benefit.

Responsibility (cf. accountability)

To be designated *'responsible'*, in a legal or moral sense, implies that one is, or can be presumed to be, an intelligent being who is capable of acting independently as a moral agent, and who can be praised or blamed for one's actions. To be *responsible for* one's own actions (*personal responsibility*) one must know what one is doing, be acting without compulsion, have the competence to perform the action required, must be aware of one's obligations, and must be capable of giving a reasoned defence of a chosen course of action. Where one exercises a duty of care for someone else (called *fiduciary responsibility*), e.g. when acting as a parent or health professional, then one is *responsible for* that person morally and legally. In both cases, and where one exercises duties delegated to one by others in an operational context, one is said to have a duty of accountability, that is a *responsibility to give an account* of one's actions, or a justification for what one has done, that is coherent, rational and ethical.

Retribution

Punishment means punishment given as punishment, not for some other perhaps well-intended reason, such as to reform the criminal, to protect others, or to deter crime.

Revelation

The belief that there are certain truths or moral rules given by God and revealed to human beings by supernatural means, or disclosed in sacred writings.

Right/wrong

Actions are defined as 'right' or 'wrong' with reference to implicit or explicit rules or agreed principles. These are terms that belong to deontological discourse, i.e. discourse about duties as required by the rules in operation in a specific context. The claim that some action is right or wrong is normally justified by appeal to a rule, or to the authority of the rule-giver.

Rights

Justified legal or moral entitlements which may be based on particular agreements (such as promises, bets, oaths, vows, covenants or contracts) or claimed universal entitlements of human beings as human beings (such as the rights embodied in the UNO Universal Declaration of Human Rights).

Rights (negative)

A right to demand that someone desist from doing something to you that harms your interests, causes you pain, damage or inconvenience. Negative rights do not make any positive demands on others. They simply require someone to stop doing something that is causing you harm.

Rights (positive)

A right that entitles you to demand that someone else (or more generally society) gives you some benefit (such as education, welfare, employment) but where the willingness and ability of the other person/s to give you your entitlements will depend on their generosity and available resources. Rights usually correlate with duties, my rights may impose duties on you and your rights impose duties on me – as would be the case with contractual agreements. (Cf. Duties/obligations.)

Role

Socially determined function, or function defined by professional status, as in the role of an actor determined by the script of the playwright.

Rule

A rule is a statement of what can, should or ought to be done (or not done). A rule is a prescription which seeks to regulate or govern what we do. Rules define our duties, and are based on some source of 'legislative' authority (e.g. parents, church, school, government). Rules create a binary universe of discourse in which only two predicates can be applied to things, actions, or opinions, i.e. they must be either 'right' or 'wrong'.

Rule deontology

The moral theory that requires that any moral rule, in order to be morally binding, must be universally applicable to all people. For example, Kant's Categorical Imperative: 'Always act so that the rule on which you act could become the basis for a universal law'. (Cf. Act deontology.)

Rule utilitarianism

The moral theory that requires that we should always act on the rule that our action should be designed to bring the greatest happiness to the greatest number, and minimise harm to the others. (Cf. Act utilitarianism.)

Russian dolls model

A description coined and used in this book to apply to an approach to corporate ethics in which we recognise several interrelated levels of ethical responsibility: at the front-line practitioner level, team level, intra-organisational level, and inter-organisational level. (Here the different levels are nested within one another in the order given like a series of Russian dolls.)

Scapegoating

When a person is made to bear the blame or punishment that rightly should fall on others (derived from the Jewish practice of symbolically laying the sins of the people on a sacrificial goat, before driving it out into the wilderness).

Second order

A statement about a statement would be a 'second order' statement, and thus moral philosophy stands in a second order relation to ethics as an exploration of the theoretical basis of everyday ethics.

Situation ethics/Situationism

The ethical theory that maintains that ethics should not have rules and that we should not be bound by rules, but respond to every situation on its own terms and apply our general principles and values as best we can to the unique circumstances. The Christian love ethic is sometimes expressed this way, namely: 'Just do what is the most loving thing in the situation'.

Social contract theory

The philosophical position which maintains that there are no natural human rights we have by virtue of being human beings, but rather that all rights and duties arise from contracts between people and between societies. Hobbes and Rousseau argued that some kind of primordial social contract was necessary to prevent anarchy and social conflict.

Sociology

The systematic study of society in general, or specific societies, in terms of people's social roles, processes of socialisation, social organisation and social structure. One line of theory has focused on the structures (e.g. social, economic, political and organisational) within which individuals live, and the extent to which these structures facilitate or constrain the actions of those individuals. Other theories take a more individualistic approach, placing emphasis on individuals and their capacity to be active and autonomous agents within their environment, or, more recently attempting a synthesis of different approaches, i.e. those that acknowledge the influence of structures on an individual's capacity to act, but at the same time accord importance to the ability of an individual's 'agency' to influence structures, even to modify or overthrow these structures.

Species being

The common nature we possess by virtue of belonging to the same species, and which distinguishes us from, say, chimpanzees and crocodiles.

Stakeholders

All those who have an interest (stake) in any enterprise, community or business, and to be distinguished from 'stockholders', namely those with a direct financial investment in a company or business.

Stakeholder analysis

A method used to brainstorm all the main individuals or groups with a stake in an organisation and the success or failure of its operations, and to determine their respective rights, roles and responsibilities. In business the shareholders form perhaps the most important, but not exclusively important, group of stakeholders, because they have a direct stake in the business in terms of their investment in stocks and shares. However, stakeholder theory, in both private and public sector organisations, has emphasised that the interests of other groups of stakeholders (e.g. customers, employees, suppliers, the community) are ignored at our peril.

Standard (cf. Norm)

An ideal example, specified level of excellence or measure of performance to which action or services or product quality should conform.

State of nature

An assumed condition of either innocence (Rousseau) or brute competition and violence (Hobbes) before people enter into a social contract to form civil or political society and accept both rights and duties to others.

Statutory duties

Duties prescribed by law or regulation.

Strategic planning

An approach to management in which corporate planning for the longer term is undertaken with a view to getting away from 'short-termism', 'ad-hockery' and 'crisis management', where setting long-term goals and objectives can help redirect operational planning and provide a framework for assessment of success in achieving the flourishing of the business as a whole.

Subjective

Usually used in a dismissive way to indicate that something is based on personal whim or fancy, without reference to public standards or without exposing your beliefs or actions to the criticism of others. However, all actions are obviously 'subjective' insofar as they are the actions of a subject.

Subjectivism

An approach to truth, beauty or ethical values which denies their objectivity, insisting that truth is relative to each individual, that 'beauty is in the eye of the beholder', and that what is good or bad is a matter of personal taste.

Subsidiarity

The principle that practical responsibility for operations, especially large organisations, should be devolved downwards to the lowest level at which required tasks can be effectively performed without the interposition of secondary or more levels of management.

Supererogatory duty

To undertake responsibilities over and above what one is asked or expected to do, to 'act over and beyond the call of duty'. By definition, supererogatory duties cannot be demanded of us, our undertaking them is an exercise of personal altruism and generosity.

SWOT exercise

An exercise commonly employed in undertaking an organisational review, either individually, or in groups, namely to identify the (S) strengths, and (W) weaknesses of the organisation and the (O) opportunities and (T) threats that it faces in its present situation.

Sympathy/Empathy (from Latin *sum* = with and *patheo* = to feel).

'Sympathy' refers to the capacity to share another person's feelings, to have feelings of pity or tenderness for someone in pain or distress. 'Empathy', derived from the Greek *em* = in and *pathos* = feeling, is a technical term used to refer to the natural capacity or learned ability to identify oneself with the predicament of another person, to 'stand in their shoes', and to see the world from their standpoint.

Systems analysis

An approach to corporate management which starts with defining the core business of an organisation and then analyses what systems are required to operate the business effectively and efficiently, including a critique of existing systems within the overall objectives of the business.

Tautology

An expression which essentially repeats in the predicate part what is already contained in the subject part of a sentence, without adding anything new, e.g. all bachelors are unmarried men; they came in succession, one after another.

Teleological ethics

Theories which focus on the goal of an action, or its consequences, to define whether actions are morally justifiable, rather than focusing on the ethical principles or means adopted to achieve the end. Teleological theories may focus either on the specific goal of an action, or maintain, like Aristotle, that all human action aims towards some end and that we are driven by a tendency to seek our own happiness or fulfilment. (From Greek *telos* = end or goal.)

Teleological eudaimonism *see* Eudaimonism.

Theonomy (cf. Autonomy and Heteronomy).

Theonomy is the belief that God rules the world, and that fundamental moral principles or laws are God-given (e.g. the Ten Commandments allegedly given by God to Moses on Mount Sinai), and that happiness is to be found in living by God's law.

Theory of structuration

Giddens's (1984) theory of structuration proposes that neither interactionism nor structuralism is adequate by itself, and that a more comprehensive sociological explanation of human behaviour should combine elements of both.

Total quality management (TQM)

An approach to corporate management which combines strategic planning with an emphasis on values as integral to defining the goals of an organisation and therefore central to the well-being of a corporation.

Transparency (cf. Openness)

While 'openness' in the sense of honesty about your thoughts and feelings is recommended for individuals, 'transparency' is recommended of organisations, particularly a requirement of evidence-based practice. The object of transparency is for the facts to be made public, so that an organisation can be judged (or defend itself) on the basis of evidence and not speculation, innuendo or rumours.

Triage

The sorting out and classification of casualties of war or disaster to determine priority of treatment and proper place of treatment. Broadly speaking, this means simply giving comfort where possible to those who are dying, leaving the 'walking wounded' to look after themselves, and concentrating efforts on those who are seriously injured, but have a chance of recovery.

Universalisability

This is a test, suggested by Kant, to determine whether a rule of action is ethical, namely, whether the maxim or rule on which you choose to act could become the basis of universal law, i.e. whether it could be universalised without conflicting with other duties.

Urbanisation

The process in rapidly developing and industrialised countries where country folk who have traditionally lived off the land move into the cities in search of employment, better opportunities and access to education.

Utilitarianism

The theory advocated in particular by Bentham and Mill that the guiding principle for all conduct should be to achieve the greatest happiness for the greatest number, and that the criterion of the rightness or wrongness of an action is whether it is useful in furthering this goal (utility principle).

Validity (logical)

A quality of arguments of the correct logical form, where it is not the truth of premises but the correct pattern or structure of an argument that validates it.

Value judgements

Judgements where an assessment has to be made of the relative importance or value of something or some action, often involving option appraisal.

Values

While beliefs do not necessarily commit us to action, values do, for we stake our lives on our choice of values. We make a commitment to values as our chosen means to attain our life goals. Values are based on beliefs, and may encourage us to change some inherited attitudes and to cultivate other attitudes, e.g. to be more tolerant of people with a different religious or cultural background. Values serve as the basis from which we make personal assessments of the worth, importance, or efficacy of things as means to achieve our life goals or the well-being of others.

Values clarification

A method of reviewing one's personal and professional values, assessing their relative importance for one's life and work, and determining one's future goals in the light of this exercise in prioritising one's values. The process can be applied to organisations as well as individuals.

Ventilatory school

An approach to the teaching of ethics that is mainly concerned with providing trainees with opportunities to share their feelings and anxieties about the exercise of ethical responsibility and making tough decisions in practice. The assumption is often made that the cathartic process will suffice to give trainees better insight into what they should do.

Vice (from Latin *vitium* = fault, imperfection).

Literally a state of imperfection due to failure to develop one's human rational potentialities, or due to culpable neglect of one's abilities, a morally bad state of being due to evil practices that have become habitual.

Virtue

A stable state of moral excellence achieved through habitual practice of appropriate dispositions and behaviours. (Cf. Vice.)

Virtue ethics

An ethical theory which focuses attention on the possession of sound moral qualities by the moral agent as necessary for consistent ethical behaviour. A theory which rejects the apparent dichotomy between deontological (duty based) and utilitarian (consequentialist) theories, in favour of emphasis on the agent as having primary responsibility for implementing principles in action.

Vision

A term used in management and strategic planning to describe the collective view of stakeholders in an organisation as to where it is going and what its goals should be.

Whistle-blowing

A term used to describe action taken by an employee to inform senior management (or some outside authority) of activity which they regard as fraudulent, dishonest, criminal or dangerous to others. There is a general requirement of the common law that one has a duty to inform the appropriate authorities if you have evidence of the commission of a crime, but protection of 'whistle-blowers' has become an issue because of the apparent inadequacy of statutory protections for public-minded individuals who disclose misconduct and who may suffer dismissal from employment as a result.

Author Index

Subject Index